Handbook of Veterinary Medicine

Handbook of Veterinary Medicine

Edited by **Andrea Santoro**

Callisto Reference
New York

Published by Callisto Reference,
106 Park Avenue, Suite 200,
New York, NY 10016, USA
www.callistoreference.com

Handbook of Veterinary Medicine
Edited by Andrea Santoro

International Standard Book Number: 978-1-63239-670-9 (Hardback)

Printed in China.

Contents

Preface

Veterinary medicine deals with the treatment and diagnosis of diseases in animals. It indirectly prevents human beings from contracting diseases from pet and farm animals in case of contact. These medicines are also applied to increase the productivity of these animals. This book provides significant information of this discipline to help develop a good understanding of veterinary science and medicine. The topics covered in this extensive book deal with the core subjects of this area of biomedical science. In this book, using case studies and examples, constant effort has been made to make the understanding of the difficult concepts as easy and informative as possible, for the readers. It includes contributions of experts and scientists which will provide innovative insights into this field.

This book is a comprehensive compilation of works of different researchers from varied parts of the world. It includes valuable experiences of the researchers with the sole objective of providing the readers (learners) with a proper knowledge of the concerned field. This book will be beneficial in evoking inspiration and enhancing the knowledge of the interested readers.

In the end, I would like to extend my heartiest thanks to the authors who worked with great determination on their chapters. I also appreciate the publisher's support in the course of the book. I would also like to deeply acknowledge my family who stood by me as a source of inspiration during the project.

Editor

1

Immune responses against classical swine fever virus: between ignorance and lunacy

*Artur Summerfield * and Nicolas Ruggli*

Institute of Virology and Immunology – IVI, Bern, Switzerland

Classical swine fever virus infection of pigs causes disease courses from life-threatening to asymptomatic, depending on the virulence of the virus strain and the immunocompetence of the host. The virus targets immune cells, which are central in orchestrating innate and adaptive immune responses such as macrophages and conventional and plasmacytoid dendritic cells. Here, we review current knowledge and concepts aiming to explain the immunopathogenesis of the disease at both the host and the cellular level. We propose that the interferon type I system and in particular the interaction of the virus with plasmacytoid dendritic cells and macrophages is crucial to understand elements governing the induction of protective rather than pathogenic immune responses. The review also concludes that despite the knowledge available many aspects of classical swine fever immunopathogenesis are still puzzling.

Keywords: classical swine fever, macrophages, dendritic cells, virulence, interferon

Edited by:
Dirk Werling, Royal Veterinary College, UK

Reviewed by:
Carol Geralyn Chitko-McKown, U.S. Meat Animal Research Center, USA
Linda Kathleen Dixon, The Pirbright Institute, UK

***Correspondence:**
Artur Summerfield, Institute of Virology and Immunology – IVI, Sensemattstrasse 293, Mittelhäusern, Bern 3147, Switzerland
artur.summerfield@ivi.admin.ch

Introduction

Classical swine fever (CSF) is a highly contagious disease of pigs caused by the classical swine fever virus (CSFV), which is a member of the genus pestivirus within the *Flaviviridae* family. CSFV is a spherical virus particle of 40–60 nm in diameter, consisting of a lipid envelope surrounded by a nucleocapsid packaging a positive-strand RNA genome of 12.3 kb. The RNA carries a single large open reading frame (ORF) which encodes a large polyprotein that is co- and post-translationally cleaved into the twelve proteins N^{pro}, C, E^{rns}, E1, E2, p7, NS2, NS3, NS4A, NS4B, NS5A, and NS5B by cellular and viral proteases. The four structural proteins C, E^{rns}, E1, and E2 are components of the virion, while the others are non-structural proteins with various functions in the viral life cycle. Virus replication is restricted to the cytoplasm and does normally not result in a cytopathic effect in cell culture. Virion assembly occurs on intracellular membranes of the endoplasmic reticulum (ER), and first progeny virus is released from the cells at 5–6 h post-infection via exocytosis (1).

Classical swine fever leads to important economic losses worldwide. In Europe, the wild boar population is an important reservoir for the virus, and represents a source for reintroduction of the disease in domestic pigs.

After oronasal infection, CSFV probably passes through the epithelial cells and M-cells of the tonsilar crypts, the primary target tissue for virus replication. Thereafter, the virus is found in the tonsils and local oropharyngeal lymph nodes (2, 3). A particular affinity of the virus for the reticuloendothelial cell system has been noted with macrophages (MΦ), dendritic cells (DC), and endothelial cells (EDC) being primary targets (2–10). From these primary sites of replication, the virus spreads to other lymphoid organs. Such secondary target organs include the spleen, lymph nodes, gut-associated lymphoid tissue, bone marrow, and thymus (2, 3, 11). CSFV has also been found in the pancreas, brain, heart, gall and urinary bladders, mandibular salivary and adrenal glands, thyroid, liver, and kidney, particularly in association with EDC and MΦ (3). More recent investigations using quantitative RT-PCR confirmed these older studies, also demonstrating a wider tissue distribution with longer durations of infection (12). This is also reflected at the level of cell tropism. For example, only in late stages of the disease, viral antigen is found in peripheral lymphocytes and immature granulocytes (7, 11, 13). Furthermore, in the skin, efficient infection of keratinocytes, hair follicle epithelial cells, and mesenchymal cells in the dermis was demonstrated at later time points after infection (14).

Highly Virulent Strains Induce a Disastrous Infection for the Immune System

Strong Peripheral and Central Lymphoid Depletion Affecting Primary and Secondary Lymphoid Tissue

The numerous field isolates and laboratory strains cover an almost continuous spectrum of virulence, from highly virulent viruses to low-virulent strains. Accordingly, the clinical outcome of CSF in pigs can vary from peracute to acute, subacute, chronic, and subclinical disease outcomes. The peracute and acute disease is characterized by pyrexia, anorexia, central nervous disorders, diarrhea, and in some cases also hemorrhages of the skin, mucosa, and various other organs. In fact, virulent CSFV can induce a typical hemorrhagic fever with immunological characteristics common to all viral hemorrhagic fevers. The disease is associated with severe lymphopenia and lymphocyte apoptosis (6, 11, 15), thrombocytopenia (3), platelet aggregation (16), bone marrow depletion affecting myelopoiesis and magakaryocytopoiesis (11, 17), and thymus atrophy as well as thymocyte apoptosis (5, 13). Lymphoid depletion is generalized, not only affecting peripheral blood and lymph nodes but also the mucosal tissue (18). At later stages, disseminated intravascular coagulation (DIC), petechial bleedings, and hemoconcentration can be found (3), which can result in a circulation failure, hypotension, and death. A recent study, however, suggests that the hemorrhagic lesions observed in the late stages of the disease are not attributable to DIC. Inhibition of diffuse fibrin and thrombi formation did not influence the extent of hemorrhagic lesions. From this, it was concluded that DIC was not the cause for the thrombocytopenia and hemorrhages observed in acute-lethal CSF (19).

Massive Induction of Interferon-α

Very high levels of serum interferon-(IFN)-α are a hallmark of the acute disease phase induced by virulent CSFV. It appears that the levels of IFN-α found in the serum correlate with disease severity and the virulence of the isolate used for infection (20, 21). Nevertheless, the association between virulence and high IFN-α levels was less clear in 6-month-old pigs (22). Our experience in younger animals clearly indicated a correlation between serum IFN-α levels and the degree of lymphopenia induced by CSFV. In fact, the onset of severe lymphopenia was concomitant with the IFN-α responses, and all animals with serum IFN-α had depleted peripheral B and T lymphocytes (21). These observations indicate that high levels of IFN-α cannot control the virus but may rather mediate aberrant responses leading to immunopathology (**Figure 1**). Microarray analyses of PBMC isolated from infected pigs confirmed not only the dominance of IFN-stimulated genes but also of cell death receptor and apoptosis pathways such as TRAIL, FAS, and TNF (23), relating to previous studies performed with peripheral blood cells using flow cytometry (15). To our knowledge, compared with other virus infections of pigs, CSFV can induce not only the most long-lasting but also the most intense systemic IFN-α responses (24).

Infection and Activation of MΦ

In vivo, MΦ infection and morphological signs of activation were found in the spleen (4, 25), the kidney (26) the lung (27), the liver (28), and the intestine (18). In addition, infection of pigs was associated with MΦ producing pro-inflammatory cytokines, such as IL-1α, IL-1β, IL-6, and TNF-α (5, 8, 25, 28). There is also evidence for macrophage activation leading to the production of vasoactive mediators including prostaglandin E2 (8) and platelet activation (16). Finally, during acute and severe CSF, an activation of the complement system has been observed (5, 25). Therefore, MΦ infection and activation have been proposed to play an important role in CSF pathogenesis, in particular, through release of pro-inflammatory and vasoactive mediators (**Figure 1**).

Infection and Activation of Dendritic Cells

It was also shown that $CD11R1^+CD172a^+$ cells, probably representing a subset of conventional DC (29), are activated *in vivo* in the blood, the tonsil, and the spleen at 24–48 h post-infection to produce TNF-α and IL-10 (10). The same study also demonstrated IFN-α and IL-12 producing $CD4^+CD172a^+$ plasmacytoid DC (pDC) in the same immunological compartments but possibly with an ever faster kinetic of response. Immunofluorescence analysis indicated that these two populations of DC do represent early target cells of CSFV (10). Only recently it became clear that the monocytic cells and DC represent two distinct lineage of cells with respect to their ontogenic development (30), and it is now also possible to clearly differentiate bona fide DC from monocytic cells in the pig (29). Although these cells do have overlapping functions, they also have a clear functional specialization. During CSF, MΦ are probably mainly responsible for the typical pro-inflammatory responses, but conventional DC appear to contribute to this response although they may also be involved in counteracting it by secretion of anti-inflammatory IL-10 (10). Finally, pDC typically secrete large quantities of IFN-α, but possibly also Th1-promoting IL-12. The impact of the virus on the antigen-presenting functions of DC is not clear but it appears that the cells are not depleted in the lymphoid tissues at least in the first 2–3 days post-infection (10).

Effects on Lymphocytes

Despite the severe lymphoid depletion, acute CSF is also associated with a pronounced anergy of T lymphocytes in the acute phase of the disease (13, 15). At later stages of severe CSF, T cell activation events (31, 32) with the detection of serum IL-2 and IFN-γ (33) have been found. Similarly, indication of B-cell activation has been described in terms of an increase in cells expressing the lambda light chain and IgM (34).

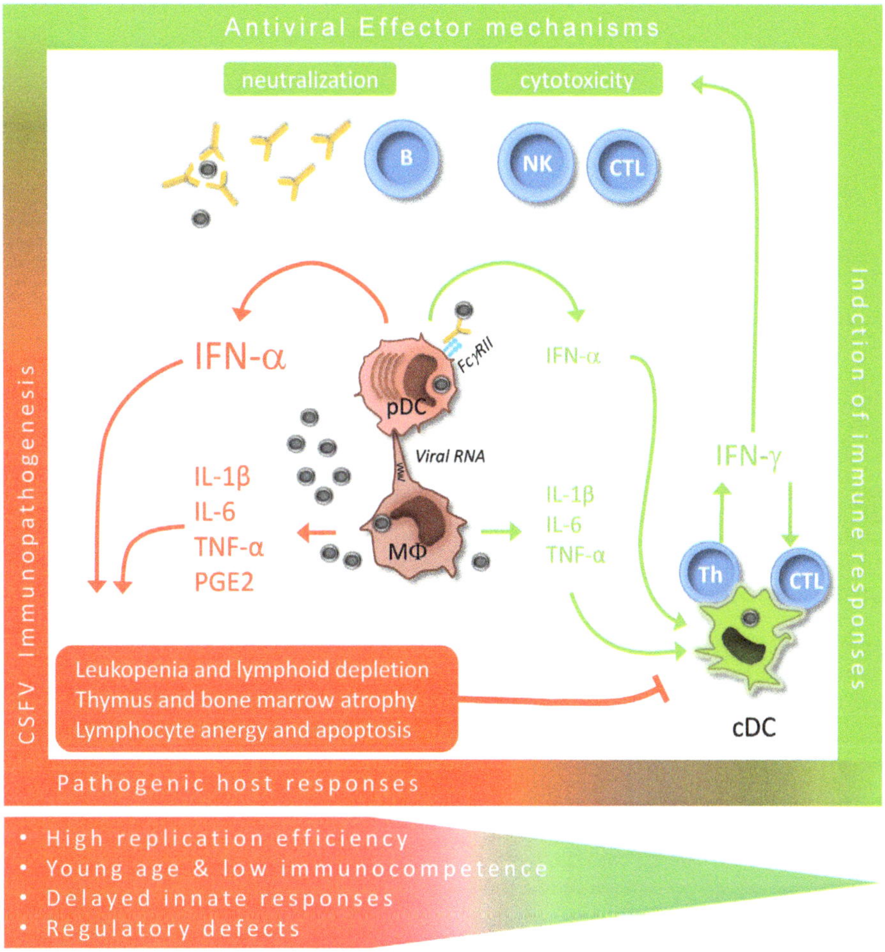

FIGURE 1 | Critical immunological pathways for protective (green) versus pathogenic (red) immune responses during acute CSFV. CSFV targets both monocytic cells with their MΦ descendants and conventional and plasmacytoid DC (cDC and pDC). MΦ are mainly responsible for the typical pro-inflammatory responses, although conventional DC may contribute to this response. We propose that the large quantities of IFN-α produced by pDC play a central role in the innate immune response to CSFV. Prolonged systemic responses are associated with pathogenic host responses while time-limited production appears to promote protective adaptive Th1 effector responses.

Low-Virulent Strains: From Controlled to Chronic Infections

In contrast to severe forms of the disease described above, infection with low-virulent strains of CSFV induces no obvious clinical symptoms or only weak and transient disease. In the serum of such animals, no or lower levels of IFN-α and pro-inflammatory cytokines can be detected (21, 22, 35). However, these animals often also develop transient lymphopenia (36, 37). If controlled, such infections result in life-long immunity against CSFV. Nevertheless, depending on the age and immune status, infection with low or moderately virulent CSFV may lead to forms of chronic disease, which can last up to 3 months before the animals die (38–40). Due to the inability of the immune system to clear the infection, these animals shed large quantities of virus and play an important role in epidemiology of the disease (41, 42). Initially, the immunopathogenic events in such animals can be similar to those described above albeit milder. At later stages, signs of lymphocyte activation and proliferation are found, which are not well defined (43, 44).

Virus–Host Interactions at the Cellular Level

CSFV Proteins Targeting Innate Immune Responses

N^pro

The N^pro is a cysteine autoprotease that cleaves itself from the viral polyprotein co-translationally and targets IRF3, an essential transcription factor for *IFNB1*. The C-terminal half of N^pro carries a zinc-binding domain that is required for interaction with IRF3 (45, 46). Through this interaction, N^pro induces efficient proteosomal degradation and depletion of IRF-3, which is the basis of the very potent antagonism of IFN type I induction by CSFV (47–51) (**Figure 2**). However, pDC are unique by constitutively expressing IRF7, and in contrast to other cells do not require

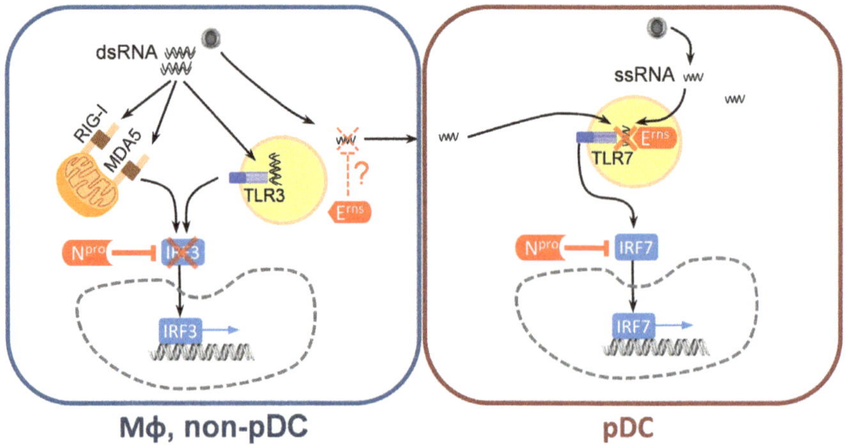

FIGURE 2 | Classical swine fever virus-encoded inhibitors of the IFN type I system. In MΦ and non-pDC target cells, N^{pro} represents the main IFN antagonist, which almost completely inhibits IRF3-mediated IFN type I induction induced by sensing viral dsRNA via RIG-I, MDA-5, and/or TLR3. In pDC, N^{pro} is also active by inhibiting IRF7-mediated IFN-α induction although this inhibition is not complete. In addition, E^{rns} represents a potent inhibitor of pDC responses through its ability to degrade viral ssRNA and thereby prevent TLR7 activation. Viral ssRNA can originate from virus replicating in pDC or in neighboring cells. The mechanism of viral RNA transfer as well as the subcellular location of RNA degradation is not clear.

IRF3 for induction of IFN-α/β (52), explaining why this cell type is exclusively able to respond to CSFV by IFN-α/β production. Nonetheless, N^{pro} was found to be also partially active in pDC, presumably through its ability to interact also with IRF7 and prevent IRF7-mediated IFN type I induction (53) (**Figure 2**). Furthermore, also in GM-CSF-driven bone marrow hematopoietic cell-derived DC, which have been induced to express IRF7 by IFN type I pre-treatment, N^{pro} was still inhibitory (54). In addition to its ability to suppress IFN type I responses, N^{pro} also mediates anti-apoptotic effects induced by synthetic double stranded (ds) RNA but not by FasL or staurosporine (48, 55, 56), preventing activation of caspases 8, 9, and 3 and inhibiting the loss of mitochondrial membrane potential and cytochrome c release (48, 55, 56). Interestingly, N^{pro} interacts with the anti-apoptotic HS-1-associated protein X-1 (HAX-1), inducing the redistribution of HAX-1 to the ER compartment. This HAX-1 redistribution to the ER during CSFV infection may increase cellular resistance to apoptosis, similar to other HAX-1 interacting proteins (56). N^{pro} also interacts with IκBα known to prevent NFκB p65 nuclear translocation but this interaction apparently has no impact on NFκB translocation (57).

Studies in pigs indicate that the N^{pro}-mediated interference with IFN type I induction contributes to pathogenicity. Single amino acid mutations specifically eliminating the ability of N^{pro} to interact with IRF3 partially attenuated moderately virulent but not highly virulent CSFV (20). On the other hand, reintroduction of functional N^{pro} into moderately virulent GPE^{-}-derived virus with unfunctional N^{pro} enhanced virulence by preventing IFN type I induction at local replication sites (58).

E^{rns}

This essential structural glycoprotein of pestiviruses has a remarkable RNase activity, with structural similarities to plant T2 RNases. The optimal catalytic activity is at acidic pH (59), with preferential cleavage of single-stranded (ss) RNA (60, 61). The protein also has an unusual membrane anchor composed of an amphipathic helix without a typical membrane anchor (62, 63), but a retention signal ensuring its association with the intracellular membrane compartments (64). Based on the observation that a minor fraction of the protein was found to be secreted from infected cells or cells expressing E^{rns} (62, 64, 65), a role for secreted E^{rns} acting in the extracellular compartment where it could degrade RNA has been postulated (66–68). In addition, E^{rns} can be rapidly endocytosed to also degrade endosomal RNA in adjacent cells (69). However, these studies were performed with recombinant E^{rns}. In the viral context, the antagonistic activity of E^{rns} on IFN-α induction was only demonstrated in pDC (70). On one side, CSFV expressing E^{rns} lacking RNase activity in contrast to wild-type virus was able to induce very strong IFN-α responses in pDC. On the other hand, cells infected with virus replicon particles lacking E^{rns} or CSFV expressing an E^{rns} without RNase activity were much more efficient at stimulating pDC than cells infected with the parent virus. This very potent stimulation of pDC by infected cells was demonstrated not to be mediated by virions but by a transfer of viral RNA to the TLR7 compartment of pDC. Based on this data it can be concluded that E^{rns} degrades viral ssRNA preventing its interaction with TLR7 in pDC. Considering that the RNase activity of E^{rns} is particularly high at acidic pH, an attractive model is that degradation would happen in the endosomal compartment (70) (**Figure 2**). We consider these findings as relevant since the stimulation of pDC by infected cells results in much higher levels of IFN-α as compared to the direct pDC stimulation by virions (70). The role of E^{rns} in other cell types expressing TLR7 and TLR8 or even TLR3 such as monocyte/MΦ, B cells, and other DC subsets still needs to be investigated. The first step would be to characterize the TLR expression in pigs. *In vivo* removal of the RNase activity results in virus attenuation (71) and abrogation of the capacity of pestiviruses to establish immunotolerance and persistent infection after infection of fetuses (72). The relationship between this inhibitory activity of Erns on the innate immune responses mediated via TLR7 and the establishment of tolerance will be an important area of future investigations.

Quiescent *In vitro* Infections

With a few exceptions, CSFV is absolutely non-cytopathogenic. In all target cells analyzed so far, except pDC, the virus does not induce IFN type I responses, and no or low cytokine responses are found. This is independent of the virulence of the strains investigated. MΦ activation following *in vitro* infection with CSFV is surprisingly weak compared to stimulation with TLR ligands such as lipopolysaccharide, and many reports confirm that CSFV only induces a minor activation of monocytic cells including monocyte-derived MΦ, monocyte-derived DC, as well as their bone marrow-derived counterparts (8, 54, 73, 74). Zaffuto et al. (75) reported microarray data showing only 11 out of 7712 genes (0.14%) induced by the virus, including arginase-1, phosphoinositide 3-kinase, chemokine receptor 4, and interleukin-1β. Obviously, these characteristics are dependent on the potent ability of N^{pro} to counteract virus sensing (76). Previous work also demonstrated that CSFV neither induces nor interferes with NFκB signaling (57). These reports with cell lines, monocyte-derived cells, and *ex vivo* isolated macrophages are remarkable, considering the replicative ability of the virus in these cells. This demonstrates that the viral innate immune system antagonist N^{pro} is most efficient in hiding the infection. For pestiviruses, it is well known that the balance of viral dsRNA accumulating during replication is regulated by a tightly controlled expression of NS3 (77). Cytopathogenic mutants typically have higher levels of dsRNA. Accordingly, such mutants do induce IFN-β and activate monocytic cells even with functional N^{pro}, indicating that evolution has driven a well-balanced relationship between N^{pro} and viral dsRNA (76). In fact, using non-functional N^{pro} mutants of CSFV, we have demonstrated that in PK-15 cells viral RNA is sensed by TLR3, RIG-I, and MDA-5 (78).

Plasmacytoid DC Responses *In vitro*

Classical swine fever virus activates pDC to produce IFN-α. This activation requires live virus and pDC infection (79). Nevertheless, compared to other viruses such as influenza virus the levels of IFN-α are relatively low (24). In fact, this can be explained by the action of N^{pro} targeting IRF7 (53) and of E^{rns} degrading viral RNA to prevent the triggering of TLR7 by viral RNA (70). A very efficient TLR7-dependent induction of IFN-α in pDC by CSFV-infected cells in the absence of virions has been demonstrated. This pathway is mediated by a transfer of RNA from an infected donor cell to pDC in a cell contact-dependent manner requiring intact lipid rafts and cytoskeleton of the donor cell. E^{rns} blocks both direct stimulation of pDC by virions and stimulation by infected cells (70). Although on a per cell basis CSFV is a weak activator of pDC, its strong tropism for lymphoid tissue and pDC is likely to result in the overall high and prolonged responses found *in vivo* (24).

Proposed Mechanisms Leading to Control

Dysregulated Responses

Published data indicate that at the initial sites of virus replication – involving principally MΦ and epithelial cells – CSFV N^{pro} inhibits virus-induced IFN-α/β allowing the virus to replicate and generate the virus load leading to viremia and spread within the organism. The speed and level by which CSFV replicates and spreads appears to be critical for the outcome of disease. The virus then infects more MΦ and pDC, resulting in massive IFN-α and pro-inflammatory cytokine release as described above (**Figure 1**). Based on the known effects of IFN-α/β on MΦ activation it is tempting to postulate that pDC activation may enhance these effects. Nevertheless, to our surprise even IFN-primed MΦ did not respond to CSFV by production of IFN-α, IL-1β, or IL-6 production (54). It is thus still puzzling to observe the discrepancy between *in vitro* and *in vivo* with regards to MΦ activation.

In vaccinated and immune animals, there are no or less immunopathological events such as development of leukopenia and systemic inflammatory responses after challenge infection (80–82). However, vaccinated animals still respond to CSFV infection with a serum IFN-α response, even in absence of viremia, but, in contrast to naïve animals, this response is lower and only of short duration (79–81, 83). A possible explanation for this observation is the fact that pDC from vaccinated pigs carry cytophilic antibodies, which mediate efficient capture of CSFV, resulting in early strong pDC stimulation (79). This observation underlines that in contrast to strong long-lasting systemic IFN-α responses, a short-lived IFN-α response is probably beneficial for the immunity against CSFV. *In vivo* administration of high levels of IFN type I is known to have comparable negative effects on the hematopoietic system (84–87). Moreover, when IFNAR knockout mice were employed in a lymphocytic choriomeningitis virus model, no induction of hematopoietic cell depletion and leukopenia was observed (88). In fact, the known antiproliferative and proapoptotic effects of IFNs (89) could be directly responsible for hematologic cytopenia (**Figure 1**).

Several attempts to shed light into host responses related to control of CSFV by the immune system have used transcriptomic profiling (23, 90, 91). In response to CSFV infection, increased expression of IFN-stimulated genes as well as other immune response genes, genes related to cell cycle, apoptosis, metabolism, and others were observed. The profiles described reflected what was expected in terms of IFN and cytokine responses measured by ELISA, apoptosis of lymphocytes, and general changes in immune cell composition described for CSF. Using a moderately virulent strain of CSFV, Hulst and co-workers compared groups of pigs able to control the infection with those developing chronic disease and excreting high quantities of virus over a period of 35 days (92). Interestingly, the animals that recovered later had a generally more robust early response in terms of genes associated with IFN type I responses and macrophage activation, whereas those developing chronic disease were found to express inhibitors of the NFκB pathway. This study also indicated a dysregulation of the complement cascade and the vitamin D3 metabolism in animals not controlling the infection. On the other hand, this work also showed that immunoregulatory molecules such as indoleamine 2,3-dioxygenase 1 (IDO1) were expressed early in controller pigs but late in non-controllers (92). Certainly, such analyses highlight the complexity of protective immune responses, which are composed of both stimulatory and regulatory elements required to prevent tissue damage at the right moment. It appears that this is a central theme in understanding the complex pathogenesis of CSF (**Figure 1**).

Protective Immune Mechanisms

It is well established that conventional live attenuated CSFV vaccines have an extraordinary protective capacity inducing protection as early as 3–5 days post vaccination (93, 94). Remarkably, transmission can even be prevented when animals are vaccinated on the day of challenge (95). Obviously, this protection is found in complete absence of neutralizing antibodies indicating alternative mechanisms of protection early post vaccination.

For this reason, several groups investigated the potential role of IFN-γ-secreting T cells (32, 35, 94, 96–98). Typically after challenge infection of pigs with virulent CSFV, only the previously vaccinated animals had circulating T cells secreting IFN-γ. In contrast, vaccination alone using C-strain based vaccine was not efficient at inducing detectable levels of activated peripheral T cells. Only in one study using three shots of a DNA vaccine, CSFV-specific IFN-γ spots were also found before infection (98). Also, in unvaccinated animals, which are challenged with a virulent strain of CSFV, no T cell activity can be detected in the peripheral blood. This is certainly caused by the severe defects in their T cell compartment which is even unable to respond to polyclonal stimulation (13, 15). Most of the IFN-γ-producing lymphocytes found in the peripheral blood belong to the $CD4^-CD8\beta^+$ T cell subset and co-express perforin indicating effector functions (82, 97) and are probably effector CTL's since they express CD107a on their surface. This is in line with previous work demonstrating cytotoxic T cell activity against CSFV-infected target cells (96). From the latter study, it appears that the ability to detect CSFV-specific cytotoxic T cell activity requires a certain level of virus replication; since in this study, CTL activity was found only in the peripheral blood of animals kept unvaccinated but challenged with a moderately virulent virus. A recent report showed induction of MHC class II on NK and $\gamma\delta$ T cells by IFN-α derived from CSFV-infected pDC *in vitro*. However, *in vivo* this was only found in tonsils and retropharygeal lymph nodes of pigs infected with virulent virus, but not following vaccination with attenuated vaccines. Furthermore, neither an increase in perforin nor IFN-γ was found both *in vitro* and *in vivo*. From this, the authors concluded that these cell types are probably not contributing to early protection induced by attenuated vaccines (99).

These studies showing an association of T cell responses with protection alone do not permit a conclusion that IFN-γ secreting T cells are a correlate of protection or even have protective value and the general contribution of T cells to protection remains unclear. A main problem is the immunopathological effects of CSFV on the T lymphocyte compartment, which if present do not permit the detection of any T cell activation. Furthermore, NS3 protein known to contain T cell epitopes (100) was not able to confer partial protection in vaccination-challenge studies (101, 102) indicating that T cell immunity alone is unlikely to control CSFV. On the other hand, neutralizing antibodies against E2 are well known to be associated with protection (83, 103–106). But E2 also contains CTL epitopes (107) whose contribution to protection is not yet clear.

Conclusion and Future Research

Despite the knowledge available on the pathogenesis of CSF, many essential aspects remain enigmatic and can only be clarified with well-defined gain- as well as loss-of-function *in vivo* experimental models. In our view, the most important questions are to identify the precise contribution of various cell types including pDC, conventional DC, and MΦ to disease pathogenesis and immunity both during the acute forms of CSF and during chronic disease. Similarly, correlates of early vaccine-induced protection remain unproven. The functions of various subsets of T cells in protection need to be defined to understand both chronic disease and vaccine-mediated early protection. Furthermore, the exact role of evolvement of viral inhibitors of the IFN type I system, targeting both non-pDC and pDC remains puzzling considering that *in vivo* IFN-α/β responses are induced. Finally, the cellular systems and the viral inhibitors described in this review need to be understood in the light of the ability of pestiviruses to induce immunotolerance, if infection occurs during certain stages of the development of the immune system.

Acknowledgments

Part of this work was supported by the Swiss National Science Foundation grants # 3100-68237, 310030-116800/1, 31003A-116608, and 310030_141045. We are grateful for the precious contributions of all present and former members of our laboratory.

References

1. Thiel H-J, Plagemann PGW, Moennig V. Pestiviruses. In: Fields BN, Knipe DM, Howley PM, editors. *Fields Virology*. Philadelphia, PA: Lippincott-Raven Publishers (1996). p. 1059–73.
2. Ressang AA. Studies on the pathogenesis of hog cholera. II. Virus distribution in tissue and the morphology of the immune response. *Zentralbl Veterinarmed B* (1973) **20**:272–88. doi:10.1111/j.1439-0450.1973.tb01127.x
3. Trautwein G, Leiss B. *Pathology and Pathogenesis of the Disease, Classical Swine Fever and Related Infections*. Boston, MA: Martinus Nijhoff Publishing (1988). p. 27–54.
4. Gomez-Villamandos JC, Ruiz-Villamor E, Bautista MJ, Sanchez CP, Sanchez-Cordon PJ, Salguero FJ, et al. Morphological and immunohistochemical changes in splenic macrophages of pigs infected with classical swine fever. *J Comp Pathol* (2001) **125**:98–109. doi:10.1053/jcpa.2001.0487
5. Sanchez-Cordon PJ, Romanini S, Salguero FJ, Nunez A, Bautista MJ, Jover A, et al. Apoptosis of thymocytes related to cytokine expression in experimental classical swine fever. *J Comp Pathol* (2002) **127**:239–48. doi:10.1053/jcpa.2002.0587
6. Susa M, Konig M, Saalmuller A, Reddehase MJ, Thiel HJ. Pathogenesis of classical swine fever: B-lymphocyte deficiency caused by hog cholera virus. *J Virol* (1992) **66**:1171–5.
7. Summerfield A, Hofmann MA, McCullough KC. Low density blood granulocytic cells induced during classical swine fever are targets for virus infection. *Vet Immunol Immunopathol* (1998) **63**:289–301. doi:10.1016/S0165-2427(98)00108-1
8. Knoetig SM, Summerfield A, Spagnuolo-Weaver M, McCullough KC. Immunopathogenesis of classical swine fever: role of monocytic cells. *Immunology* (1999) **97**:359–66. doi:10.1046/j.1365-2567.1999.00775.x
9. Carrasco CP, Rigden RC, Schaffner R, Gerber H, Neuhaus V, Inumaru S, et al. Porcine dendritic cells generated in vitro: morphological, phenotypic

and functional properties. *Immunology* (2001) **104**:175–84. doi:10.1046/j.1365-2567.2001.01299.x
10. Jamin A, Gorin S, Cariolet R, Le Potier MF, Kuntz-Simon G. Classical swine fever virus induces activation of plasmacytoid and conventional dendritic cells in tonsil, blood, and spleen of infected pigs. *Vet Res* (2008) **39**:7. doi:10.1051/vetres:2007045
11. Summerfield A, Knoetig SM, Tschudin R, McCullough KC. Pathogenesis of granulocytopenia and bone marrow atrophy during classical swine fever involves apoptosis and necrosis of uninfected cells. *Virology* (2000) **272**:50–60. doi:10.1006/viro.2000.0361
12. Liu J, Fan XZ, Wang Q, Xu L, Zhao QZ, Huang W, et al. Dynamic distribution and tissue tropism of classical swine fever virus in experimentally infected pigs. *Virol J* (2011) **8**:201. doi:10.1186/1743-422X-8-201
13. Pauly T, Konig M, Thiel HJ, Saalmuller A. Infection with classical swine fever virus: effects on phenotype and immune responsiveness of porcine T lymphocytes. *J Gen Virol* (1998) **79**(Pt 1):31–40.
14. Kaden V, Lange E, Faust A, Teifke JP. Value of skin punch biopsies for the diagnosis of acute classical swine fever. *J Vet Diagn Invest* (2007) **19**:697–701. doi:10.1177/104063870701900614
15. Summerfield A, Knotig SM, McCullough KC. Lymphocyte apoptosis during classical swine fever: implication of activation-induced cell death. *J Virol* (1998) **72**:1853–61.
16. Bautista MJ, RuizVillamor E, Salguero FJ, SanchezCordon PJ, Carrasco L, GomezVillamandos JC. Early platelet aggregation as a cause of thrombocytopenia in classical swine fever 1842. *Vet Pathol* (2002) **39**:84–91. doi:10.1354/vp.39-1-84
17. Gomez-Villamandos JC, Salguero FJ, Ruiz-Villamor E, Sanchez-Cordon PJ, Bautista MJ, Sierra MA. Classical swine fever: pathology of bone marrow. *Vet Pathol* (2003) **40**:157–63. doi:10.1354/vp.40-2-157
18. Sanchez-Cordon PJ, Romanini S, Salguero FJ, Ruiz-Villamor E, Carrasco L, Gomez-Villamandos JC. A histopathologic, immunohistochemical, and ultrastructural study of the intestine in pigs inoculated with classical swine fever virus. *Vet Pathol* (2003) **40**:254–62. doi:10.1354/vp.40-3-254
19. Blome S, Meindl-Bohmer A, Nowak G, Moennig V. Disseminated intravascular coagulation does not play a major role in the pathogenesis of classical swine fever. *Vet Microbiol* (2013) **162**:360–8. doi:10.1016/j.vetmic.2012.10.008
20. Ruggli N, Summerfield A, Fiebach AR, Guzylack-Piriou L, Bauhofer O, Lamm CG, et al. Classical swine fever virus can remain virulent after specific elimination of the interferon regulatory factor 3-degrading function of Npro. *J Virol* (2009) **83**:817–29. doi:10.1128/JVI.01509-08
21. Summerfield A, Alves M, Ruggli N, de Bruin MG, McCullough KC. High IFN-alpha responses associated with depletion of lymphocytes and natural IFN-producing cells during classical swine fever. *J Interferon Cytokine Res* (2006) **26**:248–55. doi:10.1089/jir.2006.26.248
22. von Rosen T, Lohse L, Nielsen J, Uttenthal A. Classical swine fever virus infection modulates serum levels of INF-alpha, IL-8 and TNF-alpha in 6-month-old pigs. *Res Vet Sci* (2013) **95**:1262–7. doi:10.1016/j.rvsc.2013.09.011
23. Renson P, Blanchard Y, Le Dimna M, Felix H, Cariolet R, Jestin A, et al. Acute induction of cell death-related IFN stimulated genes (ISG) differentiates highly from moderately virulent CSFV strains. *Vet Res* (2010) **41**:7. doi:10.1051/vetres/2009055
24. Summerfield A. Viewpoint: factors involved in type I interferon responses during porcine virus infections. *Vet Immunol Immunopathol* (2012) **148**:168–71. doi:10.1016/j.vetimm.2011.03.011
25. Sanchez-Cordon PJ, Nunez A, Salguero FJ, Pedrera M, Fernandez de MM, Gomez-Villamandos JC. Lymphocyte apoptosis and thrombocytopenia in spleen during classical swine fever: role of macrophages and cytokines. *Vet Pathol* (2005) **42**:477–88. doi:10.1354/vp.42-4-477
26. Gomez-Villamandos JC, Ruiz-Villamor E, Bautista MJ, Quezada M, Sanchez CP, Salguero FJ, et al. Pathogenesis of classical swine fever: renal haemorrhages and erythrodiapedesis. *J Comp Pathol* (2000) **123**:47–54. doi:10.1053/jcpa.2000.0385
27. Carrasco L, Ruiz-Villamor E, Gomez-Villamandos JC, Salguero FJ, Bautista MJ, Macia M, et al. Classical swine fever: morphological and morphometrical study of pulmonary intravascular macrophages. *J Comp Pathol* (2001) **125**:1–7. doi:10.1053/jcpa.2001.0470
28. Nunez A, Gomez-Villamandos JC, Sanchez-Cordon PJ, Fernandez de Marco M, Pedrera M, Salguero FJ, et al. Expression of proinflammatory cytokines by hepatic macrophages in acute classical swine fever. *J Comp Pathol* (2005) **133**:23–32. doi:10.1016/j.jcpa.2005.01.003
29. Summerfield A, Auray G, Ricklin M. Comparative dendritic cell biology of veterinary mammals. *Annu Rev Anim Biosci* (2014) **3**:533–57. doi:10.1146/annurev-animal-022114-111009
30. Merad M, Sathe P, Helft J, Miller J, Mortha A. The dendritic cell lineage: ontogeny and function of dendritic cells and their subsets in the steady state and the inflamed setting. *Annu Rev Immunol* (2013) **31**:563–604. doi:10.1146/annurev-immunol-020711-074950
31. Suradhat S, Sada W, Buranapraditkun S, Damrongwatanapokin S. The kinetics of cytokine production and CD25 expression by porcine lymphocyte subpopulations following exposure to classical swine fever virus (CSFV). *Vet Immunol Immunopathol* (2005) **106**:197–208. doi:10.1016/j.vetimm.2005.02.017
32. Suradhat S, Intrakamhaeng M, Damrongwatanapokin S. The correlation of virus-specific interferon-gamma production and protection against classical swine fever virus infection. *Vet Immunol Immunopathol* (2001) **83**:177–89. doi:10.1016/S0165-2427(01)00389-0
33. Sanchez-Cordon PJ, Nunez A, Salguero FJ, Carrasco L, Gomez-Villamandos JC. Evolution of T lymphocytes and cytokine expression in classical swine fever (CSF) virus infection. *J Comp Pathol* (2005) **132**:249–60. doi:10.1016/j.jcpa.2004.10.002
34. Sanchez-Cordon PJ, Romero-Trevejo JL, Pedrera M, Raya AI, Gomez-Villamandos JC. The role of B cells in the immune response to pestivirus (classical swine fever virus). *J Comp Pathol* (2006) **135**:32–41. doi:10.1016/j.jcpa.2006.04.001
35. Tarradas J, de la Torre ME, Rosell R, Perez LJ, Pujols J, Munoz M, et al. The impact of CSFV on the immune response to control infection. *Virus Res* (2014) **185**:82–91. doi:10.1016/j.virusres.2014.03.004
36. Nielsen J, Lohse L, Rasmussen TB, Uttenthal A. Classical swine fever in 6- and 11-week-old pigs: haematological and immunological parameters are modulated in pigs with mild clinical disease. *Vet Immunol Immunopathol* (2010) **138**:159–73. doi:10.1016/j.vetimm.2010.07.012
37. Summerfield A, McNeilly F, Walker I, Allan G, Knoetig SM, McCullough KC. Depletion of CD4(+) and CD8(high+) T-cells before the onset of viraemia during classical swine fever. *Vet Immunol Immunopathol* (2001) **78**:3–19. doi:10.1016/S0165-2427(00)00248-8
38. Depner KR, Hinrichs U, Bickhardt K, Greiser-Wilke I, Pohlenz J, Moennig V, et al. Influence of breed-related factors on the course of classical swine fever virus infection. *Vet Rec* (1997) **140**:506–7. doi:10.1136/vr.140.19.506
39. Moennig V, Floegel-Niesmann G, Greiser-Wilke I. Clinical signs and epidemiology of classical swine fever: a review of new knowledge. *Vet J* (2003) **165**:11–20. doi:10.1016/S1090-0233(02)00112-0
40. Van Oirschot JT, Liess B. *Description of the Virus Infection, Classical Swine Fever and Related Viral Infections*. Boston, MA: Martinus Nijhoff Publishing (1988). p. 1–18.
41. Weesendorp E, Backer J, Stegeman A, Loeffen W. Transmission of classical swine fever virus depends on the clinical course of infection which is associated with high and low levels of virus excretion. *Vet Microbiol* (2011) **147**:262–73. doi:10.1016/j.vetmic.2010.06.032
42. Weesendorp E, Stegeman A, Loeffen W. Dynamics of virus excretion via different routes in pigs experimentally infected with classical swine fever virus strains of high, moderate or low virulence. *Vet Microbiol* (2009) **133**:9–22. doi:10.1016/j.vetmic.2008.06.008
43. Korn G, Lorenz RJ. [Blood-pictures in different courses of swine fever infection concerning lymphocytic reactions, cellnecrobiosis, moving forms of lymphocytes ("lysocytes") and reactions of the bone-marrow (author's transl)]. *Zentralbl Bakteriol Orig A* (1974) **229**:299–322.
44. Narita M, Kawashima K, Shimizu M. Viral antigen and B and T lymphocytes in lymphoid tissues of gnotobiotic piglets infected with hog cholera virus. *J Comp Pathol* (1996) **114**:257–63. doi:10.1016/S0021-9975(96)80047-8
45. Szymanski MR, Fiebach AR, Tratschin JD, Gut M, Ramanujam VM, Gottipati K, et al. Zinc binding in pestivirus N(pro) is required for interferon regulatory factor 3 interaction and degradation. *J Mol Biol* (2009) **391**:438–49. doi:10.1016/j.jmb.2009.06.040
46. Gottipati K, Ruggli N, Gerber M, Tratschin JD, Benning M, Bellamy H, et al. The structure of classical swine fever virus N(pro): a novel cysteine autoprotease and zinc-binding protein involved in subversion of type I interferon induction. *PLoS Pathog* (2013) **9**:e1003704. doi:10.1371/journal.ppat.1003704

47. Bauhofer O, Summerfield A, Sakoda Y, Tratschin JD, Hofmann MA, Ruggli N. Classical swine fever virus Npro interacts with interferon regulatory factor 3 and induces its proteasomal degradation. *J Virol* (2007) **81**:3087–96. doi:10.1128/JVI.02032-06
48. Ruggli N, Bird BH, Liu L, Bauhofer O, Tratschin JD, Hofmann MA. N(pro) of classical swine fever virus is an antagonist of double-stranded RNA-mediated apoptosis and IFN-alpha/beta induction. *Virology* (2005) **340**(2):265–76. doi:10.1016/j.virol.2005.06.033
49. Seago J, Hilton L, Reid E, Doceul V, Jeyatheesan J, Moganeradj K, et al. The Npro product of classical swine fever virus and bovine viral diarrhea virus uses a conserved mechanism to target interferon regulatory factor-3. *J Gen Virol* (2007) **88**:3002–6. doi:10.1099/vir.0.82934-0
50. Chen Z, Rijnbrand R, Jangra RK, Devaraj SG, Qu L, Ma Y, et al. Ubiquitination and proteasomal degradation of interferon regulatory factor-3 induced by Npro from a cytopathic bovine viral diarrhea virus. *Virology* (2007) **366**:277–92. doi:10.1016/j.virol.2007.04.023
51. Hilton L, Moganeradj K, Zhang G, Chen YH, Randall RE, McCauley JW, et al. The NPro product of bovine viral diarrhea virus inhibits DNA binding by interferon regulatory factor 3 and targets it for proteasomal degradation. *J Virol* (2006) **80**:11723–32. doi:10.1128/JVI.01145-06
52. Honda K, Yanai H, Negishi H, Asagiri M, Sato M, Mizutani T, et al. IRF-7 is the master regulator of type-I interferon-dependent immune responses. *Nature* (2005) **434**:772–7. doi:10.1038/nature03464
53. Fiebach AR, Guzylack-Piriou L, Python S, Summerfield A, Ruggli N. Classical swine fever virus N(pro) limits type I interferon induction in plasmacytoid dendritic cells by interacting with interferon regulatory factor 7. *J Virol* (2011) **85**:8002–11. doi:10.1128/JVI.00330-11
54. Husser L, Ruggli N, Summerfield A. N(pro) of classical swine fever virus prevents type I interferon-mediated priming of conventional dendritic cells for enhanced interferon-alpha response. *J Interferon Cytokine Res* (2012) **32**:221–9. doi:10.1089/jir.2011.0068
55. Ruggli N, Tratschin JD, Schweizer M, McCullough KC, Hofmann MA, Summerfield A. Classical swine fever virus interferes with cellular antiviral defense: evidence for a novel function of N(pro). *J Virol* (2003) **77**:7645–54. doi:10.1128/JVI.77.13.7645-7654.2003
56. Johns HL, Bensaude E, La Rocca SA, Seago J, Charleston B, Steinbach F, et al. Classical swine fever virus infection protects aortic endothelial cells from pIpC-mediated apoptosis. *J Gen Virol* (2010) **91**:1038–46. doi:10.1099/vir.0.016576-0
57. Doceul V, Charleston B, Crooke H, Reid E, Powell PP, Seago J. The Npro product of classical swine fever virus interacts with IkappaBalpha, the NF-kappaB inhibitor. *J Gen Virol* (2008) **89**:1881–9. doi:10.1099/vir.0.83643-0
58. Tamura T, Nagashima N, Ruggli N, Summerfield A, Kida H, Sakoda Y. Npro of classical swine fever virus contributes to pathogenicity in pigs by preventing type I interferon induction at local replication sites. *Vet Res* (2014) **45**:47. doi:10.1186/1297-9716-45-47
59. Krey T, Bontems F, Vonrhein C, Vaney MC, Bricogne G, Rumenapf T, et al. Crystal structure of the pestivirus envelope glycoprotein E(rns) and mechanistic analysis of its ribonuclease activity. *Structure* (2012) **20**:862–73. doi:10.1016/j.str.2012.03.018
60. Hausmann Y, Roman-Sosa G, Thiel HJ, Rumenapf T. Classical swine fever virus glycoprotein E rns is an endoribonuclease with an unusual base specificity. *J Virol* (2004) **78**:5507–12. doi:10.1128/JVI.78.10.5507-5512.2004
61. Windisch JM, Schneider R, Stark R, Weiland E, Meyers G, Thiel HJ. RNase of classical swine fever virus: biochemical characterization and inhibition by virus-neutralizing monoclonal antibodies. *J Virol* (1996) **70**:352–8.
62. Fetzer C, Tews BA, Meyers G. The carboxy-terminal sequence of the pestivirus glycoprotein E(rns) represents an unusual type of membrane anchor. *J Virol* (2005) **79**:11901–13. doi:10.1128/JVI.79.18.11901-11913.2005
63. Tews BA, Schurmann EM, Meyers G. Mutation of cysteine 171 of pestivirus E rns RNase prevents homodimer formation and leads to attenuation of classical swine fever virus. *J Virol* (2009) **83**:4823–34. doi:10.1128/JVI.01710-08
64. Burrack S, Aberle D, Burck J, Ulrich AS, Meyers G. A new type of intracellular retention signal identified in a pestivirus structural glycoprotein. *FASEB J* (2012) **26**:3292–305. doi:10.1096/fj.12-207191
65. Rumenapf T, Unger G, Strauss JH, Thiel HJ. Processing of the envelope glycoproteins of pestiviruses. *J Virol* (1993) **67**:3288–94.
66. Iqbal M, Poole E, Goodbourn S, McCauley JW. Role for bovine viral diarrhea virus Erns glycoprotein in the control of activation of beta interferon by double-stranded RNA. *J Virol* (2004) **78**:136–45. doi:10.1128/JVI.78.1.136-145.2004
67. Magkouras I, Matzener P, Rumenapf T, Peterhans E, Schweizer M. RNase-dependent inhibition of extracellular, but not intracellular, dsRNA-induced interferon synthesis by Erns of pestiviruses. *J Gen Virol* (2008) **89**:2501–6. doi:10.1099/vir.0.2008/003749-0
68. Matzener P, Magkouras I, Rumenapf T, Peterhans E, Schweizer M. The viral RNase E(rns) prevents IFN type-I triggering by pestiviral single- and double-stranded RNAs. *Virus Res* (2009) **140**:15–23. doi:10.1016/j.virusres.2008.10.015
69. Zurcher C, Sauter KS, Mathys V, Wyss F, Schweizer M. Prolonged activity of the pestiviral RNase Erns as an interferon antagonist after uptake by clathrin-mediated endocytosis. *J Virol* (2014) **88**:7235–43. doi:10.1128/JVI.00672-14
70. Python S, Gerber M, Suter R, Ruggli N, Summerfield A. Efficient sensing of infected cells in absence of virus particles by plasmacytoid dendritic cells is blocked by the viral ribonuclease E(rns.). *PLoS Pathog* (2013) **9**:e1003412. doi:10.1371/journal.ppat.1003412
71. Meyers G, Saalmuller A, Buttner M. Mutations abrogating the RNase activity in glycoprotein E(rns) of the pestivirus classical swine fever virus lead to virus attenuation. *J Virol* (1999) **73**:10224–35.
72. Meyers G, Ege A, Fetzer C, von Freyburg M, Elbers K, Carr V, et al. Bovine viral diarrhea virus: prevention of persistent fetal infection by a combination of two mutations affecting Erns RNase and Npro protease. *J Virol* (2007) **81**:3327–38. doi:10.1128/JVI.02372-06
73. Alves MP, Carrasco CP, Balmelli C, Ruggli N, McCullough KC, Summerfield A. Mycoplasma contamination and viral immunomodulatory activity: dendritic cells open Pandora's box. *Immunol Lett* (2007) **110**:101–9. doi:10.1016/j.imlet.2007.04.006
74. Carrasco CP, Rigden RC, Vincent IE, Balmelli C, Ceppi M, Bauhofer O, et al. Interaction of classical swine fever virus with dendritic cells. *J Gen Virol* (2004) **85**:1633–41. doi:10.1099/vir.0.19716-0
75. Zaffuto KM, Piccone ME, Burrage TG, Balinsky CA, Risatti GR, Borca MV, et al. Classical swine fever virus inhibits nitric oxide production in infected macrophages. *J Gen Virol* (2007) **88**:3007–12. doi:10.1099/vir.0.83042-0
76. Bauhofer O, Summerfield A, McCullough KC, Ruggli N. Role of double-stranded RNA and N(pro) of classical swine fever virus in the activation of monocyte-derived dendritic cells. *Virology* (2005) **343**:93–105. doi:10.1016/j.virol.2005.08.016
77. Schweizer M, Peterhans E. Pestiviruses. *Annu Rev Anim Biosci* (2014) **2**:141–63. doi:10.1146/annurev-animal-022513-114209
78. Husser L, Alves MP, Ruggli N, Summerfield A. Identification of the role of RIG-I, MDA-5 and TLR3 in sensing RNA viruses in porcine epithelial cells using lentivirus-driven RNA interference. *Virus Res* (2011) **159**:9–16. doi:10.1016/j.virusres.2011.04.005
79. Balmelli C, Vincent IE, Rau H, Guzylack-Piriou L, McCullough K, Summerfield A. FcgammaRII-dependent sensitisation of natural interferon-producing cells for viral infection and interferon-alpha responses. *Eur J Immunol* (2005) **35**:2406–15. doi:10.1002/eji.200525998
80. Renson P, Le Dimna M, Keranflech A, Cariolet R, Koenen F, Le Potier MF. CP7_E2alf oral vaccination confers partial protection against early classical swine fever virus challenge and interferes with pathogeny-related cytokine responses. *Vet Res* (2013) **44**:9. doi:10.1186/1297-9716-44-9
81. Renson P, Le Dimna M, Gabriel C, Levai R, Blome S, Kulcsar G, et al. Cytokine and immunoglobulin isotype profiles during CP7_E2alf vaccination against a challenge with the highly virulent Koslov strain of classical swine fever virus. *Res Vet Sci* (2014) **96**:389–95. doi:10.1016/j.rvsc.2014.01.002
82. Franzoni G, Kurkure NV, Edgar DS, Everett HE, Gerner W, Bodman-Smith KB, et al. Assessment of the phenotype and functionality of porcine CD8 T cell responses following vaccination with live attenuated classical swine fever virus (CSFV) and virulent CSFV challenge. *Clin Vaccine Immunol* (2013) **20**:1604–16. doi:10.1128/CVI.00415-13
83. Rau H, Revets H, Cornelis P, Titzmann A, Ruggli N, McCullough KC, et al. Efficacy and functionality of lipoprotein OprI from *Pseudomonas aeruginosa* as adjuvant for a subunit vaccine against classical swine fever. *Vaccine* (2006) **24**:4757–68. doi:10.1016/j.vaccine.2006.03.028
84. Quesada JR, Talpaz M, Rios A, Kurzrock R, Gutterman JU. Clinical toxicity of interferons in cancer patients: a review. *J Clin Oncol* (1986) **4**:234–43.

85. Gillespie JH, Scott FW, Geissinger CM, Czarniecki CW, Scialli VT. Levels of interferon in blood serum and toxicity studies of bacteria-derived bovine alpha I1 interferon in dairy calves. *J Clin Microbiol* (1986) **24**:240–4.
86. Mann EA, Markovic SN, Murasko DM. Inhibition of lymphocyte recirculation by murine interferon: effects of various interferon preparations and timing of administration. *J Interferon Res* (1989) **9**:35–51. doi:10.1089/jir.1989.9.35
87. Heikenwalder M, Polymenidou M, Junt T, Sigurdson C, Wagner H, Akira S, et al. Lymphoid follicle destruction and immunosuppression after repeated CpG oligodeoxynucleotide administration. *Nat Med* (2004) **10**:187–92. doi:10.1038/nm987
88. Binder D, Fehr J, Hengartner H, Zinkernagel RM. Virus-induced transient bone marrow aplasia: major role of interferon-alpha/beta during acute infection with the noncytopathic lymphocytic choriomeningitis virus. *J Exp Med* (1997) **185**:517–30. doi:10.1084/jem.185.3.517
89. Chawla-Sarkar M, Lindner DJ, Liu YF, Williams BR, Sen GC, Silverman RH, et al. Apoptosis and interferons: role of interferon-stimulated genes as mediators of apoptosis. *Apoptosis* (2003) **8**:237–49. doi:10.1023/A:1023668705040
90. Durand SV, Hulst MM, de Wit AA, Mastebroek L, Loeffen WL. Activation and modulation of antiviral and apoptotic genes in pigs infected with classical swine fever viruses of high, moderate or low virulence. *Arch Virol* (2009) **154**:1417–31. doi:10.1007/s00705-009-0460-3
91. Li J, Yu YJ, Feng L, Cai XB, Tang HB, Sun SK, et al. Global transcriptional profiles in peripheral blood mononuclear cell during classical swine fever virus infection. *Virus Res* (2010) **148**:60–70. doi:10.1016/j.virusres.2009.12.004
92. Hulst M, Loeffen W, Weesendorp E. Pathway analysis in blood cells of pigs infected with classical swine fever virus: comparison of pigs that develop a chronic form of infection or recover. *Arch Virol* (2013) **158**:325–39. doi:10.1007/s00705-012-1491-8
93. Kaden V, Lange B. Oral immunisation against classical swine fever (CSF): onset and duration of immunity. *Vet Microbiol* (2001) **82**:301–10. doi:10.1016/S0378-1135(01)00400-X
94. Graham SP, Everett HE, Haines FJ, Johns HL, Sosan OA, Salguero FJ, et al. Challenge of pigs with classical swine fever viruses after C-strain vaccination reveals remarkably rapid protection and insights into early immunity. *PLoS One* (2012) **7**:e29310. doi:10.1371/journal.pone.0029310
95. Dewulf J, Laevens H, Koenen F, Mintiens K, de Kruif A. Efficacy of E2-sub-unit marker and C-strain vaccines in reducing horizontal transmission of classical swine fever virus in weaner pigs. *Prev Vet Med* (2004) **65**:121–33. doi:10.1016/j.prevetmed.2004.05.010
96. Piriou L, Chevallier S, Hutet E, Charley B, Le Potier MF, Albina E. Humoral and cell-mediated immune responses of d/d histocompatible pigs against classical swine fever (CSF) virus. *Vet Res* (2003) **34**:389–404. doi:10.1051/vetres:2003013
97. Graham SP, Haines FJ, Johns HL, Sosan O, La Rocca SA, Lamp B, et al. Characterisation of vaccine-induced, broadly cross-reactive IFN-gamma secreting T cell responses that correlate with rapid protection against classical swine fever virus. *Vaccine* (2012) **30**:2742–8. doi:10.1016/j.vaccine.2012.02.029
98. Tarradas J, Argilaguet JM, Rosell R, Nofrarias M, Crisci E, Cordoba L, et al. Interferon-gamma induction correlates with protection by DNA vaccine expressing E2 glycoprotein against classical swine fever virus infection in domestic pigs. *Vet Microbiol* (2010) **142**:51–8. doi:10.1016/j.vetmic.2009.09.043
99. Franzoni G, Edwards JC, Kurkure NV, Edgar DS, Sanchez-Cordon PJ, Haines FJ, et al. Partial activation of natural killer and gammadelta T cells by classical swine fever viruses is associated with type I interferon elicited from plasmacytoid dendritic cells. *Clin Vaccine Immunol* (2014) **21**:1410–20. doi:10.1128/CVI.00382-14
100. Armengol E, Wiesmuller KH, Wienhold D, Buttner M, Pfaff E, Jung G, et al. Identification of T-cell epitopes in the structural and non-structural proteins of classical swine fever virus. *J Gen Virol* (2002) **83**:551–60.
101. Rau H, Revets H, Balmelli C, McCullough KC, Summerfield A. Immunological properties of recombinant classical swine fever virus NS3 protein in vitro and in vivo. *Vet Res* (2006) **37**:155–68. doi:10.1051/vetres:2005049
102. Voigt H, Wienhold D, Marquardt C, Muschko K, Pfaff E, Buettner M. Immunity against NS3 protein of classical swine fever virus does not protect against lethal challenge infection. *Viral Immunol* (2007) **20**:487–94. doi:10.1089/vim.2006.0111
103. Bouma A, de Smit AJ, de Kluijver EP, Terpstra C, Moormann RJ. Efficacy and stability of a subunit vaccine based on glycoprotein E2 of classical swine fever virus 373. *Vet Microbiol* (1999) **66**:101–14. doi:10.1016/S0378-1135(99)00003-6
104. Konig M, Lengsfeld T, Pauly T, Stark R, Thiel HJ. Classical swine fever virus: independent induction of protective immunity by two structural glycoproteins. *J Virol* (1995) **69**:6479–86.
105. van Rijn PA, Bossers A, Wensvoort G, Moormann RJ. Classical swine fever virus (CSFV) envelope glycoprotein E2 containing one structural antigenic unit protects pigs from lethal CSFV challenge. *J Gen Virol* (1996) **77**(Pt 11):2737–45. doi:10.1099/0022-1317-77-11-2737
106. Terpstra C, Wensvoort G. The protective value of vaccine-induced neutralising antibody titres in swine fever. *Vet Microbiol* (1988) **16**:123–8. doi:10.1016/0378-1135(88)90036-3
107. Ceppi M, de Bruin MG, Seuberlich T, Balmelli C, Pascolo S, Ruggli N, et al. Identification of classical swine fever virus protein E2 as a target for cytotoxic T cells by using mRNA-transfected antigen-presenting cells. *J Gen Virol* (2005) **86**:2525–34. doi:10.1099/vir.0.80907-0

Conflict of Interest Statement: The authors declare that the research was conducted in the absence of any commercial or financial relationships that could be construed as a potential conflict of interest.

2

Phytogenic feed additives as an alternative to antibiotic growth promoters in broiler chickens

Ganapathi Raj Murugesan[1], Basharat Syed[2], Sudipto Haldar[3] and Chasity Pender[1]*

[1] BIOMIN America Inc., San Antonio, TX, USA, [2] BIOMIN Holding GmbH, Getzersdorf, Austria, [3] Department of Animal Nutrition, West Bengal University of Animal and Fishery Sciences, Kolkata, India

The recent trend toward reduction of antibiotic growth promoters (AGP) in North American poultry diets has put tremendous pressure on the industry to look for viable alternatives. In this context, phytogenic feed additives (PFA) are researched to improve gut health and thereby performance. An experiment was conducted with the objective to evaluate the effects of PFA as an alternative to AGP on small intestinal histomorphology, cecal microbiota composition, nutrient digestibility, and growth performance in broiler chickens. A total of 432-day-old Vencobb 400 broiler chicks were randomly assigned to one of three dietary groups, each consisting of 12 replicate pens ($n = 12$ chicks/pen). The chicks were fed a corn–soybean meal-based control (CON), CON + 500 mg/kg of AGP (bacitracin methylene disalicylate containing 450 mg active BMD/g), or CON + 150 mg/kg of proprietary blend of PFA (Digestarom® Poultry) until 39 days of age when samples were collected. Birds fed either AGP or PFA had increased villus height in all three segments of the small intestine in comparison to the birds fed CON ($P \leq 0.05$). Furthermore, the PFA-fed birds had significantly increased villus height and lower crypt depth compared to AGP fed birds ($P \leq 0.05$). Birds fed either additive also had increased total tract digestibility of dry matter, crude protein, and ether extract ($P \leq 0.05$). The strong effect of the PFA on villus height in the jejunum may suggest augmented nutrient absorption in PFA-fed birds. Although both additives reduced total cecal counts of anaerobic bacteria and *Clostridium* spp., PFA alone reduced the total coliform count while increasing the *Lactobacillus* spp. count ($P \leq 0.05$). These results suggest the establishment of beneficial microbial colonies in PFA-fed birds. Overall, both PFA and AGP increased body weight gain while lowering the feed conversion ratio ($P \leq 0.05$). Hence data from this experiment demonstrate the efficacy of PFA as a substitute to AGP in poultry diets.

Keywords: digestibility, histomorphology, microbiota, performance, poultry

Edited by:
Michael Kogut, United States Department of Agriculture – Agricultural Research Service, USA

Reviewed by:
Guillermo Tellez, University of Arkansas, USA
Morgan Brian Farnell, Mississippi State University, USA

****Correspondence:***
Ganapathi Raj Murugesan, BIOMIN America Inc., 1842 Lockhill-Selma Road, Suite 102, San Antonio, TX 78213, USA
raj.murugesan@biomin.net

Introduction

Sustaining a healthy gut environment is a prerequisite to efficient broiler performance. Antibiotic growth promoters (AGP) have been used since the mid-1940s to maintain a healthy gut environment and in turn improve the performance (1). The ban on AGP compounds from poultry diets in Europe (2) and recent moves toward reduction or termination of AGP in North America have put pressure on the poultry industry to look for viable alternatives that can improve performance, protect animal health, and maintain profit margins (3). Phytogenic feed additives (PFA) have been gaining considerable interest lately due to their ability to improve performance by sustaining a healthy gut environment.

According to European Union legislation (EC 1831/2003) (4), PFA are categorized as sensory and flavoring compounds, which consist mainly of plant extracts (essential oils, oleoresins, and flavonoids) and their active principles (5). The essential oils present in PFA, which contain most of the active substances of the plant, have been suggested to increase the growth performance (6, 7), nutrient digestibility (8), and gut health (6, 9) in poultry species. The numerous beneficial qualities of PFA are predominantly derived from their bioactive molecules including carvacrol, thymol, capsaicin, cineole, etc. (10). It is these properties of PFA that project them as suitable alternatives to AGP.

The primary mode of action of PFA is controlling potential pathogens and beneficially modulating the intestinal microbiota. Several plant extracts are known to have antimicrobial, antiviral, anticoccidial, fungicidal, and/or antioxidant properties (11). Studies conducted in broilers have demonstrated the antimicrobial efficacy of PFA against pathogenic bacteria, such as *Escherichia coli* and *Clostridium perfringens*, potentially indicating a reduced risk for the development of colibacillosis and necrotic enteritis (8, 12). Alleviation of coccidiosis symptoms, including reduction in lesion severity and oocyst shedding, by PFA has also been documented (6). The antimicrobial effects of PFA are primarily attributed to their phenolic components and their action on pathogenic cells (13, 14).

It has been suggested that PFA augment nutrient utilization in the gastrointestinal tract (GIT) by enhancing production of digestive secretions and enzymatic activity (11, 15). Furthermore, several studies have observed positive effects of PFA on the morphology of small intestinal tissues, such as increased villus height, decreased crypt depth, and increased goblet cell counts (16–18). Such effects on gastrointestinal morphology have been postulated to increase the nutrient digestibility in poultry (19). PFA, like AGP, may also reduce mucosal thickness, thus contributing to the diffusion of nutrients to the apical surface of epithelial cells and increased absorption and feed efficiency (20).

Overall, PFA are capable of reducing microbial threat and promoting intestinal health, which is imperative for optimal bird performance and profitability. The objective of this study was to evaluate the efficacy of PFA as an alternative to AGP in broiler production by determining their effects on cecal microbiota composition, small intestinal histomorphology, nutrient digestibility, and growth performance.

Materials and Methods

Animals and Housing

All animal procedures were conducted according to the ethical norm of West Bengal University of Animal and Fishery Sciences. An experiment of 39 days duration was conducted using a total of 432-day-old Vencobb 400 broiler chicks, which were randomly assigned to one of three dietary groups at the start of experiment. The 3 groups consisted of 12 replicate pens of 12 chicks, each resulting in 144 birds per group.

Diets and Groups

The dietary groups were (i) control (CON), (ii) basal diet + AGP (AGP), and (iii) basal diet + PFA (PFA). The CON diet consisted of a corn–soybean meal-based basal diet, and was formulated to meet or exceed breeder recommendations [**Table 1**; "Nutrient Levels," Venky's Ltd. (21)]. The AGP used was bacitracin methylene disalicylate containing 450 mg active BMD/g at the inclusion rate of 500 mg/kg of diet. The PFA used was Digestarom® Poultry (Biomin Holding GmbH, Austria) at the inclusion rate of 150 mg/kg of diet. The PFA contains a combination of over 30 essential oils and phytogenic compounds. Neither exogenous polysaccharide-degrading enzymes nor anticoccidial drugs were added in the diets as these might partly mask the effects of the PFA, but a mycotoxin binder was used.

Measurements of Production Traits

Birds were monitored twice daily and any mortality was removed, weighed, and recorded. Birds were individually weighed at 7, 21, and 39 days, which designated the end of pre-starter, starter, and grower periods, respectively. Total feed intake (FI) per pen was also measured on the same days. Body weight gain (BWG), average daily feed intake (ADFI), and feed conversion rate (FCR) were calculated per pen for each period and for the overall period. Mortality BWG data were used to correct the FCR.

Determination of Apparent Total Tract Nutrient Digestibility

Two birds were randomly selected from each pen and were distributed to cages at 30 days of age (eight cages per group, three birds per cage) to provide an acclimatization period of 6 days. Total excreta collection was done for three consecutive days from

TABLE 1 | Formulation and composition (gram/kilogram) of the experimental diets.

	Starter (1–7 days)	Grower (8–21 days)	Finisher (22–39 days)
Ingredients			
Ground corn	540.7	567.2	583.4
Soybean meal (46% CP)	396.0	362.5	328.0
Soybean oil	27.0	33.7	51.1
Calcite powder	12.45	12.45	12.45
Di-calcium phosphate	16.5	16.5	17.0
D-methionine	0.55	0.95	1.35
Lysine hydrochloride	0.3	0.2	0.2
Sodium bicarbonate	2	2	2
Salt	2	2	2
Premix[a]	2	2	2
Toxin binder	0.05	0.5	0.5
Calculated composition (g/kg as-fed)			
ME_N (MJ/kg)	11.85	12.14	12.65
Crude protein	223.5	210.4	196.3
Ether extract	52.7	59.8	7.33
Crude fiber	2.5	2.4	2.4
Calcium	9.57	9.47	9.38
Available P	3.18	3.16	3.13
Digestible lysine	11.02	10.19	9.39
Digestible methionine	3.51	3.76	3.99
Digestible methionine + cysteine	6.87	6.73	6.77

[a]*Including vitamins and trace minerals.*

36 to 39 days of age at 2 h intervals. Samples were mixed, weighed, and a 10% aliquot was frozen at −20°C. The sampled excreta were again pooled by cage at the end of the collection period, and a 10% aliquot was taken and dried. Feed samples were collected daily for the same 3-day period (36–39 days) and pooled to produce a single composite of each diet. Diet and excreta samples were analyzed to determine the apparent total tract digestibility of dry matter (DM), crude protein (CP), and ether extract (EE) (22, 23).

Histomorphology of the Small Intestine

One bird per replicate pen was euthanized via carbon dioxide asphyxiation at the end of the experiment on day 39. The entire GIT tract was removed aseptically before separating into sections of duodenum, jejunum, ileum, cecum, and colon. The small intestinal segments (duodenum, jejunum, and ileum) were processed for histomorphological analysis (24). Segments measuring 2-cm in length from the mid-points of the duodenum, jejunum, and ileum were cut, flushed with cold saline, fixed in 10% buffered formalin, and stained with hematoxylin–eosin. Histological sections were examined with a phase contrast microscope coupled with a deconvolution imaging analysis system [VayTek®, Fairfield, IA, USA; (25)]. Villus height (VH, from the tip of the villus to the top of the lamina propria), crypt depth (CD, from the base to the region of transition between the crypt and villus), and the thickness of the muscularis mucosae in the duodenum, jejunum, and ileum were determined. Measurements of 10 complete villi for VH and associated crypts for CD were taken from each segment, and the average of these values was used for statistical analysis.

Caecal Microbiota Composition

The ceca with contents were stored at 4°C for determination of cecal microbiota. The cecal digesta was processed within 24 h (5). Each cecal digesta homogenate was serially diluted from 10-1 to 10-8. Coliforms were cultured using HiCrome *E. coli* HiVeg Agar (Product code: MV1295; Hi-Media Laboratories, Mumbai, India), anaerobic bacteria were cultured using Wilkins Chalgren Anaerobic Agar (Product code: M832; Hi-Media Laboratories), *Staphylococcus aureus* was cultured using HiCrome Staph Agar (Product code: M1837; Hi-Media Laboratories), *Lactobacillus* spp. were cultured using *Lactobacillus* MRS Agar (Product code: M641; Hi-Media Laboratories), *Pseudomonas aeruginosa* was cultured using Cetrimide Agar (Product code: M024; Hi-Media Laboratories), and the *Clostridium* were cultured in Reinforced Clostridial Agar (Product code: M154; Hi-Media Laboratories). Diluted digesta samples were streaked onto the agar plates and incubated at 37°C for 48 h, while the clostridia plates were incubated anaerobically at similar temperature. Visible colonies were enumerated using a colony counter and the results were expressed as $\log_{10}$ CFU/g of cecal digesta.

Statistical Analysis

The data were analyzed as a complete randomized design using General Linear Model procedure of SPSS (version 17.0). Repeated measures ANOVA was used to analyze performance parameters, which were measured over the course of the experiment. Means were separated using Tukey-WSD following ANOVA. Values were considered statistically different at $P \leq 0.05$. The replicate pens were used as experimental units for all parameters except apparent total tract nutrient digestibility where the cages were used as experimental units.

Results

Production Performance

Body Weight Gain

Mortalities for the groups were statistically insignificant at 4.22, 2.22, and 2.78% for the CON, AGP, and PFA groups, respectively, for the 1–39 days period. No significant differences in BWG were noted during the 1–7 days pre-starter phase (**Table 2**). There was an effect of dietary treatment on BWG during the starter phase (8–21 days; $P = 0.03$), grower phase (22–39 days; $P < 0.01$), and during the overall period (1–39 days; $P < 0.01$). During the starter phase, birds-fed AGP had significantly increased BWG compared to CON-fed birds ($P \leq 0.05$), while the BWG for PFA-fed birds was not significantly different from either CON or AGP groups. During the grower phase, birds-fed PFA had significantly increased BWG in comparison to both CON ($P \leq 0.05$) and AGP groups ($P \leq 0.05$), which did not differ from each other. Supplementation of either AGP ($P \leq 0.05$) or PFA ($P \leq 0.05$) to the basal diet significantly increased BWG for the overall experimental period.

Feed Intake

No significant differences in FI were noted among the groups throughout the experimental period, except during the starter phase (8–21 days; $P = 0.01$) when the FI of PFA-fed birds was significantly lower in comparison to both AGP- ($P \leq 0.05$) and CON-fed birds ($P \leq 0.05$; **Table 2**).

TABLE 2 | Performance of broilers supplemented with either an antibiotic or a phytogenic feed additive during 1–39 days of age*.

	Dietary treatments†			SEM	*P* value
	Control	AGP	PFA		
Pre-starter period (1–7 days)					
Body weight gain (g)	140.5	144.3	142.3	1.20	0.44
Feed intake (g)	185.4	185.9	185.5	1.03	0.98
Feed conversion‡	1.323	1.292	1.305	0.012	0.57
Starter period (8–21 days)					
Body weight gain (g)	823.4^{b}	860.3^{a}	835.1^{ab}	5.93	0.03
Feed intake (g)	1004.5^{a}	1007.8^{a}	975.3^{b}	4.96	0.01
Feed conversion‡	1.221^{a}	1.173^{ab}	1.169^{b}	0.089	0.02
Grower period (22–39 days)					
Body weight gain (g)	1073.5^{b}	1109.2^{b}	1183.1^{b}	12.49	<0.01
Feed intake (g)	2599.6	2606.5	2590.6	7.56	0.71
Feed conversion‡	2.431^{a}	2.355^{a}	2.195^{b}	0.028	<0.01
Overall period (1–39 days)					
Body weight gain (g)	1896.9^{b}	1969.5^{a}	2018.2^{a}	14.41	<0.01
Feed intake (g)	3789.5	3800.2	3751.5	9.81	0.10
Feed conversion‡	2.002^{a}	1.931^{ab}	1.860^{b}	0.015	<0.01

Means with dissimilar letters in a row varied significantly.

**Means of 12 replicate pens (n = 12 birds per pen).*

†Supplemented with either an antibiotic growth promoter, bacitracin methylene disalicylate, 500 mg/kg (AGP), or a phytogenic feed additive (Digestarom® Poultry) 150 mg/kg (PFA). The control group received the unsupplemented basal diet.

‡Corrected for mortality.

Mortality-Corrected Feed Conversion Ratio

No significant differences in FCR were present during the 1–7 days pre-starter phase (**Table 2**). There was an effect of treatment on FCR during the 8–21 days starter phase ($P = 0.02$), 22–39 days grower phase ($P < 0.01$), and for the overall period (1–39 days; $P < 0.01$). Supplementation of PFA lowered the FCR in comparison to CON-fed birds during all time periods ($P \leq 0.05$). The FCR for birds-fed AGP did not differ significantly from either the CON or PFA groups for the starter phase as well as for the overall period. During the grower phase, however, PFA-fed birds had significantly lower FCR in comparison to the AGP-fed group ($P \leq 0.05$).

Nutrient Digestibility

There was a significant effect of dietary treatment on apparent total tract digestibility of DM ($P < 0.01$), CP ($P = 0.04$), and EE ($P = 0.02$; **Table 3**). The apparent total tract DM digestibility for the PFA-fed group was increased in comparison to the CON group ($P \leq 0.05$), while the AGP group was not different from either the CON or PFA groups. Supplementation of either AGP or PFA to the basal diet significantly increased the apparent total tract digestibility of CP and EE when compared to the CON group ($P \leq 0.05$).

Histomorphology of Small Intestine

Dietary treatment had a significant effect on VH in the duodenum ($P = 0.02$), jejunum ($P < 0.01$), and ileum ($P < 0.01$; **Table 4**). The VH was significantly increased by AGP supplementation in the duodenum in comparison to the CON group ($P \leq 0.05$), while PFA was not different from either AGP or CON. In the jejunum, both AGP and PFA significantly increased the VH in comparison to CON ($P \leq 0.05$); however, the PFA group had significantly increased VH compared to AGP-fed birds ($P \leq 0.05$). Additionally, both AGP and PFA significantly increased the ileal VH in comparison to the CON group ($P \leq 0.05$). Overall, the supplementation of either AGP or PFA increased the VH across the small intestine.

No significant differences in CD were noted in any dietary group in the duodenum or ileum (**Table 4**). There was a significant effect of dietary treatment in the jejunum ($P < 0.01$), where inclusion of PFA in the basal diet lowered the CD in the jejunum when compared to both CON and AGP groups ($P \leq 0.05$).

Additionally, there was a significant effect of treatment on mucosal thickness in the duodenum ($P < 0.01$) and ileum ($P < 0.01$; **Table 4**). Both AGP and PFA significantly lowered the mucosal thickness in the duodenum and ileum in comparison to the CON group ($P \leq 0.05$), but no differences were present in the jejunal mucosal thickness.

Cecal Microbiota Composition

The composition of cecal microbiota at 39 days of age in $\log_{10}$ CFU/g of wet cecal digesta is provided in **Table 5**. There was a significant effect of dietary treatment on total coliform ($P < 0.01$), anaerobic bacteria ($P < 0.01$), *Lactobacillus* spp. ($P < 0.01$), and *Clostridium* spp. ($P = 0.01$) counts. Supplementation of PFA significantly decreased the total coliform count in comparison to the CON and the AGP groups ($P \leq 0.05$). The CFU of total anaerobic bacteria and total *Clostridium* were decreased with the supplementation of either AGP or PFA ($P \leq 0.05$). Supplementation of either AGP or PFA tended to decrease *Staphylococcus aureus* in comparison to the CON group ($P = 0.06$). No effect of dietary treatment on the cecal population of *Pseudomonas aeruginosa* was noted; however, supplementation of PFA significantly increased the number of cecal *Lactobacillus* in comparison to the CON and AGP groups ($P \leq 0.05$).

TABLE 3 | Nutrient digestibility of broilers supplemented with either an antibiotic or a phytogenic feed additive during 1–39 days of age*.

	Dietary treatments†			SEM	*P* value
	Control	AGP	PFA		
Nutrient digestibility (g/g intake)					
Dry matter	0.674[b]	0.711[ab]	0.744[a]	0.007	<0.01
Crude protein	0.761[b]	0.784[a]	0.794[a]	0.005	0.04
Ether extract	0.736[b]	0.781[a]	0.782[a]	0.005	0.02

Means with dissimilar letters in a row varied significantly.

**Digestibility trial was conducted at 36 days of age for three consecutive days. Randomly selected birds were placed in metabolism cages. There were eight cages per treatment with three birds in each cage.*

†Supplemented with either an antibiotic growth promoter, bacitracin methylene disalicylate, 500 mg/kg (AGP), or a phytogenic feed additive (Digestarom® Poultry) 150 mg/kg (PFA). The control group received the unsupplemented basal diet.

TABLE 4 | Villus height, crypt depth, and thickness of muscularis mucosae (micrometer) of broilers supplemented with either an antibiotic or a phytogenic feed additive during 1–39 days of age*.

	Dietary treatments†			SEM	*P* value
	Control	AGP	PFA		
Duodenum					
Villus height	2549.1[b]	3481.1[a]	2903.4[ab]	140.23	0.02
Crypt depth	45.3	42.7	32.8	2.55	0.10
Mucosa thickness	387.1[a]	183.9[b]	230.4[b]	22.69	<0.01
Jejunum					
Villus height	2583.6[c]	2969.9[b]	3290.1[a]	280.51	<0.01
Crypt depth	29.8[a]	31.1[a]	20.2[b]	1.31	<0.01
Mucosa thickness	206.8	215.6	212.9	6.85	0.88
Ileum					
Villus height	2050.1[b]	2736.4[a]	2839.9[a]	94.03	<0.01
Crypt depth	34.1	30.9	31.6	1.04	0.45
Mucosa thickness	320.3[a]	233.9[b]	211.8[b]	14.31	<0.01

Means with dissimilar letters in a row varied significantly.

**Means of 12 birds per treatment. Birds were randomly selected and euthanized at 39 days of age.*

†Supplemented with either an antibiotic growth promoter, bacitracin methylene disalicylate, 500 mg/kg (AGP), or a phytogenic feed additive (Digestarom® Poultry) 150 mg/kg (PFA). The control group received the unsupplemented basal diet.

Discussion

Supplementation of PFA significantly lowered the overall FCR by 3.6% (7 points) and 7.0% (14 points) in comparison to the AGP and CON groups, respectively. This was in agreement with earlier reports (5), which indicated improvement in final BW and FCR with PFA supplementation without any effect on the FI. The growth promoting effects of the PFA and the AGP in this experiment may be correlated with the significant increase in apparent total tract digestibility of nutrients. Furthermore, a significant

TABLE 5 | Cecal microbiota composition ($\log_{10}$ CFU/g wet cecal digesta) of broilers supplemented with either an antibiotic or a phytogenic feed additive during 1–39 days of age*.

	Dietary treatments†			SEM	*P* value
	Control	AGP	PFA		
Coliforms	5.54^{a}	5.62^{a}	5.10^{b}	0.07	<0.01
Anaerobic bacteria	5.91^{a}	5.64^{b}	5.53^{b}	0.04	<0.01
Staphylococcus aureus	2.61	1.24	1.14	0.49	0.06
Pseudomonas aeruginosa	4.81	4.74	4.84	0.06	0.27
Lactobacillus spp.	4.96^{b}	5.01^{b}	5.35^{a}	0.04	<0.01
Clostridium spp.	5.17^{a}	4.95^{b}	4.97^{b}	0.03	0.01

Means with dissimilar letters in a row varied significantly.

**Means of 12 birds per treatment. Birds were randomly selected and euthanized at 39 days of age.*

†Supplemented with either an antibiotic growth promoter, bacitracin methylene disalicylate, 500 mg/kg (AGP), or a phytogenic feed additive (Digestarom® Poultry) 150 mg/kg (PFA). The control group received the unsupplemented basal diet.

decrease in FI in the PFA group was noted during the starter phase, perhaps suggesting that the bird's nutrient requirements are being satisfied with a smaller quantity of feed (26). It has been well documented that AGP-increased nutrient digestibility is mostly due to their effects on the intestinal microbiota (27). Increased nutrient digestibility with the addition of PFA and growth performance similar to Avilamycin was reported by Hernandez et al. (19). It has been noted that extracts from spices and herbs may stimulate digestive secretions and enzymatic activity, thus exerting beneficial actions within the digestive tract (28). The present findings further support the idea that PFA favorably modulate gut functions and digestive activities to stimulate growth in broilers.

Morphological changes in the GIT caused by PFA may provide further information on possible benefits to the digestive tract. In general, PFA and AGP significantly increased the VH across the small intestine. In the absence of any inflammation, this ought to increase absorptive surface area and efficiency of digestion and absorption (29). A similar effect of PFA on VH has been reported by Namkung et al. (17). The positive effect of PFA in the present experiment in increasing the VH in the jejunum could increase the efficiency of absorptive process considering the fact that the majority of absorption occurs in the jejunum. Furthermore, greater VH increases the activities of mucosal digestive enzymes, resulting in improved digestibility (30, 31). As intestinal crypts are the source of epithelial cells for villi and CD is directly correlated with epithelial cell turnover, the shallower crypts in the jejunum due to PFA supplementation may be indicative of decreased cellular turnover and improved intestinal health. Moreover, cellular turnover is an energy consuming process that uses resources that might otherwise be utilized toward growth; thus, shallower crypts are also related to improved performance (32). In the current study, mucosa thickness was significantly reduced in the duodenums and ileums of AGP and PFA supplemented birds. Gordon and Bruckner-Kardoss (33) reported that germ-free birds had thinner muscularis mucosa than the birds reared under conventional management systems, indicating that thinning of the mucosa might spare nutrients for productive processes and this was reflected in the BWG of the birds.

Literature depicting antimicrobial role of PFA is ample (8, 12, 14, 34, 35), while very few explore the mode of action by which the PFA may facilitate the proliferation of beneficial bacteria, such as *Lactobacillus* spp. (5, 8). In the present experiment, PFA significantly reduced the cecal population of coliforms and fortified the gut microbiota with beneficial bacteria, such as *Lactobacillus* spp. Once the *Lactobacillus* spp. are established, they might selectively exclude the pathogens from adhering due to their fast colonization, proliferation, and acidification properties in the GIT (9). The inhibitory effect of PFA on *Clostridium* spp. is encouraging and paves the way for removal of the AGP from poultry diets. The essential oils present in PFA have been shown to inhibit the growth of *Clostridia* (34). Mitsch et al. (12) opined that PFA stabilizes the gut microbiota and thereby reduces the colonization of *Clostridia* in gut. Evaluation of the cecal microbiota population in this study has revealed that AGP and PFA alike reduced total bacterial load in the gut. This inhibitory effect of PFA on bacterial load may alleviate pressure on the immune system, thus allowing the reallocation of energy toward improving performance. Overall from the gut perspective, the PFA purportedly favored a healthy gut, which in turn could be concomitant with the growth enhancement.

In conclusion, supplementation of either AGP or PFA increased the apparent total tract nutrient digestibility by increasing the VH throughout the small intestine. In comparison to the AGP, the PFA supported establishment of a favorable gut microbiota composed of higher numbers of *Lactobacillus* spp. and less *Clostridium* spp. Furthermore, supplementation of PFA to a corn–soybean meal-based coccidiostat free diet increased the BWG and lowered the FCR in 39 days, which was comparable to the AGP used in this experiment. Overall, the present work demonstrated the efficacy of PFA utilization and confirms the importance of considering the inclusion of PFA in poultry diets as an alternative to AGP.

Author Note

Presented in the Gut Health Symposium held at St. Louis, MO, USA on November 12, 2014.

References

1. Dibner JJ, Richards JD. Antibiotic growth promoters in agriculture: history and mode of action. *Poult Sci* (2005) **84**:634–43. doi:10.1093/ps/84.4.634
2. Castanon JI. History of the use of antibiotic as growth promoters in European poultry feeds. *Poult Sci* (2007) **86**:2466–71. doi:10.3382/ps.2007-00249
3. Yegani M, Korver DR. Factors affecting intestinal health in poultry. *Poult Sci* (2008) **87**:2052–63. doi:10.3382/ps.2008-00091
4. EC (European Commission). Regulation 1831 of the European Parliament and of the Council of 22 September 2003 on additives for use in animal nutrition. *Off J Eur Union L* (2003) **268**:29.
5. Mountzouris KC, Paraskevas V, Tsirtsikos P, Palamidi I, Stenier T, Schatzmayr G, et al. Assessment of a phytogenic feed additive effect on broiler growth performance, nutrient digestibility and caecal micro flora composition. *Anim Feed Sci Technol* (2011) **168**:223–31. doi:10.1016/j.anifeedsci.2011.03.020
6. Giannenas I, Florou Paneri P, Papazahariadou M, Christaki E, Botsoglou NA, Spais AB. Effect of dietary supplementation with oregano essential oil on performance of broilers after experimental infection with *Eimeria tenella*. *Arch Anim Nutr* (2003) **57**:99–106. doi:10.1080/0003942031000107299
7. Isabel B, Santos Y. Effects of dietary organic acids and essential oils on growth performance and carcass characteristics of broiler chickens. *J Appl Poult Res* (2009) **18**:472–6. doi:10.3382/japr.2008-00096

8. Jamroz D, Wiliczkiewicz A, Wertelecki T, Orda J, Scorupinska J. Use of active substances of plant origin in chicken diets based on maize and domestic grains. *Br Poult Sci* (2005) **46**:485–93. doi:10.1080/00071660500191056
9. McReynolds C, Waneck C, Byrd J, Genovese K, Duke S, Nisbet D. Efficacy of multistrain direct-fed microbial and phytogenetic products in reducing necrotic enteritis in commercial broilers. *Poult Sci* (2009) **88**:2075–80. doi:10.3382/ps.2009-00106
10. Mountzouris KC, Paraskevas V, Fegeros K. Phytogenic compounds in broiler nutrition. In: Steiner T, editor. *Phytogenics in Animal Nutrition: Natural Concepts to Optimize Gut Health and Performance*. Nottingham, UK: Nottingham University Press (2010). p. 97–110.
11. Applegate TJ, Klose V, Steiner T, Ganner A, Schatzmayr G. Probiotics and phytogenics for poultry: myth or reality? *J Appl Poult Res* (2010) **19**:194–210. doi:10.3382/japr.2010-00168
12. Mitsch P, Zitterl-Eglseer K, Kohler B, Gabler C, Losa R, Zimpernik I. The effect of two different blends of essential oil components on the proliferation of *Clostridium perfringens* in the intestines of broiler chickens. *Poult Sci* (2004) **83**:669–75. doi:10.1093/ps/83.4.669
13. Burt S. Essential oils: their antibacterial properties and potential application in foods – a review. *Int J Food Microbiol* (2004) **94**:223–53. doi:10.1016/j.ijfoodmicro.2004.03.022
14. Si W, Gong J, Tsao R, Zhou T, Yu H, Poppe C, et al. Antimicrobial activity of essential oils and structurally related synthetic food additives towards selected pathogenic and beneficial gut bacteria. *J Appl Microbiol* (2006) **100**:296–305. doi:10.1111/j.1365-2672.2005.02789.x
15. Windisch W, Schedle K, Plitzner C, Kroismayr A. Use of phytogenic products as feed additives for swine and poultry. *J Anim Sci* (2007) **86**:E140–8. doi:10.2527/jas.2007-0459
16. Jamroz D, Wertelecki T, Houszka M, Kamel C. Influence of diet type on the inclusion of plant origin active substances on morphological and histochemical characteristics of the stomach and jejunum walls in chicken. *J Anim Physiol Anim Nutr* (2006) **90**:255–68. doi:10.1111/j.1439-0396.2005.00603.x
17. Namkung H, Li M, Gong J, Yu H, Cottrill M, de Lange CFM. Impact of feeding blends of organic acids and herbal extracts on growth performance, gut microbiota and digestive function in newly weaned pigs. *Can J Anim Sci* (2004) **84**:697–704. doi:10.4141/A04-005
18. Reisinger N, Steiner T, Nitsch S, Shatzmayr G, Applegate T. Effects of a blend of essential oils on broiler performance and intestinal morphology during coccidial vaccine exposure. *J Appl Poult Res* (2011) **20**:272–83. doi:10.3382/japr.2010-00226
19. Hernandez F, Madrid J, Garcia V, Orengo J, Megias MD. Influence of two plant extracts on broilers performance, digestibility, and digestive organ size. *Poult Sci* (2004) **83**:169–74. doi:10.1093/ps/83.2.169
20. Yang C, Kabir Chowdhurry MA, Hou Y, Gong J. Phytogenic compounds as alternatives to in-feed antibiotics: potentials and challenges in application. *Pathogens* (2015) **4**:137–56. doi:10.3390/pathogens4010137
21. Venky's Ltd. *Nutrient Levels*. Available from: http://www.venkys.com/vh-breeds/vencobb-broiler-broiler-breeder/vencobb-broiler-management-guide/nutrient-levels/. (accessed June 12, 2015).
22. AOAC. *Official Methods of Analysis*. 15th ed. Washington, DC: AOAC (1990).
23. Murugesan GR, Persia ME. Validation of the effects of small differences in dietary ME and feed restriction in first-cycle laying hens. *Poult Sci* (2013) **92**:1238–43. doi:10.3382/ps.2012-02719
24. Haldar S, Ghosh TK, Toshiwati, Bedford MR. Effects of yeast (*Saccharomyces cerevisiae*) and yeast protein concentrate on production performance of broiler chickens exposed to heat stress and challenged with Salmonella enteritidis. *Anim Feed Sci Technol* (2011) **168**:61–71. doi:10.1016/j.anifeedsci.2011.03.007
25. Murugesan GR, Wesley IV, Remus J, Plumstead PW, Persia ME. Interactions of exogenous enzymes and direct-fed microbial on intestinal energy metabolism, integrity, pathogen shedding and performance in first cycle laying hens. *Austr Poult Sci* (2013) **24**:148–51.
26. Richards MP, Proszkowiec-Weglarz M. Mechanisms regulating feed intake, energy expenditure, and body weight in poultry. *Poult Sci* (2007) **86**:1478–90. doi:10.1093/ps/86.7.1478
27. Bedford M. Removal of antibiotic growth promoters from poultry diets: implications and strategies to minimise subsequent problems. *World Poult Sci J* (2000) **56**:349–64. doi:10.1079/WPS20000024
28. Platel K, Srinivasan K. Digestive stimulant action of spices: a myth or reality? *Indian J Med Res* (2004) **119**:167–79.
29. Murugesan GR, Gabler NK, Persia ME. Effects of direct-fed microbial supplementation on broiler performance, intestinal nutrient transport and integrity under experimental conditions with increased microbial challenge. *Br Poult Sci* (2014) **55**:89–97. doi:10.1080/00071668.2013.865834
30. Baurhoo B, Phillip L, Ruiz-Feria CA. Effects of purified lignin and mannan oligosaccharides on intestinal integrity and microbial populations in the ceca and litter of broiler chickens. *Poult Sci* (2007) **86**:1070–8. doi:10.1093/ps/86.6.1070
31. Murugesan GR, Romero LF, Persia ME. Effects of protease, phytase and a Bacillus sp. direct-fed microbial on nutrient and energy digestibility, ileal brush border digestive enzyme activity and cecal short-chain fatty acid concentration in broiler chickens. *PLoS One* (2014) **9**:e101888. doi:10.1371/journal.pone.0101888
32. Markovic R, Sefer D, Krstic M, Petrujkic B. The effect of different growth promotors on broiler performance and gut morphology. *Arch Med Vet* (2009) **41**:163–9. doi:10.4067/S0301-732X2009000200010
33. Gordon HA, Bruckner-Kardoss E. Effect of normal microflora on intestinal surface area. *Am J Physiol* (1961) **201**:175–8.
34. Dorman HJD, Deans SG. Antimicrobial agents from plants: antibacterial activity of plant volatile oils. *J Appl Microbiol* (2000) **88**:308–16. doi:10.1046/j.1365-2672.2000.00969.x
35. Jamroz D, Orda I, Kamel C, Wiliczkiewicz A, Wertelecki T, Skorupinska I. The influence of phytogenic extracts on performance, nutrient digestibility, carcass characteristics, and gut microbial status in broiler chickens. *J Anim Feed Sci* (2003) **12**:583–96.

Conflict of Interest Statement: The authors declare that the research was conducted in the absence of any commercial or financial relationships that could be construed as a potential conflict of interest.

3

Objects in contact with classical scrapie sheep act as a reservoir for scrapie transmission

Timm Konold[1], Stephen A. C. Hawkins[2], Lisa C. Thurston[3], Ben C. Maddison[4], Kevin C. Gough[5], Anthony Duarte[1] and Hugh A. Simmons[1]*

[1] Animal Sciences Unit, Animal and Plant Health Agency Weybridge, Addlestone, UK, [2] Pathology Department, Animal and Plant Health Agency Weybridge, Addlestone, UK, [3] Surveillance and Laboratory Services, Animal and Plant Health Agency Penrith, Penrith, UK, [4] ADAS UK, School of Veterinary Medicine and Science, University of Nottingham, Sutton Bonington, UK, [5] School of Veterinary Medicine and Science, University of Nottingham, Sutton Bonington, UK

Edited by:
Scott Napper,
University of Saskatchewan, Canada

Reviewed by:
Franck Carbonero,
University of Arkansas, USA
Jason Kindrachuk,
National Institutes of Health, USA

Correspondence:
Timm Konold,
Animal and Plant Health Agency Weybridge, New Haw, Addlestone, Surrey KT15 3NB, UK
timm.konold@apha.gsi.gov.uk

Classical scrapie is an environmentally transmissible prion disease of sheep and goats. Prions can persist and remain potentially infectious in the environment for many years and thus pose a risk of infecting animals after re-stocking. *In vitro* studies using serial protein misfolding cyclic amplification (sPMCA) have suggested that objects on a scrapie-affected sheep farm could contribute to disease transmission. This *in vivo* study aimed to determine the role of field furniture (water troughs, feeding troughs, fencing, and other objects that sheep may rub against) used by a scrapie-infected sheep flock as a vector for disease transmission to scrapie-free lambs with the prion protein genotype *VRQ/VRQ*, which is associated with high susceptibility to classical scrapie. When the field furniture was placed in clean accommodation, sheep became infected when exposed to either a water trough (four out of five) or to objects used for rubbing (four out of seven). This field furniture had been used by the scrapie-infected flock 8 weeks earlier and had previously been shown to harbor scrapie prions by sPMCA. Sheep also became infected (20 out of 23) through exposure to contaminated field furniture placed within pasture not used by scrapie-infected sheep for 40 months, even though swabs from this furniture tested negative by PMCA. This infection rate decreased (1 out of 12) on the same paddock after replacement with clean field furniture. Twelve grazing sheep exposed to field furniture not in contact with scrapie-infected sheep for 18 months remained scrapie free. The findings of this study highlight the role of field furniture used by scrapie-infected sheep to act as a reservoir for disease re-introduction although infectivity declines considerably if the field furniture has not been in contact with scrapie-infected sheep for several months. PMCA may not be as sensitive as *VRQ/VRQ* sheep to test for environmental contamination.

Keywords: classical scrapie, prion, transmissible spongiform encephalopathy, sheep, field furniture, reservoir, serial protein misfolding cyclic amplification

Introduction

Classical scrapie is a transmissible spongiform encephalopathy (TSE) of sheep and goats, which is caused by infection with a proteinacious infectious particle, the prion (1). Prions are particularly resistant to commonly used disinfectants and inactivating methods and can remain biologically active, which increases the risk of re-infection after re-stocking.

Soil has been implicated as plausible reservoir of scrapie prions because laboratory studies have shown that scrapie-associated prion protein (PrP^{Sc}) can bind to soil particles, which may remain close to the surface where it was released so that it is accessible to grazing animals (2). Indeed, pastures not used by a scrapie-infected flock for more than a month remained contaminated and led to infection of genetically fully susceptible "clean" sheep, even if exposed for only 6 weeks (3). However, the scrapie agent was reportedly also able to re-infect sheep in a building that had not been used for 16 years (4); thus, reservoirs other than soil contribute to scrapie transmission.

While contamination of the environment had historically been mainly attributed to prions in placentae from scrapie-infected ewes (5), it has now been established by PrP^{Sc} detection methods that various sources may contribute to environmental contamination, such as urine (6), feces (7), saliva (8), and possibly rubbed off skin (9), which explains the lateral transmission of scrapie to sheep where no lambing has occurred (10, 11). However, less is known about the vectors that facilitate disease transmission, particularly in buildings that have previously housed scrapie-infected sheep.

Prions were detected by serial protein misfolding cyclic amplification (sPMCA) in swabs taken from water troughs and fences that had been present on a scrapie-infected sheep farm, and it was hypothesized that they could act as environmental reservoirs to contribute to scrapie transmission (12). The current study was designed to investigate the persistence of environmental scrapie infectivity using a sheep bioassay. As there was surprisingly little evidence of environmental contamination on pastures used previously by a scrapie-infected flock after re-introduction of new sheep, this study aimed to confirm the relevance of field furniture as a vector for scrapie transmission by exposing sheep to objects that had been in contact with a scrapie-infected flock.

Materials and Methods

All procedures were in accordance with the United Kingdom (UK) Animal (Scientific Procedures) Act 1986, under license from the UK Government Home Office (project licenses 70/6774 and 70/7782) following approval by the institutional ethical review process.

Scrapie-Infected Flock

A scrapie research flock was established in 1998 by purchasing clinically healthy sheep from scrapie-affected flocks with scrapie-susceptible genotypes and maintained through breeding sheep of susceptible genotypes (10). At the time of the project, more than 50% of the sheep in the flock were homozygous *VRQ* (valine at codon 136, arginine at 154, and glutamine at 171 of the ovine prion protein gene), which is associated with high susceptibility to classical scrapie (13), and developed clinical disease from 18 months of age. Sheep were kept on pastures for many years, being kept in sheds just before lambing and occasionally in severe weather. The pasture was managed on a rotation basis and was plowed and reseeded as required. Manure and composted bedding from the lambing sheds was incinerated and not spread on the pasture. For logistical reasons, sheep with clinical signs suggestive of scrapie were predominantly kept on one particular pasture to enable closer monitoring until cull at clinical end-stage.

Classical Scrapie-Free Flock

Testing for infectivity was carried out using Cheviot sheep from a flock that was originally generated from imported sheep from New Zealand and kept free of classical scrapie through strict biosecurity measures (14), which was confirmed routinely by testing of culled sheep's brains for TSEs (Bio-Rad TeSeE; Bio-Rad Laboratories, UK). All sheep were homozygous *VRQ*.

Level of Contamination of Field Furniture in Clean Housing

Field furniture that had been in contact with the scrapie flock 8 weeks earlier was used. Selection of items was to some degree influenced by the results from an earlier study where environmental sources of scrapie prions were investigated by sPMCA and which had demonstrated the presence of PrP^{Sc} on a fire extinguisher box (referred to as plastic scratching post in Reference 12), wooden fence post, and fencing (12) 2 years earlier. Sample extractions from objects and sPMCA methodology were carried out as described previously (12). Briefly, eight swabs were taken for each surface, a swab sample consisted of a wetted foam swab that had been rubbed 10 times over an area of approximately 10 cm × 2 cm, and these were stored frozen at −80°C until extraction. Samples were extracted using a silicon dioxide enrichment methodology (15), the extracts from two swabs being finally eluted in 200 µl of 0.1% w/v SDS solution, of which 10 µl was then used to seed each sPMCA reaction. Each extracted sample was amplified in triplicate or duplicate reactions for nine sPMCA rounds using a substrate consisting of a 10% healthy *VRQ/VRQ* sheep brain homogenate [a different brain substrate to that used in Ref. (12)]. The 0.2-ml PCR tubes containing the extracts and substrate were placed in an ultrasonicating water bath (model S4000; Misonix, USA) at 37°C. Sonications were performed for 10 s at 200 W and these were repeated once every 30 min for 24 h (one PMCA round). After each PMCA round, the samples were diluted 1 in 3 with fresh substrate in a final volume of 100 µl and the process repeated up to a total of nine rounds. Reaction products were then digested with 50 µg/ml proteinase K (PK) with the addition of 0.045% (wt/vol) SDS for 1 h at 37°C before western blot analysis using 12% (wt/vol) NuPAGE precast Bis-Tris gels. Reactions were scored positive if a PK-resistant triplet was visible on the western blot after probing with the antibody SHa31- and HRP-based chemiluminescent detection.

For *in vivo* testing of the infectivity of objects from pastures grazed by the scrapie flock, 24 *VRQ/VRQ* lambs 1–5 days of age (83% aged 2 days) were housed in a building that had never been used for any classical scrapie-infected sheep. The lambs, which were kept with their dams until 3–4 months of age, were housed in four pens with group sizes determined by availability of sheep and housing capacity as follows:

Pen 1. Five lambs in a pen with clean furniture (building controls).

Pen 2. Six lambs in a pen with a water trough from a pasture used mainly by subclinically infected sheep of the scrapie flock.

Pen 3. Six lambs in a pen with a water trough from a pasture, which was used by clinically affected sheep prior to cull.

Pen 4. Seven lambs in a pen with a wooden fence post, fencing with traces of fleece from sheep attached to it and a fire extinguisher box. This box had been fixed outside an area where the sheep from the scrapie-infected flock would gather just before entering the handling area and had been used by sheep to rub their backs and head.

None of the items were cleaned but the water troughs were emptied and filled with new water in the animal accommodation. All items placed into pens 2–4 were swabbed and analyzed by sPMCA in triplicate before arrival of the sheep. Swabs were taken from analogous surfaces to the scrapie-contaminated farm, e.g., water troughs, metal hurdles, etc., at the farm housing the classical scrapie-free flock to serve as control samples, which were tested in parallel with the samples from the scrapie-contaminated objects.

The pens shared common air space but were separated by 3 m high concrete walls, and each pen had its own entrance and separate equipment and protective clothing to avoid cross-contamination.

Scrapie infection was monitored by rectal biopsy at approximately 6, 9, 13, and 19 months post exposure (mpe). Biopsies were taken under local anesthesia with a prilocaine and lidocaine mixture (EMLA cream; AstraZeneca, UK) and the recto-anal mucosa-associated lymphoid tissue (RAMALT) examined for presence of disease-associated prion protein (PrP^{Sc}) with rat monoclonal antibody R145 (APHA, UK) according to previously published methods (16). For the rectal biopsy at 6 mpe, lambs were sedated with 0.8 ml acepromazine (ACP injection 2 mg/ml; Novartis Animal Health, UK) given intramuscularly approximately 30 min prior to the biopsy due to their restlessness. Sheep were examined for signs of scrapie according to a short clinical protocol (17) prior to cull from 23 mpe, whereby sheep were assessed by a veterinarian for signs of abnormal behavior (e.g. separation from others), gait (e.g. ataxia), and sensation (e.g. reaction to scratching with head or lip movements, impaired menace response) and – depending on the display of signs – classified as clinical suspect, inconclusive, or clinically healthy with regards to scrapie.

Scrapie infection was determined postmortem by immunohistochemical examination of lymphoreticular tissue (RAMALT, distal ileum, mesenteric lymph node) in all animals and – in all sheep over 12 months of age – additional examination of brain tissue (right and left half of the obex) for PrP^{Sc} by immunohistochemistry (18) and for the proteinase-resistant form of PrP^{Sc} (PrP^{res}) by ELISA (Bio-Rad TeSeE; Bio-Rad Laboratories, UK) according to the manufacturer's instructions.

Exposure of Sheep to Contaminated Furniture on Pasture in Paddock 1

For the field study, a 5.4 ha-sized pasture that had been occupied by scrapie sheep was divided into four equal paddocks, with two paddocks (termed 1 and 2) used for the reported study. Each paddock, measured approximately 13,000 m^2, was double fenced with new fencing, with a minimum of 2 m between the fences to prevent nose-to-nose contact between sheep in different paddocks. Each paddock had its own set of protective clothing for farm workers and equipment.

Contamination of the soil in both paddocks used for the reported study was previously investigated by moving groups of six 2-day-old lambs with their dams to these paddocks, each equipped with a new water trough. None of the six lambs in each group had detectable PrP^{Sc} in a rectal biopsy taken at 6 and 9 mpe and although they were subsequently moved to a different paddock at 10 mpe, none of the sheep presented with detectable PrP^{Sc} in brain and lymphoid tissue when culled at 34 months of age.

Contaminated field furniture added to paddock 1, which by that time had not been grazed by scrapie-affected sheep for 40 months, were metal hurdles, a metal lamb creep and a water trough, replacing the previous one, which all had been in contact with the scrapie flock 8 weeks earlier.

The paddock was occupied by 24 lambs aged 1–4 days (67% aged 2 days) with their dams, with the exception of one ewe that arrived with a 14-day-old lamb delivered by cesarean section. Dams were removed 3–4 months later and not tested for scrapie. Rectal biopsies were taken at approximately 9 mpe and examined as described above. Based on the RAMALT results (see Results), all sheep were culled from 11 mpe and examined for scrapie by postmortem tests as before.

Swabs were taken as described above from water trough, fence, wooden post, hurdles, and lamb creep 5 days after the first sheep were introduced in the paddock and examined for PrP^{Sc} by sPMCA in duplicate reactions.

Effect of Replacement of Contaminated Furniture on Pasture in Paddock 1

Twelve 18- to 28-day-old lambs (median 21 days) were moved with their dams to paddock 1, which had been occupied up to 7 days previously by sheep to test for infectivity of contaminated furniture (see above), but clean furniture was now provided (water trough from a paddock not used by scrapie sheep before, fencing replaced). The increase in age was due to poor weather conditions at the time of lambing. Dams were removed as before after 3–4 months. The sheep were culled from 11 mpe and tissues examined by TSE postmortem tests, as described above.

Exposure of Sheep to Weathered Contaminated Furniture on Pasture in Paddock 2

Concurrently with the furniture replacement study, 13 12- to 25-day-old lambs (median 21 days) moved with their dams to paddock 2, which had been grazed by the natural scrapie flock 53 months previously, and contained a water trough and additional objects (lamb creep and hurdles used during lambing of the scrapie flock) from the scrapie-infected flock, which had not been used by these sheep for 18 months. Removal of dams and TSE testing protocol was identical to the furniture replacement study.

Statistical Tests

Where appropriate infection rates between groups were compared by Fisher's exact test (Prism 6, GraphPad Software, USA), with $P < 0.05$ classified as statistically significant (adjusted in the case of multiple comparisons by multiplying the P value following each test by the number of comparisons).

Results

The results of the sheep studies are summarized in **Table 1**.

TABLE 1 | Summary of the results in each sheep study.

Location	Exposure to	Rate of infection (*N* positive/*N* total)
Level of contamination of field furniture not used by scrapie flock for 8 weeks		
Pen 1	Clean furniture (control)	0/5
Pen 2	Water trough (used by predominantly pre-clinical scrapie sheep)	0/6
Pen 3	Water trough (used also by clinically affected scrapie sheep)	4/5[a]
Pen 4	Scratch post, fence, fire extinguisher box	4/7
Exposure of sheep to contaminated furniture on pasture		
Paddock 1[b]	Metal hurdles, metal lamb creep, water trough not used by scrapie flock for 8 weeks on pasture not used by scrapie flock for 40 months	20/23[c]
Effect of replacement of contaminated furniture on pasture		
Paddock 1	Water trough not used by scrapie sheep before and new fencing on pasture not occupied by pre-clinical scrapie sheep for a week	1/12
Exposure of sheep to weathered contaminated furniture on pasture		
Paddock 2[b]	Water trough, lamb creep and hurdles, not used by the scrapie flock for 18 months on pasture not occupied by the scrapie flock for 53 months	0/13

[a]*One lamb was excluded, which died 28 days post exposure and was not TSE tested.*
[b]*No scrapie infection demonstrated in groups of six lambs occupying these paddocks for up to 10 months, after they had been used by the scrapie flock 5 months earlier.*
[c]*One lamb was excluded, which was culled 7 days post exposure due to joint infection and not TSE tested.*

Level of Contamination of Field Furniture in Clean Housing

Infection of sheep was first demonstrated in RAMALT at 9 mpe in a water trough-exposed group (water trough previously exposed to clinically infected sheep) and at 13 mpe in the rubbing objects-exposed group. Scrapie was confirmed in four sheep on brain examination by immunohistochemistry (three exposed to the water trough, one to rubbing objects) but only one was also confirmed by ELISA. This sheep was the only sheep that presented with clinical signs prior to cull at 23 mpe. Evidence of infection in the other sheep was based on presence of PrP^{Sc} in lymphoid tissue only.

Despite evidence of infection in the sheep exposed to one of the water troughs and the scratch objects, the difference compared to the control group was statistically not significant ($P = 0.14$ and $P = 0.24$, respectively, after adjusting for multiple comparisons).

PrP^{Sc} was detected by sPMCA in swabs taken from water trough and fencing (see **Table 2**) in an assay that could consistently detect PrP^{Sc} within 10 pg of ovine brain from a clinically affected animal. However, PrP^{Sc} was also detected in 2 out of 139 reactions from environmental swab samples taken from the classical scrapie-free farm, and the difference in the sPMCA results between scrapie-affected and scrapie-free farm was statistically not significant ($P = 0.124$).

TABLE 2 | Detection of PrP^{Sc} by sPMCA in swabs from objects placed in clean housing and on pasture.

Location	Object	sPMCA result (*N* positive/*N* total)
Level of contamination of field furniture not used by scrapie flock for 8 weeks		
Pen 2	Water trough used mainly by pre-clinical scrapie cases	
	Sample 1	0/3
	Sample 2	0/3
Pen 3	Water trough used by clinically affected scrapie cases	
	Sample 1	0/3
	Sample 2	1/3
Pen 4	Fire extinguisher box	0/3
	Fencing with traces of fleece attached to it	
	Sample 1	0/3
	Sample 2	1/3
	Fence post	
	Sample 1	0/3
	Sample 2	0/3
Exposure of sheep to contaminated furniture on pasture		
Paddock 1	Water trough	0/2
	Fence	0/2
	Wooden post	0/2
	Hurdles	0/2
	Lamb creep	0/2

Exposure of Sheep to Contaminated Furniture on Pasture in Paddock 1

PrP^{Sc} was first detected in RAMALT of 18 (78%) sheep. When the sheep were culled 3 months later at 11–12 mpe, scrapie was confirmed by postmortem tests on lymphoid tissue in 20 (87%), six of which also had PrP^{Sc} in the obex (no detectable PrP^{res} by ELISA). **Figure 1** gives an example of a sheep with confirmed scrapie infection compared to a sheep in the same paddock with no evidence of infection.

None of the swabs taken from the furniture yielded detectable PrP^{Sc} by sPMCA (**Table 2**), even though other analogous environmental samples (from inside farm buildings) run concurrently for a different study yielded positive results (data not presented).

Effect of Replacement of Contaminated Furniture on Pasture in Paddock 1

Scrapie infection was confirmed in a single sheep (8%), which presented with PrP^{Sc} in lymphoid tissue only. Compared with exposure of sheep to contaminated furniture in the same paddock, this was a significant reduction in the infection rate ($P < 0.0001$).

Exposure of Sheep to Weathered Contaminated Furniture on Pasture in Paddock 2

Exposure to objects not used by scrapie-infected sheep for 18 months did not result in any infection.

Discussion

Classical scrapie is an environmentally transmissible disease because it has been reported in naïve, supposedly previously unexposed sheep placed in pastures formerly occupied by

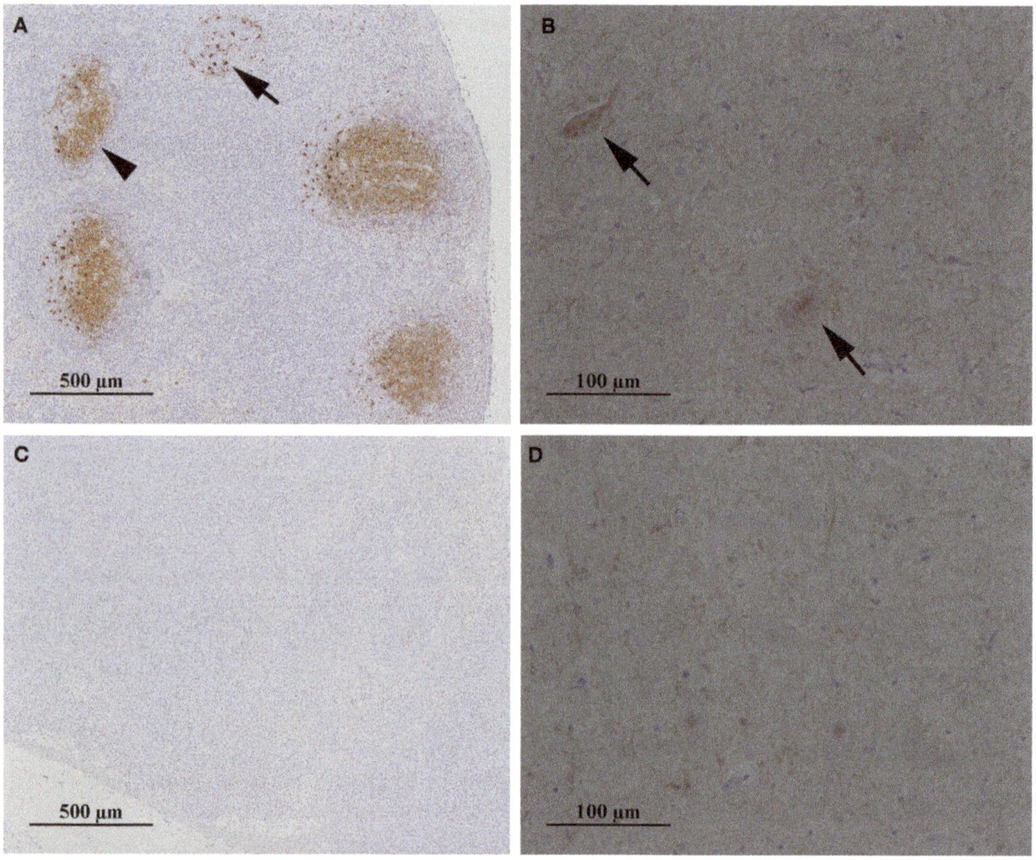

FIGURE 1 | Presence and absence of PrP^{Sc} in the lymph node and brainstem of two sheep exposed to contaminated furniture on pasture in paddock 1. Immunohistochemical examination of mesenteric lymph node **(A,C)** and brainstem at the level of the obex **(B,D)** taken from sheep 25/13 **(A,B)** and 38/13 **(C,D)**, respectively. Antibody: R145. Sheep 25/13 presents with PrP^{Sc} in tingible body macrophages **(A)**, black arrow, and the network of follicular dentritic cells **(A)**, black arrowhead, in follicles of the lymph node and also in neurons in the dorsal motor nucleus (parasympathetic nucleus) of the vagus nerve **(B)**, black arrows, whereas PrP^{Sc} is neither detectable in lymph node **(C)** nor in brainstem **(D)** of sheep 38/13.

scrapie-infected sheep (4, 19, 20). Although the vector for disease transmission is not known, soil is likely to be an important reservoir for prions (2) where – based on studies in rodents – prions can adhere to minerals as a biologically active form (21) and remain infectious for more than 2 years (22). Similarly, chronic wasting disease (CWD) has re-occurred in mule deer housed in paddocks used by infected deer 2 years earlier, which was assumed to be through foraging and soil consumption (23).

Our study suggested that the risk of acquiring scrapie infection was greater through exposure to contaminated wooden, plastic, and metal surfaces via water or food troughs, fencing, and hurdles than through grazing. Drinking from a water trough used by the scrapie flock was sufficient to cause infection in sheep in a clean building. Exposure to fences and other objects used for rubbing also led to infection, which supported the hypothesis that skin may be a vector for disease transmission (9). The risk of these objects to cause infection was further demonstrated when 87% of 23 sheep presented with PrP^{Sc} in lymphoid tissue after grazing on one of the paddocks, which contained metal hurdles, a metal lamb creep and a water trough in contact with the scrapie flock up to 8 weeks earlier, whereas no infection had been demonstrated previously in sheep grazing on this paddock, when equipped with new fencing and field furniture. When the contaminated furniture and fencing were removed, the infection rate dropped significantly to 8% of 12 sheep, with soil of the paddock as the most likely source of infection caused by shedding of prions from the scrapie-infected sheep in this paddock up to a week earlier.

This study also indicated that the level of contamination of field furniture sufficient to cause infection was dependent on two factors: stage of incubation period and time of last use by scrapie-infected sheep. Drinking from a water trough that had been used by scrapie sheep in the predominantly pre-clinical phase did not appear to cause infection, whereas infection was shown in sheep drinking from the water trough used by scrapie sheep in the later stage of the disease. It is possible that contamination occurred through shedding of prions in saliva, which may have contaminated the surface of the water trough and subsequently the water when it was refilled. Contamination appeared to be sufficient to cause infection only if the trough was in contact with sheep that included clinical cases. Indeed, there is an increased risk of bodily fluid infectivity with disease progression in scrapie (24) and CWD (25) based on PrP^{Sc} detection by sPMCA. Although ultraviolet light and heat under natural conditions do not inactivate prions (26), furniture in contact with the scrapie flock, which was assumed to be sufficiently contaminated to cause infection, did not act as vector for disease if not used for 18 months, which suggest that the weathering process alone was sufficient to inactivate prions.

PrP^{Sc} detection by sPMCA is increasingly used as a surrogate for infectivity measurements by bioassay in sheep or mice. In this reported study, however, the levels of PrP^{Sc} present in the environment were below the limit of detection of the sPMCA method, yet were still sufficient to cause infection of in-contact animals. In the present study, the outdoor objects were removed from the infected flock 8 weeks prior to sampling and were positive by sPMCA at very low levels (2 out of 37 reactions). As this sPMCA assay also yielded 2 positive reactions out of 139 in samples from the scrapie-free farm, the sPMCA assay could not detect PrP^{Sc} on any of the objects above the background of the assay. False positive reactions with sPMCA at a low frequency associated with *de novo* formation of infectious prions have been reported (27, 28). This is in contrast to our previous study where we demonstrated that outdoor objects that had been in contact with the scrapie-infected flock up to 20 days prior to sampling harbored PrP^{Sc} that was detectable by sPMCA analysis [4 out of 15 reactions (12)] and was significantly more positive by the assay compared to analogous samples from the scrapie-free farm. This discrepancy could be due to the use of a different sPMCA substrate between the studies that may alter the efficiency of amplification of the environmental PrP^{Sc}. In addition, the present study had a longer timeframe between the objects being in contact with the infected flock and sampling, which may affect the levels of extractable PrP^{Sc}. Alternatively, there may be potentially patchy contamination of this furniture with PrP^{Sc}, which may have been missed by swabbing. The failure of sPMCA to detect CWD-associated PrP in saliva from clinically affected deer despite confirmation of infectivity in saliva-inoculated transgenic mice was associated with as yet unidentified inhibitors in saliva (29), and it is possible that the sensitivity of sPMCA is affected by other substances in the tested material. In addition, sampling of amplifiable PrP^{Sc} and subsequent detection by sPMCA may be more difficult from furniture exposed to weather, which is supported by the observation that PrP^{Sc} was detected by sPMCA more frequently in indoor than outdoor furniture (12). A recent experimental study has demonstrated that repeated cycles of drying and wetting of prion-contaminated soil, equivalent to what is expected under natural weathering conditions, could reduce PMCA amplification efficiency and extend the incubation period in hamsters inoculated with soil samples (30). This seems to apply also to this study even though the reduction in infectivity was more dramatic in the sPMCA assays than in the sheep model. Sheep were not kept until clinical end-point, which would have enabled us to compare incubation periods, but the lack of infection in sheep exposed to furniture that had not been in contact with scrapie sheep for a longer time period supports the hypothesis that prion degradation and subsequent loss of infectivity occurs even under natural conditions.

In conclusion, the results in the current study indicate that removal of furniture that had been in contact with scrapie-infected animals should be recommended, particularly since cleaning and decontamination may not effectively remove scrapie infectivity (31), even though infectivity declines considerably if the pasture and the field furniture have not been in contact with scrapie-infected sheep for several months. As sPMCA failed to detect PrP^{Sc} in furniture that was subjected to weathering, even though exposure led to infection in sheep, this method may not always be reliable in predicting the risk of scrapie infection through environmental contamination. These results suggest that the VRQ/VRQ sheep model may be more sensitive than sPMCA for the detection of environmentally associated scrapie, and suggest that extremely low levels of scrapie contamination are able to cause infection in susceptible sheep genotypes.

Author Contributions

TK analyzed the data and drafted the manuscript. HS designed and managed the study, supported by SH, LT, and TD who participated in the coordination of different parts of the study. BM and KG were responsible for the sPMCA investigations. All authors contributed to the final draft of this manuscript and read and approved the final manuscript.

Funding

The study was funded by the UK Department for Environment, Food and Rural Affairs (project SE1861).

Acknowledgments

We are grateful to present and past members of staff at the Animal Sciences Unit at APHA Weybridge who cared for the animals, and to staff at the Pathology Department and Prion unit at APHA Weybridge who provided the scrapie diagnostic results. We thank staff at ADAS-UK for provision of classical scrapie-free lambs.

References

1. Prusiner SB. Novel proteinaceous infectious particles cause scrapie. *Science* (1982) **216**:136–44. doi:10.1126/science.6801762
2. Smith CB, Booth CJ, Pedersen JA. Fate of prions in soil: a review. *J Environ Qual* (2011) **40**:449–61. doi:10.2134/jeq2010.0412
3. Dexter G, Tongue SC, Heasman L, Bellworthy SJ, Davis A, Moore SJ, et al. The evaluation of exposure risks for natural transmission of scrapie within an infected flock. *BMC Vet Res* (2009) **5**:38. doi:10.1186/1746-6148-5-38
4. Georgsson G, Sigurdarson S, Brown P. Infectious agent of sheep scrapie may persist in the environment for at least 16 years. *J Gen Virol* (2006) **87**:3737–40. doi:10.1099/vir.0.82011-0
5. Detwiler LA, Baylis M. The epidemiology of scrapie. *Rev Sci Tech Off Int Epiz* (2003) **22**:121–43.
6. Rubenstein R, Chang B, Gray P, Piltch M, Bulgin MS, Sorensen-Melson S, et al. Prion disease detection, PMCA kinetics, and IgG in urine from sheep naturally/experimentally infected with scrapie and deer with preclinical/clinical chronic wasting disease. *J Virol* (2011) **85**:9031–8. doi:10.1128/JVI.05111-11
7. Terry LA, Howells L, Bishop K, Baker CA, Everest S, Thorne L, et al. Detection of prions in the faeces of sheep naturally infected with classical scrapie. *Vet Res* (2011) **42**:65. doi:10.1186/1297-9716-42-65
8. Tamgüney G, Richt JA, Hamir AN, Greenlee JJ, Miller MW, Wolfe LL, et al. Salivary prions in sheep and deer. *Prion* (2012) **6**:52–61. doi:10.4161/pri.6.1.16984

9. Thomzig A, Schulz-Schaeffer W, Wrede A, Wemheuer W, Brenig B, Kratzel C, et al. Accumulation of pathological prion protein PrPSc in the skin of animals with experimental and natural scrapie. *PLoS Pathog* (2007) **3**:e66. doi:10.1371/journal.ppat.0030066
10. Ryder S, Dexter G, Bellworthy S, Tongue S. Demonstration of lateral transmission of scrapie between sheep kept under natural conditions using lymphoid tissue biopsy. *Res Vet Sci* (2004) **76**:211–7. doi:10.1016/j.rvsc.2003.11.007
11. Konold T, Moore SJ, Bellworthy SJ, Simmons HA. Evidence of scrapie transmission via milk. *BMC Vet Res* (2008) **4**:14. doi:10.1186/1746-6148-4-14
12. Maddison BC, Baker CA, Terry LA, Bellworthy SJ, Thorne L, Rees HC, et al. Environmental sources of scrapie prions. *J Virol* (2010) **84**:11560–2. doi:10.1128/JVI.01133-10
13. Warner RG, Morris D, Dawson M. PrP genotype progression in flocks participating in the National scrapie plan for Great Britain. *Vet Rec* (2006) **159**:473–9. doi:10.1136/vr.159.15.473
14. Simmons HA, Simmons MM, Spencer YI, Chaplin MJ, Povey G, Davis A, et al. Atypical scrapie in sheep from a UK research flock which is free from classical scrapie. *BMC Vet Res* (2009) **5**:8. doi:10.1186/1746-6148-5-8
15. Rees HC, Maddison BC, Owen JP, Whitelam GC, Gough KC. Concentration of disease-associated prion protein with silicon dioxide. *Mol Biotechnol* (2009) **41**:254–62. doi:10.1007/s12033-008-9129-5
16. González L, Dagleish MP, Martin S, Dexter G, Steele P, Finlayson J, et al. Diagnosis of preclinical scrapie in live sheep by the immunohistochemical examination of rectal biopsies. *Vet Rec* (2008) **162**:397–403. doi:10.1136/vr.162.13.397
17. Konold T, Phelan L. Clinical examination protocol to detect atypical and classical scrapie in sheep. *J Vis Exp* (2014) (83):e51101. doi:10.3791/51101
18. Ryder S, Dexter G, Heasman L, Warner R, Moore SJ. Accumulation and dissemination of prion protein in experimental sheep scrapie in the natural host. *BMC Vet Res* (2009) **5**:9. doi:10.1186/1746-6148-5-9
19. Greig JR. Scrapie. Observations on the transmission of the disease by mediate contact. *Vet J* (1940) **96**:203–6.
20. Hourrigan JL, Klingsporn AL. Scrapie: studies on vertical and horizontal transmission. In: Gibbs CJ Jr, ed. *Bovine Spongiform Encephalopathy. The BSE Dilemma*. New York, NY: Springer (1996). p. 59–83.
21. Johnson CJ, Phillips KE, Schramm PT, Mckenzie D, Aiken JM, Pedersen JA. Prions adhere to soil minerals and remain infectious. *PLoS Pathog* (2006) **2**:e32. doi:10.1371/journal.ppat.0020032
22. Seidel B, Thomzig A, Buschmann A, Groschup MH, Peters R, Beekes M, et al. Scrapie Agent (Strain 263K) can transmit disease via the oral route after persistence in soil over years. *PLoS One* (2007) **2**:e435. doi:10.1371/journal.pone.0000435
23. Miller MW, Williams ES, Hobbs NT, Wolfe LL. Environmental sources of prion transmission in mule deer. *Emerg Infect Dis* (2004) **10**:1003–6. doi:10.3201/eid0905.020660
24. Gough KC, Baker CA, Rees HC, Terry LA, Spiropoulos J, Thorne L, et al. The oral secretion of infectious scrapie prions occurs in preclinical sheep with a range of PRNP genotypes. *J Virol* (2012) **86**:566–71. doi:10.1128/JVI.05579-11
25. Haley NJ, Mathiason CK, Carver S, Zabel M, Telling GC, Hoover EA. Detection of chronic wasting disease prions in salivary, urinary, and intestinal tissues of deer: potential mechanisms of prion shedding and transmission. *J Virol* (2011) **85**:6309–18. doi:10.1128/jvi.00425-11
26. Taylor DM. Inactivation of transmissible degenerative encephalopathy agents: a review. *Vet J* (2000) **159**:10–7. doi:10.1053/tvjl.1999.0406
27. Maddison BC, Rees HC, Baker CA, Taema M, Bellworthy SJ, Thorne L, et al. Prions are secreted into the oral cavity in sheep with preclinical scrapie. *J Infect Dis* (2010) **201**:1672–6. doi:10.1086/652457
28. Morales R, Duran-Aniotz C, Diaz-Espinoza R, Camacho MV, Soto C. Protein misfolding cyclic amplification of infectious prions. *Nat Protoc* (2012) **7**:1397–409. doi:10.1038/nprot.2012.067
29. Haley NJ, Seelig DM, Zabel MD, Telling GC, Hoover EA. Detection of CWD prions in urine and saliva of deer by transgenic mouse bioassay. *PLoS One* (2009) **4**:e4848. doi:10.1371/journal.pone.0004848
30. Yuan Q, Eckland T, Telling G, Bartz J, Bartelt-Hunt S. Mitigation of prion infectivity and conversion capacity by a simulated natural process – repeated cycles of drying and wetting. *PLoS Pathog* (2015) **11**:e1004638. doi:10.1371/journal.ppat.1004638
31. Hawkins SA, Simmons HA, Gough KC, Maddison BC. Persistence of ovine scrapie infectivity in a farm environment following cleaning and decontamination. *Vet Rec* (2015) **176**:99. doi:10.1136/vr.102743

Conflict of Interest Statement: The authors declare that the research was conducted in the absence of any commercial or financial relationships that could be construed as a potential conflict of interest.

4

Identification of potential biomarkers for gut barrier failure in broiler chickens

Juxing Chen[1], Guillermo Tellez[2], James D. Richards[1] and Jeffery Escobar[1]*

[1] *Novus International, Inc., St. Charles, MO, USA,* [2] *Department of Poultry Science, University of Arkansas, Fayetteville, AR, USA*

The objective of the present study was to identify potential biomarkers for gut barrier failure in chickens. A total of 144 day-of-hatch Ross 308 male broiler chickens were housed in 24 battery cages with six chicks per cage. Cages were randomly assigned to either a control group (CON) or gut barrier failure (GBF) group. During the first 13 days, birds in CON or GBF groups were fed a common corn–soy starter diet. On day 14, CON chickens were switched to a corn grower diet, and GBF chickens were switched to rye–wheat–barley grower diet. In addition, on day 21, GBF chickens were orally challenged with a coccidiosis vaccine. At days 21 and 28, birds were weighed by cage and feed intake was recorded to calculate feed conversion ratio. At day 28, one chicken from each cage was euthanized to collect intestinal samples for morphometric analysis, blood for serum, and intestinal mucosa scrapings for gene expression. Overall performance and feed efficiency was severely affected ($P < 0.05$) by a GBF model when compared with CON group at days 21 and 28. Duodenum of GBF birds had wider villi, longer crypt depth, and higher crypt depth/villi height ratio than CON birds. Similarly, GBF birds had longer crypt depth in jejunum and ileum when compared with CON birds. Protein levels of endotoxin and 1-acid glycoprotein (AGP) in serum, as well as mRNA levels of interleukin (IL)-8, IL-1 , transforming growth factor (TGF)- 4, and fatty acid-binding protein (FABP) 6 were increased ($P < 0.05$) in GBF birds compared to CON birds; however, mRNA levels of FABP2, occludin, and mucin 2 (MUC2) were reduced by 34% ($P < 0.05$), 24% ($P = 0.107$), and 29% ($P = 0.088$), respectively, in GBF birds compared to CON birds. The results from the present study suggest that serum endotoxin and AGP, as well as, gene expression of FABP2, FABP6, IL-8, IL-1 , TGF- 4, occludin, and MUC2 in mucosa may work as potential biomarkers for gut barrier health in chickens.

Keywords: gut barrier function, morphometric analysis, endotoxin, AGP, gene expression, biomarker

Edited by:
Michael Kogut,
USDA Agricultural Research Service, USA

Reviewed by:
Jason Kindrachuk,
National Institute of Allergy and Infectious Diseases, USA
Wolfgang Ludwig Köster,
University of Saskatchewan, Canada

Correspondence:
Juxing Chen,
Novus International, Inc., 20 Research Park Drive, St. Charles, MO 63304, USA
juxing.chen@novusint.com

Abbreviations: AGP, 1-acid glycoprotein; AJ, adherens junctions; BW, body weight; BWG, body weight gain; CON, control; ERK, extracellular signal-regulated kinase; FABP, fatty acid-binding protein; FCR, feed conversion ratio; FI, feed intake; GBF, gut barrier failure; GIT, gastrointestinal tract; IEC, intestinal epithelial cells; IL, interleukin; JAM, junctional adhesion molecule; MUC2, mucin 2; NSP, non-starch polysaccharide; PAMP, pathogen-associated molecular pattern; PRR, pattern recognition receptor; TGF, transforming growth factor; TJ, tight junction; TLR, toll-like receptor; TNF, tumor necrosis factor; ZO, zonula occluden.

Introduction

Barrier function is a critical aspect of gut heath. Oxidative stress, poorly digestible protein, and coccidiosis are some examples that can cause gut barrier failure (1–5). Nevertheless, as a consequence of the removal of anti-microbial growth promoters, new multi-factorial diseases causing enteritis and gut disorders of unknown origin have emerged in broilers, causing negative impacts in health and performance (6–9). Among them, dysbacteriosis, defined as the presence of a qualitatively and/or quantitatively abnormal microbiota in the proximal parts of the small intestine, associated with reduced nutrient digestibility, impaired intestinal barrier function, bacterial translocation, and inflammatory responses have been reported (4, 5, 10). However, more recently, poor gut health has also been associated with bacterial chondronecrosis with osteomyelitis in broiler chickens and breeders (11–13). As the largest organ in the body, the gut serves as a selective barrier to take up nutrients and fluids into the body, while excluding undesirable molecules and pathogens (3, 14, 15). Therefore, proper gut barrier function is essential to maintain optimal health and balance throughout the body, and represents a key line of defense against foreign antigens from the environment (16). The first layer of gut barrier is the extrinsic mucus layer comprised an outer layer associated with bacteria and an inner layer with high concentrations of secretory IgA and mucin. The outer layer is loosely attached to epithelium. The inner layer is adherent to the second layer of gut barrier, the intestinal epithelial cells (IEC). IEC are a single layer of epithelial cells that separate the intestinal lumen from underlying lamina propria (17–19). These epithelial cells must be able to rapidly regenerate in the event of tissue damage (14, 20, 21). The enterocytes in the apical epithelium are responsible for absorption of nutrients. Tight junctions (TJ) seal the paracellular space between adjacent epithelial cells and regulate the permeability of intestinal barrier by preventing diffusion of microorganisms and antigens (22, 23). Since IEC are the primary cell type coming into contact with the external environment, they act as the host's first line of the defense. In spite of their non-hematopoietic derivation, IEC represent a core element of innate immunity within the gut-associated lymphoid tissue, displaying a wide array of immune functions. In fact, IEC are able to recognize pathogens through the expression of innate immune receptors, release of anti-microbial molecules, and secretion of a wide number of hormones, neuro transmitters, enzymes, as well as cytokines and chemokines that link innate and adaptive immune responses (24–26). Hence, any direct or indirect damage on IEC may cause a breakdown in gut barrier and consequently, disruption of normal mucosal immune homeostasis that can potentially lead to uncontrolled chronic intestinal and systemic inflammation (27, 28).

Several investigators have described the pathways associated with the disruption of the protein networks that connect epithelial cells by inflammatory mediators, such as hormones, oxygen free radical species, enzymes, as well as multiple proinflammatory cytokines (27, 29, 30). Feeding oxidized/unpreserved fat has been also shown to increase intestinal epithelial turnover rates and increase apoptosis at villus tips in poultry and swine (31). Non-starch polysaccharides (NSP), such as -glucans and pentosans have been shown to have a detrimental influence on the utilization of nutrients in broilers by increasing digesta viscosity and reducing digestibility of nutrients (e.g., fat and protein) (32, 33), which could cause dysbacteriosis. Currently, no biomarkers have been described as tools to evaluate gut inflammation or gut barrier failure in broiler chickens. The objective of the present study was not to determine the individual effects of diet ingredients or coccidia challenge on gut health, rather to identify potential biomarkers for gut barrier failure. Therefore, we attempted to exacerbate gut barrier failure by feeding a high NSP diet containing rye, wheat, and barley to induce high digesta viscosity (4, 5) in combination with a 2× coccidiosis vaccination to induce gut health challenge.

Materials and Methods

Animal Source and Diets

A total of 144 day-of-hatch Ross 308 male broiler chickens were randomly housed in 24 battery cages with six chicks per cage in environmentally controlled rooms. To avoid cross contamination of coccidiosis vaccine, birds in control group (CON) and gut barrier failure (GBF) group were housed in two separate but identically controlled rooms. Temperature was maintained at 34°C for the first 5 days and then gradually reduced according to normal management practices, until a temperature of 23°C was achieved. Lighting was provided for 24 h/day. During the first 13 days, birds in CON or GBF groups were fed common corn–soy starter diet (**Table 1**). On day 14, birds in CON group were switched to a corn–soy grower diet (14–28 days) and the GBF group was switched to rye–wheat–barley diet (**Table 1**). The experimental diets were formulated to approximate the nutritional requirements of broiler chickens (34). On day 21, birds in GBF treatment were orally challenged with 2× dose of Advent™ coccidiosis vaccine, a mixture of *Eimeria acervulina*, *Eimeria maxima*, and *Eimeria tenella* (Huvepharma Sofia, Bulgaria). All research procedures were reviewed and approved by a licensed veterinarian and also followed the protocols described previously (5, 35), which were approved by IACUC at University of Arkansas. All studies performed by Novus International, Inc. are in accordance to the standards of the Guide for the Care and Use of Agricultural Animals in Research and Teaching (35).

Experimental Design

The 144 day-of-hatch chickens were randomly allotted to one of two groups; CON or GBF on the basis of initial body weight (BW). Each treatment was comprised of 12 replicates of six chicks each ($n = 72$/group). At 21 and 28 days, BW, body weight gain (BWG), and feed intake (FI) were recorded in each cage to calculate feed conversion ratio (FCR).

Sample Collection

At 28 days of age, one chicken from each cage was euthanized by CO_2 asphyxiation for sample collection. Blood sample was taken from cardiac puncture using a syringe, kept at room temperature for 3 h to allow clotting, and centrifuged (1,000 × g for 15 min at 4°C) to separate serum. Following euthanasia, a 1-cm section of duodenum was collected from the middle of the descending duodenum; a 1-cm section of jejunum was collected at the Meckel's diverticulum; a 1-cm section of ileum was collected 2 cm before the ceca. All of intestinal sections were rinsed with

TABLE 1 | Ingredient composition and nutrient content of common, control, and gut barrier failure (GBF) diets, as-is basis.

Ingredient	Common starter, 0–13 days (%)	Control grower, 14–28 days (%)	GBF grower, 14–28 days (%)
Corn	60.6	60.6	0
Rye	0	0	33.95
Wheat	0	0	20
Barley	0	0	10
SBM, 47.5% CP	32.56	32.56	28.8
Soybean oil	1.08	1.08	2.96
L-lysine HCl	1.48	1.48	0.14
MHA®	0.3	0.3	0.42
L-threonine	0.01	0.01	0.05
L-tryptophan	0.14	0.14	0.11
Dicalcium phosphate, 18.5%	1.59	1.59	1.57
Limestone	1.09	1.09	1
Salt	0.25	0.25	0.25
Choline chloride, 60%	0.25	0.25	0.25
Sodium bicarbonate	0.2	0.2	0.2
Mineral premix[a]	0.2	0.2	0.2
Vitamin premix[b]	0.1	0.1	0.1
Santoquin™ Mixture 6	0.02	0.02	0
MycoCURB™	0.05	0.05	0
Coban® 90	0.05	0.05	0
BMD® 60	0.03	0.03	0
Calculated nutrients			
ME, kcal/kg	3,031	3,152	3,152
SID Lysine, %	1.27	1.1	1.1
SID TSAA, %	0.94	0.84	0.84
Total CP, %	22	20.7	21.8
Ca, %	1.05	0.9	0.9
Available P, %	0.5	0.45	0.45

[a]*Mineral premix supplied per kilogram of diet: Mn, 120 mg; Zn, 100 mg; Fe, 40 mg; Cu, 10 mg, I, 1.25 mg, Se, 0.30 mg.*

[b]*Vitamin premix supplied per kilogram of diet: retinol, 9.2 mg; cholecalciferol, 100 µg; dl- -tocopherol, 90 mg; menadione, 6 mg; thiamine, 6.2 mg; riboflavin, 26.5 mg; pantothenic acid, 39.7 mg; niacin, 100 mg; pyridoxine, 11 mg; folic acid, 4 mg; biotin, 0.3 mg; cyanocobalamin, 0.1 mg.*

10% neutral buffered formalin and then fixed in 20× volume of 10% neutral buffered formalin. A 10-cm section of jejunum was rinsed with ice cold phosphate buffered saline (pH 7.4) and cut open to scrape mucosa using RNAse-free glass slides into 2-ml tubes with 1 ml RNAlater (Applied Biosystems, NY, USA). The mucosal scrapings were stored at 4°C for 24 h and then at −20°C until total RNA isolation.

Histological Sample Preparation and Intestinal Morphometry Measurement

Intestinal segments were trimmed, processed, and embedded in paraffin. A 5-µm section of each sample was placed on a glass slide and stained with hematoxylin and eosin for morphometry examination and measurement under Olympus light microscope using Olympus MicroSuite™ Imaging software (Center Valley, PA, USA). Five replicate measurements for each variable studied were taken from each sample, and the average values were used in statistical analyses. Villi height was measured from the top of the villi to the top of the submucosa. Crypt depth was measured from the base upwards to the region of transition between the crypt and villi. Villi width was measured at the middle of each villus, whereas crypt/villi ratio was determined as the ratio of crypt depth to villi height (36).

Serum Endotoxin and Serum 1 Acute Phase Protein Determination

Endotoxin was measured using a chicken Endotoxin Elisa kit from Amsbio (Cambridge, MA, USA). Acute phase protein, 1-acid glycoprotein (AGP) was measured using chicken 1-acid glycoprotein measurement kit from The Institute for Metabolic Ecosystem (Miyagi, Japan). The Optical Density for both kits was determined at 450 nm using a BIO-TEK ELx800 (BIO-TEK Instrument, Winooski, VT, USA).

Quantitative Reverse Transcription Polymerase Chain Reaction (qRT–PCR)

Total RNA was isolated from mucosa scraping samples using Clontech Total RNA isolation NucleoSpin® RNA II kit (Clontech Laboratories, Inc., CA, USA). One microgram of total RNA, 11mer oligo mix from Fluoresentric, and M-MLV Reverse Transcriptase (Life Technologies, Grand Island, NY, USA) were used to synthesize cDNA according to the manufacturers' instructions. The relative mRNA levels of mucin 2 (MUC2), fatty acid-binding protein (FABP) 2, FABP6, interleukin (IL)-8, IL-1 , transforming growth factor (TGF)- 4, occludin, zonula occluden (ZO)-1, junctional adhesion molecule (JAM) 2, JAM3, catenin, tumor necrosis factor (TNF) , Toll-like receptor (TLR) 2 , TLR4, and claudin 1 were measured by quantitative PCR using Applied Biosystems® SYBR® Green PCR Master Mix, the 7500 Fast Real-Time PCR System, and primers in **Table 2**. Results were expressed as the level relative to the corresponding housekeeping gene *actin*. All primers were verified for the efficiency and linearity of amplification.

Statistical Analyses

All data were tested for normality and subjected to one-way ANOVA as a completely randomized design using the GLM procedure of SAS (37). Each cage was used as the experimental unit for the analysis. Growth performance including BW, BWG, FI, and FCR used the average data per cage. Gut morphometric measurements, serum endotoxin, AGP, and qRT–PCR used individual measurement from one randomly chosen bird per cage. Data are expressed as mean ± SE.

Results

Growth Performance

The results of the growth performance parameters between CON and GBF groups are summarized in **Table 3**. BW, FI per bird, BWG and FCR at 21 and 28 days of age were dramatically reduced in GBF chickens when compared with CON chickens ($P < 0.05$), indicating that GBF model substantially compromised the growth performance of chickens.

Histomorphometric Analysis

The results of the histomorphometric analysis of duodenum, jejunum, and ileal tissue between CON and GBF chickens at 28 days of age are summarized in **Table 4**. The duodenum, jejunum, and ileum all showed increased ($P < 0.05$) crypt depth

TABLE 2 | List of primers used for qRT–PCR.

Genes	Forward primer	Reverse primer	Fragment size (bp)
Actin	CAACACAGTGCTGTCTGGTGGTA	ATCGTACTCCTGCTTGCTGATCC	205
MUC2	GCCTGCCCAGGAAATCAAG	CGACAAGTTTGCTGGCACAT	59
FABP2	AAAGATAATGGAAAAGTACTCACAGCAT	CCTTCGTACACGTAGGTCTGTATGA	77
FABP6	CGGTCTCCCTGCTGACAAGA	CCACCTCGGTGACTATTTTGC	59
IL-8	TCCTGGTTTCAGCTGCTCTGT	CGCAGCTCATTCCCCATCT	52
TGF- 4	CGGCCGACGATGAGTGGCTC	CGGGGCCCATCTCACAGGGA	113
Occludin	GAGCCCAGACTACCAAAGCAA	GCTTGATGTGGAAGAGCTTGTTG	68
ZO1	CCGCAGTCGTTCACGATCT	GGAGAATGTCTGGAATGGTCTGA	63
JAM2	AGCCTCAAATGGGATTGGATT	CATCAACTTGCATTCGCTTCA	59
JAM3	CCGACGGCTGTTTGTGTTT	GGCGGTGCAAAGTTTTGG	56
Catenin	CGACAACTGCTCCCTCTTTGA	GCGTTGTGTCCACATCTTCCT	63
TNF	TGTTCTATGACCGCCCAGTTC	GACGTGTCACGATCATCTGGTT	63
TLR2	CGCTTAGGAGAGACAATCTGTGAA	GCCTGTTTTAGGGATTTCAGAGAATTT	90
TLR4	AGTCTGAAATTGCTGAGCTCAAAT	GCGACGTTAAGCCATGGAAG	190
Claudin 1	TGGCCACGTCATGGTATGG	AACGGGTGTGAAAGGGTCATAG	62
IL-4	GCCAGCACTGCCACAAGA	GGAGCTGACGCGTGTTGAG	54
IL-6	GAGGGCCGTTCGCTATTTG	ATTGTGCCCGAACTAAAACATTC	67
IL-1	CAGCCCGTGGGCATCA	CTTAGCTTGTAGGTGGCGATGTT	59

TABLE 3 | Performance parameters between control and gut barrier failure grower groups (GBF).

Treatments and growing phase	BW (g)	FI per bird (g)	BWG (g)	FCR during each phase
21 days				
CON	866.25 ± 11.87^{a}	617.25 ± 8.76^{a}	390.58 ± 6.21^{a}	1.58 ± 0.02^{b}
GBF	642.58 ± 10.50^{b}	480.67 ± 11.85^{b}	203.17 ± 11.27^{b}	2.42 ± 0.09^{a}
28 days				
CON	$1,302.75 \pm 26.45^{a}$	729.50 ± 26.17^{a}	436.50 ± 19.04^{a}	1.67 ± 0.03^{b}
GBF	895.50 ± 21.58^{b}	578.17 ± 9.5^{b}	252.92 ± 20.30^{b}	2.42 ± 0.17^{a}

Data are expressed as mean ± SE.
^{a,b}Superscripts within columns indicate difference at $P < 0.05$.

(shown as * in **Figure 1**) in GBF chickens compared to CON chickens. GBF chickens also had wider villi in duodenum and jejunum, and higher crypt/villi ratio in duodenum compared to CON chickens; however, the crypt/villi ratio was not different in jejunum ($P = 0.064$) and ileum ($P = 0.208$) because the villus height in jejunum and ileum was also increased ($P < 0.03$) in GBF birds compared to CON birds. The increase of crypt depth and/or the crypt/villi ratio is an indication of greater need of cell proliferation to maintain proper gut health, which suggests that GBF model generated unhealthy gut barrier.

TABLE 4 | Histomorphometric analysis of duodenum, jejunum, and ileum in control (CON) and gut barrier failure (GBF) groups in chickens at 28 days of age.

Tissue	CON	GBF
Duodenum		
Villus height, μm	2324.7 ± 123.84^{a}	2649.8 ± 156.21^{a}
Villus width, μm	172.81 ± 5.24^{b}	214.08 ± 13.04^{a}
Crypt depth, μm	104.51 ± 4.76^{b}	201.74 ± 17.10^{a}
Crypt/villi ratio	0.04 ± 0.01^{b}	0.08 ± 0.01^{a}
Jejunum		
Villus height, μm	1883.40 ± 141.54^{b}	2273.80 ± 77.17^{a}
Villus width, μm	170.57 ± 9.17^{b}	190.02 ± 12.08^{a}
Crypt depth, μm	112.84 ± 9.32^{b}	172.78 ± 10.59^{a}
Crypt/villi ratio	0.06 ± 0.01^{a}	0.07 ± 0.01^{a}
Ileum		
Villus height, μm	1005.70 ± 45.77^{b}	1334.13 ± 79.61^{a}
Villus width, μm	163.80 ± 4.97^{a}	166.25 ± 7.85^{a}
Crypt depth, μm	113.63 ± 7.91^{b}	174.70 ± 14.11^{a}
Crypt/villi ratio	0.11 ± 0.01^{a}	0.13 ± 0.01^{a}

Values are expressed as means ± SE.
^{a,b}Superscripts within rows indicate difference at $P < 0.05$.

Serum Endotoxin and AGP

Table 5 shows the comparison of serum AGP and endotoxin levels between CON and GBF groups of broiler chickens at 28 days of age. AGP, a marker for systemic inflammation, was increased ($P < 0.05$) by 3.8-fold in GBF birds compared to CON birds (**Table 5**), suggesting that systemic inflammation was occurring in GBF birds. Endotoxin, a toxin released by gram-negative bacteria in the gut, was increased ($P < 0.05$) by 2.1-fold in serum of GBF birds compared to CON birds (**Table 5**), which suggests that greater amount of endotoxin was translocated from intestinal lumen into blood.

Gene Expression in Jejunal Mucosa by qRT–PCR

The relative mRNA levels of genes that are possibly involved in gut barrier function and inflammation in jejunal mucosa of broilers chickens at 28 days of age are shown in **Table 6**. The relative mRNA levels of IL-8, IL-1 , TGF- 4, and FABP6 were increased ($P < 0.04$) by 3-, 1.5-, 2.2-, and 7-fold, respectively, in GBF chickens compared to CON chickens. However, FABP2, occludin, and MUC2 mRNA levels were decreased by 34%

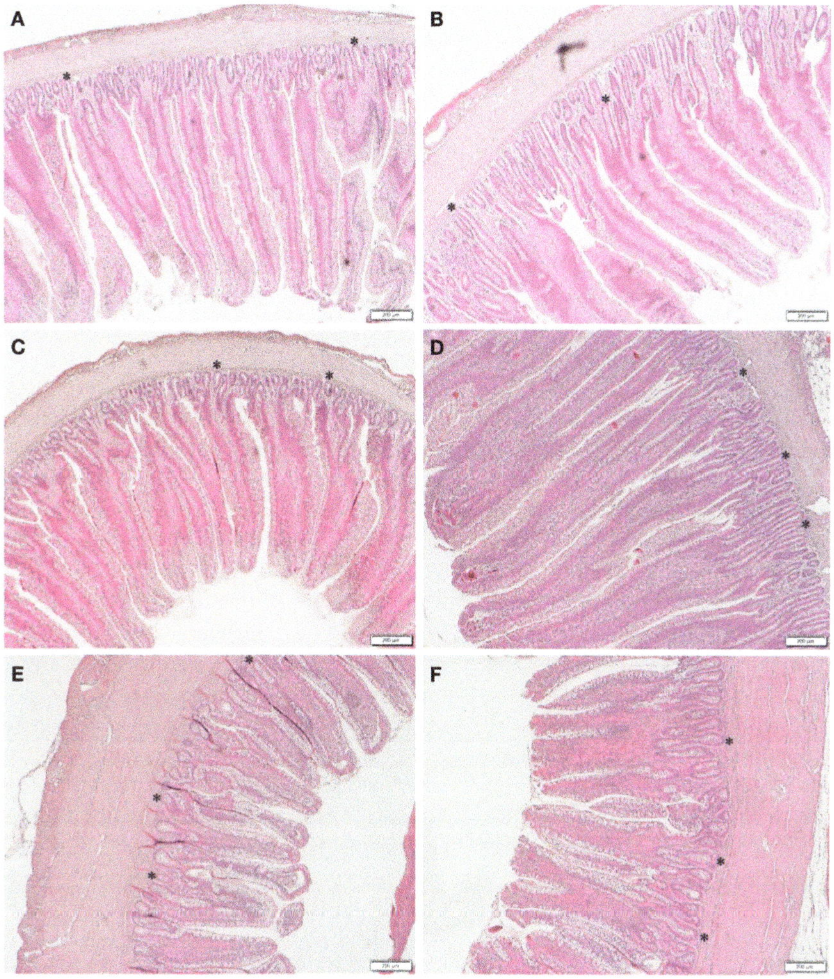

FIGURE 1 | Representative images of duodenum (A,B), jejunum (C,D), and ileum (E,F) in control (A,C,E) and gut barrier failure (B,D,F) groups of broilers chickens at 28 days of age. The representative crypts are shown as *.

TABLE 5 | Comparison of serum endotoxin and 1 acute phase protein (AGP) values between control and gut barrier failure groups in chickens at 28 days of age.

Treatment	Endotoxin pg/ml	α1 Acute phase protein (AGP) μg/ml
CON	159.03 ± 8.56^{b}	174.40 ± 28.95^{b}
GBF	331.84 ± 80.46^{a}	655.30 ± 6.38^{a}

Data are expressed as mean ± SE.
^{a,b}Superscripts within columns indicate difference at $P < 0.05$.

($P = 0.005$), 24% ($P = 0.107$), and 29% ($P = 0.088$), respectively, in GBF birds compared to CON birds. The mRNA levels of catenin, claudin 1, ZO1, JAM2, JAM3, IL-4, IL-6, TLR4, TLR2 , and TNF- were not different ($P > 0.1$) between CON and GBF chickens (data not shown).

Discussion

It is well known that poor gut health causes negative impacts in the health and growth performance of broiler chickens in poultry industry. Alternative grains, such as wheat, barley, and rye that are high in NSP, have been reported to cause a significant reduction in performance (38–40). Several mechanisms of the action of NSP on nutrient absorption have been described including an increased digesta viscosity due to reduced digestibility, thickening of the mucous layer on the intestinal mucosa, epithelial cell apoptosis, and inflammation caused by dysbacteriosis (10, 31, 39). Poultry have little or no intrinsic enzymes capable of hydrolyzing these NSP, so high concentrations of NSP in wheat, barley, or rye lead to reduced nutrient digestibility. The undigested feed ingredients in the gut provide nutrients for bacteria overgrowth in the hind gut, leading to dysbacteriosis. High NSP diets have also been associated with necrotic enteritis, a multifactorial disease caused by *Clostridium perfringens* that is probably the most important bacterial disease in terms of economic implications in broiler chickens (41). The nutritional and economic consequences of mounting an inflammatory response in poultry are inversely related to BWG and overall performance (42, 43). In the present study, a wheat-barley-rye diet in combination with a coccidia challenge was used to induce gut barrier failure in broiler chickens. The overall growth performance and feed efficiency

TABLE 6 | Relative mRNA levels of genes in jejunal mucosa between control and gut barrier failure groups of broilers chickens at 28 days of age.

Treatment	mRNA TGF-β4	mRNA IL-1β	mRNA IL-8	mRNA FABP2	mRNA FABP6	mRNA MUC2	mRNA occludin
CON	81.98 ± 4.55[a]	25.6 ± 4.52[a]	0.04 ± 0.01[a]	26.72 ± 1.99[b]	0.01 ± 0.001[a]	123.30 ± 15.51[b]	2.23 ± 0.26[b]
GBF	182.03 ± 18.09[b]	43.89 ± 6.65[b]	0.13 ± 0.01[b]	17.66 ± 1.89[a]	0.07 ± 0.01[b]	87.11 ± 12.16[b]	1.69 ± 0.16[b]
P-value	0.0001	0.040	<0.0001	0.0005	0.020	0.088	0.107

Data are normalized by actin mRNA and expressed as mean ± SE.
[a,b]Superscripts within columns indicate difference at $P < 0.05$.

were severely reduced by this GBF model. These results are in agreement with previous studies that high NSP diets compromised growth performance in chickens (4, 5, 44, 45).

The morphometry of duodenum, jejunum, and ileum in CON and GBF chickens at 28 days of age was measured under microscope to confirm whether the rye–barley–wheat diet and coccidia challenge generated gut barrier failure. GBF birds had longer crypt depth than CON birds in duodenum, jejunum, and ileum and also higher crypt/villi height ratio in duodenum than CON birds. Crypt depth and the ratio of crypt depth to villus height are measures of efficiency because the increase of crypt depth and/or crypt/villi ratio indicates greater need of cell proliferation to maintain gut barrier integrity (46–48). In addition to longer crypt depth, duodenum and jejunum of GBF birds also had wider villi. Narrow villi have greater nutrient absorption area. Widening of villus indicates less nutrient absorption area and probably also greater amount of gut-associated immune tissue proliferation and accumulation in the villus, which is another indication of compromised gut heath. The structural change in GBF birds confirmed that gut barrier failure was occurring in GBF birds, which may be associated with the poor performance in this study and is consistent with a previous study (49).

The gastrointestinal tract (GIT) is repeatedly challenged by foreign antigens and the intestinal mucosa must have the capability of fast restoration in the event of tissue damage (50). Impairment of this fragile barrier leads to enteritis and other inflammatory diseases (9). The intestinal mucosa contains different types of epithelial cells with specific functions. IEC control surface-associated bacterial populations without upsetting the microbiome that are vital for host health (51), and play an essential role in maintaining gut homeostasis and barrier function (52, 53). As a single-cell layer, IEC serve as a protective barrier against the external environment and maintain a defense against intraluminal toxins and antigens in addition to support nutrients and water transport (54). IEC are sealed together by adherens junctions (AJ) and TJ that are composed of cadherins, claudins, occludins, and JAM (29, 55–57). Upon injury, IEC undergo a wound healing process that is reliant on three cellular events: restitution, proliferation, and differentiation (27). Previous studies have shown that various regulatory peptides, including growth factors and cytokines, are capable of influencing the restoration of damaged IEC (58).

Gram-negative bacteria in the gut release endotoxin during growth, division, and death, and luminal endotoxin can translocate to circulation via two routes: (1) non-specific paracellular transport through TJ of epithelial cells, and (2) transcellular transport through lipid raft membrane domains and receptor-mediated endocytosis (2, 59). TLR4 is involved in the latter route (60). The lack of difference of TLR4 mRNA levels between CON and GBF birds suggests that endotoxin probably did not enter into circulation via transcellular transport. Pathogens, such as *Escherichia coli* or *C. perfringens*, as well as their elaborated toxins (e.g., endotoxin or entertoxin) have been reported to alter epithelial TJ and gut barrier function (23). Poor integrity of gut barrier or opening of TJ has been reported to facilitate paracellular transport of endotoxin, which will increase proinflammatory cytokine secretion and activate innate and adaptive immune response (61, 62). Secreted cytokines may enter the IEC through the basolateral side, resulting in further increased inflammation, disruption of TJ complexes, and increased paracellular endotoxin transport (63). Interestingly, there were detectable levels of endotoxin in CON chickens, which are actually not the background noise detected by ELISA kit. In this study, the CON chickens were much healthier than GBF chickens, the endotoxin in the serum of CON chickens could be non-specific paracellular diffusion of endotoxin from intestinal lumen into circulation. The increase of endotoxin levels in GBF birds indicates that gut barrier failure increased the transport of endotoxin from intestinal lumen into circulation, which could further negatively affect the integrity of TJ as evidenced by the decrease of occludin mRNA levels in GBF birds. Occludin, one of the major components of TJ, is involved in the regulation of inter-membrane diffusion and paracellular diffusion of small molecules (64). Occludin is down-regulated in patients with Crohn's Disease and ulcerative colitis, two common types of inflammatory bowel disease in humans (57, 64), suggesting the important role of occludin in intestinal health. However, no differences were detected between GBF and CON chickens in the expression of other TJ components, such as claudin 1, ZO1, JAM2, and JAM3. Claudin 1 is a member of multiple-span transmembrane protein called claudins, a protein family with more than 20 members, JAM2 and JAM3 are single-span transmembrane protein (51, 65, 66). ZO1 is a plaque protein that acts as adaptors to connect transmembrane proteins to the perijunctional actomyosin ring (23). These results indicate that GBF model impaired TJ integrity by reducing occludin expression, which facilitates the transport of endotoxin from intestinal lumen into blood for systemic circulation.

Endotoxin was also reported to increase satiety peptide secretion, which will reduce FI (20). The decreased growth performance in GBF birds could be partially associated with the increase of satiety peptide resulting from the elevated endotoxin levels, although satiety peptide was not measured in this study.

1-Acid glycoprotein, an acute phase protein, has been used as a marker for systemic inflammation in poultry (67). Increase of AGP in GBF birds confirms that systemic inflammation was occurring in GBF birds, which led us to investigate the local inflammation status in the gut. Changes in the gut microbiota have been reported to negatively affect gut barrier integrity, leading to increased leakage of endotoxin and fatty acids, which can act upon TLR4 to activate systemic inflammation (68). Activation of macrophages via TLR is important for inflammation and host defense against pathogens; however, recent studies suggest that non-pathogenic molecules are able to induce inflammation via TLR2 and TLR4 (16, 69–71). The capacity to detect tissue injury and to initiate adequate repair mechanisms is indispensable for the survival of all higher species. A common aspect of all types of injury - caused by infectious, physical, chemical, or immune processes - is a compositional change of the cellular environment leading to the presence of novel molecular patterns. These patterns are recognized by a group of receptors termed pattern recognition receptors (PRR) and trigger specific responses that promote the restoration of tissue function, including inflammation and wound healing (20, 72). Pathogen recognition is critical to survive in an essentially hostile environment that is full of potentially infective microorganisms. Detection systems for molecular patterns characteristic for pathogens (pathogen-associated molecular patterns, PAMP) develop early in evolution, and are present in most species including plants and invertebrates (69). As a group of highly conserved PRR, TLR signals the presence of various PAMP to cellular constituents of the innate and adaptive immune (69, 73), therefore acting as gatekeepers for several highly efficient response systems that regulate tissue homeostasis and protect the host after acute injury (60, 74). Upon injury, the intestinal epithelium undergoes a wound healing process (69). Recent studies have revealed the activation of TLR by the microbiota during the healing process (20). In addition, several cytokines, such as TGF- , TGF- , IL-1 , and IL-2, are also increased during healing process (16, 75). In this study, the mRNA levels of TGF- and IL-1 in GBF chickens were increased, but TLR4, TLR2 , TGF- , IL-4, and IL-6 mRNA levels were not different compared to CON chickens. These results suggest that the inflammation occurred in GBF birds in this study is likely not mediated by TLR2 or TLR4 pathway. However, TLR3 mRNA and protein levels of TLR2, TLR4, and TLR3 were not measured in this study. Therefore, we are not able to exclude the possibility that TLR pathway is involved in the inflammation in GBF birds. IL-1 is an important mediator of the inflammatory response and is involved in a variety of cellular activities, including cell proliferation, differentiation, and apoptosis (76). TGF- , a key mediator of mucosal immune homeostasis, mediates IgA production, retains lymphocytes in the gut and promotes wound healing of intestinal epithelium and mucosa (75). TGF- also promotes IEC proliferation through the activation of extracellular signal-regulated kinase (ERK) 1/ERK2 mitogen-activated protein kinase during wound healing (20). IL-8 is secreted basolaterally by intestinal epithelium in response to pathogenic bacteria or specific inflammory cytokines, and triggers neutrophil migration and inflammation in intestine (73). The increase of systemic AGP, and mucosal TGF- , IL-8, and IL-1 in GBF birds indicate that GBF model increased intestinal inflammation and activated intestinal innate immune response and wound healing.

Mucins are large glycoproteins that cover epithelial surfaces of the intestine and form a mucus layer to protect epithelial cells from gut health challenge. There are two major types of mucins, membrane-bound and secreted (77, 78). In chickens (*Gallus gallus*), three transmembrane mucins (MUC4, MUC13, and MUC16) and four gel-forming mucins (MUC6, MUC2, MUC5ac, and MUC5b) have been identified (79). In mammals, MUC2, the mucin secreted by goblet cells, is the most abundant mucin in the intestine, and its deficiency has been reported to increase bacterial translocation and inflammation (18, 80). Evolutionary studies suggest that mucins share a common ancestor, since their domain structures are well conserved in metazoans (71, 81). All mucins (MUC) contain at least one PTS domain, a region rich in proline, threonine, and serine (18, 82). Chicken MUC2 has been reported to be remarkably similar to human and mouse outside of the central PTS domain, but is highly divergent within this central repetitive structure (82, 83). Although the physiological implications and disease associations of MUC on various mucosal surfaces are well understood, there are still many questions as to how and why the gene architecture of this family contributes to diverse protein modifications that show diverse biological effects between metazoans in health and disease (18, 84–87). MUC2 gene expression has been used as a marker for gut health in poultry and other species (85, 88, 89). For example, Li et al. found that zinc supplementation in breeder diets improved morphometry, increased the number of goblet cell per villus, and MUC2 gene expression, and reduced mRNA levels of proinflammatory cytokines, such as IL-6 and IL-1 in the jejunum of their offspring (89). In the present study, MUC2 gene expression was reduced by 29% in GBF birds compared to CON birds, suggesting that GBF model reduced mucus layer protection in jejunum.

Intracellular lipid chaperones known as FABP are a group of molecules that coordinate lipid response and metabolism in cells (90). FABP are found across species, from *Drosophila melanogaster* and *Caenorhabditis elegans* to mice and humans, demonstrating strong evolutionary conservation (90). FABP-mediated lipid metabolism is closely linked to both metabolic and inflammatory processes through modulating critical lipid sensitive pathways in target cells, especially adipocytes and macrophages (90, 91). Nine FABP have been identified so far in intestine, liver, brain, adipose, and muscle, the organs that show high rates of lipid metabolism, in vertebrates (92, 93). Intestinal FABP, FABP2, and FABP6, are expressed at high levels in the small intestine and ileum, respectively, and in addition to mediate lipid metabolism, they are also involved in intestinal inflammatory conditions by modulating critical lipid-sensitive pathways in adipocytes and macrophages in human (94, 95). FABP2 is down-regulated in patients with ischemia/reperfusion-induced intestinal barrier injury (93), suggesting the important role of FABP2 in gut barrier health. FABP2 has been identified as a specific marker for the relative amount of epithelium in humans and pigs (96). Several FABP (FABP1, FABP2, FABP6, and FABP10) have been identified to be predominantly expressed in the digestive tract of chickens (97, 98); however, much remains to be determined regarding their expression and biological functions in poultry. FABP10 plays an important hepatic role in in response to FI in chicken (98). FABP2 is involved in lipogenesis and fatty acids transport, and plays an important role in abdominal fat content in broiler chickens (98–100). In the present study, GBF model reduced FABP2 gene expression, suggesting that, like the role of FABP2 in human intestinal barrier health, FABP2 can be used as a marker of gut barrier function in chicken. Reduction of FABP2 expression indicates the loss of epithelial cell content and occurrence of intestinal barrier failure in GBF birds.

The ileal lipid binding protein (ILBP; human gene FABP6) was recently shown to be needed for the efficient transport of bile acids from the apical side to the basolateral side of enterocytes in the distal portion of murine intestine (101). Bile acids are synthesized by the liver and released into the lumen of the small intestine via bile, and the majority of bile acids are recovered in the distal end of the small intestine and then returned to the liver for reuse (102). Bile acid has emerged as important biological molecules that emulsify lipids and liposoluble dietary nutrients to facilitate their digestion and absorption (103, 104). It has strong anti-microbial activity and therefore is emerging as a host factor that regulates the composition of microbiota in the gut (105, 106). Reduced bile acid levels in the gut are reported to be associated with bacterial overgrowth and inflammation (106). Gut inflammation in GBF birds may have resulted in lower levels of bile acids, which unfortunately were not measured in this study. The substantial increase of FABP6 by four fold in GBF birds indicates high demand of bile acids as an anti-microbial to promote the recovery of dysbacteriosis and barrier failure in the gut of GBF birds.

In conclusion, the purpose of this study was not to determine the individual effects of diet ingredients or coccidia challenge but rather to determine the potential biomarkers that may be used to define gut barrier failure in future studies. We attempted to exacerbate gut barrier failure with the tools available for us, and the results obtained in the present study suggest that the combination of high NSP diet and a coccidia challenge induced gut barrier failure and inflammation in broilers characterized by the increase of endotoxin and AGP in serum, as well as increase of IL-8, IL-1 , TGF- 4, and FABP6 mRNA, and reduction of FABP2, MUC2, and occludin mRNA in jejunal mucosa of GBF birds compared to CON birds. These parameters may be utilized as potential biomarkers for gut barrier health in chickens. Now that we have a better understanding of what biomarkers are relevant in gut barrier failure models in chickens, further studies will be conducted to evaluate the effects of chicken enteropathogens, different dietary ingredients or feed additives, such as probiotics and prebiotics, on gut barrier function in broiler chickens.

Acknowledgments

We would like to acknowledge Terra Wineman, Cindy Atwell, and Beaver Wuelling for the technical assistance, and Dr. Karen Wedekind for critical reading of manuscript. The study was financially supported by Novus International Inc.

References

1. Williams R. Intercurrent coccidiosis and necrotic enteritis of chickens: rational, integrated disease management by maintenance of gut integrity. *Avian Pathol* (2005) **34**:159–80. doi:10.1080/03079450500112195
2. Sharma R, Tepas JJ III, Hudak ML, Mollitt DL, Wludyka PS, Teng R-J, et al. Neonatal gut barrier and multiple organ failure: role of endotoxin and proinflammatory cytokines in sepsis and necrotizing enterocolitis. *J Pediatr Surg* (2007) **42**:454–61. doi:10.1016/j.jpedsurg.2006.10.038
3. Pastorelli L, De Salvo C, Mercado JR, Vecchi M, Pizarro TT. Central role of the gut epithelial barrier in the pathogenesis of chronic intestinal inflammation: lessons learned from animal models and human genetics. *Front Immunol* (2013) **4**:280. doi:10.3389/fimmu.2013.00280
4. Latorre JD, Hernandez-Velasco X, Kogut MH, Vicente JL, Wolfenden R, Wolfenden A, et al. Role of a *Bacillus subtilis* direct-fed microbial on digesta viscosity, bacterial translocation, and bone mineralization in turkey poults fed with a rye-based diet. *Front Vet Sci* (2014) **1**:26. doi:10.3389/fvets.2014.00026
5. Tellez G, Latorre JD, Kuttappan VA, Kogut MH, Wolfenden A, Hernandez-Velasco X, et al. Utilization of rye as energy source affects bacterial translocation, intestinal viscosity, microbiota composition, and bone mineralization in broiler chickens. *Front Genet* (2014) **5**:339. doi:10.3389/fgene.2014.00339
6. Dahiya J, Wilkie D, Van Kessel AG, Drew M. Potential strategies for controlling necrotic enteritis in broiler chickens in post-antibiotic era. *Anim Feed Sci Technol* (2006) **129**:60–88. doi:10.1016/j.anifeedsci.2005.12.003
7. Gholamiandehkordi AR, Timbermont L, Lanckriet A, Broeck WV, Pedersen K, Dewulf J, et al. Quantification of gut lesions in a subclinical necrotic enteritis model. *Avian Pathol* (2007) **36**:375–82. doi:10.1080/03079450701589118
8. Castanon J. History of the use of antibiotic as growth promoters in European poultry feeds. *Poult Sci* (2007) **86**:2466–71. doi:10.3382/ps.2007-00249
9. Yegani M, Korver D. Factors affecting intestinal health in poultry. *Poult Sci* (2008) **87**:2052–63. doi:10.3382/ps.2008-00091
10. Teirlynck E, Gussem M, Dewulf J, Haesebrouck F, Ducatelle R, Van Immerseel F. Morphometric evaluation of "dysbacteriosis" in broilers. *Avian Pathol* (2011) **40**:139–44. doi:10.1080/03079457.2010.543414
11. Wideman RF, Prisby RD. Bone circulatory disturbances in the development of spontaneous bacterial chondronecrosis with osteomyelitis: a translational model for the pathogenesis of femoral head necrosis. *Front Endocrinol (Lausanne)* (2011) **3**:183. doi:10.3389/fendo.2012.00183
12. Wideman R, Hamal K, Stark J, Blankenship J, Lester H, Mitchell K, et al. A wire-flooring model for inducing lameness in broilers: evaluation of probiotics as a prophylactic treatment. *Poult Sci* (2012) **91**:870–83. doi:10.3382/ps.2011-01907
13. Wideman R, Al-Rubaye A, Kwon Y, Blankenship J, Lester H, Mitchell K, et al. Prophylactic administration of a combined prebiotic and probiotic, or therapeutic administration of enrofloxacin, to reduce the incidence of bacterial chondronecrosis with osteomyelitis in broilers. *Poult Sci* (2015) **94**:25–36. doi:10.3382/ps/peu025
14. Groschwitz KR, Hogan SP. Intestinal barrier function: molecular regulation and disease pathogenesis. *J Allergy Clin Immunol* (2009) **124**:3–20. doi:10.1016/j.jaci.2009.05.038
15. Sharma R, Young C, Neu J. Molecular modulation of intestinal epithelial barrier: contribution of microbiota. *J Biomed Biotechnol* (2010) **2010**:305879. doi:10.1155/2010/305879
16. Jeon MK, Klaus C, Kaemmerer E, Gassler N. Intestinal barrier: molecular pathways and modifiers. *World J Gastrointest Pathophysiol* (2013) **4**:94–9. doi:10.4291/wjgp.v4.i4.94
17. Sakamoto K, Hirose H, Onizuka A, Hayashi M, Futamura N, Kawamura Y, et al. Quantitative study of changes in intestinal morphology and mucus gel on total parenteral nutrition in rats. *J Surg Res* (2000) **94**:99–106. doi:10.1006/jsre.2000.5937
18. Kim YS, Ho SB. Intestinal goblet cells and mucins in health and disease: recent insights and progress. *Curr Gastroenterol Rep* (2010) **12**:319–30. doi:10.1007/s11894-010-0131-2
19. Johansson ME, Gustafsson JK, Sjöberg KE, Petersson J, Holm L, Sjövall H, et al. Bacteria penetrate the inner mucus layer before inflammation in the dextran sulfate colitis model. *PLoS One* (2010) **5**:e12238. doi:10.1371/journal.pone.0012238
20. Iizuka M, Konno S. Wound healing of intestinal epithelial cells. *World J Gastroenterol* (2011) **17**:2161–71. doi:10.3748/wjg.v17.i17.2161
21. Audy J, Mathieu O, Belvis J, Tompkins T. Transcriptomic response of immune signalling pathways in intestinal epithelial cells exposed to lipopolysaccharides, Gram-negative bacteria or potentially probiotic microbes. *Benef Microbes* (2012) **3**:273–86. doi:10.3920/BM2012.0027
22. Sander GR, Cummins AG, Powell BC. Rapid disruption of intestinal barrier function by gliadin involves altered expression of apical junctional proteins. *FEBS Lett* (2005) **579**:4851–5. doi:10.1016/j.febslet.2005.07.066

23. Ulluwishewa D, Anderson RC, McNabb WC, Moughan PJ, Wells JM, Roy NC. Regulation of tight junction permeability by intestinal bacteria and dietary components. *J Nutr* (2011) **141**:769–76. doi:10.3945/jn.110.135657
24. Ballard ST, Hunter JH, Taylor AE. Regulation of tight-junction permeability during nutrient absorption across the intestinal epithelium. *Annu Rev Nutr* (1995) **15**:35–55. doi:10.1146/annurev.nutr.15.1.35
25. Alverdy J, Zaborina O, Wu L. The impact of stress and nutrition on bacterial-host interactions at the intestinal epithelial surface. *Curr Opin Clin Nutr Metab Care* (2005) **8**:205–9. doi:10.1097/00075197-200503000-00016
26. Edelblum KL, Turner JR. The tight junction in inflammatory disease: communication breakdown. *Curr Opin Pharmacol* (2009) **9**:715–20. doi:10.1016/j.coph.2009.06.022
27. Schulzke JD, Ploeger S, Amasheh M, Fromm A, Zeissig S, Troeger H, et al. Epithelial tight junctions in intestinal inflammation. *Ann N Y Acad Sci* (2009) **1165**:294–300. doi:10.1111/j.1749-6632.2009.04062.x
28. Ilan Y. Leaky gut and the liver: a role for bacterial translocation in nonalcoholic steatohepatitis. *World J Gastroenterol* (2012) **18**:2609–18. doi:10.3748/wjg.v18.i21.2609
29. Steed E, Balda MS, Matter K. Dynamics and functions of tight junctions. *Trends Cell Biol* (2010) **20**:142–9. doi:10.1016/j.tcb.2009.12.002
30. Hu Y-J, Wang Y-D, Tan F-Q, Yang W-X. Regulation of paracellular permeability: factors and mechanisms. *Mol Biol Rep* (2013) **40**:6123–42. doi:10.1007/s11033-013-2724-y
31. Dibner J, Atwell C, Kitchell M, Shermer W, Ivey F. Feeding of oxidized fats to broilers and swine: effects on enterocyte turnover, hepatocyte proliferation and the gut associated lymphoid tissue. *Anim Feed Sci Technol* (1996) **62**:1–13. doi:10.1016/S0377-8401(96)01000-0
32. Friesen OD, Guenter W, Marquardt RR, Rotter BA. The effect of enzyme supplementation on the apparent metabolizable energy and nutrient digestibilities of wheat, barley, oats, and rye for the young broiler chick. *Poult Sci* (1992) **71**:1710–21. doi:10.3382/ps.0711710
33. Knudsen KE. Fiber and nonstarch polysaccharide content and variation in common crops used in broiler diets. *Poult Sci* (2014) **93**:2380–93. doi:10.3382/ps.2014-03902
34. National Research Council. *Nutrient Requirements of Poultry*. 9th ed. Washington, DC: National Academic Press (1994).
35. FASS. *Guide for the Care and Use of Agricultural Animals in Research and Teaching*. 3rd ed. Champaign, IL. Federation of Animal Science Societies (2010).
36. Biloni A, Quintana CF, Menconi A, Kallapura G, Latorre J, Pixley C, et al. Evaluation of effects of EarlyBird associated with FloraMax-B11 on *Salmonella* Enteritidis, intestinal morphology, and performance of broiler chickens. *Poult Sci* (2013) **92**:2337–46. doi:10.3382/ps.2013-03279
37. SAS Institute Inc. *SAS User Guide. Version 9.1*. Cary, NC: SAS Institute Inc. (2002).
38. Choct M, Hughes RJ, Trimble RP, Angkanaporn K, Annison G. Non-starch polysaccharide-degrading enzymes increase the performance of broiler chickens fed wheat of low apparent metabolizable energy. *J Nutr* (1995) **125**:485–92.
39. Murphy T, McCracken J, McCann M, George J, Bedford M. Broiler performance and in vivo viscosity as influenced by a range of xylanases, varying in ability to effect wheat in vitro viscosity. *Br Poult Sci* (2009) **50**:716–24. doi:10.1080/00071660903389950
40. Kiarie E, Romero LF, Nyachoti CM. The role of added feed enzymes in promoting gut health in swine and poultry. *Nutr Res Rev* (2013) **26**:71–88. doi:10.1017/S0954422413000048
41. Timbermont L, Haesebrouck F, Ducatelle R, Van Immerseel F. Necrotic enteritis in broilers: an updated review on the pathogenesis. *Avian Pathol* (2011) **40**:341–7. doi:10.1080/03079457.2011.590967
42. Van Leeuwen P, Mouwen J, Van Der Klis J, Verstegen M. Morphology of the small intestinal mucosal surface of broilers in relation to age, diet formulation, small intestinal microflora and performance. *Br Poult Sci* (2004) **45**:41–8. doi:10.1080/00071660410001668842
43. Shirzadi H, Moravej H, Shivazad M. Influence of non starch polysaccharide-degrading enzymes on the meat yield and viscosity of jejunal digesta in broilers fed wheat/barley-based diet. *Afr J Biotechnol* (2010) **9**:1517–22.
44. Bedford M, Classen H, Campbell G. The effect of pelleting, salt, and pentosanase on the viscosity of intestinal contents and the performance of broilers fed rye. *Poult Sci* (1991) **70**:1571–7. doi:10.3382/ps.0701571
45. Bedford M, Classen H. An *in vitro* assay for prediction of broiler intestinal viscosity and growth when fed rye-based diets in the presence of exogenous enzymes. *Poult Sci* (1993) **72**:137–43. doi:10.3382/ps.0720137
46. Uni Z, Ganot S, Sklan D. Posthatch development of mucosal function in the broiler small intestine. *Poult Sci* (1998) **77**:75–82. doi:10.1093/ps/77.1.75
47. Awad W, Ghareeb K, Abdel-Raheem S, Böhm J. Effects of dietary inclusion of probiotic and synbiotic on growth performance, organ weights, and intestinal histomorphology of broiler chickens. *Poult Sci* (2009) **88**:49–56. doi:10.3382/ps.2008-00244
48. Awad W, Ghareeb K, Böhm J. Evaluation of the chicory inulin efficacy on ameliorating the intestinal morphology and modulating the intestinal electrophysiological properties in broiler chickens. *J Anim Physiol Anim Nutr* (2011) **95**:65–72. doi:10.1111/j.1439-0396.2010.00999.x
49. Ozdogan M, Topal E, Paksuz EP, Kirkan S. Effect of different levels of crude glycerol on the morphology and some pathogenic bacteria of the small intestine in male broilers. *Animal* (2013) **8**:36–42. doi:10.1017/S1751731113001833
50. Savage DC. Microbial ecology of the gastrointestinal tract. *Annu Rev Microbiol* (1997) **31**:107–33. doi:10.1146/annurev.mi.31.100177.000543
51. Tellez G. Prokaryotes versus eukaryotes: who is hosting whom? *Front Vet Sci* (2014) **1**:3. doi:10.3389/fvets.2014.00003
52. Sharma R, Tepas JJ III. Microecology, intestinal epithelial barrier and necrotizing enterocolitis. *Pediatr Surg Int* (2010) **26**:11–21. doi:10.1007/s00383-009-2536-2
53. Lamprecht M, Frauwallner A. Exercise, intestinal barrier dysfunction and probiotic supplementation. *Med Sport Sci* (2012) **59**:47–56. doi:10.1159/000342169
54. Loehry C, Creamer B. Three-dimensional structure of the human small intestinal mucosa in health and disease. *Gut* (1969) **10**:6–12. doi:10.1136/gut.10.1.6
55. Schneeberger EE, Lynch RD. Structure, function, and regulation of cellular tight junctions. *Am J Physiol* (1992) **262**:L647–61.
56. Matter K, Balda MS. Epithelial tight junctions, gene expression and nucleo-junctional interplay. *J Cell Sci* (2007) **120**:1505–11. doi:10.1242/jcs.005975
57. Assimakopoulos SF, Papageorgiou I, Charonis A. Enterocytes' tight junctions: from molecules to diseases. *World J Gastrointest Pathophysiol* (2011) **2**:123–37. doi:10.4291/wjgp.v2.i6.123
58. Bethune MT, Khosla C. Parallels between pathogens and gluten peptides in celiac sprue. *PLoS Pathog* (2008) **4**.e34. doi.10.1371/journal.ppat.0040034
59. Awad W, Aschenbach J, Khayal B, Hess C, Hess M. Intestinal epithelial responses to *Salmonella enterica* serovar Enteritidis: effects on intestinal permeability and ion transport. *Poult Sci* (2012) **91**:2949–57. doi:10.3382/ps.2012-02448
60. Mollen KP, Anand RJ, Tsung A, Prince JM, Levy RM, Billiar TR. Emerging paradigm: toll-like receptor 4-sentinel for the detection of tissue damage. *Shock* (2006) **26**:430–7. doi:10.1097/01.shk.0000228797.41044.08
61. Steverink P, Salden H, Sturk A, Klein W, van der Velden M, Németh F. Laboratory and clinical evaluation of a chromogenic endotoxin assay for horses with acute intestinal disorders. *Vet Q* (1994) **16**:117–21. doi:10.1080/01652176.1994.9694517
62. Senior J, Proudman C, Leuwer M, Carter S. Plasma endotoxin in horses presented to an equine referral hospital: correlation to selected clinical parameters and outcomes. *Equine Vet J* (2011) **43**:585–91. doi:10.1111/j.2042-3306.2010.00328.x
63. Heller F, Florian P, Bojarski C, Richter J, Christ M, Hillenbrand B, et al. Interleukin-13 is the key effector Th2 cytokine in ulcerative colitis that affects epithelial tight junctions, apoptosis, and cell restitution. *Gastroenterology* (2005) **129**:550–64. doi:10.1016/j.gastro.2005.05.002
64. Saleh M, Elson CO. Experimental inflammatory bowel disease: insights into the host-microbiota dialog. *Immunity* (2011) **34**:293–302. doi:10.1016/j.immuni.2011.03.008
65. Al-Sadi R, Boivin M, Ma T. Mechanism of cytokine modulation of epithelial tight junction barrier. *Front Biosci* (2009) **14**:2765–8. doi:10.2741/3413
66. Wijtten PJ, van der Meulen J, Verstegen MW. Intestinal barrier function and absorption in pigs after weaning: a review. *Br J Nutr* (2011) **105**:967–81. doi:10.1017/S0007114510005660
67. Adler KL, Peng PH, Peng RK, Klasing KC. The kinetics of hemopexin and 1-acid glycoprotein levels induced by injection of inflammatory agents in chickens. *Avian Dis* (2001) **45**(2):289–96. doi:10.2307/1592967

68. Velloso LA, Folli F, Saad MJ. TLR4 at the crossroads of nutrients, gut microbiota and metabolic inflammation. *Endocr Rev* (2015) **26**:er20141100. doi:10.1210/er.2014-1100
69. Ozinsky A, Underhill DM, Fontenot JD, Hajjar AM, Smith KD, Wilson CB, et al. The repertoire for pattern recognition of pathogens by the innate immune system is defined by cooperation between toll-like receptors. *Proc Natl Acad Sci U S A* (2000) **97**:13766–71. doi:10.1073/pnas.250476497
70. Kigerl KA, Lai W, Rivest S, Hart RP, Satoskar AR, Popovich PG. Toll-like receptor (TLR)-2 and TLR-4 regulate inflammation, gliosis, and myelin sparing after spinal cord injury. *J Neurochem* (2007) **102**:37–50. doi:10.1111/j.1471-4159.2007.04524.x
71. Kimbrell DA, Beutler B. The evolution and genetics of innate immunity. *Nat Rev Genet* (2001) **2**:256–67. doi:10.1038/35066006
72. Huebener P, Schwabe RF. Regulation of wound healing and organ fibrosis by toll-like receptors. *Biochim Biophys Acta* (2013) **1832**:1005–17. doi:10.1016/j.bbadis.2012.11.017
73. Berkes J, Viswanathan V, Savkovic S, Hecht G. Intestinal epithelial responses to enteric pathogens: effects on the tight junction barrier, ion transport, and inflammation. *Gut* (2003) **52**:439–51. doi:10.1136/gut.52.3.439
74. Dasu MR, Ramirez SR, La TD, Gorouhi F, Nguyen C, Lin BR, et al. Crosstalk between adrenergic and toll-like receptors in human mesenchymal stem cells and keratinocytes: a recipe for impaired wound healing. *Stem Cells Transl Med* (2014) **3**:745. doi:10.5966/sctm.2013-0200
75. Konkel JE, Chen W. Balancing acts: the role of TGF- in the mucosal immune system. *Trends Mol Med* (2011) **17**:668–76. doi:10.1016/j.molmed.2011.07.002
76. Ojeda MO, van't Veer C, Fernandez Ortega CB, Araña Rosainz Mde J, Buurman WA. Dialyzable leukocyte extract differentially regulates the production of TNF , IL-6, and IL-8 in bacterial component-activated leukocytes and endothelial cells. *Inflamm Res* (2005) **54**:74–81. doi:10.1007/s00011-004-1326-5
77. Williams SJ, Wreschner DH, Tran M, Eyre HJ, Sutherland GR, McGuckin MA. Muc13, a novel human cell surface mucin expressed by epithelial and hemopoietic cells. *J Biol Chem* (2001) **276**:18327–36. doi:10.1074/jbc.M008850200
78. Toribara N, Roberton A, Ho S, Kuo W, Gum E, Hicks J, et al. Human gastric mucin. Identification of a unique species by expression cloning. *J Biol Chem* (1993) **268**:5879–85.
79. Lang T, Hansson GC, Samuelsson T. An inventory of mucin genes in the chicken genome shows that the mucin domain of Muc13 is encoded by multiple exons and that ovomucin is part of a locus of related gel-forming mucins. *BMC Genomics* (2006) **7**:386–95. doi:10.1186/1471-2164-7-197
80. Wei X, Yang Z, Rey FE, Ridaura VK, Davidson NO, Gordon JI, et al. Fatty acid synthase modulates intestinal barrier function through palmitoylation of mucin 2. *Cell Host Microbe* (2012) **11**:140–52. doi:10.1016/j.chom.2011.12.006
81. Lang T, Hansson GC, Samuelsson T. Gel-forming mucins appeared early in metazoan evolution. *Proc Natl Acad Sci U S A* (2007) **104**:16209–14. doi:10.1073/pnas.0705984104
82. Jiang Z, Applegate TJ, Lossie AC. Cloning, annotation and developmental expression of the chicken intestinal MUC2 gene. *PLoS One* (2013) **8**:e53781. doi:10.1371/journal.pone.0053781
83. Zhang Q, Eicher SD, Applegate TJ. Development of intestinal mucin 2, IgA, and polymeric Ig receptor expressions in broiler chickens and Pekin ducks. *Poult Sci* (2015) **94**(2):172–80. doi:10.3382/ps/peu064
84. Clark JA, Doelle SM, Halpern MD, Saunders TA, Holubec H, Dvorak K, et al. Intestinal barrier failure during experimental necrotizing enterocolitis: protective effect of EGF treatment. *Am J Physiol Gastrointest Liver Physiol* (2006) **291**:G938–49. doi:10.1152/ajpgi.00090.2006
85. Forder RE, Nattrass GS, Geier MS, Hughes RJ, Hynd PI. Quantitative analyses of genes associated with mucin synthesis of broiler chickens with induced necrotic enteritis. *Poult Sci* (2012) **91**:1335–41. doi:10.3382/ps.2011-02062
86. Liu D, Guo S, Guo Y. Xylanase supplementation to a wheat-based diet alleviated the intestinal mucosal barrier impairment of broiler chickens challenged by *Clostridium perfringens*. *Avian Pathol* (2012) **41**:291–8. doi:10.1080/03079457.2012.684089
87. Hollingsworth MA, Swanson BJ. Mucins in cancer: protection and control of the cell surface. *Nat Rev Cancer* (2004) **4**:45–60. doi:10.1038/nrc1251
88. Dkhil MA, Delic D, Al-Quraishy S. Goblet cells and mucin related gene expression in mice infected with *Eimeria papillata*. *ScientificWorldJournal* (2013) **2013**:439865. doi:10.1155/2013/439865
89. Li C, Guo S, Gao J, Guo Y, Du E, Lv Z, et al. Maternal high-zinc diet attenuates intestinal inflammation by reducing DNA methylation and elevating H3K9 acetylation in the A20 promoter of offspring chicks. *J Nutr Biochem* (2015) **26**(2):173–83. doi:10.1016/j.jnutbio.2014.10.005
90. Furuhashi M, Hotamisligil GS. Fatty acid-binding proteins: role in metabolic diseases and potential as drug targets. *Nat Rev Drug Discov* (2008) **7**:489–503. doi:10.1038/nrd2589
91. Storch J, Corsico B. The emerging functions and mechanisms of mammalian fatty acid-binding proteins. *Annu Rev Nutr* (2008) **28**:73–95. doi:10.1146/annurev.nutr.27.061406.093710
92. Schaap FG, van der Vusse GJ, Glatz JF. Evolution of the family of intracellular lipid binding proteins in vertebrates. *Mol Cell Biochem* (2002) **239**:69–77. doi:10.1023/A:1020519011939
93. Albala C, Santos JL, Cifuentes M, Villarroel AC, Lera L, Liberman C, et al. Intestinal FABP2 A54T polymorphism: association with insulin resistance and obesity in women. *Obes Res* (2004) **12**:340–5. doi:10.1038/oby.2004.42
94. Levy E, Ménard D, Delvin E, Stan S, Mitchell G, Lambert M, et al. The polymorphism at codon 54 of the FABP2 gene increases fat absorption in human intestinal explants. *J Biol Chem* (2001) **276**:39679–84. doi:10.1074/jbc.M105713200
95. Ohmachi T, Inoue H, Mimori K, Tanaka F, Sasaki A, Kanda T, et al. Fatty acid binding protein 6 is overexpressed in colorectal cancer. *Clin Cancer Res* (2006) **12**:5090–5. doi:10.1158/1078-0432.CCR-05-2045
96. Schroyen M, Stinckens A, Verhelst R, Geens M, Cox E, Niewold T, et al. Susceptibility of piglets to enterotoxigenic *Escherichia coli* is not related to the expression of MUC13 and MUC20. *Anim Genet* (2012) **43**:324–7. doi:10.1111/j.1365-2052.2011.02241.x
97. Zhang Q, Shi H, Liu W, Wang Y, Wang Q, Li H. Differential expression of L-FABP and L-BABP between fat and lean chickens. *Genet Mol Res* (2013) **12**:4192–206. doi:10.4238/2013.October.7.5
98. Hughes AL, Piontkivska H. Evolutionary diversification of the avian fatty acid-binding proteins. *Gene* (2011) **490**:1–5. doi:10.1016/j.gene.2011.09.016
99. Hu G, Wang S, Tian J, Chu L, Li H. Epistatic effect between ACACA and FABP2 gene on abdominal fat traits in broilers. *J Genet Genomics* (2010) **37**:505–12. doi:10.1016/S1673-8527(09)60070-9
100. Guo S, Liu D, Zhao X, Li C, Guo Y. Xylanase supplementation of a wheat-based diet improved nutrient digestion and mRNA expression of intestinal nutrient transporters in broiler chickens infected with *Clostridium perfringens*. *Poult Sci* (2014) **93**:94–103. doi:10.3382/ps.2013-03188
101. Praslickova D, Torchia EC, Sugiyama MG, Magrane EJ, Zwicker BL, Kolodzieyski L, et al. The ileal lipid binding protein is required for efficient absorption and transport of bile acids in the distal portion of the murine small intestine. *PLoS One* (2012) **7**:e50810. doi:10.1371/journal.pone.0050810
102. Zwicker BL, Agellon LB. Transport and biological activities of bile acids. *Int J Biochem Cell Biol* (2013) **45**:1389–98. doi:10.1016/j.biocel.2013.04.012
103. Iritani N, Fukuda E, Ibamoto K. Effect of fat intake on cholesterol turnover and bile acid formation. *J Nutr Sci Vitaminol* (1977) **23**:35–42. doi:10.3177/jnsv.23.35
104. Hofmann AF. Bile acids: the good, the bad, and the ugly. *News Physiol Sci* (1999) **14**:24–9.
105. Yokota A, Fukiya S, Islam KB, Ooka T, Ogura Y, Hayashi T. Is bile acid a determinant of the gut microbiota on a high-fat diet? *Gut Microbes* (2012) **3**:455–9. doi:10.4161/gmic.21216
106. Ridlon JM, Kang DJ, Hylemon PB, Bajaj JS. Bile acids and the gut microbiome. *Curr Opin Gastroenterol* (2014) **30**:332–8. doi:10.1097/MOG.0000000000000057

Conflict of Interest Statement: The authors declare that the research was conducted with financial support of Novus International Inc. Mention of trade names or commercial products in this article is solely for the purpose of providing specific information and does not imply recommendations or endorsement by Novus International Inc.

5

Tuberculosis and One Health – What is in a Name?

*Susanna Sternberg Lewerin**

Department of Biomedical Sciences and Veterinary Public Health, Swedish University of Agricultural Sciences (SLU), Uppsala, Sweden

Keywords: zoonotic, tuberculosis, epidemiology, nomenclature, terminology

Edited by:
Guillermo Tellez, University of Arkansas, USA

Reviewed by:
Kaori Sakamoto, University of Georgia, USA
Sherry Layton, Vetanco, Argentina

Correspondence:
Susanna Sternberg Lewerin
susanna.sternberg-lewerin@slu.se

INTRODUCTION

Most control programs for bovine tuberculosis include reporting to both veterinary and public health authorities, and measures to prevent transmission from animals to humans. On the other hand, reporting of human cases to veterinary authorities is rare, unless an animal source is suspected. Exchange of data and strategic discussions between veterinary and public health authorities would strengthen tuberculosis surveillance in both animal and human populations.

A One Health approach is clearly warranted for tuberculosis. The disease has similarly serious consequences for humans and a broad range of animal species, and it has been strongly advocated as a One Health issue (1). Yet, tuberculosis cases in humans and animals are commonly treated as separate problems (2, 3).

Tuberculosis is caused by bacteria within the *Mycobacterium tuberculosis* complex (MTBC). "Bovine tuberculosis" usually means infection in cattle with *Mycobacterium bovis* (3, 4). However, this definition may be too restrictive, and the term bovine tuberculosis has been proposed to signify infection in cattle with any bacteria in the MTBC (5, 6). Similarly, "human tuberculosis" usually refers to infection in humans with *M. tuberculosis*, while "zoonotic tuberculosis" refers to human infection with *M.* bovis (7). However, for control and monitoring purposes, as well as a One Health approach, it would be preferable to use the terms "human tuberculosis" and "bovine tuberculosis" for infection with all bacteria within the MTBC in humans and cattle, respectively. Consequently, infections in other host species could be named after the host species, complemented by specifying the infecting bacterial species. In the following, the term "tuberculosis" is used for infection with bacteria within the MTBC, regardless of host species.

TUBERCULOSIS IN DIFFERENT HOST POPULATIONS

Bacteria within the MTBC have a broad host range, although there are differences in host susceptibility as well as in the detailed pathophysiology of the infection (4, 8, 9). Factors such as host species, individual immunity, route of infection, and infectious dose have a strong impact on the course of the disease, regardless of bacterial species (8, 10), and it may be difficult to discern the exact pathogenic peculiarities of each species.

Differences in the infectious dose for a certain host species via a certain route are reflected in the epidemiology of the disease in different populations (8, 10). In a high prevalence environment, the probability of exposure and infection is high for any susceptible host as seen in sporadic cases or outbreaks of tuberculosis in species, such as sheep, pigs, and horses.

Infection by *M. bovis* has been reported in a wide range of domesticated and wild animals. Although not as frequent a cause as *M. tuberculosis*, a substantial number of humans with tuberculosis are infected with *M. bovis*. The prevalence of *M. bovis* in human tuberculosis is generally higher in low-income regions with a high prevalence in cattle. However, it has been proposed that the global prevalence of *M. bovis* in humans is underestimated (11–15). In the absence of immunosuppression, human-to-human transmission of *M. bovis* is rare but has been observed (15, 16). *Mycobacterium caprae*, previously regarded as a caprine subtype of *M. bovis*, has also been identified as the causative agent of tuberculosis in domestic and wild animals, as well as humans.

Mycobacterium tuberculosis is most commonly isolated from people, but in regions with a high prevalence in the human population, the infection may spill over to animals. Most animal isolates of *M. tuberculosis* originate from cattle, pigs, dogs, and Indian elephants, but the infection has also been demonstrated in captive and free-living wildlife. Molecular epidemiology has demonstrated transmission between humans and animals, in both directions (17–20). Other MTBC species, such as *Mycobacterium microti*, *Mycobacterium pinnipedii*, and *Mycobacterium africanum*, have also been isolated from various host species. Genomic studies into bacterial evolution suggest that sea mammals, in addition to human dispersals, may have played a role in transmitting tuberculosis across the ocean in Pre-Columbian times, illustrating the complexity of the host–pathogen relationship (21).

EPIDEMIOLOGY OF TUBERCULOSIS IN DIFFERENT POPULATIONS

Infectious dose and route of infection are important factors for the pathogenesis of the disease in individual hosts. Consequently, population dynamics, spatial distribution, contact patterns, and population sizes influence disease epidemiology. Efforts to categorize host species as "maintenance hosts" and "spillover hosts" are sometimes contradictory (8, 10, 22), probably due to the fact that the populations of these species differ between regions and ecological systems. The maintenance population may consist of one or several host species, depending on how the effective critical community size is achieved in different ecosystems (23).

Detailed data, sufficient to demonstrate the epidemiology of different MTBC species in different host populations, are difficult to obtain. The epidemiology of the infection differs regionally as well as within different populations in the same region (8, 12, 24).

A crucial aspect of epidemiological data collection is case definition. A case of human tuberculosis may be a patient with a smear-positive sputum sample, a tuberculin reactor, a patient from whom *M. tuberculosis* has been isolated, or a patient with samples positive for any bacteria within the MTBC. Similarly, animal cases may be defined as tuberculin reactors, animals with visible lesions *post mortem*, animals with histological lesions indicative of tuberculosis, or individuals with samples yielding *M. bovis* (or MTBC) in culture. Furthermore, the tuberculin test in animals may be performed as a single or comparative test in the skin of the neck or in the caudal fold, and the interpretation may be different in different situations (e.g., regarding all inconclusive reactions as positive, if a higher test sensitivity is prioritized above specificity) (25). Different case definitions may be used for different purposes, and this must be taken into account when drawing conclusions from data.

OTHER ASPECTS AFFECTING PREVALENCE FIGURES

Isolation of bacteria from each case would enable species identification and molecular typing to support epidemiological investigations. This is, however, not always feasible, and zoonotic transmission (in either direction) of tuberculosis may be overlooked.

In most regions of the world where the prevalence of tuberculosis in animals and humans is high, lack of resources means that diagnostics are insufficient for bacterial identification to species level. Even in high-income countries, diagnostics may rely on microscopy of sputum smears, histological examination of formalin-fixed tissue, culture on media not suitable for all MTBC species, or the use of DNA probes unable to distinguish between MTBC species (7, 13, 22). For example, the addition of glycerol in culture media will enhance growth of *M. tuberculosis* but inhibit growth of *M. bovis*, while culture media for *M. bovis* should preferably include pyruvate (4, 13, 22). Most diagnostic methods require some presumption about expected findings, and this will affect disease monitoring across different populations and geographical regions.

In the absence of bacteriological results, the clinical presentation of tuberculosis cases is sometimes used as an indicator of the causative agent. The primary manifestation of *M. bovis* in humans is usually extrapulmonary, but the proportion of pulmonary cases appears to be increasing (12, 26). Occupational exposure among farmers and abattoir workers usually leads to aerosol infection, this type of exposure may be more frequent in low-income countries with a high prevalence of tuberculosis in animals but where detailed data are scarce (8, 10, 16, 22, 26, 27). Site of infection is, therefore, not a solid basis for conclusions about the causative agent.

WHAT IS IN A NAME?

Terminology affects risk perception and behavior (28), a fact that is well known in the commercial world but not as commonly discussed in the scientific arena (29). The use of terms like bovine and human tuberculosis would be better applied to mean infection with MTBC in the respective host species. While acknowledging the difference between the species within MTBC and the need to identify each one in each case, it is important not to let the definition of the disease lead to too narrow a perspective, with possible lapses in tracing and control of the infection. Despite public awareness campaigns to combat human tuberculosis, knowledge of the risk presented by infected animals and vice versa can be poor (30), perhaps reflecting a failure in communication and or/awareness among the medical and veterinary professions. The use of terms like "human tuberculosis" and "zoonotic tuberculosis" (2, 3, 26) as contrasting events is not helping disease control, although it may be seen as formally correct.

PUBLIC HEALTH AND ANIMAL DISEASE CONTROL

The primary reason for tuberculosis control in animals is to protect public health. As cattle infected with members of the MTBC can shed the bacteria in milk, unpasteurized dairy products represent a public health risk. In many parts of the world, milk is heat-treated, but other dairy products may be made with raw milk. While pasteurization of all dairy products is crucial, tuberculosis control in cattle and other animals remain important for human and animal health (1, 10, 12, 22, 24). However, all stakeholders may not support disease control efforts, which are perceived as too costly and cumbersome, and therefore, not justifiable, when milk is pasteurized anyway (31). There may be a risk that the progress of tuberculosis control in animals, in combination with pasteurization of milk, has made professionals in human and veterinary medicine less aware, or even ignorant, of the fact that tuberculosis does not restrict itself to one host population. A stronger collaboration between veterinary and public health is often called for, and this call for collaboration must be repeated until taken for granted, and fully implemented in surveillance and control activities.

Many of the most heavily infected regions in the world lack the resources and infrastructure needed to control tuberculosis in animals and humans, while the epidemiology may be entirely different from what has been seen in countries where the disease has been eradicated from the animal population (10, 12, 24). This presents new challenges.

CONCLUSION

A systematic collaboration between different professions and control systems, and a common nomenclature clearly separating the name of the host species from the infecting bacterial species are the first steps toward effective tuberculosis surveillance and control.

We should learn from history and not repeat the mistake of those who, upon Koch's discovery of different MTBC species, first assumed that bovine tuberculosis did not affect humans, leading to the pasteurization of milk for calves long before it was applied to milk for human consumption. The more careful attitude of some early scientists, proposing to omit the host designation of the different bacterial species in order to anticipate assumptions that they are limited to the host whose name they bear (32), should be remembered as we make scientific progress. Understanding the complex ecosystem of the multi-host pathogens within the MTBC is necessary for disease control. There is an urgent need for scientific advances in order to meet the need for global tuberculosis control in all host populations, but this will require a new thinking as regards the ecology of tuberculosis and a practical application of the One Health concept.

REFERENCES

1. Kaneene J, Miller RA, Kaplan B, Steele JH, Thoen CO. Preventing and controlling zoonotic tuberculosis: a one health approach. *Vet Ital* (2014) **50**:7–22. doi:10.12834/VetIt.1302.08
2. OIE. *Terrestrial Code. Chapter 11.5 Bovine Tuberculosis* (2015). Available from: http://www.oie.int/index.php?id=169&L=0&htmfile=chapitre_bovine_tuberculosis.htm [Accessed August, 2015]
3. WHO. *Factsheet N 104 Reviewed March 2015: Tuberculosis* (2015). Available from: http://www.who.int/mediacentre/factsheets/fs104/en/ [Accessed August, 2015]
4. Quinn PJ, Markey BK, Leonard FC, FitzPatrick ES, Fanning S, Hartigan PJ. *Veterinary Microbiology and Microbial Disease*. 2nd ed. Oxford: Blackwell Science Ltd (2011).
5. SANCO/7059/2013. *European Commissison Health & Consumers Directorate-General, Unit G2. Working Document on Causal Agents of Bovine Tuberculosis*. Available from: https://www.visavet.es/bovinetuberculosis/data/wd/SANCO-7059-2013_M.tuberculosis_complex.pdf [Accessed August, 2015]
6. SANCO/10067/2013. *European Commissison Health & Consumers Directorate-General, Unit G5. Working Document on Eradication of Bovine Tuberculosis in the EU*. Available from: http://ec.europa.eu/food/animal/diseases/eradication/tb_workingdoc2006_en.pdf [Accessed August, 2015]
7. Müller B, Dürr S, Alonso S, Hattendorf J, Laisse CJM, Parsons SDC, et al. Zoonotic *Mycobacterium bovis*-induced tuberculosis in humans. *Emerg Infect Dis* (2013) **19**:899–908. doi:10.3201/eid1906.120543
8. Biet F, Boschiroli ML, Thorel MF, Guilloteau LA. Zoonotic aspects of *Mycobacterium bovis* and *Mycobacterium intracellulare* complex (MAC). *Vet Res* (2005) **36**:411–36. doi:10.1051/vetres:2005001
9. García-Jiménez WL, Benítez-Medina JM, Fernández-Llario P, Abecia JA, García-Sánchez A, Martínez R, et al. Comparative pathology of the natural infections by *Mycobacterium bovis* and by *Mycobacterium caprae* in wild boar (*Sus scrofa*). *Transbound Emerg Dis* (2013) **60**:102–9. doi:10.1111/j.1865-1682.2012.01321.x
10. Michel AL, Müller B, van Helden PD. *Mycobacterium bovis* at the animal-human interface: a problem or not? *Vet Microbiol* (2010) **140**:371–81. doi:10.1016/j.vetmic.2009.08.029
11. Ritacco V, de Kantor IN. Zoonotic tuberculosis in Latin America. *J Clin Microbiol* (1992) **30**:3299–300.
12. Cosivi O, Grange JM, Daborn JC, Raviglione MC, Fujikura T, Cousins D, et al. Zoonotic tuberculosis due to *Mycobacterium bovis* in developing countries. *Emerg Infect Dis* (1998) **4**:59–70. doi:10.3201/eid0401.980108
13. Drobniewski F, Strutt M, Smith G, Magee J, Flanagan P. Audit of scope and culture techniques applied to samples supplied for the diagnosis of *Mycobacterium bovis* by hospital laboratories in England and Wales. *Epidemiol Infect* (2003) **130**:235–7. doi:10.1017/S0950268802008105
14. Smith RMM, Drobniewski F, Gibson A, Montague JDE, Logan MN, Hunt D, et al. *Mycobacterium bovis* infection, United Kingdom. *Emerg Infect Dis* (2004) **10**:539–41. doi:10.3201/eid1003.020819
15. Pérez-Lago L, Navarro Y, García-de-Viedma D. Current knowledge and pending challenges in zoonosis caused by *Mycobacterium bovis*: a review. *Res Vet Sci* (2014) **97**:S94–100. doi:10.1016/j.rvsc.2013.11.008
16. Sunder S, Lanote P, Godreuil S, Martin C, Boschiroli ML, Besnier JM. Human-to-human transmission of tuberculosis caused by *Mycobacterium bovis* in immunocompetent patients. *J Clin Microbiol* (2009) **47**:1249–51. doi:10.1128/JCM.02042-08
17. Ocepek M, Pate M, Zolnir-Dovc M, Poljak M. Transmission of *Mycobacterium tuberculosis* from human to cattle. *J Clin Microbiol* (2005) **43**:3555–7. doi:10.1128/JCM.43.7.3555-3557.2005
18. Regassa A, Medhin G, Ameni G. Bovine tuberculosis in cattle owned by farmers with active tuberculosis in central Ethiopia. *Vet J* (2008) **178**:119–25. doi:10.1016/j.tvjl.2007.06.019
19. Chen Y, Chao Y, Deng Q, Liu T, Xiang J, Chen J, et al. Potential challenges to the stop TB plan for humans in China; cattle maintain *M. bovis* and *M. tuberculosis*. *Tuberculosis* (2009) **89**:95–100. doi:10.1016/j.tube.2008.07.003
20. Mittal M, Chakravarti S, Sharma V, Sanjeeth BS, Churamani CP, Kanwar NS. Evidence of presence of *Mycobacterium tuberculosis* in bovine tissue samples by multiplex PCR: possible relevance to reverse zoonosis. *Transbound Emerg Dis* (2014) **61**:97–104. doi:10.1111/tbed.12203
21. Bos KI, Harkins KM, Herbig A, Coscolla M, Weber N, Comas I, et al. Pre-Columbian mycobacterial genomes reveal seals as a source of new world human tuberculosis. *Nature* (2014) **514**:494–7. doi:10.1038/nature13591

22. de la Rua-Domenech R. Human *Mycobacterium bovis* infection in the United Kingdom: incidence, risks, control measures and review of the zoonotic aspects of bovine tuberculosis. *Tuberculosis* (2006) **86**:77–109. doi:10.1016/j.tube.2005.05.002
23. Haydon DT, Cleaveland S, Taylor LH, Laurenson MK. Identifying reservoirs of infection: a conceptual and practical challenge. *Emerg Infect Dis* (2002) **8**:1468–73. doi:10.3201/eid0812.010317
24. Miller M, Olea-Popelka F. One health in the shrinking world: experiences with tuberculosis at the human-livestock-wildlife interface. *Comp Immunol Microbiol Infect Dis* (2013) **36**:263–8. doi:10.1016/j.cimid.2012.07.005
25. OIE. *Terrestrial Manual. Bovine Tuberculosis* (2009). Available from: http://www.oie.int/fileadmin/Home/eng/Health_standards/tahm/2.04.07_BOVINE_TB.pdf [Accessed August, 2015]
26. Dürr S, Müller B, Alonso S, Hattendorf J, Laisse CJM, van Helden PD, et al. Differences in primary sites of infection between zoonotic and human tuberculosis: results from a worldwide systematic review. *PLoS Negl Trop Dis* (2013) **7**:e2399. doi:10.1371/journal.pntd.0002399
27. Pal M, Zenebe N, Rahman MT. Growing significance of *Mycobacterium bovis* in human health. *Microbes Health* (2014) **3**:29–34. doi:10.3329/mh.v3i1.19779
28. Buckton CH, Lean MEJ, Comber E. 'Language is the source of misunderstandings'-impact of terminology on public perceptions of health promotion messages. *BMC Public Health* (2015) **15**:579. doi:10.1186/s12889-015-1884-1
29. Dohle S, Siegrist M. Fluency of pharmaceutical drug names predicts perceived hazardousness, assumed side effects and willingness to buy. *J Health Psychol* (2014) **19**:1241–9. doi:10.1177/1359105313488974
30. Kidane AH, Sifer D, Aklilu M, Pal M. Knowledge, attitude and practice towards human and bovine tuberculosis among high school students in Addis Ababa, Ethiopia. *Int J Livest Res* (2015) **5**:1–11. doi:10.5455/ijlr.20150202104134
31. Torgerson P, Torgerson D. Benefits of stemming bovine TB need to be demonstrated. *Nature* (2009) **457**:657. doi:10.1038/457657d
32. Smith T. A comparative study of bovine tubercle *Bacilli* in man in relation to cattle. *J Exp Med* (1898) **3**:451–511. doi:10.1084/jem.3.4-5.451

Conflict of Interest Statement: The author declares that the research was conducted in the absence of any commercial or financial relationships that could be construed as a potential conflict of interest.

6

Effect of dietary exogenous enzyme supplementation on enteric mucosal morphological development and adherent mucin thickness in Turkeys

*Ayuub A. Ayoola, Ramon D. Malheiros, Jesse L. Grimes and Peter R. Ferket**

Prestage Department of Poultry Science, North Carolina State University, Raleigh, NC, USA

Edited by:
Michael Kogut,
USDA-ARS, USA

Reviewed by:
Lisa Bielke,
Ohio State University, USA
Ryan Arsenault,
University of Delaware, USA

****Correspondence:***
Peter R. Ferket
peter_ferket@ncsu.edu

Anti-nutritional factors (ANFs) in feed ingredients can challenge gut health and reduce nutrient utilization. Birds typically activate their innate immune system as a protective response against the adverse effects of ANF, which often involves the secretion of mucin. Although dietary supplementation of exogenous enzymes are commonly used to alleviate the adverse effects of ANF on apparent nutrient digestibility, little is known about how they affect gut health, particularly in relation to the morphological development and mucin secretion of enteric mucosa. We carried out two trials to examine the effect of dietary supplementation of different types of exogenous enzymes on gut health of by accessing the effect of jejunum morphological development and ileal enteric adherent mucin thickness layer in turkeys. Dietary β-mannanase supplementation reduced ileal adherent mucin thickness layer (804 vs 823 μg/g; $p < 0.05$), while a commercial blend of xylanase, amylase, and protease (XAP) reduced ileal adherent mucin layer thickness (589 vs 740 μg/g; $p < 0.05$); thus reducing the apparent endogenous loss of nutrients. Both enzyme supplements also affected gut morphological characteristics. In comparison to the control treatment, dietary β-mannanase supplementation improved the jejunum tip width (219 vs 161; $p < 0.05$), base width (367 vs 300; $p < 0.05$), surface area (509,870 vs 380, 157; $p < 0.05$) and villi height/crypt depth ratio (7.49 vs 5.70; $p < 0.05$), and XAP improved the crypt depth ($p < 0.05$). In conclusion, dietary supplementation of exogenous enzymes may help alleviate the adverse effects of ANF on nutrient utilization by directly or indirectly removing the mucosal irritation that stimulates enteric mucin secretion.

Keywords: supplemental enzymes, gut health, enteric mucosal morphology, mucin, turkeys

INTRODUCTION

The gut is a very complex and diverse ecosystem, and maintenance of gut health is a high nutrient-consuming task. Croom et al. (1) reported that energy required for gut maintenance accounts for about 25% of the total basal metabolic needs of an animal. The requirements may even be higher during an event of enteric distress or microbial pathogen challenge, which can significantly impact the partitioning of energy and other nutrients away from growth, thus reducing the overall feed conversion efficiency. Gut health can be maintained by a balance between the protective function of intestinal mucosa mucin secretion and the symbiotic community of microorganisms that competitively exclude pathogenic microbes (2).

Dietary composition plays an important role in maintaining the healthy gut ecosystem. Non-starch polysaccharides (NSPs), such as arabinoxylan and β-mannan, are one of the dietary components that influence the gut ecosystem. Their complex water-soluble structure increases digesta viscosity (3), which may entrap macronutrients, such as fat, protein, and starch, and reduces digestive enzyme–substrate interactions (4). Consequently, digestion and nutrient absorption in the foregut is impeded, which adversely effects nutrient supply for growth and reduces feed conversion efficiency. Furthermore, viscous β-mannan and arabinoxlyan may carry undigested nutrients from foregut into the hindgut where they become substrate for the fermentation of competitive microflora that alters the enteric ecosystem stability (5).

Excessive NSPs in the diet, such as arabinoxylan and β-mannan, may lead to the proliferation of undesirable pathogenic intestinal microflora, such as *E. coli* and *Clostridium spp.* (5–7). These enteric pathogens initiate a mucosal inflammatory response, leading to enteric distress, and suppressed gut morphological development. Consequently, this could have a biological effect on intestinal health by changing the mucosal morphological architecture and diverting more nutrients away from productive purposes toward intestinal maintenance. Enteric inflammation, due to enteric pathogen challenge, is associated with the activation of the innate immune system, which is positively associated with the stimulation of intestinal mucous secretion (8). Mucin, which is secreted by the goblet cells, is the protein-rich component of mucous. Although, little information is available on the influence of dietary arabinoxylan and β-mannan on enteric mucosa morphological development and health, atrophic shortening and thickening of jejunum villi, along with increased number of goblet cells per villus, has been observed in broilers fed a diet containing β-glucans which is a similar NSPs (9).

To our knowledge, there are limited published data available on the influence of enzymes on intestinal health, particularly as it affects gut morphology and intestinal adherent mucin secretion in turkey poults. This paper is a report of results from two experiments that evaluated the influence of dietary enzyme supplementation of turkeys fed high and low-energy diets, modified by dietary fat supplementation, on gut health as assessed by changes in mucosa morphometric characteristics and adherent ileal mucosa mucin layer thickness.

MATERIALS AND METHODS

Experiment 1

Experimental diet

The experiment was designed as a 2 × 2 factorial arrangement of two dietary inclusion levels of β-mannanase (0 and 0.05% CTCzyme®, CTCBio, Inc., Korea), supplying 0 and ~500 U endo-beta-D-mannanase/kg of diet, respectively, and two dietary levels of metabolizable energy (high and low) that differed by 150 kcal ME/kg by the addition of supplemental beef tallow fat. All experimental diets were corn-SBM based formulations. The high-energy basal diet was made and divided into two lots, and each was mixed with either 0.05% of vermiculite, or 0.05% of β-mannanase. A second low-energy basal diet (150 kcal/kg less than the high-energy basal diet) was also made and divided into two parts, each was also mixed with either 0.05% of vermiculite or 0.05% of β-mannanase. Vermiculite was added as a non-nutritional filler in place of the enzyme in the experimental control diets. All experimental diets were formulated to meet or exceed NRC (10) requirements for turkeys (**Table 1**). All diets were supplemented with 2.0% Celite® (Celite Corp., Lompar, CA, USA) which served as an acid insoluble ash indigestible reference marker for the determination of digestibility coefficients. The calculated and analyzed composition of the experimental diets, including the supplemental enzymes, is reported in **Table 1**. All diets were produced at the North Carolina State University Feed Mill Educational Unit (Raleigh, NC, USA).

Bird Husbandry and Tissue Sampling

Four hundred thirty-two Nicholas hen poults were obtained from a commercial hatchery (Prestage Farms Hatchery, Clinton, NC, USA) and randomly assigned to one of 48 wire-floored cages with nine poults per cage (Alternative Design cages, Alternative Design Manufacturing and Supply, Inc., Siloam Springs, AR, USA). Each bird was identified with a numbered neck-tag in sequence for each replicate cage group. Four experimental treatment groups were randomly assigned among 48 cages. Feed and water was available *ad libitum*. Birds were reared until 28 days of age. From 1 to 7 days, the birds were provided 23 h of light to 1 h darkness, and 14 L:10 D after 7 days. On 7, 14, and 21 days, a 3-cm segment of the jejunum, from the end of the duodenal loop toward the Meckel's diverticulum, was sampled from each of four poults per cage, gently flushed with saline, and fixed in 10% formalin solution for subsequent histological analysis. Another gut segment, representing 1 cm into the ileal section from the Meckel's diverticulum, was collected from each of the same four poults per cage for mucin histochemical analysis.

Experiment 2

Experimental Diets

The objective of the second experiment was to determine the effect of the dietary supplementation of an experimental blend of xylanase, amylase, and protease (XAP) and a direct-fed microbial (DFM) product (DuPont, St. Louis, MO, USA) on gut morphological development and ileal adherent mucin layer thickness in turkeys. The experiment was designed as a 2 × 4 factorial, with two inclusion levels of DDGS and four levels of different type of feed supplements [negative control (NC), 2% supplemental fat, XAP, and XAP + DFM]. Two experimental corn-soybean meal basal diets, containing 6 or 18% DDGS, were pelleted and crumbled and subsequently divided into four lots. The first lot was retained as the NC, the second lot was supplemented with 2% supplemental fat, the third lot was supplemented with the enzyme blend XAP, and the fourth lot was supplemented with the combination of XAP + DFM. The enzyme activities per gram of the XAP blend was 2000 FTU of xylanase, 200 FTU of amylase, and 5000 FTU of protease, and the XAP + DFM also

TABLE 1 | Dietary ingredient composition and nutrient composition of starter diets fed to turkey hens from 1 to 28 days of age.

Ingredients	High energy		Low energy	
	% Dietary β-mannanase supplementation			
	0	0.05	0	0.05
	(% of Diet)			
Corn	30.56	30.56	34.98	34.98
Soybean meal	44.84	44.84	44.24	44.24
Soy hulls	6.11	6.11	6.03	6.03
Poultry meal	5.00	5.00	5.00	5.00
Fat beef tallow	5.82	5.82	2.09	2.09
Dical phosphate	3.03	3.03	3.03	3.03
Limestone	0.95	0.95	0.95	0.95
DL-Methionine	0.44	0.44	0.43	0.43
Sodium chloride	0.32	0.32	0.32	0.32
L-Lysine-HCl	0.26	0.26	0.27	0.27
Choline chloride	0.22	0.22	0.22	0.22
Trace mineral[a]	0.20	0.20	0.20	0.20
Vitamin premix[b]	0.15	0.15	0.15	0.15
Selenite premix[c]	0.05	0.05	0.05	0.05
Celite™	2.00	2.00	2.00	2.00
CTCzyme[d]	0.00	0.05	0.00	0.05
Filler (vermiculite)	0.05	0.00	0.05	0.00
Calculated chemical composition				
Dry matter (%)	93.34	93.34	92.72	92.72
ME poultry (kcal/kg)	2850	2850	2700	2700
Crude protein (%)	30.06	30.06	30.19	30.19
Crude fat (%)	8.04	8.04	4.92	4.92
Crude fiber (%)	4.34	4.34	4.37	4.37
Calcium (%)	4.34	4.34	4.37	4.37
Total phosphorus (%)	1.40	1.40	1.40	1.40
Avail. phosphorus poultry (%)	1.09	1.09	1.09	1.09

[a]Each kilogram of mineral premix (0.1% inclusion) supplied the following per kg of complete feed: 60 mg Zn as $ZnSO_4 \cdot H_2O$; 60 mg Mn as $MnSO_4 \cdot H_2O$; 40 mg Fe as $FeSO_4 \cdot H_2O$; 5 mg Cu as $CuSO_4$; 1.25 mg I as $Ca(IO_3)_2$; and 1 mg Co as $CoSO_4$.
[b]Each kilogram of vitamin premix (0.1% inclusion) supplied the following per kg of complete feed: vitamin A, 13,200 IU; cholecalciferol, 4000 IU; alpha-tocopherol, 66 IU; niacin, 110 mg; pantothenic acid, 22 mg; riboflavin, 13.2 mg; pyridoxine, 8 mg; menadione, 4 mg; folic acid, 2.2 mg; thiamin, 4 mg; biotin, 0.253 mg; vitamin B_{12}, 0.04 mg; ethoxyquin, 100 mg.
[c]$NaSeO_3$ premix provided 0.3 mg Se/kg of complete feed.
[d]Enzyme provided 0.05% of beta-mannanase in diet.

contained 75,000 cfu of *Bacillus subtilis* per gram of diet. This same experimental diet preparation procedure was used for all feed phases. All experimental diets were formulated to meet or exceed the NRC (10) nutritional recommendations for turkeys (**Table 2**). All diets were manufactured at the North Carolina State University Feed Mill Educational Unit (Raleigh, NC, USA).

Bird Husbandry and Tissue Sampling

Eight hundred sixty-four 1-day old female poults (Hybrid Converter Hens, Cold Springs Farm, Thamesford, Ontario, Canada) were randomly assigned to 48 litter floor pens containing 18 poults per pen. Six replicate pens were randomly assigned per dietary treatment. The poults had access to *ad libitum* feed and water and raised according to standard commercial practices. At 42 days of age, six birds per treatments were euthanized by cervical dislocation to collect tissue for histological assessment. A 6-cm section from the mid-portion of the jejunum was taken from each bird, gently flushed with saline, and fixed in 10% formalin solution for subsequent morphometric analysis. Ileal sections were also taken each of the euthanized birds for mucosal adherent mucin secretion as previously described.

Histological and Histochemical Analysis

Histological Analyses

The tissue samples were immediately rinsed with saline, and fixed in 10% neutral-buffered formalin solution for at least 72 h before processing. A total of four sections of about 2–3 mm in length were taken from a 3-cm fixed jejunum section collected from each sampled bird. These smaller sections were placed in tissue cassettes and submerged in 10% buffered formalin solution until processed at the Histopathology Laboratory (NC State University, College of Veterinary Medicine, Raleigh, NC, USA). The fixed jejunum sections were embedded in paraffin wax, and 5 μm thick transverse sections were cut with a microtome. The 5 μm-cut sections were placed on slides and were stained with Lilee Meyer hematoxylin and counter-stained with eosin yellow. A light-microscope (LEICA-DMR light-microscope, Leica Camera AG, Solms, Germany) was used to visualize the transverse sections placed on slides. The images were captured using a Spot-LTCR digital camera (Diagnostic Instruments, Inc., Sterling Heights, MI, USA) and analyzed using Image Tool software (UTHSCSA Image Tool Software, Version 3.0, the University of Texas, San Antonio, TX, USA). Villus height, villus apical width at the tip of the villus, villus basal width at the crypt-villus junction, crypt depth, and muscularis depth were measured on 10 villi per sampled poult. The villi height:crypt depth ratio for each poult was calculated by dividing the average of the 10 villi heights measured per poult by the average of the 10 crypt depths measured on the same poult. The following mathematical formula was used to determine apparent villus surface area {[(villus tip + villus base)/2] × villus height}, according to Iji et al. (11).

Histochemical Analyses – Measurement of Adherent Ileal Mucin Layer Thickness

The epithelial-adherent mucin layer thickness was assessed histochemically with Alcian blue stain, based on the affinity of the stain for mucin (12). The thickness of the ileal mucus adherent layer was estimated based on the modification of Parman's method (13). A 1-cm section of ileal tissue from each sampled bird was removed and placed in 10 g/L Alcian blue dye solution in buffer containing 160 mmol/L sucrose and 50 mmol/L sodium acetate, pH 5.8. After 6 h of incubation, excess dye was extracted with 250 mmol/L sucrose. The absorbed dye was extracted from the tissue by incubation in 10 g/L docusate sodium salt solution overnight at room temperature. Samples were centrifuged at 700 g, plated on 96-well plate, and the optical densities were measured at 620 nm using Alcian blue solution as a standard. The amount of absorbed dye was reported as micrograms of Alcian blue per gram of ileal tissue.

TABLE 2 | Dietary ingredients and nutrients composition fed to turkey hens in experiment 2.

Ingredients	Starter		Grower 1		Grower 2	
	6% DDGS	18% DDGS	6% DDGS	18% DDGS	6% DDGS	18% DDGS
	(% of Diet)					
Soybean meal	42.65	44.37	35.59	31.07	31.99	26.65
Corn	39.25	28.74	46.43	38.83	50.44	43.74
DDGS	6.00	18.00	6.00	18.00	6.00	18.00
Poultry meal (60% CP)	5.00	3.00	5.00	5.00	5.00	5.00
Poultry fat	1.53	2.85	2.17	2.40	2.32	2.45
Dical P 18.5	2.39	2.60	1.92	1.64	1.51	1.25
Limestone	1.23	1.48	1.28	1.46	1.24	1.42
Alimet	0.55	0.53	0.41	0.37	0.38	0.35
L-Lysine HCl	0.35	0.39	0.29	0.37	0.22	0.33
Micro salt	0.32	0.33	0.30	0.26	0.27	0.24
Trace mineral premix[a]	0.20	0.20	0.20	0.20	0.20	0.20
Choline chloride 60%	0.19	0.16	0.19	0.14	0.18	0.14
Vitamin premix[b]	0.15	0.15	0.15	0.15	0.15	0.15
L-Threonine	0.11	0.13	0.02	0.02	0.02	0.02
Sodium selenite premix[c]	0.05	0.05	0.05	0.05	0.05	0.05
Feed supplement/filler[d]	0.02	0.02	0.02	0.02	0.02	0.02
Phytase	0.01	0.01	0.01	0.01	0.01	0.01
Chemical analysis						
Dry matter* (%)	88.3	89.97	90.35	90.5	90.3	89.38
ME poultry (kcal/kg)	2900	2900	3000	3000	3050	3050
Crude protein* (%)	29.6	29.1	26.01	26.49	24.4	23.5
Crude fat* (%)	5.91	6.18	6.63	7.25	6.13	7.7
Crude fiber (%)	2.68	3.33	2.55	3.04	2.49	2.97
Arabinoxylan (%)	1.80	2.75	2.02	3.04	2.12	3.18
Calcium* (%)	1.16	0.8	1.18	1.33	1.13	1.16
Total phosphorus* (%)	0.79	10.98	0.74	0.74	0.76	0.72
Avail. phosphorus poultry	0.8	0.8	0.7	0.7	0.62	0.62
Lysine (%)	1.889	1.894	1.648	1.669	1.4917	1.5119

[a]Each kilogram of mineral premix (0.1% inclusion) supplied the following per kg of complete feed: 60 mg Zn as $ZnSO_4{\cdot}H_2O$; 60 mg Mn as $MnSO_4{\cdot}H_2O$; 40 mg Fe as $FeSO_4{\cdot}H_2O$; 5 mg Cu as $CuSO_4$; 1.25 mg I as $Ca(IO_3)_2$; and 1 mg Co as $CoSO_4$.

[b]Each kilogram of vitamin premix (0.1% inclusion) supplied the following per kg of complete feed: vitamin A, 13,200 IU; cholecalciferol, 4000 IU; alpha-tocopherol, 66 IU; niacin, 110 mg; pantothenic acid, 22 mg; riboflavin, 13.2 mg; pyridoxine, 8 mg; menadione, 4 mg; folic acid, 2.2 mg; thiamin, 4 mg; biotin, 0.253 mg; vitamin B_{12}, 0.04 mg; ethoxyquin, 100 mg.

[c]$NaSeO_3$ premix provided 0.3 mg Se/kg of complete feed.

[d]Feed supplements include XAP, XAP + DFM, and supplemental fat. Approximately 2% supplemental fat was added to create ME difference of 150 kcal/kg. Filler was added in diets that had no feed supplement.

**As determined by chemical analysis.*

Statistical Analysis

The experiments were analyzed as completely randomized designs. Pen or cage means were respectively used as the experimental unit for the statistical analysis of adherent ileal mucin secretion. For histological analysis, 10 villi measurements were averaged per tissue sample collected, and this average number served as the experimental unit for the statistical analysis. Data were analyzed using JMP software (Version 10, SAS Institute, Cary, NC, USA). ANOVA was used to examine the main effect of dietary treatment factors, and their interaction on parameters evaluated. Means were separated using the LS Means at $P < 0.05$.

Animal Ethics

Care of the birds used in all experiments conformed to the Guide for Care and Use of Agricultural Animals in Research and Teaching (14). Moreover, all animal husbandry practices and euthanasia performed during the conduct of these experiments were conducted according to protocol # 12-014-A approved by Institutional Animal Care and Use Committee at North Carolina State University.

RESULTS

Experiment 1

Table 3 summarizes the effect of dietary energy level and β-mannanase supplementation on villi morphological characteristics and ileal adherent mucin thickness layer of turkey hens at 21 days of age.

Gut Morphological Development

There were no significant treatment effects observed on jejunum mucosa morphology at 7 and 14 days; however, there was a significant treatment effect observed at 28 days. Increasing dietary energy level was associated with an 18% decrease in the villus base width and a 21% decrease in villus surface area ($P < 0.05$). In contrast, dietary supplementation of β-mannanase increased

TABLE 3 | Effect of dietary energy level and β-mannanase supplementation on jejunum villi morphological characteristics and ileal adherent mucin thickness layer of turkey hens at 28 days of age.[c]

Main effect		Tip width	Villi height	Base width	Crypt depth	Muscularis thickness	Surface area	Villi height/crypt depth	Ileal adherent mucin thickness layer
		Micron					Micron[d]		μg/g tissue
Energy level									
High energy		173	1661	301^{b}	244	256	393,523^{b}	6.19	752
Low energy		207	1768	366^{a}	222	266	496,505^{a}	6.97	804
β-Mannanase level (%)									
0.05		219^{a}	1714	367^{a}	224	251	509,870^{a}	7.49^{a}	804^{b}
0.00		161^{b}	1715	300^{b}	242	269	380,157^{b}	5.70^{b}	832^{a}
Interactions									
Energy level	**β-Mannanase level (%)**								
High energy	0.05	204	1733^{a,b}	335	232	266	468,246	6.97^{a,b}	631^{b}
High energy	0.00	143	1588^{b}	266	255	243	318,800	5.43^{b}	977^{a}
Low energy	0.05	235	1694^{a,b}	399	215	236	551,495	7.94^{a}	791^{a,b}
Low energy	0.00	179	1842^{a}	334	228	296	441,514	5.92^{a,b}	873^{a,b}
Source of variations									
		P-values							
Energy		0.141	0.097	0.011	0.373	0.586	0.003	0.149	0.1616
β-Mannanase		0.017	0.983	0.009	0.470	0.383	0.001	0.006	0.0466
Energy × β-mannanase		0.909	0.030	0.928	0.831	0.060	0.501	0.025	0.0261
SEM(40)[d]		10	29	11	11	10	14,242	0.35	27.51

[a,b]*Means with different letter superscripts within a column are significantly different (P < 0.05).*
[c]*Values are means of four replicates each treatment.*
[d]*SEM(40), standard error of the mean with 40 degrees of freedom.*

the villus tip width by 36% and villus height/crypt depth by 32% ($P < 0.05$), while the villus base width and surface area was increased by about 22.5 and 34%, respectively ($P < 0.05$).

Ileal Adherent Mucin Layer Thickness

There was no significant main effect of dietary energy; however, poults fed the β-mannanase supplemented diet had a 4% reduction in ileal adherent mucin layer thickness as compared to the unsupplemented control diet. Furthermore, the supplementation of β-mannanase to the high-energy diet reduced the ileal adherent mucin layer thickness by about 36% as compared to the high-energy diet without supplementation ($P < 0.05$), but neither of these diets were significantly different from the results observed among birds fed the low-energy diets with or without the enzyme supplementation ($P > 0.05$).

Experiment 2

Table 4 summarizes the influence of dietary DDGS level, and XAP and DFM supplementation on the morphological measurements of jejunum villi and mucosa of turkey hens at 42 days.

Gut Morphological Development

Some effects were observed on mucosa morphology development at 42 days of age. Dietary inclusion of 18% DDGS was associated with a 15% decrease in villus tip width ($P < 0.05$) and 11% decrease in villi surface area ($P < 0.05$) relative to the 6% DDGS treatment. However, the 18% dietary inclusion of DDGS treatment had a 13% increase in muscularis thickness ($P < 0.05$) relative to the 6% DDGS inclusion. DDGS inclusion did not have significant effect on the villi height, crypt depth, villi height/crypt depth, and villi base width. The dietary supplements did not have any effect on villi tip width, height, villi height/crypt depth, villi base width, muscularis thickness, and villi surface area, although they did affect the crypt depth. Poults-fed diets supplemented with XAP alone or in combination with DFM had reduced crypt depth by about 12 and 11%, respectively, when compared with the supplemental fat and NC ($P < 0.05$).

Ileal Adherent Mucin Layer Thickness

The results of the ileal adherent mucin layer thickness are also presented in **Table 4**. Increasing the dietary level of DDGS increased the ileal adherent mucin layer thickness observed in poults at 42 days of age ($P < 0.05$). However, in comparison to the supplemental fat and NC treatments, dietary supplementation of XAP reduced the ileal adherent mucin layer thickness by 24 and 20%, respectively ($P < 0.05$); but neither response was different from XAP + DFM.

DISCUSSION

Gut Morphological Development

Dietary soluble and insoluble β-mannans and arabinoxylans have been reported to exhibit some anti-nutritional properties and adverse effects on growth performance of poultry. The high arabinoxylan content in DDGS along with its inferior amino acid digestibility and variability of other nutrients limits the dietary inclusion of DDGS in poultry feed to <6%. Likewise, the viscous nature of β-mannan in diets, that contain a lot of soybean meal, has been observed to cause physiological and morphological changes to the gastrointestinal tract in poultry, which can impede efficient nutrients utilization (15, 16).

TABLE 4 | Influence of dietary DDGS level, and XAP and DFM supplementation on the morphological measurements of jejunum villi and mucosa of turkey hens at 42 days.[c]

Main effect		Tip width	Crypt depth	Muscularis thickness	Surface area	Ileal adherent mucin thickness layer
		Micron			Micron[d]	μg/g tissue
DDGS level (%)						
6		275[a]	166	251[b]	684,224[a]	679[b]
18		233[b]	169	294[a]	606,656[b]	705[a]
Feed supplements						
Negative control (NC)		264	176[a]	285	670,514	740[a]
~2% Supplemental fat (suppl. fat)		267	180[a]	274	639,138	770[a]
XAP		240	157[c]	266	618,222	589[b]
XAP + DFM		246	159[c]	264	653,887	670[a,b]
Interactions						
DDGS level (%)	Feed supplement					
6	NC	296	177	268	735,289	737
6	Suppl. fat	295	185	255	660,544	726
6	XAP	252	145	244	630,957	576
6	XAP + DFM	260	157	238	710,104	679
18	NC	232	176	303	605,737	744
18	Suppl. fat	239	174	293	617,733	814
18	XAP	228	167	288	605,486	603
18	XAP + DFM	233	161	291	597,670	661
Source of variations						
				P-values		
DDGS		0.002	0.614	<0.01	0.037	0.045
Feed supplement		0.373	0.037	0.334	0.740	0.032
DDGS x feed supplement		0.576	0.423	0.885	0.664	0.871
SEM(40)[d]		12	6.519	13	34,110	46

[a,b]*Means with different letter superscripts within a column are significantly different ($P < 0.05$).*

[c]*Values are means of six replicates per treatment.*

[d]*SEM(40), standard error of the mean with 40 degrees of freedom.*

The general hypothesis tested in the two studies reported herein was that the supplementation with β-mannanase, XAP, or a combination of XAP + DFM will reduce the anti-nutritional effects and improve apparent nutrient utilization by reducing endogenous nutrient losses associated with enteric mucin secretion, enhancing gut morphological development, and improving gut health. Because dietary inclusion of the enzymes may help degrade the NSPs, their anti-nutritional effects may, thereby, be diminished and thus improve nutrient utilization, as residual enteric substrates are altered to positively favor symbiotic microflora and microbial diversity over the pro-inflammatory pathogenic ones in the hindgut ecosystem, consequently improving the gut health.

Measured changes in intestinal morphology, such as shorter villi and deeper villi crypts, have been used as indicators of gut health and enteric distress (17). Tall mucosal villi increase the surface area available for nutrients absorption (18, 19). There is correlation between the crypt depth and the rate of proliferation of the epithelial cells (20, 21). Epithelial regeneration starts from the villi crypt, so a deep crypt is an indication of rapid enterocyte turnover and increased mucosal tissue maintenance requirements (17, 22). The rapid enterocyte proliferation and the epithelial cell turnover rate greatly impacts protein and energy requirements of the small intestine mucosa (23). Diet composition may produce microscopic alterations in the intestinal mucosa, and it is possible that the change in morphology of the gastrointestinal tract may be associated with dietary NSP levels (24).

Some studies have demonstrated that enzyme treatment can influence the morphological development of intestinal villi (19, 25, 26). In the first trial, we observed that dietary inclusion of β-mannanase had a positive effect on jejunum mucosal morphology among poults sampled at 28 days: villus surface area and tip and base widths were all increased. Although there are few publications demonstrating the effect of β-mannanase on gut morphology, the work of Mehri et al. (27) corroborated our findings. There was an increase in the villi surface area and jejunum villi height/crypt depth ratio by dietary β-mannanase supplementation. Mehri et al. (27) observed an increase in villus height and crypt depth in the duodenum when β-mannanase was supplemented to corn–soy diets at 700 and 900 g/ton.

In the second experiment, the level of arabinoxylan, a NSP anti-nutritional factor (ANF), was calculated to increase by about 50% as the dietary inclusion level DDGS increased from 6 to 18% (**Table 2**). Choct and Annison (28) have shown anti-nutritional effects of depressed apparent metabolizable energy when 3% pentosans, primarily comprised of arabinoxylans, was added to broiler diets. Relative to the 6% DDGS treatment, dietary inclusion of 18% DDGS adversely affected jejunum mucosal morphology as indicated by reduced villi surface area, tip width and increased thickness of the villi muscularis. The poor jejunum morphological development may be associated with relatively higher NSP content in the 18% DDGS diet. Iji (29) reported that NSP can negatively impact gut morphology by increasing crypt depth of both the jejunum and ileum, thus accelerating enterocyte turnover. Although we evaluated the effects of a blend of supplemental enzymes containing xylanase in the second experiment, xylanase supplementation alone has been reported to increase villus height of the duodenum, jejunum, and ileum, and the villus height/crypt depth of these three segments (19). Furthermore, the dietary inclusion of DFM may also impact the gut morphology by increasing the jejunum and ileal villi heights (30, 31). Dietary supplementation of the enzyme blend of XAP and XAP + DFM combination had a beneficial effect on gut morphology development. The addition of the enzyme blend with or without the DFM reduced the crypt depth, indicating reduced mucosal distress, in comparison to the NC or fat-supplemented diet.

Apparently, the effects observed on enteric mucosa morphology in both trials may have been associated with the changes in the substrate characteristics within the enteric ecosystem by the dietary supplementations (β-mannanase, XAP, and XAP + DFM), which in turn altered the fermentation of resident enteric microflora (32).

Adherent Ileal Mucin Secretion

Establishment of a symbiotic enteric ecosystem minimizes the inflammatory symptoms of enteric distress caused by the proliferation of enteric pathogens, which is associated with increased intestinal mucin secretion (33, 34). Parsaie et al. (35) reported that distressed intestinal morphology, as indicated by the shortened villi and deepened crypts, may cause increased mucosal secretions, primarily as mucin. Indeed, some research reports have shown that the dietary inclusion of enzymes reduce the mucosal blanket secretions in monogastric animals (36, 37).

In addition to the improved gut morphological development observed in this study, a reduction in the ileal adherent mucin layer thickness was observed with dietary β-mannanase supplementation, especially in the high-energy (fat) diets. Few studies have been reported on the influences of β-mannanase on mucin secretion. However, research results reported trial by Mehri et al. (27) indirectly validated our observation. They reported that dietary β-mannanase supplementation reduced the number of mucosal goblet cells per unit of epithelial surface area in broilers. Since mucin is secreted by the epithelial goblet cells, this observation agrees with our observations that dietary β-mannanase supplementation significantly reduces intestinal adherent mucin layer thickness.

We also observed that the addition of XAP reduced ileal mucin thickness layer. Bedford et al. (36) also noted that xylanase supplementation improved the apparent digestibility of threonine, which was associated with a decrease in intestinal mucin secretion. Pirgozliev et al. (37) also observed a decrease in the quantity of threonine excreted by the birds fed with a xylanase-supplemented diet, which he attributed to less secretion of intestinal mucin.

CONCLUSION

Improved gut morphological development of the mucosa villi in the jejunum and ileum and the reduced adherent ileal mucin thickness layer could likely contribute to the improved apparent nutrient utilization, which reflects in the better growth performance in poultry often observed when their diets are supplemented with exogenous enzymes. Enteric microflora profile has been demonstrated to be influenced by nutrient abundance (32). Digesta viscosity increases as dietary anti-nutritional NSPs increases, which impairs foregut digestion and absorption of fats, starches, and proteins, and causes more of these nutrients to pass to the hindgut where they "feed" competitive pathogenic bacteria. Proliferation of pathogenic bacteria, like *C. perfringens*, causes enteric tissue inflammation, mucosal leakage, and increased mucin secretion as a protective innate immune response. With protein being a major component of mucin, this increase in mucin secretion can further exacerbate the proliferation of putrefying bacterial pathogens and also contribute to the significantly reduced apparent nitrogen retention. Dietary supplementation of NSP enzymes can be an effective means to counter the adverse effects of high digesta viscosity and cause the hind gut microflora to shift toward a more symbiotic ecosystem.

The research results reported herein demonstrate that dietary supplementation of either β-mannanase, XAP, or XAP + DFM can improve gut health in turkey poults as indicated by improved morphological development of the enteric mucosa and reduction in adherent ileal mucin secretion, thereby increasing productive use of nutrients toward better growth performance. Further studies are still needed to evaluate the effect of other supplemental enzymes on gut health, especially as the trend of limiting the use of antibiotic growth promoters in animal feed continues.

FUNDING

Funding was provided by the NC Agricultural Foundation, Inc., Raleigh, NC, USA, and National Institute of Food and Agriculture Project Number NC06343, United State Department of Agriculture.

REFERENCES

1. Croom J, Edens FW, Ferket PR. The impact of nutrient digestion and absorption on poultry performance and health. In: Ferket PR, editor. *Proceedings of the 27th Annual Carolina Poultry Nutrition Conference*. Raleigh, NC: Carolina Feed Industry Association, Research Triangle Park (2000). p. 65 73.
2. Ferket PR. Alternatives to antibiotics in poultry production: responses, practical experience and recommendations. In: Lyons TP, Jacques KA, editors. *Nutritional Biotechnology in the Feed and Food Industries: Proceedings of Alltech's 20th Annual Symposium*. Lexington, KY: Nottingham University Press (2004). p. 56–67.
3. Lee JT, Bailey CA, Cartwright AL. β-Mannanase ameliorates viscosity-associated depression of growth in broiler chickens fed guar germ and hull fractions. *Poult. Sci* (2003) **82**:1925–31.
4. Smits CH, Veldman NA, Verstegen MWA, Beynen AC. Dietary carboxymethylcellulose with high instead of low viscosity reduces macronutrient digestion in broiler chickens. *J Nutr* (1997) **127**:483–7.
5. Choct M, Hughes RJ, Wang J, Bedford MR, Morgan AJ, Annison G. Increased small intestinal fermentation is partly responsible for the anti-nutritive activity

of non-starch polysaccharides in chickens. *Br Poult Sci* (1996) **37**:609–21. doi:10.1080/00071669608417891
6. Apajalahti J, Bedford MR. Improve bird performance by feeding its microflora. *World Poult* (1999) **15**:20–3.
7. Choct M, Dersjant-Li Y, McLeish J, Peisker M. Soy oligosaccharides and soluble non-starch polysaccharides: a review of digestion, nutritive and anti-nutritive effects in pigs and poultry. *Asian-Aust J Anim Sci* (2010) **23**(10):1386–98. doi:10.5713/ajas.2010.90222
8. Deplancke B, Gaskins HR. Microbial modulation of innate defense: goblet cells and the intestinal mucus layer. *Am J Clin Nutr* (2001) **73**(l):1131S–41S.
9. Viveros A, Brenes A, Pizarro M, Castario M. Effect of enzyme supplementation of a diet based on barley, and autoclave treatment, on apparent digestibility, growth performance and gut morphology of broilers. *Ani Feed Sci Tech* (1994) **48**:237–51. doi:10.1016/0377-8401(94)90175-9
10. NRC. *Nutrient Requirements of Poultry*. 9th rev. ed. Washington, DC: National Academy Press (1994).
11. Iji PA, Saki A, Tivey DR. Body and intestinal growth of broiler chicks on a commercial starter diet. 1. Intestinal weight and mucosal development. *Br Poult Sci* (2001) **42**:505–13. doi:10.1080/00071660120073151
12. McManusi FA, Mowry RW. *Staining Methods Histology and Histochemical*. New York: Paul B. Hoeber, Inc. (1960). 423 p.
13. Parman NS, Desai JK. A review of the current methodology for the evaluation of gastric and duodenal anti-ulcer agents. *Indian J Pharmacol* (1993) **25**:120–35.
14. FASS. *Guide for the Care and Use of Agricultural Animals in Research and Teaching*. 3rd ed. Champaign, IL: Federation of Animal Science Society (2010).
15. Cassidy MM, Lightfoot FG, Grau LE, Story JA, Kritchevsky D, Vahouny GH. Effect of chronic intake of dietary fibers on the ultra-structural topography of rat jejunum and colon: a scanning electron microscopy study. *Am J Clin Nutr* (1981) **34**:218–28.
16. Jacobs LR. Effects of dietary fiber on mucosal growth and cell proliferation in the small intestine of the rat: a comparison of oat bran, pectin, and guar with total fiber deprivation. *Am J Clin Nutr* (1983) **37**:954–60.
17. Yason CV, Summers BA, Schat KA. Pathogenesis of rotavirus infection in various age groups of chickens and turkeys: pathology. *Am J Vet Res* (1987) **6**:927–38.
18. Awad W, Ghareeb K, Böhm J. Intestinal structure and function of broiler chickens on diets supplemented with a symbiotic containing *Enterococcus faecium* and oligosaccharides. *Int J Mol Sci* (2008) **9**:2205–16. doi:10.3390/ijms9112205
19. Luo D, Yanga F, Yang X, Yao J, Shi B, Zhou Z. Effects of xylanase on performance, blood parameters, intestinal morphology, microflora and digestive enzyme activities of broilers fed wheat-based diets. *Asian-Aust J Anim Sci* (2009) **22**(9):1288–95. doi:10.5713/ajas.2009.90052
20. Brunsgaard G. Weaning and the weaning diet influence the villous height and crypt depth in the small intestine of pigs and alter the concentrations of short chain fatty acids in the large intestine and blood. *J Nutr* (1998) **128**:947–53.
21. Yasar S, Forbes JM. Performance and gastro-intestinal response of broiler chickens fed on cereal grain-based foods soaked in water. *Br Poult Sci* (1999) **40**:65–76. doi:10.1080/00071669987854
22. Paulus U, Potten CS, Loeffler M. A model of the control of cellular regeneration in the intestinal crypt after perturbation based solely on local stem cell regulation. *Cell Prolif* (1992) **25**:559–78. doi:10.1111/j.1365-2184.1992.tb01460.x
23. Simon O. Metabolism of proteins and amino acids. In: Bock HD, Eggum BO, Low AG, Simon O, Zebrowska T, editors. *Protein Metabolism and Farm Animals. Evaluation, Digestion, Absorption and Metabolism*. Berlin, Germany: Oxford University Press and VEB Dt Landwirtschaftsverlag (1989). p. 271–336.
24. Yamauchi K. Review of chicken intestinal villus histological alterations related with intestinal function. *J Poult Sci* (2002) **39**:229–42. doi:10.2141/jpsa.39.229
25. Brenes A, Smith M, Guenter W, Marquardt RR. Effect of enzyme supplementation on the performance and digestive tract size of broiler chickens fed wheat and barley based diets. *Poult Sci* (1993) **72**:1731–9. doi:10.3382/ps.0721731
26. Amat C, Planas JM, Moretó M. Kinetics of hexose uptake by the small and large intestine of the chicken. *Am J Physiol* (1996) **271**(4 Pt 2):R1085–9.
27. Mehri M, Adibmoradi M, Samie A, Shivazad M. Effects of β-Mannanase on broiler performance, gut morphology and immune system. *African J Biotech* (2010) **9**(37):6221–8. doi:10.5897/AJB09.1371
28. Choct M, Annison G. Anti-nutritive activity of wheat pentosans in broiler diets. *Br Poult Sci* (1990) **31**:811–21. doi:10.1080/00071669008417312
29. Iji PA. The impact of cereal non-starch polysaccharides on intestinal development and function in broiler chickens. World's Poult. *Sci J* (1999) **55**:375–87.
30. Chichowski M, Croom WJ, Edens FW, MacBride BW, Qiu R, Chiang CC, et al. Microarchitecture and spatial relationship between bacteria and ileal, cecal and colonic epithelium in chicks fed a direct-fed microbial, PrimaLac, and Salinomycin. *Poult Sci* (2007) **86**:1121–32. doi:10.1093/ps/86.6.1121
31. Samli HE, Senkoylu N, Koc F, Kante M, Agma A. Effects of Enterococcus faecium and dried whey on broiler performance, gut histomprphology and microbiota. *Arch Anim Nutr* (2007) **61**:42–9. doi:10.1080/17450390601106655
32. Knarreborg A, Simon R, Engberg M, Jensen BB, Tannock GW. Effects of dietary fat source and subtherapeutic levels of antibiotic on the bacterial community in the ileum of broiler chickens at various ages. *Appl Environ Microb* (2002) **68**:5918–24. doi:10.1128/AEM.68.12.5918-5924.2002
33. Fukata T, Sasai K, Miyamoto T, Baba E. Inhibitory effects of competitive exclusion and fructooligosaccharide, singly and in combination, on Salmonella colonization of chicks. *J Food Protect* (1999) **62**:229–33.
34. Grizard D, Barthomeuf C. Non-digestible oligosaccharides used as prebiotic agents: mode of production and beneficial effects on animal and human health. *Reprod Nutr Dev* (1999) **39**:563–88. doi:10.1051/rnd:19990505
35. Parsaie S, Shariatmadari F, Zamiri MJ, Khajeh K. Influence of wheat-based diets supplemented with xylanas, bile acid and antibiotics on performance, digestive tract measurements and gut morphology of broilers compared with a maize-based diet. *Br Poult Sci* (2007) **48**:594–600. doi:10.1080/00071660701615788
36. Bedford MR, Scott TA, Silversides FG, Classen HL, Swift ML, Pack M. The effect of wheat cultivar, growing environment, and enzyme supplementation on digestibility of amino acids by broilers. *Can J Anim Sci* (1998) **78**:335–42. doi:10.4141/A98-012
37. Pirgozliev V, Acamovic T, Bedford MR. The effect of dietary xylanase on energy, amino acid and mineral metabolism and egg production and quality in laying hens. *Br Poult Sci* (2010) **51**(05):639–47. doi:10.1080/00071668.2010.514325

Conflict of Interest Statement: The authors declare that the research was conducted in the absence of any commercial or financial relationships that could be construed as a potential conflict of interest.

7

Preliminary analysis of modified low-density lipoproteins in the serum of healthy and obese dogs and cats

Nobuko Mori, Yuki Okada, Naoto Tsuchida, Yutaka Hatano, Makoto Habara, Shingo Ishikawa, Ichiro Yamamoto and Toshiro Arai*

Department of Basic Veterinary Medicine, School of Veterinary Medicine, Nippon Veterinary and Life Science University, Tokyo, Japan

Edited by:
Koichi Orino, Kitasato University, Japan

Reviewed by:
Kaori Sakamoto, University of Georgia, USA
Takeshi Ohkubo, Ibaraki University, Japan

***Correspondence:**
Nobuko Mori, Department of Basic Veterinary Medicine, School of Veterinary Medicine, Nippon Veterinary and Life Science University, 1-7-1 Kyonan-cho, Musashino-city, Tokyo 180-8602, Japan
d0908@nvlu.ac.jp

Oxidized low-density lipoprotein (LDL) is thought to play an important role in the inflammatory response associated with human obesity. The purpose of this preliminary study was to determine oxidized LDL concentrations in healthy dogs and cats, and to evaluate whether obesity affects oxidized LDL concentration, using 39 cats and 19 dogs that had visited two different veterinary clinics in Japan. We hypothesized that oxidized LDL concentrations measured against body condition score (BCS) may have a potential value in evaluating the qualities of accumulated or circulating lipids in obese dogs and cats that do not show signs of metabolic diseases. The mean oxidized LDL value in BCS3 dogs ($2.4 \pm 0.9\,\mu g/dl$) was very similar to that of BCS5 dogs ($2.2 \pm 0.3\,\mu g/dl$). The mean oxidized LDL value of BCS4 dogs was $7.2 \pm 10.3\,\mu g/dl$ and the highest among three groups. BCS4 dogs included two dogs whose oxidized LDL values were higher than the mean oxidized LDL value of healthy humans ($11.2 \pm 0.3\,\mu g/dl$). On the other hand, the mean oxidized LDL value of BCS3 cats was $2.5 \pm 0.9\,\mu g/dl$, and those of BCS4 and 5 cats were higher than that of BCS3, but there was no significant difference. The BCS4 cat group included one cat with a higher oxidized LDL value, and the BCS5 group also included two cats with oxidized LDL values higher than the mean oxidized LDL value of healthy humans. Interestingly, the oxidized LDL values in two obese dogs and three obese cats were indeed higher than the mean oxidized LDL value of humans with coronary artery disease ($20.1 \pm 1.1\,\mu g/dl$). In conclusion, this preliminary study showed reference ranges of oxidized dogs and cats against BCS. Obesity alone does not appear to have any direct effect on serum oxidized LDL values in healthy dogs and cats.

Keywords: oxidized LDL, dog, cat, ELISA, electrophoresis

Introduction

Hyperlipidemia can be characterized by quantitative increases in circulating lipoproteins or by higher lipid concentrations of various lipoproteins classes. Obesity in dogs and cats is commonly associated with hyperlipidemia. Generally, the treatment of hyperlipidemia in dogs and cats is to reduce the intake of cholesterol and/or triglycerides (TG). Recently, the modification of lipids has been identified as an important factor in human hyperlipidemia; therefore, it has been considered more effective to inhibit the oxidization of low-density lipoprotein (LDL) rather than to reduce the amount of cholesterol in humans (1). For instance, oxidized LDL is thought to play an important role in the inflammatory response. Oxidized LDL alters the biological properties of growth factors, cytokines, monocytes, and T lymphocytes by modulating their production (2–8). Acute coronary syndrome is triggered by the activation of immune-mediated inflammatory processes with atherothrombosis (9–11). Some reports indicated that highly oxidized LDL has been detected in the plasma of coronary heart disease (CHD) patients (12–14). Studies in laboratory animals and humans have shown that oxidized LDL is a better predictor of atherosclerosis and cardiovascular disease. In animal studies, administration of antioxidant drugs, like probucol, inhibits LDL oxidation and arterial plaque formation, even when there is no change in blood cholesterol levels (15–18). In fact, administration of the antioxidant butylated hydroxytoluene (BHT) significantly reduces the degree of atherosclerosis in the aorta of rabbits, even though it raises LDL cholesterol levels (19).

By immunoassays, using murine monoclonal antibodies prepared against malondialdehyde-modified LDL (MDA-LDL) found in human plasma, higher concentrations of MDA-LDL were found in the patients with CHD (13, 20). Elevated concentrations of oxidized LDL are predictive of future CHD events in apparently healthy men (21). Because CHD is the leading cause of human death, there are many studies of oxidized LDL causing CHD and/or arteriosclerosis. It was shown that an increase in oxidized LDL level is the most important factor associated with CHD (22).

It is commonly considered that dogs and cats rarely develop atherosclerosis in the absence of metabolic disease (23). This is due to the fact that high-density lipoprotein (HDL) levels in dogs and cats are higher than LDL, VLDL, and chylomicron levels. They are considered to be HDL-dominant animals unlike humans (24). Therefore, many veterinarians do not test for oxidized LDL levels in dogs and cats. There are no oxidized LDL data of dogs and cats with/without disease. There is no data available to evaluate whether high concentrations of LDL or oxidized LDL are risk factors for CHD.

However, this does not mean that dogs and cats do not develop atherosclerosis. It has been reported that dogs develop severe atherosclerosis when a plasma cholesterol concentration of over 750 mg/dl persists for more than 6 months (25). Some veterinarians feel that as obesity in animals has increased in developed countries, so will atherosclerosis, as seen in humans.

A retrospective report by Hess (26) showed that dogs with atherosclerosis were over 53 times more likely to have concurrent diabetes mellitus than dogs without atherosclerosis. By the same token, dogs with atherosclerosis were over 51 times more likely to have concurrent hypothyroidism than dogs without atherosclerosis (26). Other studies have shown that glomerulopathy is more prevalent in dogs with atherosclerosis compared to dogs without atherosclerosis (27). If we could accurately measure and understand oxidized LDL concentrations in dogs and cats, it may become a preventive marker for metabolic syndrome, diabetes mellitus, hypothyroidism, and glomerulopathy. The purpose of this preliminary study was to investigate oxidized LDL concentrations and develop the normal ranges of oxidized LDL concentration in healthy dogs and cats, and to evaluate how obesity affects the concentrations of oxidized LDL.

Obesity is a clinical sign that develops as the first sign of metabolic disease. When dogs and cats gain weight, their lipoprotein fractions are modified as well. Previously, we showed a specific elevation in HDL_1 fraction, which plays an important role in reverse cholesterol transport similar to LDL, in obese dogs, and increased LDL concentrations of all fractions in obese cats (24). Therefore, we hypothesized that oxidized LDL concentration measured against body condition score (BCS) may have a potential value in evaluating the qualities of accumulated or circulating lipids in obese dogs and cats that do not show clinical signs of metabolic diseases.

We selected the following two methods to measure and analyze oxidized LDL: one was to determine the quantity of oxidized LDL by ELISA, and the second method was to validate modified LDL (modified charged LDL) by lipoprotein electrophoresis customized for dogs and cats.

Materials and Methods

Animals

This study consisted of 19 dogs and 39 cats that had visited two different veterinary clinics (Ibaraki and Kanagawa) during a 2-month period from the middle of November 2014 to the middle of January 2015. The dogs utilized in the study included 8 females and 11 males, ages 1–16 years old, and the cat group consisted of 22 females and 17 males, ages 0–15 years old. The dog breeds represented were American cocker spaniel [female (F) $n = 1$, male (M) $n = 2$], Chihuahua (F-1, M-1), Labrador retriever (M-1), Maltese (M-1), Miniature dachshund (F-1, M-2), Shiba (F-1), Shih tzu (F-1, M-1), Toy poodle (F-2), Yorkshire Terrier (M-1), and Mixed breed (F-1, M-2). The cat group included American shorthair (M-1), British shorthair (M-1), Norwegian (F-2, M-1), Scottish Fold (M-1), and Mixed breed (F-20, M-13). The subjects were diagnosed to be clinically healthy, according to the physical examination, clinical signs, and biochemical data evaluated by the attending veterinarians. These subjects did not have hypothyroidism or diabetes mellitus. They received a BCS of 1–5 (28) based on palpation and inspection. The BCS applies a 5-point scale: (1, very thin; 2, underweight; 3, ideal; 4, overweight; 5, obese). The resultant groups of dogs and cats were classified as Normal (BCS3) and Obese (BCS4, 5).

This study was approved by the Nippon Veterinary and Life Science University Animal Research Committee.

Blood Sampling

Postprandial blood samples (at least 4 h after the last meal) were collected from the cephalic veins into serum separator plastic tubes (Venoject II, Terumo Corporation, Tokyo, Japan). They were centrifuged at approximately 300 rpm for 15 min. In accordance with an Ox LDL ELISA kit protocol, all samples were aliquotted for oxidized LDL measurement to avoid loss of bioactivity and contamination, and were stored at −20°C for no more than 2 months. They were not processed through repeated freeze–thaw cycles.

Analysis of Serum Parameters

Serum lipid metabolites and enzyme activities were measured. Glucose (GLU), TG, total cholesterol (T-Cho), alanine

TABLE 1 | Comparison of parameters in normal and obese animals.

Dog	Normal	Obesity		High oxidized LDL dogs in obesity (*n* = 2)
	BCS3 dog (*n* = 9)	BCS4 dog (*n* = 8)	BCS5 dog (*n* = 2)	
Age (years)	6.5 ± 3.6	9.0 ± 6.4	12.5 ± 0.7	13.5 ± 0.7
BW (kg)	5.6 ± 2.8	13.1 ± 10.2	14.0 ± 7.0	18.9 ± 13.9
BCS (/5)	3.2 ± 0.3	4.0 ± 0.0[a]	5.0 ± 0.0[a]	4.0 ± 0.0
Glucose (mg/dl)	91.4 ± 43.2	77.7 ± 33.1	54.5 ± 6.4	62.5 ± 44.5
Triglyceride (mg/dl)	72.4 ± 64.1	127.1 ± 106.3	489.0 ± 367.7	195.5 ± 77.1
Total cholesterol (mg/dl)	183.0 ± 50.8	212.8 ± 39.1	288.0 ± 72.1[a]	226.0 ± 19.8
Oxidized LDL (μg/dl)	2.4 ± 0.9	7.2 ± 10.3	2.2 ± 0.3	22.4 ± 11.0
ALT (IU/l)	56.1 ± 31.0	63.0 ± 53.6	50.5 ± 44.5	112.5 ± 98.3
AST (IU/l)	35.2 ± 8.3	33.4 ± 14.8	23.5 ± 3.5	33.5 ± 12.0
Total protein (g/dl)	7.1 ± 0.7	7.4 ± 0.8	7.9 ± 0.9	7.6 ± 0.6
BUN (mg/dl)	17.2 ± 6.4	17.0 ± 4.4	17.5 ± 4.9	19.0 ± 9.9
Creatinine (mg/dl)	0.8 ± 0.2	1.0 ± 0.4	1.1 ± 0.6	1.2 ± 0.5

Values are presented as means ± SD. BCS, body condition score.
High oxidized LDL dogs in obesity is animals with mean value of oxidized LDL greater than that of humans (11.2 ± 0.3 μg/dl)
[a]Indicates significance (Holm–Sidak One-way ANOVA, $p < 0.05$) when BCS4 or 5 High ox LDL dogs were compared pairwise against BCS3 dog.

Cat	Normal	Obesity		High oxidized LDL cats in obesity (*n* = 3)
	BCS3 cat (*n* = 10)	BCS4 cat (*n* = 15)	BCS5 cat (*n* = 14)	
Age (years)	1.0 ± 1.2	6.9 ± 5.1[a]	8.7 ± 4.7[a]	12.3 ± 3.8
BW (kg)	3.1 ± 0.7	4.7 ± 0.8[a]	6.7 ± 2.2[a]	6.0 ± 2.0
BCS (/5)	3.0 ± 0.0	4.0 ± 0.0[a,b]	5.0 ± 0.0[a]	4.7 ± 0.6
Glucorse (mg/dl)	168.4 ± 43.0	130.2 ± 57.9	122.5 ± 70.9	153.0 ± 35.4
Triglyceride (mg/dl)	37.5 ± 19.3	66.1 ± 41.8	152.6 ± 218.3	71.7 ± 11.6
Total cholesterol (mg/dl)	96.7 ± 24.9	158.5 ± 55.9[a]	168.1 ± 50.0[a]	128.3 ± 11.6
Oxidized LDL (μg/dl)	2.5 ± 0.9	7.5 ± 17.0	9.5 ± 17.1	52.0 ± 10.6
ALT (IU/l)	73.0 ± 38.9	36.7 ± 18.8[a]	47.8 ± 30.4	54.5 ± 7.8
AST (IU/l)	32.4 ± 17.4	24.4 ± 19.0	31.1 ± 20.4	23.5 ± 2.1
Total protein (g/dl)	7.3 ± 0.4	7.9 ± 0.6[a]	8.2 ± 0.9[a]	8.9 ± 0.1
BUN (mg/dl)	22.4 ± 4.3	25.0 ± 4.0	28.4 ± 18.1	20.5 ± 2.1
Creatinine (mg/dl)	1.2 ± 0.3	1.5 ± 0.3[a]	1.4 ± 0.3	1.6 ± 0.1

Values are presented as means ± SD. BCS, body condition score.
High oxidized LDL cats in obesity is animals with mean value of oxidized LDL greater than that of humans (11.2 ± 0.3 μg/dl)
[a]Indicates significance (Holm–Sidak One-way ANOVA, $p < 0.05$) when BCS4 or 5 cats were compared pairwise against BCS3 cat.
[b]Indicates significance (Holm–Sidak One-way ANOVA, $p < 0.05$) when BCS4 cat were compared pairwise against BCS5 cat.

aminotransferase (ALT), aspartate aminotransferase (AST), total protein, blood urea nitrogen (BUN), and creatinine (CRE) were determined using a biochemical auto analyzer (JCA-BM2250, JEOL Ltd., Tokyo, Japan) with the manufacturer's reagents. Oxidized LDL was determined using a Dog Oxidized low-density lipoprotein ELISA (Kameyama Biomedical Company, WA, USA). This ELISA kit uses a mouse monoclonal antibody for all of malondialdehyde (MDA)-LDL, Nepsilon (carboxymethyl) lysine (CML)-LDL, and detects advanced glycosylation end product (AGE)-LDL; it cannot distinguish between them. We constructed a calibration curve by plotting the average optical density for each calibrator on the horizontal (X) axis against the concentration on the vertical (Y) axis, and drawing the best-fit curve to generate a four parameter logistic (4-PL) curve-fit.

Electrophoresis of Lipoprotein Cholesterol

Serum lipoprotein cholesterol profiles were measured by the biphasic agarose gel electrophoresis method using a commercial kit, Quick gel LIPO gels (Helena Laboratories, Saitama, Japan). Agarose gel fraction bands were analyzed using customized Epalyzer 2 Electrophoresis Processing Analyzer (Helena Laboratories, Saitama, Japan). In brief, 30 μl of each sample was loaded onto the gel, and run with a 14-min migration time at 250 V and 20°C. After migration, the gels underwent a 15-min reaction time, followed by a 12-min decolorizing and a 30-s fixing time. Cholesterol lipoprotein fractions were assessed and analyzed using Edbank III analysis software (Helena Laboratories, Saitama, Japan).

The band of modified LDL on electrophoresis migrates toward the positive electrode when the charge of apo-lipoprotein in LDL is modified. We set normal animals (BCS3) as control and compared the band position of obese animals against each control group.

Statistical Analysis

Values are expressed as mean ± SD. Statistical significance was determined by Holm–Sidak One-way ANOVA. All tests were performed using Sigmaplot version.11.2 (Systat Software Inc., San Diego, CA, USA). The significance level was set at $p < 0.05$. The correlations were determined by Pearson's product-moment

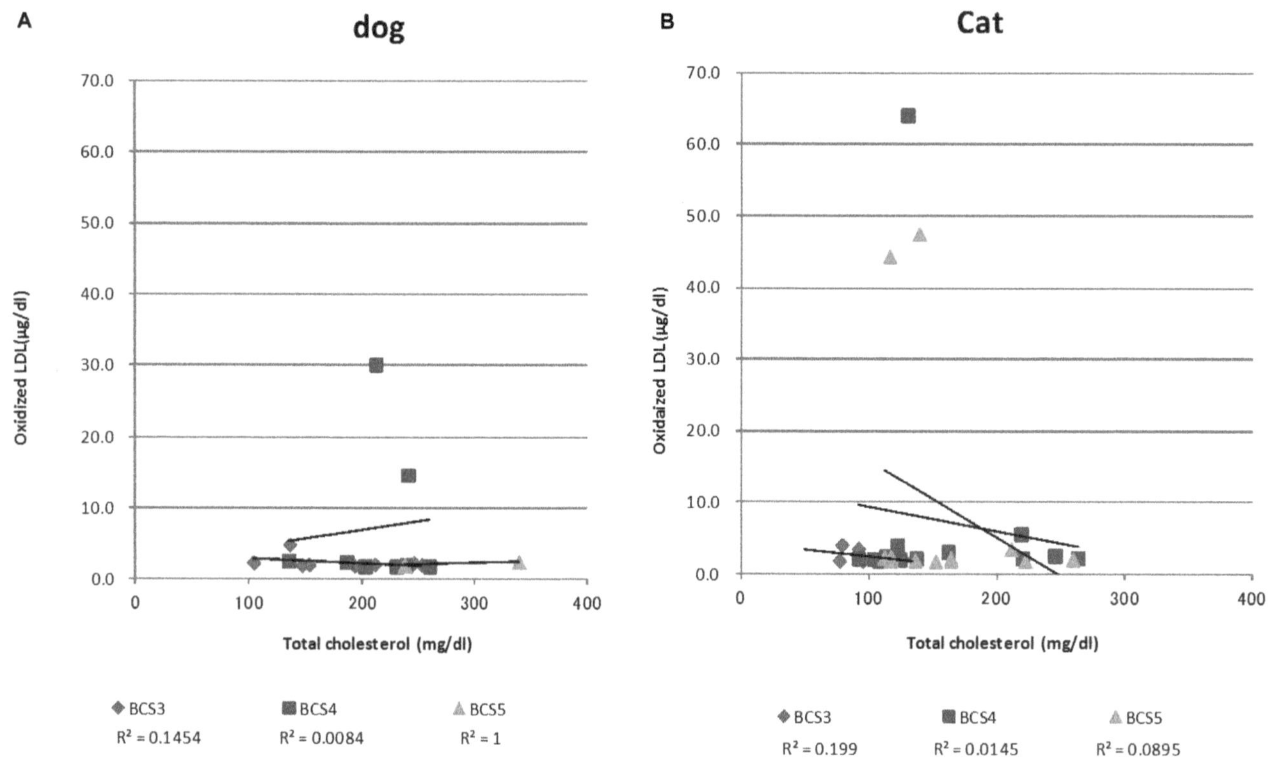

FIGURE 1 | Serum oxidized LDL and total cholesterol concentrations among all dogs (A) and cats (B). This graph shows a correlation between total cholesterol levels and oxidized LDL levels by Pearson's product-moment correlation.

correlation coefficients, *r*, and are displayed as $p < 0.05$. The Electrophoresis bands were assessed and analyzed using Edbank III analysis software (Helena Laboratories, Saitama, Japan).

Results

The parameters measured in normal (BCS3) and obese (BCS4 and 5) animals are shown in **Table 1**. The T-Cho of BCS5 dogs was significantly higher than that of BCS3 dogs, but other parameters did not show significant differences. On the other hand, cats showed significant differences in certain parameters. Age, BW, T-Cho, and total protein of BCS4 and 5 cats were higher than those of BCS3 cats. The ALT of BCS4 cats was significantly lower than that of BCS3 cats, whereas the CRE value of BCS4 cats was higher than that of BCS3 cats. **Figure 1** shows the correlations of T-Cho and oxidized LDL with BCS groups. Dog oxidized LDLs that correlated with T-Cho were BCS3 ($r = -0.4$), BCS4 ($r = 0.1$), and BCS5 ($r = 1.0$). Cat oxidized LDLs that correlated with T-Cho were BCS3 ($r = -0.4$), BCS4 ($r = -0.1$), and BCS5 ($r = -0.3$).

The oxidized LDL value in BCS3 dogs (2.4 ± 0.9 μg/dl) was similar to BCS5 dogs (2.2 ± 0.3 μg/dl). The oxidized LDL value of BCS4 dogs (7.2 ± 10.3 μg/dl) tended to be higher than other BCS groups. The BCS4 group included two dogs whose oxidized LDL values were higher than that of healthy humans (11.2 ± 0.3 μg/dl) (29). The group consisted of one Mixed breed (14-year-old female) and one Miniature dachshund (13-year-old male).

On the other hand, the mean oxidized LDL value of BCS3 cats was 2.5 ± 0.9 μg/dl, BCS4 was 7.5 ± 17.0 μg/dl, and BCS5 was 9.5 ± 17.1 μg/dl; however, these increases were not significant. BCS4 and 5 cats also included three cats with oxidized LDL values that were higher than that of healthy humans. These cats were Mixed breed (8-year-old male, 14-year-old male, 15-year-old female). **Figure 1** also shows the list of oxidized LDL dogs and cats that were extremely high.

When we examined the lipoprotein fractions by electrophoresis, one obese dog and six obese cats had LDL peaks migrating toward the positive electrode, unlike that of the controls. Representative examples of degeneration fraction graphs with the LDL migration of dogs and cats were as seen in **Figure 2**. The results were not consistent with the quantitative measurement of oxidized LDL. In fact, seven animals that had LDL fractions migrating toward the positive side on electrophoresis did not have higher oxidized LDL values on ELISA.

Discussion

Previous studies have shown that thyroid dysfunction is accompanied by changes in caloric intake and body weight, as well as changes in the lipid profile. Hypothyroid rats showed significantly decreased oxidized LDL levels, whereas hyperthyroid rats showed significantly increased oxidized LDL levels (30). Another report showed that oxidized LDL levels in 125 obese human patients were positively correlated with body mass index and T-Cho concentration (31). The most recent report showed the presence of oxidized

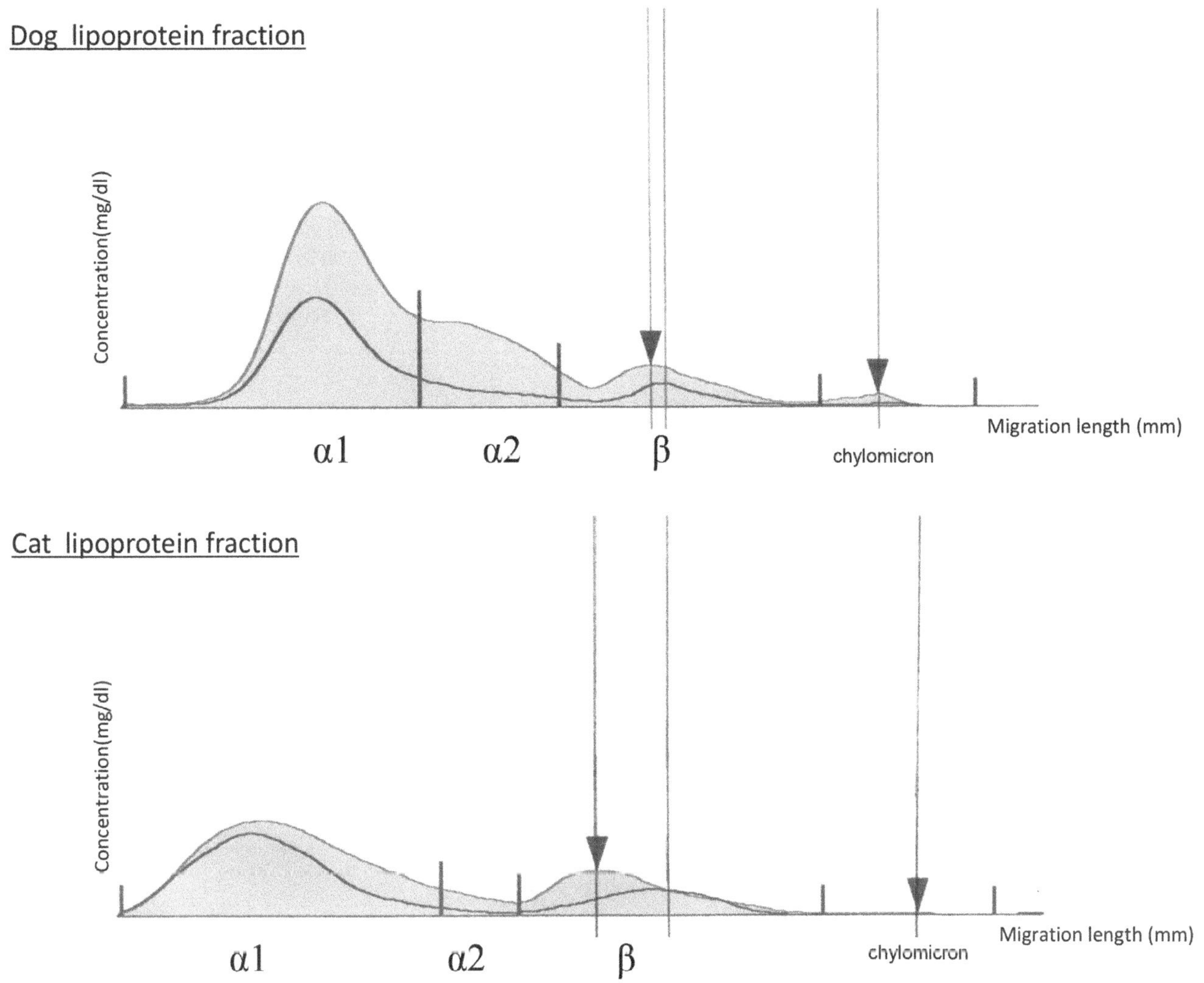

FIGURE 2 | Graphs of lipoprotein cholesterol separated by electrophoresis in obese dogs and cats. The upper curve represents the obese animal lipoprotein cholesterol fraction, and the lower curve represents a normal animal lipoprotein cholesterol fraction. Left ▼ is the LDL peak of obese animals. Right ▼ represents the origin. The electrophoresis bands were assessed and analyzed using Edbank III analysis software (Helena Laboratories, Saitama, Japan) and shown graphically.

LDL in human salivary samples and highlighted a correlation between salivary and serum oxidized LDL levels. Moreover, salivary oxidized LDL levels were higher in overweight/obese subjects than in control subjects (32).

In this study, we were able to quantify oxidized LDL levels in dogs and cats that had been diagnosed as healthy by their veterinarians. These levels were approximately one-quarter of the oxidized LDL value of healthy humans (11.2 ± 0.3 μg/dl) (29). Dogs and cats are known as high HDL animals, in that HDL is dominant, and the total amount of LDL is typically lower than that of humans. Naturally, oxidized LDL levels in dogs and cats are lower than that seen in humans. However, some obese dogs and cats showed extremely high oxidized LDL values. The oxidized LDL values in two obese dogs and three obese cats were indeed higher than the mean value in humans (20.1 ± 1.1 μg/dl) with coronary artery disease (29). Interestingly, the two high oxidized LDL dogs were in the BCS4 group, not the BCS5 group. The three high oxidized LDL cats were composed of one BCS4 cat and two BCS5 cats, and the highest oxidized LDL cat was in BCS4 group. This result suggests that BCS is not correlated with oxidized LDL levels.

Limitations of this study include a small sample size for the determination of reference ranges. Furthermore, the result of the LDL fraction migration by electrophoresis was not consistent with the ELISA results. In humans, migration of the LDL fraction peak toward the positive electrode is determined by the charge of the LDL particle, reflecting both glycation and oxidation. This is because the negative charge of apo B100 in LDL increases by modifications, such as oxidation and glycation (33). A previous human study reported that plasma could be separated into LDL sub-fractions [modified LDL (=oxidized LDL) and native slow-migrating LDL] by capillary electrophoresis, and oxidized LDL was shown as modified LDL. In this study, migration was not clearly visible via this electrophoresis method, and further studies using an appropriate electrophoresis method need to be performed.

Atherosclerosis is characterized by the accumulation of lipids and cholesterol in the inner membrane and tunica media of arteries (34). There are variations in lipoprotein metabolism among animal species, and dogs are less likely to develop atherosclerosis when compared to humans (35). Atherosclerosis is a cardiovascular and fibroproliferative inflammatory disease commonly associated with age- and dietary-related factors in humans (36). In a retrospective study of 21 dogs diagnosed with atherosclerosis on postmortem examinations, Miniature Schnauzer, Doberman pinscher, and Golden Retriever breeds were overrepresented, possibly owing to the increased risk for dyslipoproteinemia in these three breeds (37). Unfortunately, our obese high oxidized LDL dogs were Miniature dachshund and Mixed breed. In order to verify the breed predilection, more samples are needed.

Atherosclerosis in dogs occurs secondary to chronic inflammatory diseases, such as hypothyroidism (38), diabetes mellitus (39), hyperlipidemia (40), and dyspnea associated with obesity (34). These diseases usually affect the brain, eyes, spinal cord, heart, spleen, kidneys, lungs, pancreas, alimentary tract, and urogenital organs, such as prostate and urinary bladder (41). The association between atherosclerosis and glomerular disease is well established in humans (42). Interestingly, canine glomerulopathy is more prevalent in dogs with atherosclerosis as compared to dogs without atherosclerosis. Furthermore, canine atherosclerosis accompanied by glomerulopathy contributes to an elevation in serum cholesterol concentrations (27).

In this study, there was no significant difference in oxidized LDL values between normal and obese animals, whereas there were significant differences in T-Cho among BCS groups of dogs and cats. The correlation between T-Cho and oxidized LDL did not clearly show any trend. It suggests that obesity alone does not have a direct effect on serum oxidized LDL values in healthy dogs and cats. On measuring oxidized LDL by electrophoresis, we found that it is difficult to verify the migration of LDL fractions as modified LDL. In future studies, oxidized LDL will be analyzed by capillary electrophoresis, which will separate the LDL fractions more clearly.

The association between atherosclerosis and glomerular disease in humans is multifactorial. Human arteriosclerosis with renal failure is shown to progress rapidly and has not been fully understood. When renal failure is progressing, enhanced expression of LOX-1 (receptor for oxidized LDL) is involved in the formation of interstitial lesions in particular (43). However, oxidized LDL may be a risk factor for chronic diseases in animals, such as renal failure and diabetes mellitus. As a future study, we plan to investigate whether inflammatory diseases (i.e., diabetes mellitus, hypothyroidism, renal failure) can influence or induce different changes in oxidized LDL and/or cholesterol lipoprotein fraction ratios.

Unfortunately, this study has limitations. Only a small number of dogs and cats could be included in each group; hence, results and conclusions need to be interpreted with care. In order to validate our results, a larger sample pool is needed.

Acknowledgments

We would like to thank the two veterinary clinics (Kanagawa, Ibaraki) in Japan for their assistance in obtaining blood samples from client-owned dogs and cats. This work was supported by Grant-in-Aid for Scientific Research (C) of JSPS KAKENHI Grant Number 26450435.

References

1. Trpkovic A, Resanovic I, Stanimirovic J, Radak D, Mousa SA, Cenic-Milosevic D, et al. Oxidized low-density lipoprotein as a biomarker of cardiovascular diseases. *Crit Rev Clin Lab Sci* (2015) **2**:70–85. doi:10.3109/10408363.2014.992063
2. Berliner JA, Territo MC, Sevanian A, Ramin S, Kim JA, Bamshad B, et al. Minimally modified low density lipoprotein stimulates monocyte endothelial interactions. *J Clin Invest* (1990) **85**:1260–6. doi:10.1172/JCI114562
3. Cushing SD, Berliner JA, Valente AJ, Territo MC, Navab M, Parhami F, et al. Minimally modified low density lipoprotein induces monocyte chemotactic protein 1 in human endothelial cells and smooth muscle cells. *Proc Natl Acad Sci U S A* (1990) **87**:5134–8. doi:10.1073/pnas.87.13.5134
4. Deckert V, Persegol L, Viens L, Lizard G, Athias A, Lallemant C, et al. Inhibitors of arterial relaxation among components of human oxidized low-density lipoproteins: cholesterol derivatives oxidized in position 7 are potent inhibitors of endothelium-dependent relaxation. *Circulation* (1997) **95**:723–31. doi:10.1161/01.CIR.95.3.723
5. Hamilton TA, Ma G, Chisolm GM. Oxidized low density lipoprotein suppresses the expression of tumor necrosis factor- mRNA in stimulated murine peritoneal macrophages. *J Immunol* (1990) **144**:2343–50.
6. Kugiyama K, Sakamoto T, Misumi I, Sugiyama S, Ohgushi M, Ogawa H, et al. Transferable lipids in oxidized low-density lipoprotein stimulate plasminogen activator inhibitor-1 and inhibit tissue-type plasminogen activator release from endothelial cells. *Circ Res* (1993) **73**:335–43. doi:10.1161/01.RES.73.2.335
7. McMurray HF, Parthasarathy S, Steinberg D. Oxidatively modified low density lipoprotein is a chemoattractant for human T lymphocytes. *J Clin Invest* (1993) **92**:1004–8. doi:10.1172/JCI116605
8. Rajavashisth TB, Andalibi A, Territo MC, Berliner JA, Navab M, Fogelman AM, et al. Induction of endothelial cell expression of granulocyte and macrophage colony-stimulating factors by modified low-density lipoproteins. *Nature* (1990) **344**:254–7. doi:10.1038/344254a0
9. Ross R. Atherosclerosis: an inflammatory disease. *N Engl J Med* (1999) **340**:115–26. doi:10.1056/NEJM199901143400207
10. Haverkate F, Thompson SG, Pyke SDM, Gallimore JR, Pepys MB; European Concerted Action on Thrombosis and Disabilities Angina Pectoris Study Group. Production of C-reactive protein and risk of coronary events in stable and unstable angina. *Lancet* (1997) **349**:462–6. doi:10.1016/S0140-6736(96)07591-5
11. Koenig W. Atherosclerosis involves more than just lipids: focus on inflammation. *Eur Heart J Suppl* (1999) **1**(Suppl T):T19–26.
12. Holvoet P, Stassen JM, Van Cleemput J, Collen D, Vanhaecke J. Oxidized low density lipoproteins in patients with transplant-associated coronary artery disease. *Arterioscler Thromb Vasc Biol* (1998) **18**:100–7. doi:10.1161/01.ATV.18.1.100
13. Holvoet P, Vanhaecke J, Janssens S, Van de Werf F, Collen D. Oxidized LDL and malondialdehyde-modified LDL in patients with acute coronary syndromes and stable coronary artery disease. *Circulation* (1998) **98**:1487–94. doi:10.1161/01.CIR.98.15.1487
14. Toshima S, Hasegawa A, Kurabayashi M, Itabe H, Takano T, Sugano J, et al. Circulating oxidized low density lipoprotein levels: a biochemical risk marker for coronary heart disease. *Arterioscler Thromb Vasc Biol* (2000) **20**:2243–7. doi:10.1161/01.ATV.20.10.2243
15. Sasahara M, Raines EW, Chait A, Carew TE, Steinberg D, Wahl PW, et al. Inhibition of hypercholesterolemia induced atherosclerosis in the non human primate by probucol, I: is extent of atherosclerosis related to resistance of LDL to oxidation? *J Clin Invest* (1994) **94**:155–64. doi:10.1002/jsfa.4163

16. Tangirala RK, Casanada F, Miller E, Witztum JL, Steinberg D, Palinski W. Effect of the antioxidant N,N'-diphenyl 1,4-phenylenediamine (DPPD) on atherosclerosis in apo E deficient mice. *Arterioscler Thromb Vasc Biol* (1995) **5**:1625–30. doi:10.1161/01.ATV.15.10.1625
17. Carew TE, Schwenke DC, Steinberg D. Antiatherogenic effect of probucol unrelated to its hypocholesterolemic effect: evidence that antioxidants in vivo can selectively inhibit low density lipoprotein degradation in macrophage-rich fatty streaks and slow the progression of atherosclerosis in the Watanabe-heritable hyperlipidemic rabbit. *Proc Natl Acad Sci U S A* (1987) **84**:7725–9.
18. Bjorkhem I, Henriksson-Freyschuss A, Breuer O, Diczfalusy U, Berglund L, Henriksson P. The antioxidant butylated hydroxytoluene protects against atherosclerosis. *Arterioscler Thromb* (1991) **11**:15–22. doi:10.1161/01.ATV.11.1.15
19. Daugherty A, Zweifel BS, Schonfeld G. Probucol attenuates the development of aortic atherosclerosis in cholesterol-fed rabbits. *Br J Pharmacol* (1989) **98**:612–8. doi:10.1111/j.1476-5381.1989.tb12635.x
20. Holvoet P, Donck J, Landeloos M, Brouwers E, Luijtens K, Arnout J, et al. Correlation between oxidized low density lipoproteins and von Willebrand factor in chronic renal failure. *Thromb Haemost* (1996) **76**:663–9.
21. Meisinger C, Baumert J, Khuseyinova N, Loewel H, Koenig W. Plasma oxidized low-density lipoprotein, a strong predictor for acute coronary heart disease events in apparently healthy, middle-aged men from the general population. *Circulation* (2005) **112**:651–7. doi:10.1161/CIRCULATIONAHA.104.529297
22. Grundy SM. Oxidized LDL and atherogenesis: relation to risk factors for coronary heart disease. *Clin Cardiol* (1993) **16**:I3–5. doi:10.1002/clc.4960161303
23. Bailhache E, Nguyen P, Krempf M, Siliart B, Magot T, Ouguerram K. Lipoproteins abnormalities in obese insulin-resistant dogs. *Metabolism* (2003) **52**:559–64. doi:10.1053/meta.2003.50110
24. Mori N, Lee P, Kondo K, Kido T, Saito T, Arai T. Potential use of cholesterol profile to confirm obesity states in dogs. *Vet Res Commun* (2011) **35**:223–35. doi:10.1007/s11259-011-9466-x
25. Mahley RW, Weisgraber KH, Innerarity T. Canine lipoproteins and atherosclerosis. II. Characterization of the plasma lipoproteins associated with atherogenic and nonatherogenic hyperlipidemia. *Circ Res* (1974) **35**:722–33. doi:10.1161/01.RES.35.5.722
26. Hess RS, Kass PH, Van Winkle TJ. Association between diabetes mellitus, hypothyroidism or hyperadrenocorticism, and atherosclerosis in dogs. *J Vet Intern Med* (2003) **17**:489–94. doi:10.1111/j.1939-1676.2003.tb02469.x
27. Hess RS, Kass PH, Van Winkle TJ. Association between atherosclerosis and glomerulopathy in dogs. *Int J Appl Res Vet Med* (2006) **4**:224–31.
28. Laflamme D. Nutritional management. *Vet Clin North Am Small Anim Pract* (1997) **27**:1561–77. doi:10.1016/S0195-5616(97)50139-2
29. Kosaki J, Koyama C. The turning point hyperlipidemia treatment. *Nikkei Med* (1997) **6**:60–9.
30. Zelzer S, Mangge H, Pailer S, Ainoedhofer H, Kieslinger P, Stojakovic T, et al. Oxidized LDL is strictly limited to hyperthyroidism irrespective of fat feeding in female Sprague Dawley rats. *Int J Mol Sci* (2015) **16**:11689–98. doi:10.3390/ijms160511689
31. Nascimento H, Alves AI, Coimbra S, Catarino C, Gomes D, Bronze-da-Rocha E, et al. Bilirubin is independently associated with oxidized LDL levels in young obese patients. *Diabetol Metab Syndr* (2015) **7**:4. doi:10.1186/1758-5996-7-4
32. De Giuseppe R, Cossellu G, Vigna L, Dicorato F, De Vita C, Venturelli G, et al. Correlation between salivary and serum oxidized LDL levels: a pilot study on overweight/obese subjects. *J Oral Pathol Med* (2015). doi:10.1111/jop.12322
33. Saku K. The role of LDL in the metabolic syndrome. *J Jpn Coll Angiol* (2006) **46**:465–73.
34. Liu SK, Tilley LP, Tappe JP, Fox PR. Clinical and pathologic findings in dogs with atherosclerosis: 21 cases (1970-1983). *J Am Vet Med Assoc* (1986) **189**:227–32.
35. Mahley RW, Innerarity TL, Weisgraber KH, Fry DL. Canine hyperlipoproteinemia and atherosclerosis. Accumulation of lipid by aortic medial cells in vivo and in vitro. *Am J Pathol* (1977) **87**:205–26.
36. Singh RB, Mengi SA, Xu YJ, Arneja AS, Dhalla NS. Pathogenesis of atherosclerosis: a multifactorial process. *Exp Clin Cardiol* (2002) **7**:40–53.
37. Wong VM, Kidney BA, Snead EC, Myers SL, Jackson ML. Serum C-reactive protein concentrations in healthy Miniature Schnauzer dogs. *Vet Clin Pathol* (2011) **40**:380–3. doi:10.1111/j.1939-165X.2011.00336.x
38. Indrieri RJ, Whalen LR, Cardinet GH, Holliday TA. Neuromuscular abnormalities associated with hypothyroidism and lymphocytic thyroiditis in three dogs. *J Am Vet Med Assoc* (1987) **190**:544–8.
39. Bennett N. Monitoring techniques for diabetes mellitus in the dog and the cat. *Clin Tech Small Anim Pract* (2002) **17**:65–9. doi:10.1053/svms.2002.33044
40. Xenoulis PG, Steiner JM. Lipid metabolism and hyperlipidemia in dogs. *Vet J* (2010) **183**:12–21. doi:10.1016/j.tvjl.2008.10.011
41. Kagawa Y, Hirayama K, Uchida E, Izumisawa Y, Yamaguchi M, Kotani T, et al. Systemic atherosclerosis in dogs: histopathological and immunohistochemical studies of atherosclerotic lesions. *J Comp Pathol* (1998) **118**:195–206. doi:10.1016/S0021-9975(05)80126-4
42. Sarnak MJ, Levey AS, Schoolwerth AC, Coresh J, Culleton B, Hamm LL, et al. Kidney disease as a risk factor for development of cardiovascular disease: a statement from the American heart association councils on kidney in cardiovascular disease, high blood pressure research, clinical cardiology, and epidemiology and prevention. *Hypertension* (2003) **42**:1050–65. doi:10.1161/01.HYP.0000102971.85504.7c
43. Chen M, Masaki T, Sawamura T. LOX-1, the receptor for oxidized low-density lipoprotein identified from endothelial cells: implications in endothelial dysfunction and atherosclerosis. *Pharmacol Ther* (2002) **95**:89–100. doi:10.1016/S0163-7258(02)00236-X

Conflict of Interest Statement: The authors declare that the research was conducted in the absence of any commercial or financial relationships that could be construed as a potential conflict of interest.

8

A role for the non-canonical Wnt-β-Catenin and TGF-β signaling pathways in the induction of tolerance during the establishment of a *Salmonella enterica* serovar Enteritidis persistent cecal infection in chickens

Michael H. Kogut* and Ryan J. Arsenault

Southern Plains Agricultural Research Center (SPARC), Agricultural Research Service (ARS), United States Department of Agriculture (USDA), College Station, TX, USA

Edited by:
Dirk Werling,
Royal Veterinary College, UK

Reviewed by:
Filip Boyen,
Ghent University, Belgium
Sherry Layton,
Vetanco, Argentina

****Correspondence:***
Michael H. Kogut,
Southern Plains Agricultural Research Center (SPARC), Agricultural Research Service (ARS), United States Department of Agriculture (USDA), College Station, TX 77845, USA
mike.kogut@ars.usda.gov

Non-typhoidal *Salmonella enterica* induce an early pro-inflammatory response in chickens. However, the response is short-lived, asymptomatic of disease, resulting in a persistent colonization of the ceca, and fecal shedding of bacteria. The underlying mechanisms that control this persistent infection of chickens by *Salmonella* are unknown. Recently, we found an expansion of the Treg population and subsequent increased *in vitro* immunosuppressive functions of the $CD4^+CD25^+$ cells isolated from the ceca of the *Salmonella*-infected chickens by day 4 post-infection that increased steadily throughout the course of the 14 days of infection, whereas the number of $CD4^+CD25^+$ cells in the non-infected controls remained steady throughout the study. $CD4^+CD25^+$ cells from cecal tonsils of *S. enteritidis*-infected birds had greater expression of IL-10 mRNA content than the $CD4^+CD25^+$ cells from the non-infected controls at all the time points studied. These results suggest the development of a tolerogenic immune response in the cecum of *Salmonella*-infected chickens may contribute to the persistance of *Salmonella* cecal colonization. Using a chicken-specific kinome peptide immune array, we have analyzed the signaling pathways altered during the establishment of this tolerogenic state. This analysis has revealed a role for the non-canonical Wnt signaling pathway in the cecum at 4 days post-infection. Infection induced the significant ($p < 0.01$) phosphorylation of the G-protein-coupled transmembrane protein, Frizzled 1 (FZD1), resulting in an influx of intracellular Ca^{2+} and the phosphorylation of the Ca^{2+}-dependent effector molecules calcium/calmodulin-dependent kinase II (CamKII), β-catenin, protein kinase C, and the activation of the transcription factor, NFAT. Nuclear translocation of NFAT resulted in a significant increase in the expression of the anti-inflammatory cytokines IL-10 and TGF-β. Increased expression of TGF-β4 mRNA activates the TGF-β signaling pathway that phosphorylates the receptor-activated Smads, Smad2 and Smad3. Combined with the results from our Treg studies, these studies describe kinome-based phenotypic changes in the cecum of chickens during *Salmonella* Enteritidis infection starting 4 days post-infection that leads to an anti-inflammatory, tolerogenic local environment, and results in the establishment of persistent intestinal colonization.

Keywords: *Salmonella*, chickens, kinome array, Wnt signaling pathway, tolerance

Introduction

Salmonellosis is a zoonotic disease produced by the Gram-negative enteric bacterium *Salmonella*. *Salmonella* are not restricted to particular host species, with more than 2500 serotypes having been described mostly belonging to the species *Salmonella enterica* (1), with most having asymptomatic colonization of the gastrointestinal tract of animals. The most prevalent serovars, *S. enterica* serovar Typhimurium (S. Typhimurium) and serovar Enteritidis (S. Enteritidis) are major causes of intestinal infections in a wide range of host species worldwide (2, 3). Both serovars have a broad host range able to infect poultry, livestock, and humans (4). S. Typhimurium and S. Enteritidis infections of humans, cattle, and pigs cause self-limiting gastroenteritis manifested by abdominal pain, vomiting, and inflammatory diarrhea (5); whereas, infection of birds more than a few days old with either serovar produces asymptomatic cecal colonization with persistent shedding of bacteria that may persist for months, causing carcass contamination at slaughter with potential human food safety issues (6–10).

The host responds to infection with pathogens by activating the innate and adaptive immune mechanisms. However, some pathogens, such as *Salmonella*, have evolved the ability to survive the initial host immune response and persist. The interactions between the host and pathogen during this persistent phase are multifaceted and reflect the co-evolution of bacterial virulence mechanisms and host immune responses. Very little is known about the regulatory interactions between the host immune response and virulence mechanisms that lead to *S. enterica* persistence in the avian intestine. Chronic colonization of the intestinal tract is an important aspect of persistent *Salmonella* infection in poultry because it results in propagation of bacteria in the birds due to the impossibility to isolate contaminated animals (11).

A better comprehension of the host factors that are exploited by the bacteria in order to establish a persistent infection would be invaluable for the identification and development of therapeutic targets. Recently, Chausse and colleagues (12) found that genes involved in the inflammatory response were down-regulated during the carrier state, suggesting a bias toward a Th2 response in susceptible chickens. Furthermore, in a murine model of long-term S. *typhimurium* infection, the bacteria preferentially associated with anti-inflammatory/M2 macrophages during the later stages of infection (13). Lastly, the immune-suppression role of regulatory T cells has been shown to play a role in *Salmonella* persistence in a murine model (14). All told, we speculate that the bacterium is involved in redirecting the host response toward immune tolerance. The present study was designed to address the question on the induction of immune tolerance during a persistent paratyphoid *Salmonella* infection in chickens.

When considering the effects of an infection on a host, such as asymptomatic salmonellosis in poultry, studying the protein level as opposed to the gene or transcript level reduces complicating variables. The proteome contains the final effectors resulting in the organism's phenotype. Such studies can provide a dramatically different perspective on the avian host's biochemical and physiological properties to this asymptomatic enteric bacterial pathogen. Our recent report of the development of chicken species-specific peptide arrays for kinome analysis of host signaling responses to *Salmonella* provided us with the prospect to characterize a more detailed understanding of the host–pathogen interactions in the chicken (15). Using a metabolism kinome array, we have documented altered metabolic signaling pathways in the skeletal muscle of S. Typhimurium-infected chickens that affected fatty acid and glucose metabolism through the AMPK and the mTOR signaling pathways over the first 3 weeks post-infection (16). Additionally, using a chicken-specific immune array, we have detailed the toll-like receptor (TLR) signaling pathways stimulated in monocytes by TLR ligands, CpG (TLR 21) and poly I:C (TLR3), but also identified a unique signaling pathway stimulated by the combination of CpG/poly I:C treatment that was not observed by treatment with the individual ligands (17).

Therefore, in the present study we hypothesized that *S. enterica* serovar Enteritidis (S. Enteritidis) induces an immune tolerance in chickens that results in the bacteria's ability to persistently colonize the cecum of poultry. To test this hypothesis, we analyzed temporal chicken-specific kinomic immune peptide arrays anti-inflammatory cytokine gene transcription of avian cecal tissue during a persistent infection by S. Enteritidis. Using these approaches, we were able to begin to characterize the specific immune post-translational signaling events during a persistent *Salmonella* colonization in chickens. Furthermore, we characterized the cellular and cytokine profiles that provide confirmation for the transition of an early pro-inflammatory mucosal response to the development of an immune tolerogenic mucosal response.

Materials and Methods

Experimental Animals

Experiments were conducted according to the regulations established by the U.S. Department of Agriculture Animal Care and Use Committee. Straight-run broiler chickens used in this study were obtained from a commercial breeder and were all of the same genetic background and were not vaccinated at any time. Chicks were placed in floor pens containing wood shavings, provided supplemental heat, water, and a balanced, unmedicated corn and soybean meal-based chick starter diet *ad libitum* that met or exceeded the levels of critical nutrients recommended by the National Research Council (18). *Salmonella* was not detected in the feed or from the paper tray liners using standard procedures (19).

S. Enteritidis Challenge

A poultry isolate of *S. enterica* serovar Enteritidis [*S.* Enteritidis; (ID 9711771, part 24)] was obtained from the National Veterinary Services Laboratory (Ames, IA, USA), and was selected for resistance to nalidixic acid and novobiocin and maintained in tryptic soy broth (Difco Laboratories, Sparks, MD, USA) containing antibiotics (20 µg/ml nalidixic acid and 25 µg/ml novobiocin; Sigma Chemical Co., St. Louis, MO, USA). A stock culture was prepared in sterile PBS and adjusted to a concentration of 1×10^9 colony forming units (cfu)/ml. The viable cell concentration of the challenge dose for each experiment was determined by colony counts on XLT4 agar base plates with XLT4 supplement (Difco) and nalidixic acid and novobiocin (XLT-NN).

Experimental Design

One-day-old broiler chickens were randomly distributed into either non-infected control or infected groups each with 50 birds per group. The birds were fed a balanced, unmedicated corn and soybean meal-based diet. At 4 days post-hatch, all chickens were orally challenged with 1 ml of either 5×10^6 CFU/ml *S.* Enteritidis or mock challenged with 1 ml sterile PBS. Four, 7, 10, and 14 days after challenge, 10 chickens from each group were humanely euthanized, cecal contents were analyzed for *S.* Enteritidis colonization, cecal tonsils were collected for quantitative real-time PCR (qRTPCR), and cecal tissue from 3 of the 10 chickens per treatment was flash frozen in liquid nitrogen and stored for use in the peptide arrays (see below).

All experiments were replicated three times. Therefore, for the mRNA expression, the ceca from a total of 40 chickens for each of the two groups (10 chickens at each of four time points) were used to prepare the mRNA for the qRT-PCR assays. RNA from each bird ($n = 10$) was isolated and assayed separately and not pooled. Each RNA sample was replicated three times per immune gene per experiment).

Sample Collection for Peptide and Antibody Arrays

At 4, 7, 10, and 14 days post-infection, a 25 cm^2 section from one cecum (from the middle of the cecal pouch) was removed from each of the three randomly selected birds from each group (non-infected and infected) and immediately flash frozen in liquid nitrogen to preserve kinase enzymatic activity, and then transferred to a −80°C freezer until used in the peptide array. Following microbiological analysis of the cecal contents (see below), the cecal tissues from three confirmed non-infected and three confirmed infected chickens (out of the 10 birds per group peer time point) were used for the peptide and antibody arrays.

Peptide Arrays

At each of the time points and under each condition (infected and uninfected), three cecal samples from three different animals were taken from storage for analysis (24 samples total). Cecal tissue samples were weighed to obtain a consistent 40 mg sample for the array protocol. Samples were homogenized in lysis buffer and the homogenates were used in the peptide array protocol as described previously (19, 20).

Antibody Array

The Wnt pathway antibody array assay kit was obtained from Full Moon BioSystems (Sunnyvale, CA, USA) and the protocol was carried out as per the manufacturer's instructions. The antibody array was used as an alternative to performing several western blot assays.

Data Analysis for Peptide and Antibody Arrays

Data normalization and PCA analysis were performed for both the peptide and antibody microarrays as described previously (21). Gene ontology (GO) and Kyoto encyclopedia of genes and genomes (KEGG) pathway analysis were performed by uploading the statistically significant peptide lists to the search tool for the retrieval of interacting genes (STRING) (22).

Sample Collection for Bacterial Contents

The ceca from each chicken were removed aseptically and the contents (0.25 g) from one cecal pouch was serially diluted in sterile saline to 1:100, 1:1000, or 1:10,000 and spread onto XLT-NN plates. The plates were incubated at 37°C for 24 h, and the number of NN-resistant *S.* Enteritidis cells per gram of cecal contents was determined. The data from each experimental group were pooled from three separate trials for statistical analysis.

Sample Collection for mRNA

Chickens from each experimental group were euthanized at 4, 7, 10, and 14 days post-infection. A 25-mg piece of tissue was removed from the cecal tonsils and was washed in PBS, placed in a 2-ml microcentrifuge tube with 1 ml of RNAlater (Qiagen, Inc., Valencia, CA, USA), and stored at −20°C until processed. In addition, for comparison purposes, a 25 mg piece of ceca from the 10 extra birds from each group (see above 50 birds total per group, 10 used per time point = 40) was collected at 2 days post-infection.

RNA Isolation

Tissues (25 mg) were removed from RNAlater and transferred to pre-filled 2 ml tubes containing Triple-Pure™ 1.5 mm zirconium beads. RLT lysis buffer (600 µl) from the RNeasy mini kit (Qiagen) was added and the tissue was homogenized for 1–2 min at 4,000 rpm in a Bead Bug microtube homogenizer (Benchmark Scientific, Inc., Edison, NJ, USA). Total RNA was extracted from the homogenized lysates according to the manufacturer's instructions, eluted with 50 µl RNase-free water, and stored at −80°C until qRT-PCR analyses were performed. RNA was quantified and the quality evaluated using a spectrophotometer (NanoDrop Products, Wilmington, DE, USA). Total RNA (300 ng) from each sample was prepared.

Quantitative Real-Time PCR

Primer and probe sets for the cytokines and 28S rRNA were designed using the Primer Express Software program (Applied Biosystems, Foster City, CA, USA) have been described (23, 24) and are provided in **Table 1**. The qRT-PCR was performed using the TaqMan fast universal PCR master mix and one-step RT-PCR

TABLE 1 | Real-time quantitative RT-PCR probes and primers for IL-6 and TGF-β4.

RNA target		Probe/primer sequence	Accession number[a]
28S	Probe	5′-(FAM[d])-AGGACCGCTACGGACCTCCACCA-(TAMRA)-3′	X59733
	F[b]	5′-GGCGAAGCCAGAGGAAACT-3′	
	R[c]	5′-GACGACCGATTGCACGTC-3′	
IL-6	Probe	5′-(FAM)-AGGAGAAATGCCTGACGAAGCTCTCCA-(TAMRA)-3′	AJ250838
	F	5′-GCTCGCCGGCTTCGA-3′	
	R	5′-GGTAGGTCTGAAAGGCGAACAG-3′	
TGF-β4	Probe	5′-(FAM)-ACCCAAAGGTTATATGGCCAACTTCTGCAT-(TAMRA)-3′	M31160
	F	5′-AGGATCTGCAGTGGAAGTGGAT-3′	
	R	5′-CCCCGGGGTTGTGTGTTGGT-3′	

[a]*Genomic DNA sequence.*
[b]*Forward.*
[c]*Reverse.*
[d]*5-carboxyfluorescein.*

master mix reagents (Applied Biosystems). Amplification and detection of specific products were performed using the Applied Biosystems 7500 Fast real-time PCR system with the following cycle profile as described previously (23, 24). Quantification was based on the increased fluorescence detected by the 7500 Fast sequence detection system due to hydrolysis of the target-specific probes by the 5-nuclease activity of the r*Tth* DNA polymerase during PCR amplification. Normalization was carried out using 28S rRNA as a housekeeping gene. To correct for differences in RNA levels between samples within the experiment, the correction factor for each sample was calculated by dividing the mean threshold cycle (*CT*) value for 28S rRNA-specific product for each sample by the overall mean *CT* value for the 28S rRNA-specific product from all samples. The corrected cytokine mean was calculated as follows: (average of each replicate × cytokine slope)/(28S slope × 28S correction factor). Fold changes in mRNA levels were calculated from mean 40 *CT* values by the formula $2^{(40\ CT\ \text{of infected group} - 40\ CT\ \text{in non-infected group})}$.

Calcium Detection

Intracellular Ca^{2+} in cecal lysates from non-infected and infected chickens was measured with a colorimetric Ca^{2+} Detection Kit (Abcam, Inc., Cambridge, MA, USA). Preparation of cell extracts was done according to the manufacturer's instructions. Total amount of Ca^{2+} was determined using a standard curve.

Statistical Analysis

The data from these replicated experiments were pooled for presentation and statistical analysis. The mean and SEM were calculated and differences between groups were determined by analysis of variance. Significant differences were further separated using Duncan's multiple-range test (23). A p value of <0.05 was considered statistically significant.

Results

S. Enteritidis Infection

Infection status of the chickens was confirmed by *S.* Enteritidis culturing of cecal contents and feces from each bird with and without enrichment. Cultures confirmed that greater than 70% of the chickens in the infected group displayed *S.* Enteritidis throughout the experiment while *Salmonella* was not isolated from the birds in the control group (**Tables 2** and **3**).

TABLE 2 | Number of chickens positive for *Salmonella* Enteritidis ceca colonization for 2 weeks following challenge.

	Percent positive for *Salmonella* Enteritidis cecal colonization (total positive/total challenged)			
	Days post-challenge			
Treatment groups	4	7	10	14
Non-infected control	0 (0/30)	0 (0/30)	0 (0/30)	0 (0/30)
Infected	100 (30/30)	100 (30/30)	85 (26/30)	70 (21/30)

Results shown are pooled from three separate experiments.

TABLE 3 | Cecal *Salmonella* Enteritidis for 2 weeks following challenge.

	CFU of *Salmonella* Enteritidis in cecum (log 10)			
	Days post-challenge			
Treatment groups	4	7	10	14
Non-infected control	0	0	0	0
Infected	4.11 ± 1.37	4.79 ± 1.28	5.23 ± 1.41	4.36 ± 1.78

Results are expressed as the mean ± SEM of three separate experiments.

Altered Expression of Cytokines

Characteristically, during an acute infection (within 24 h) by paratyphoid strains of *Salmonella* in chickens, there is an up-regulation of pro-inflammatory cytokines mRNA expression in the cecum (25). Few, if any, studies have measured the comparative expression of mRNA between anti-inflammatory cytokines and pro-inflammatory cytokines during persistent *Salmonella* infections. In the present studies, we profiled the pro-inflammatory (IL-6) and anti-inflammatory (TGF-β4) cytokine mRNA expression in the cecum of chickens over the first 14 days post-infection with *S.* Enteritidis and compared the results to the non-infected control birds. Initially, at 48 h post-infection, as expected, IL-6 (14.21-fold change) mRNA expression in the ceca from *S.* Enteritidis-infected chickens was up-regulated when compared to the expression in the cecum from the non-infected birds (**Figure 1**). However, by 4 days post-infection, there was a dramatic reduction in IL 6 mRNA expression (1.45 fold change)

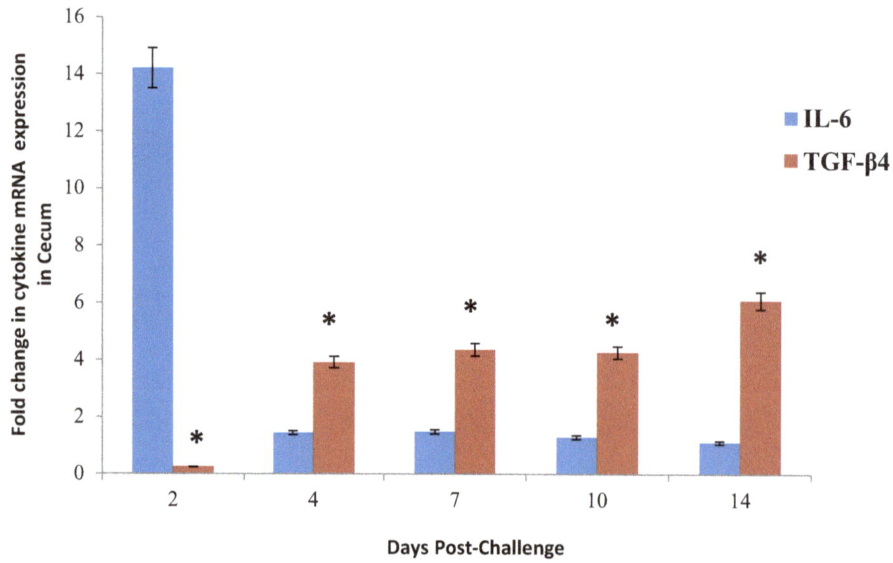

FIGURE 1 | Expression of pro-inflammatory (IL-6) or anti-inflammatory TGF-β4) cytokine mRNA in the ceca from experimental chickens with persistent colonization by *Salmonella* Enteritidis. The expression of cytokine mRNA was determined by quantitative RT-PCR. Data represent the fold change in mRNA expression in the cecum from infected chickens when compared to the mRNA expression in the cecum from non-infected chickens. Data represent the mean ± SEM from three separate experiments.

TABLE 4 | KEGG pathways generated by STRING.

		4 days		7 days		10 days		14 days	
GO ID	**Pathway**	**# peptides**	***p*-Value (FDR)**	**# peptides**	***p*-Value (FDR)**	**# peptides**	***p*-Value (FDR)**	**# peptides**	***p*-Value (FDR)**
hsa04141	Protein processing in endoplasm reticulum pathway	4	0.07	13	0.073	1	1.00	3	0.071
hsa05130	Pathogenic *Escherichia coli* infection	–	N/S	2	N/S	4	N/S	4	N/S
hsa04250	TGF-β4 signaling pathway	12	0.016	–	N/S	–	N/S	–	N/S
hsa04310	Wnt signaling pathway	16	0.0004	2	N/S	–	N/S	5	0.024
hsa04623	Cytosolic DNA-sensing pathway	4	7.01×10^{-2}	5	N/S	4	N/S	–	N/S
hsa05217	Basal cell carcinoma	–	N/S	–	N/S	2	0.338	–	N/S
hsa04672	Intestinal immune response for IgA production	1	1.00	5	N/S	–	N/S	–	N/S

Peptides that displayed a significant change in phosphorylation state were input into the STRING database for each time point. Generated pathways involved in immune activation/suppression that displayed p-value of less than 0.05 (FDR corrected) are listed. N/S indicates that the pathway is non-significant.

that remained low throughout the 14 days post-infection. In fact, there was no statistical difference in IL-6 mRNA expression between the infected and non-infected cecal tissues.

Alternatively, as the pro-inflammatory IL-6 mRNA expression was decreasing, the *S.* Enteritidis infection persisted, and the expression of the anti-inflammatory cytokine TGF-β4 mRNA were significantly up-regulated over the course of the 14-day infection period with the most profound up-regulation of both between 7 and 10 days post-infection when compared to the non-infected controls birds (**Figure 1**).

Peptide Arrays

Chicken-specific peptide arrays designed for the study of chicken immune signaling pathways were used to analyze the cecal samples from the non-infected and infected control chickens. To account for any changes in phosphorylation state that were not due to the infection, the results at each time point were corrected using their respective time matched controls.

The KEGG pathway results generated from STRING showed a large number of pathways implicated by the data at a statistically significant level [$p < 0.05$ false discovery rate (FDR) corrected]. Of particular interest were those pathways that showed a large number of statistically significant peptides that were phosphorylated at different times over the course of the study. These pathways are shown in **Table 4**. Of note are the Wnt signaling and TGF-β4 signaling pathways that were dramatically altered by the infection. Both of the pathways had multiple significantly altered peptide phosphorylation events at multiple time points post-infection; however, a total of 20 differentially phosphorylated peptides were found within these two pathways in chickens on the fourth day post-infection with *S.* Enteritidis (**Table 4**), signifying a dramatic local post-translational modification of the infected cecum. Of the 20 peptides that were differentially phosphorylated, 13 belong to the Wnt signaling pathway and 7 to the TGF-β4 pathway. Interestingly, only nine more total peptides were found to be differentially phosphorylated within these two specific pathways over days 7–14 post-infection (**Table 4**).

Phosphorylation Events Within Specific Pathways

Wnt Signaling Pathway

Frizzled is a family of G protein-coupled receptor proteins that serves as receptors in the Wnt signaling pathway. We found frizzled 1 (FZD1) to be significantly phosphorylated in the ceca of *S.* Enteritidis-infected chickens (**Table 5**), providing us with the first indication of the involvement of the Wnt pathway. Further analysis of the peptide alterations in the Wnt signaling pathway revealed other significant changes in phosphorylation events: (1) the serine/threonine kinase, glycogen synthase kinase 3β (GSK3β), was significantly dephosphorylated in the *S.* Enteritidis-infected cecal tissue at 4 days post-infection when compared to the non-infected control cecal tissue, while β-catenin was significantly phosphorylated; (2) both protein kinase C (PKC) alpha isoforma (PRKCA) and calcium/calmodulin-dependent protein kinase type II alpha chain (CaMK2A) are significantly phosphorylated in the *S.* Enteritidis-infected cecal tissue at 4 days post-infection when compared to the non-infected control cecal tissue; (3) the serine–threonine protein calcineurin (PPSCA), an inhibitor of the canonical Wnt signaling pathway, was significantly phosphorylated in the *S.* Enteritidis-infected cecal tissue at 4 days post infection; and (4) nuclear factor of activated T cells (NFAT), a family of transcription factors that play a pivotal role in the transcription of cytokine genes and other genes critical for the immune response were found to be significantly phosphorylated in the ceca of *S.* Enteritidis-infected chickens (**Table 5**).

TGF-β Signaling Pathway

The TGF-β signaling pathway showed statistically significant changes in the cecal tissue from chickens 4 days post-infection with *S.* Enteritidis (**Table 6**). Smad proteins 1–3 were all significantly phosphorylated in the infected cecal tissue. Smads are intracellular proteins that transduce extracellular signals from TGF-β ligands and activate gene transcription. Smads 1–3 are receptor-regulated proteins that associate with receptor kinases and are phosphorylated. These proteins then typically bind to the common mediator Smad or co-Smad, Smad4. Smad complexes then accumulate in the cell nucleus where they regulate transcription of specific target genes.

In addition to Smad signaling, which directly impacts transcription, TGF-β induces mTORC1 (the mammalian target of rapamycin complex 1) signaling through phosphoinositide 3-kinase (PI3K) and Akt (26). Further analysis of the TGF-β signaling pathway showed a significant phosphorylation of p70S6 kinase, a serine–theonine kinase that is a target for the S6 ribosomal protein (**Table 6**). P70S6 kinase is in a signaling pathway that includes the mammalian target of rapamycin (mTOR). mTOR can be activated in distinct ways, thereby activating p70S6K.

Validation of Kinome Analysis with Antibody Array

Despite the scarcity of chicken-specific antibodies, the key proteins of interest based on the peptide array results were relatively well conserved between humans and chickens, giving us confidence that we would observe significant cross-reactivity

TABLE 5 | Peptides from the Wnt signaling pathway that displayed a statistically significant change in phosphorylation.

	Wnt signaling pathway							
	Days post-infection							
	4		7		10		14	
Peptide	Fold change	*p*-Value	Fold change	*p*-Value	Fold change	*p*-Value	Fold change	*p*-Value
CAMK2A	2.789	0.008	–		–		–	
β-catenin	1.657	0.044	1.538	0.035	–		–	
EP300	1.954	0.017	–		–		1.804	0.047
Jun	3.604	0.001	–		–		–	
Jun	3.389	0.0003	–		–		–	
GSK-3β	−2.254	0.002	–		2.448	0.018	–	
NFATC1			–		–		1.957	0.009
NFATC2	1.779	0.045	–		–		–	
NFATC3	2.239	0.006	–		–		1.655	0.020
Calcineurin	2.447	0.003	–		–		–	
PRKCA Thr638	1.744	0.042	–		–		–	
PRKCA Tyr657	2.555	0.011	–		–		1.927	0.024
RAC1	1.740	0.008	–		–		–	
SMAD2 Ser345	3.434	0.008	1.756	0.013	–		–	
SMAD2 Thr255	4.532	0.006						
SMAD3	1.442	0.033	–		–		–	
FZD1	2.712	0.034	–		–	–	1.844	0.008

Peptides that displayed a p-value of less than 0.05 are listed.

TABLE 6 | Peptides from the TGF-β4 signaling pathway that displayed a statistically significant change in phosphorylation.

	TGF-β4 signaling pathway							
	Days post-infection							
	4		7		10		14	
Peptide	**Fold change**	***p*-Value**	**Fold change**	***p*-Value**	**Fold change**	***p*-Value**	**Fold change**	***p*-Value**
EP300	1.954	0.017	–		–		–	
MAP3K7 (TAK1)	2.709	0.016	–		–		–	
MAPK8 (JNK1)	2.207	0.022	–		–		1.167	0.013
MAPK3 (ERK1)	4.269	0.001	–		–		–	
p70S6K	1.145	0.023	–		–		–	
P70S6K	3.005	0.012	–		–		–	
P70S6K	3.759	0.009	–		–		–	
SMAD1	2.698	0.021	–		–		–	
SMAD1	2.916	0.00	–		–		–	
SMAD2 Ser345	3.434	0.008	–		–		–	
SMAD2 Thr255	4.532	0.006	–		–		–	
SMAD3	1.441	0.032	–		–		–	

Peptides that displayed a p-value of less than 0.05 are listed.

TABLE 7 | Antibody array results.

	Antibody array		Peptide array			Homology
ID	**Fold change**	***p*-value**	**ID**	**Fold change**	***p*-value**	
Calmodulin (phospho-Thr286)	1.31	0.003	Calmodulin T185	2.99	0.008	100
CAMK2-beta (phospho-Ser33)	1.18	0.002	CAMK2-beta Ser33	1.66	0.044	100
MAP3K7 (TAK1) (phospho-431)	1.49	0.001	MAP3K7 (TAK1) Ser446	2.71	0.016	100
MAP3K7 (TAK1) (phospho-Thr187)	1.50	0.005	MAP3K7 (TAK1) T177	1.85	0.05	100
NFATC2 (phospho-Ser168/170)	1.05	0.009	NFATC2	1.76	0.045	100
NFATC4 (phospho-Ser203)	2.21	0.006	NFATC4 Ser203	2.24	0.01	100
PPP2CA (phospho-Ser307)	1.91	0.03	PPP2CA Ser304	2.45	0.003	93
SMAD1 (phospho-Ser206)	2.70	0.021	SMAD1 Ser206	2.09	0.02	100
SMAD1 (phospho-Ser462)	2.92	0.004	SMAD1 Ser462	3.43	0.008	100
SAMD2 (phospho-Thr220)	1.68	0.025	SMAD2 Thr255	4.53	0.006	93
SMAD2 (Ser350)	1.21	0.004	SMAD2 Ser345	3.43	0.008	100
SAMD3 (phospho-Thr199)	1.36	0.001	SAMD3 Thr180	1.44	0.006	93
PKCA (phosphor-Thr640)	1.18	0.036	PKCA Thr640	2.55	0.01	100
PKCA (phospho-Ser657)	1.34	0.0009	PKCA Ser659	1.74	0.04	100
PLCB (phospho-Tyr783)	−1.19668	0.03417	PLCG1 Y675	−2.78738	0.00067	86

Statistically significant ($p < 0.05$) phosphospecific antibody array results of Salmonella Entertidis cecal samples. Four days post-infection samples were compared to non-infected control samples to find changes in infected cecal tissue over time. Antibodies bound to phosphorylated protein having a statistically significant difference in fluorescent signal are shown. Fold Change Antibody Array is the change in fluorescent signal when comparing the infected samples to control samples. Homology indicates the % similarity between human and chicken at the 15 amino acid region flanking the phosphorylation residue. Fold Change Peptide Array is the change in fluorescent signal as indicated by the peptide array.

from the antibodies. The percent orthology between the human and chicken at the 15 amino acid phosphorylation target sites as determined by NCBI Protein Blast analysis is shown in **Table 7**. Following the data normalization, the results pointed to a similar pattern to that observed with the peptide arrays (**Table 7**).

Verification of Increased Ca^{2+} in Infected Cecal Tissues

Using a commercial ELISA kit to measure intracellular Ca^{2+} levels, we found almost five times more intracellular Ca^{2+} in the cecal tissue from chickens 4 days post-infection with S. Enteritidis (**Figure 2**). These results provide further proof of the activation of the non-canonical Wnt-Ca^{2+} signaling pathway during the establishment of a persistent *Salmonella* infection in the cecum.

Discussion

In chickens, *Salmonella* have evolved the capacity to survive the initial immune response and persist. Very little is known about the regulatory interactions between the host immune response and virulence mechanisms that lead to *S. enterica* persistence in the avian intestine. The carrier state, corresponding to a persistent colonization of the gut, is established, and *Salmonella* is able to stay in the ceca for months without clinical signs (10). Chronic colonization of the intestinal tract is an important aspect of persistent *Salmonella* infection because it results in a silent propagation of bacteria in poultry stocks due to the impossibility to isolate contaminated animals (11).

Collectively, the results from the current experiments demonstrate the phenotypic plasticity of the avian immune system in

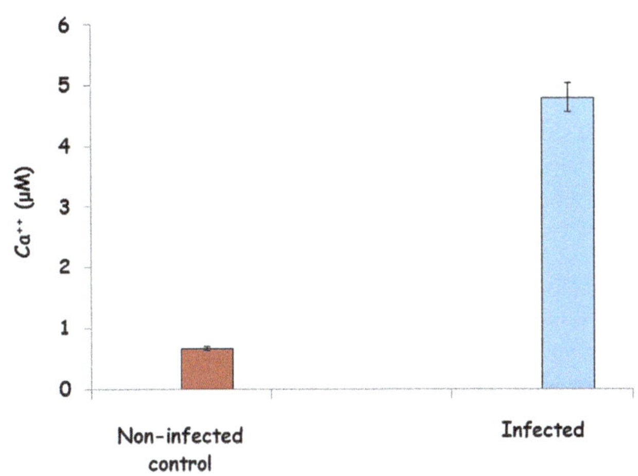

FIGURE 2 | Ca^{2+} levels in the ceca of *Salmonella*-infected and non-infected chickens 4 days post-challenge. Intracellular Ca^{2+} in cecal lysates from non-infected and infected chickens was measured with a colorimetric Ca^{2+} Detection Kit. Data represents the amount of Ca^{2+} measured in the cecal tissue from infected and non-infected chickens and are expressed as the mean micromoles of Ca^{2+} ± SEM from three separate experiments.

the gastrointestinal tract as it first orchestrates an inflammatory response against a primary *Salmonella* infection followed by a dramatic change in the immune microenvironment during the establishment of a persistent *Salmonella* infection.

The 4-day post-infection time period is the initiation of a transitional period between the acute inflammatory response to a primary *Salmonella* infection and the establishment of an "immune *status quo*" (27). As described in the present experiments, by 4 days post infection, we see a dramatic down-regulation of pro-inflammatory cytokine expression that coincides with the up-regulation of anti-inflammatory cytokine expression (**Figure 1**). Further, by day 4 post-infection, a dramatic increase in Tregs ($CD4^+CD25^+$) in the cecum and remains elevated through the 14-day post-infection time period (27). This coordinated production of pro- versus anti-inflammatory responses is fundamental for the development of an effective initial inflammatory response and subsequent return to tissue homeostasis. Finally, we used the power of kinomics to highlight the mechanisms used by *S.* Enteritidis to alter the avian inflammatory responses and uncover host signaling events that are manipulated by the bacteria in order to establish a persistent infection. Our experiments have identified multiple effects on the host kinome during the establishment of a *Salmonella* persistent infection in the avian cecum. This comparative immune kinome analysis between the *S.* Enteritidis-infected avian cecum versus non-infected cecum provides unique information on host molecular signaling cascades that are mobilized during the establishment of *Salmonella* persistence. Additionally, the relative lack of differential phosphorylation events found in the host signaling pathways between the infected and non-infected ceca 7–14 days post-infection are suggestive that a level of homeostasis was achieved and that the *Salmonella* were no longer recognized as "foreign" and were part of the commensal population. Future experiments are planned to characterize and compare this homeostasis to that of the non-infected controls. Lastly, the identified tissue protein kinases represent potential targets for future antimicrobial compounds for decreasing *Salmonella* loads from the intestines of food animals before going to market.

TGF-β Signaling Pathway

The purpose of these studies was to begin to understand and characterize the biological and molecular mechanisms that regulate the mucosal phenotype of the chicken cecum during the establishment of a persistent infection by *Salmonella*. $CD4^+CD25^+$ regulatory T cells (Tregs) are potent regulators of immune homeostasis (28). We have recently described a dramatic increase in the number of Tregs in the chicken cecum 4 days post-infection with *Salmonella* Enteritidis, and that the number of T regs remains elevated through the 14 days post-infection (29). Understanding the signals necessary for this generation and expansion of Tregs is important for understanding persistence of *Salmonella* in poultry. The pleotropic cytokine, TGF-β, plays a major role in the regulation of inflammation, with T cells being a key target (30). TGF-β suppresses T cell proliferation and T effector cell function (30) while promoting the generation and function of Treg cells (31). Here, we show a dramatic increase in TGF-β mRNA expression between 2 and 4 days after *Salmonella* challenge that remained elevated through 14 days post-infection (**Figure 1**). Simultaneously, using our chicken-specific immune kinome array, for the first time, we have characterized dramatic changes in phosphorylation events where we observed a significant increase in phosphorylation events within the TGF-β signaling pathway (**Table 6**). The TGF-β signaling pathway is mediated by a Smad transcription factor-dependent pathway (21). Upon ligand binding, the TGF-β receptor phosphorylates and activates receptor-associated Smad2 and Smad3, which then associate with Smad4 to control TGF-β-targeted gene expression (32). Both Smad2 and Smad3 are significantly phosphorylated in the ceca from *Salmonella*-infected chickens at 4 days post-infection (**Table 6**). Mitogen-activated protein kinases can also mediate TGF-β signaling through Smad-independent pathways, including TGF-β-activated kinase (TAK1 and MAP3K7), extracellular signal-regulated kinase (ERK and MAPK3), Jun-N-terminal-3-kinase (JNK and MAPK8) (33, 34), all of which are significantly phosphorylated in the ceca from the *Salmonella*-infected chickens at 4 days post-infection. Therefore, the establishment of a persistent cecal colonization in chickens by *Salmonella* initiates the activation of both the canonical (Smad-dependent) and non-canonical (Smad-independent) TGF-β signaling pathways. Smad-dependent and -independent TGF-β signaling appear to separately control Treg and non-Treg function (35). Specifically, Smad-dependent pathways appear to be required to mediate TGF-β functions in non-Treg cells, including non-T cells, whereas Smad-independent pathways are important for Treg function (35, 36). Further, Smad 2/3 are involved in the suppression of pro-inflammatory cytokines by inhibiting the activation of different signal transducers and activators of transcription (STAT) proteins, including STAT1 and 4 to inhibit IFN-γ production (37). Therefore, it is reasonable to speculate that the change in the cecal mucosal phenotype from pro-inflammatory to tolerance is at least partially mediated by the increased expression of TGF-β that results in the activation of both Smad-dependent and -independent TGF-β pathways and the increase differentiation and function of Tregs that provide the environment essential for *Salmonella* to establish a persistent infection.

Wnt Signaling Pathway

The Wnt signaling pathway system is evolutionarily conserved system that regulates a diverse series of essential functions (38, 39). There are three distinct pathways in Wnt signaling: the canonical Wnt/β-catenin and two non-canonical pathways, Wnt/Planar Cell Polarity and Wnt/Ca^{2+} pathways (39). Based on the results from the kinome array, a number of peptides from the Wnt signaling pathway exhibited statistically significant changes in their phosphorylation (**Table 5**). Further observation of these results indicates that two of the Wnt signaling pathways had significant changes in phosphorylation events, namely the canonical Wnt/β-catenin and the non-canonical Wnt/Ca^{2+} pathways.

Bacterial Effect on Canonical Wnt Signaling

The phosphorylation of two peptides in the canonical Wnt pathway was significantly altered at the 4 days after *Salmonella*-infection time point: glycogen synthase kinase 3β (GSK-3β) and β-catenin (**Table 5**). GSK-3β was significantly dephosphorylated, whereas β-catenin was significantly phosphorylated in these experiments. GSK-3β is a constitutively active serine/threonine kinase that regulates the phosphorylation and degradation of β-catenin (40). In response to external stimuli, GSK-3β is regulated by phosphorylation, inactivated by dephosphorylation of Tyr216 or activated by dephosphorylation of Ser9. The results found here determined that GSK-3β was dephosphorylated at Ser9. This site-specific phosphorylation of GSK-3β results in the activation of its kinase activity (41). In its activated form, GSK-3β forms a catalytically active complex that phosphorylates β-catenin inducing ubiquitylation and proteasomal degradation of β-catenin (39). In these studies, β-catenin was phosphorylated at Ser33 (**Tables 5** and **6**). This phosphorylation site promotes ubiquitylation and targeted destruction of β-catenin (39).

Bacterial Effect on Non-Canonical Wnt Signaling

Non-canonical Wnt signaling controls nuclear localization of nuclear factor of activated T cell (NFAT) transcriptional factor though Ca^{2+} and suppresses canonical Wnt signaling (42, 43). Using the chicken-specific kinome array (**Table 5**), Wnt antibody array (**Table 6**), and a Ca^{2+} ELISA assay (**Figure 2**), we have outlined the activation of the entire non-canonical Wnt/Ca^{2+} pathway in the cecum of chickens as *Salmonella* establishes a persistent infection beginning 4 days after infection (**Figure 3**). The Wnt5A (fold change = 1.82696, $p < 0.0001$)/frizzled 1 receptor complex induces the influx of intracellular Ca^{2+} that, in turn, phosphorylates calcinuerin, a Ca^{2+}, calmodulin-dependent serine/threonine protein phosphatase. Phosphorylated calcinuerin phosphorylates both calmodulin-dependent kinase II (CaMK2A)

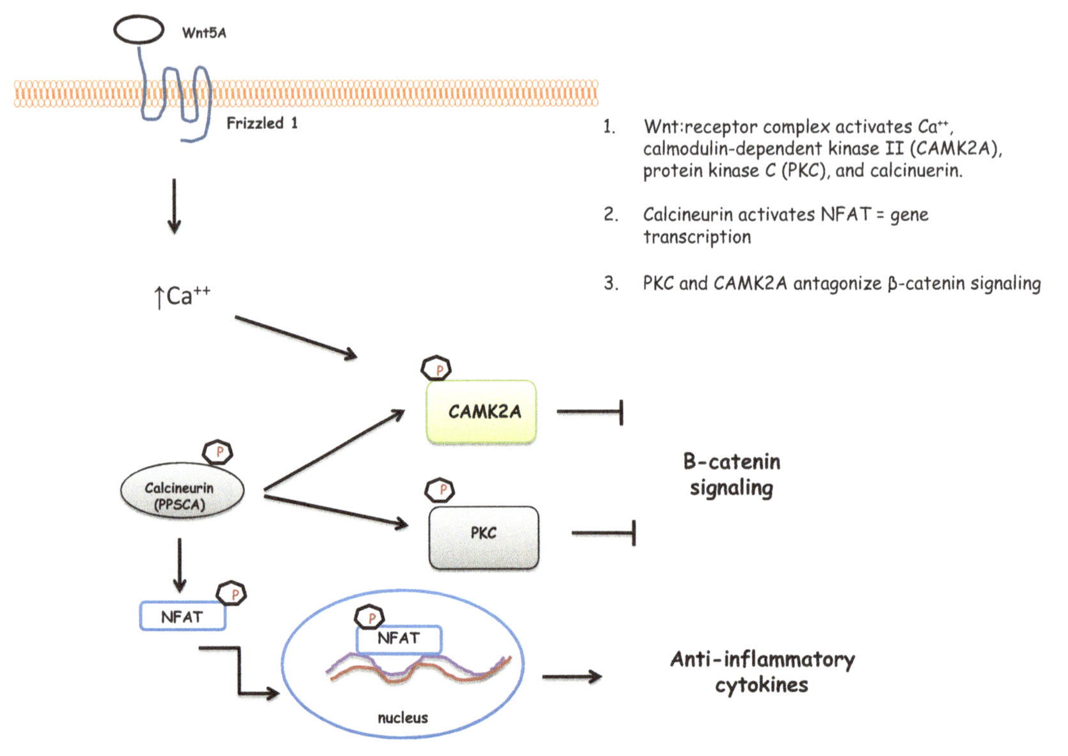

FIGURE 3 | A schematic of the proposed non-canonical Wnt signaling pathway induced in the ceca from experimental chickens with persistent colonization by *Salmonella* Enteritidis.

and PKC and activates NFAT, which can then translocate to the nuclease to induce gene transcription (44). NFAT functions to regulate the interaction of the innate immune cells with acquired immunity and to promote anti-inflammatory programs (45). Thus, the increased phosphorylation of NFAT peptides would suggest the initiation of anti-inflammatory signals. Further, Ca^{2+}/calcineurin/NFAT pathway is crucial for both development and function of regulatory T cells (46). Lastly, NF-κB (nuclear factor kappa-light-chain-enhancer of activated B cells) is a transcription factor that plays a key role in regulating the pro-inflammatory response whose activity is triggered in response to infectious agents and pro-inflammatory cytokines via the IκB kinase (IKK) complex (47, 48). Thus, dephosphorylation of both IKK (Thr37, fold change = −1.63995, $p < 0.0024$; Ser194, fold change = −2.86736, $p < 5 \times 10^5$) and NF-κB (NF-κB1 p105, Ser342, fold change = −31.2387, $p < 0.025$) would result in a down-regulation of pro-inflammatory cytokines, as we observed in the present experiments (**Figure 1**).

In summary, the results from the present studies, taken together with our previous studies with Treg, provide solid evidence of a phenotypic change in the mucosal microenvironment that allows for the establishment of a persistent infection by *S.* Enteritidis in the avian cecum. The phenotype alteration appears to be partially mediated due to the targeting of signaling cascades, such as the non-canonical Wnt/Ca^{2+} and the TGF-β signaling pathways that inhibit the transcription of pro-inflammatory responses that provide an appropriate local environment for the generation and expansion of Tregs.

References

1. CDC (Centers for Disease Control and Prevention). *National Salmonella Surveillance Overview 2011* (2011). Available from: http://www.cdc.gov/ncezid/dfwed/PDFs/salmonella-annual-summary-2009-508c.pdf
2. Rodrigue DC, Tauxe RV, Rowe B. International increase in *Salmonella enteritidis*: a new pandemic? *Epidemiol Infect* (1990) **105**:21–7. doi:10.1017/S0950268800047609
3. Barrow PA. The paratyphoid *Salmonellae*. *Rev Sci Tech* (2000) **19**:351–75.
4. Gopinath S, Carden S, Monack D. Shedding light on *Salmonella* carriers. *Trends Immunol* (2012) **20**:320–7. doi:10.1016/j.tim.2012.04.004
5. Santos RL, Raffatellu M, Bevins CL, Adams LG, Tükel C, Tsolis RM, et al. Life in the inflamed intestine, *Salmonella* style. *Trends Microbiol* (2009) **17**:498–506. doi:10.1016/j.tim.2009.08.008
6. Smith HW, Tucker JF. The virulence of *Salmonella* strains for chickens: their excretion by infected chickens. *J Hyg (Lond)* (1975) **84**:479–88. doi:10.1017/S0022172400027017
7. Barrow PA, Lovell MA. Experimental infection of egg-laying hens with *Salmonella enteritidis*. *Avian Pathol* (1991) **20**:339–52. doi:10.1080/03079459108418769
8. Barrow PA, Huggins MB, Lovell MA, Simpson JM. Observations on the pathogenesis of experimental *Salmonella typhimurium* infection in chickens. *Res Vet Sci* (1987) **42**:194–9.
9. Guillot J, Beaumont C, Bellatif F, Mouline C, Lantier F, Colin P, et al. Comparison of resistance of various poultry lines to infection by *Salmonella enteritidis*. *Vet Res* (1995) **26**:81–6.
10. Duchet-Suchaux M, Léchopier P, Marly J, Bernardet P, Delaunay R, Pardon P. Quantification of experimental *Salmonella enteritidis* carrier state in B13 leghorn chicks. *Avian Dis* (1995) **39**:796–803. doi:10.2307/1592416
11. Lawley TD, Bouley DA, Hoy YE, Gerke C, Relman DA, Monack DM. Host transmission of *Salmonella enterica* serovar Typhimurium is controlled by virulence factors and indigenous intestinal microbiota. *Infect Immun* (2008) **76**:403–16. doi:10.1128/IAI.01189-07
12. Chausse A-M, Grepinet O, Bottreau E, Robert V, Hennequet-Antier C, Lalmanach A-C, et al. Susceptibility to *Salmonella* carrier-state: a possible Th2 response un susceptible chicks. *Vet Immunol Immunopathol* (2014) **159**:16–28. doi:10.1016/j.vetimm.2014.03.001
13. Eisele NA, Ruby T, Jacobson A, Manzanillo PS, Cox JS, Lam L, et al. *Salmonella* require the fatty acid regulator PPARδ for the establishment of a metabolic environment essential for long-term persistence. *Cell Host Microbe* (2013) **14**:171–82. doi:10.1016/j.chom.2013.07.010
14. Johanns TM, Ertelt JM, Rowe JH, Way SS. Regulatory T cell suppressive potency dictates the balance between bacterial proliferation and clearance during persistent *Salmonella* infection. *PLoS Pathog* (2010) **6**:e1001043. doi:10.1371/journal.ppat.1001043
15. Arsenault R, Kogut MH. Chicken-specific peptide arrays for kinome analysis: flight for the flightless. *Curr Top Biotechnol* (2013) **7**:79–89.
16. Arsenault R, Napper S, Kogut MH. *Salmonella enterica* Typhimurium infection causes metabolic changes in chicken muscle involving AMPK, fatty acid and insulin/mTOR signaling. *Vet Res* (2013) **44**:35. doi:10.1186/1297-9716-44-35
17. Arsenault R, Kogut MH, He H. Combined CpG and poly I:C stimulation of monocytes results in unique signaling activation not observed with the individual ligands. *Cell Signal* (2013) **2**:2246–54. doi:10.1016/j.cellsig.2013.07.014
18. National Research Council. *Nutritional Requirements of Poultry*. 9th ed. Washington, DC: National Academy Press (1994).
19. Andrews WH, Poelma PL, Wilson CR, Romero A. Isolation and identification of *Salmonella*. 5th ed. *Bacteriological Analytical Manual*. Washington, DC: Association of Analytical Chemists (1978). p. 1–29.
20. Jalal S, Arsenault R, Potter AA, Babiuk LA, Griebel PJ, Napper S. Genome to kinome: species-specific peptide arrays for kinome analysis. *Sci Signal* (2009) **2**:l1. doi:10.1126/scisignal.254pl1
21. Li Y, Arsenault RJ, Trost B, Slind J, Griebel PJ, Napper S, et al. A systematic approach for analysis of peptide array kinome data. *Sci Signal* (2012) **5**:l2. doi:10.1126/scisignal.2002429
22. Szklarczyk D, Franceschini A, Kuhn M, Simonovic M, Roth A, Minguez P, et al. The STRING database in 2011: functional interaction networks of proteins, globally integrated and scored. *Nucleic Acids Res* (2011) **39**(Suppl 1):D561–8. doi:10.1093/nar/gkq973
23. Kaiser P, Rothwell L, Galyov EE, Barrow PA, Burnside J, Wigley P. Differential cytokine expression in avian cells in response to invasion by *Salmonella typhimurium*, *Salmonella enteritidis* and *Salmonella gallinarum*. *Microbiology* (2000) **146**:3217–26. doi:10.1099/00221287-146-12-3217
24. Kogut MH, Rothwell L, Kaiser P. Differential regulation of cytokine gene expression by avian heterophils during receptor-mediated phagocytosis of opsonized and nonopsonized *Salmonella enteritidis*. *J Interferon Cytokine Res* (2003) **23**:319–27. doi:10.1089/107999003766628160
25. Wathanage GS, Kaiser P, Wigley P, Powers C, Mastroeni P, Brooks H, et al. Rapid expression of chemokines and pro-inflammatory cytokines in newly hatched chickens infected with *Salmonella enterica* serovar Typhimurium. *Infect Immun* (2004) **72**:2152–9. doi:10.1128/IAI.72.4.2152-2159.2004
26. Lamouille S, Derynck R. Cell size and invasion in TGF-β-induced epithelial to mesenchymal transition is regulated by activation of tem TOR pathway. *J Cell Biol* (2007) **178**:437–51. doi:10.1083/jcb.200608033
27. Ruby T, McLaughlin L, Gopinath S, Monack D. *Salmonella's* long-term relationship with its host. *FEMS Microbiol Rev* (2012) **36**:600–15. doi:10.1111/j.1574-6976.2012.00332.x
28. Belkaid Y. Regulatory T cells and infection: a dangerous necessity. *Nat Rev Immunol* (2007) **7**:875–88. doi:10.1038/nri2189
29. Shanmugasundarm R, Kogut MH, Arsenault RJ, Swaggerty CL, Cole K, Reddish MJ, et al. Effect of *Salmonella* infection on cecal tonsil T regulatory T cell properties in the chicken. *Poult Sci* (2015) **94**(8):1828–35. doi:10.3382/ps/pev161
30. Sakaguchi S. Naturally arising CD4+ regulatory T cells for immunologic self-tolerance and negative control of immune responses. *Annu Rev Immunol* (2004) **22**:531–62. doi:10.1146/annurev.immunol.21.120601.141122
31. Rubtsov YP, Rudesky AY. TGFbeta signaling in control of T-cell-mediated self-reactivity. *Nat Rev Immunol* (2007) **7**:443–53. doi:10.1038/nri2095
32. Li MO, Wan YY, Sanjabi S, Robertson AK, Flavell RA. Transforming growth factor-beta regulation of immune responses. *Annu Rev Immunol* (2006) **24**:99–146. doi:10.1146/annurev.immunol.24.021605.090737

33. Derynck R, Zhang YE. Smad-dependent and Smad-independent pathways in TGF-beta family signaling. *Nature* (2003) **425**:577–84. doi:10.1038/nature02006
34. Yu L, Hebert MC, Zhang YE. TGF-β receptor-activated p38 MAP kinase mediates Smad-independent TGF-β responses. *EMBO J* (2002) **21**:3749–59. doi:10.1093/emboj/cdf366
35. Gu AD, Wang Y, Lin L, Zhang SS, Wan YY. Requirements of transcription factor Smad-dependent and -independent TGF-β signaling to control discrete T-cell functions. *Proc Natl Acad Sci U S A* (2012) **109**:905–10. doi:10.1073/pnas.1108352109
36. Shi Y, Massague J. Mechanisms of TGF-beta signaling from cell membrane to the nuclease. *Cell* (2003) **113**:685–700. doi:10.1016/S0092-8674(03)00432-X
37. Yoshimura A, Wakabayashi Y, Mori T. Cellular and molecular basis for the regulation of inflammation by TGF-β. *J Biochem* (2010) **147**:781–92. doi:10.1093/jb/mvq043
38. Angers J, Moon RT. Proximal events in Wnt signal transduction. *Nat Rev Mol Cell Biol* (2009) **10**:468–77. doi:10.1038/nrm2717
39. Gordon MD, Nusse R. Wnt signaling, multiple pathways, multiple receptors, and multiple transcription factors. *J Biol Chem* (2006) **281**:22429–33. doi:10.1074/jbc.R600015200
40. Doble BW, Woodgett JD. GSK-3L tricks of the trade for a multi-tasking kinase. *J Cell Sci* (2003) **116**:1175–86. doi:10.1242/jcs.00384
41. Cross DA, Alessi DR, Cohen P, Andjelkovich M, Hemmigs BA. Inhibition of glycogen synthase kinase-3 by insulin mediated by protein kinase B. *Nature* (1995) **178**:785–9. doi:10.1038/378785a0
42. Mikels AJ, Nusse R. Purified Wnt5a protein activates or inhibits beta-catenin-TCF signaling depending on receptor context. *PLoS Biol* (2006) **4**:e115. doi:10.1371/journal.pbio.0040115
43. Murphy LL, Hughes CC. Endothelial cells stimulate T cell NFAT nuclear translocation in the presence of cyclosporin A: involvement of the wnt/glycogen synthase kinase-3 beta pathway. *J Immunol* (2002) **169**:3717–25. doi:10.4049/jimmunol.169.7.3717
44. Baine I, Abe BT, Macian F. Regulatory T-cell tolerance by calcium/NFT signaling. *Immunol Rev* (2009) **231**:225–40. doi:10.1111/j.1600-065X.2009.00817.x
45. Zanoni I, Granucci F. Regulation and dysregulation of innate immunity by NFAT signaling downstream of pattern recognition receptors (PRRs). *Eur J Immunol* (2012) **42**:1924–31. doi:10.1002/eji.201242580
46. Oh-hora M, Rao A. The calcium/NFAT pathway: role in development and function of regulatory T cells. *Microbes Infect* (2009) **11**:612–9. doi:10.1016/j.micinf.2009.04.008
47. Dev A, Iywe S, Razani B, Cheng G. NF-kappaB and innate immunity. *Curr Top Microbiol Immunol* (2011) **349**:115–43. doi:10.1007/82_2010_102
48. Hacker H, Karin M. Regulation and function of IKK and IKK-related kinases. *Sci STKE* (2006) **2006**:re13. doi:10.1126/stke.3572006re13

Conflict of Interest Statement: The authors declare that the research was conducted in the absence of any commercial or financial relationships that could be construed as a potential conflict of interest.

9

Temporal Relationships Exist Between Cecum, Ileum, and Litter Bacterial Microbiomes in a Commercial Turkey Flock, and Subtherapeutic Penicillin Treatment Impacts Ileum Bacterial Community Establishment

*Jessica L. Danzeisen[1], Jonathan B. Clayton[1], Hu Huang[2], Dan Knights[2,3,4], Brian McComb[5], Shivdeep S. Hayer[1] and Timothy J. Johnson[1,6]**

[1] *Department of Veterinary and Biomedical Sciences, University of Minnesota, Saint Paul, MN, USA,* [2] *Department of Biomedical Informatics and Computational Biology, University of Minnesota, Minneapolis, MN, USA,* [3] *Department of Computer Science and Engineering, University of Minnesota, Minneapolis, MN, USA,* [4] *Biotechnology Institute, University of Minnesota, Saint Paul, MN, USA,* [5] *Willmar Poultry Company, Willmar, MN, USA,* [6] *Mid-Central Research and Outreach Center, University of Minnesota, Willmar, MN, USA*

Edited by:
Ryan Arsenault,
University of Delaware, USA

Reviewed by:
Carl James Yeoman,
Montana State University, USA
Filip Boyen,
Ghent University, Belgium

***Correspondence:**
Timothy J. Johnson
joh04207@umn.edu

Gut health is paramount for commercial poultry production, and improved methods to assess gut health are critically needed to better understand how the avian gastrointestinal tract matures over time. One important aspect of gut health is the totality of bacterial populations inhabiting different sites of the avian gastrointestinal tract, and associations of these populations with the poultry farm environment, since these bacteria are thought to drive metabolism and prime the developing host immune system. In this study, a single flock of commercial turkeys was followed over the course of 12 weeks to examine bacterial microbiome inhabiting the ceca, ileum, and corresponding poultry litter. Furthermore, the effects of low-dose, growth-promoting penicillin treatment (50 g/ton) in feed on the ileum bacterial microbiome were also examined during the early brood period. The cecum and ileum bacterial communities of turkeys were distinct, yet shifted in parallel to one another over time during bird maturation. Corresponding poultry litter was also distinct yet more closely represented the ileal bacterial populations than cecal bacterial populations, and also changed parallel to ileum bacterial populations over time. Penicillin applied at low dose in feed significantly enhanced early weight gain in commercial poults, and this correlated with predictable shifts in the ileum bacterial populations in control versus treatment groups. Overall, this study identified the dynamics of the turkey gastrointestinal microbiome during development, correlations between bacterial populations in the gastrointestinal tract and the litter environment, and the impact of low-dose penicillin on modulation of bacterial communities in the ileum. Such modulations provide a target for alternatives to low-dose antibiotics.

Keywords: poultry, avian, Turkey, bacteria, penicillin, microbiome, antibiotic, growth promoter

INTRODUCTION

Turkey meat is one of the leanest meat sources of protein available, and its production is a multibillion dollar per year U.S. industry (1). Nearly 250 million turkeys are grown each year, making the U.S. the world's largest producer of turkeys and the biggest exporter of turkey products. The U.S. produces 7.5 billion pounds of turkey meat per year, and this number is steadily increasing.

The gastrointestinal health of an animal is key to its successful growth and development. For many years, gut health and development in U.S. commercial poultry has been routinely managed through the use of low-dose levels of antibiotics in feed to prevent diseases, improve overall flock consistency, and increase final body weights (2). Even with the use of low-dose antibiotics, gut health issues still occur. For example, turkey flocks are still plagued by a condition known as "Light Turkey Syndrome," or LTS (3, 4). LTS has not been attributed to any known pathogen or management practice (3), yet some farms yield market weights 1–3 pounds below the national average, using the same source of poults as farms achieving these weight goals. Higher doses of some antibiotics can alleviate these problems, but they present their own set of problems related to the development of antibiotic resistant bacterial pathogens that threaten both human and animal health. With an ongoing movement to withdraw the use of low-dose antibiotics on poultry farms, alternatives to antibiotics are greatly needed to sustain health and performance in commercial turkey flocks.

In the avian intestinal bacterial community, it is well established that great differences exist from a spatial (proximal to distal) standpoint (5). The chicken ileum and ceca alone are thought to harbor at least 10^8 and 10^{11} organisms per gram of digesta, respectively (6), and this density is achieved within days after hatch (6). However, the taxonomic composition of these microbes changes rapidly during the first week of development. Early studies involving denaturing gradient gel electrophoresis (DGGE) revealed that the chicken cecal microbiome, while quite diverse, is dominated by a small subset of conserved bacterial species in mature birds (7, 8). In general, the cecal microbiome is dominated by Clostridiales, and the small intestine is dominated by Lactobacillales (9). However, the avian microbiome is highly dependent on bird age, and there is great diversity at the bacterial species level (10). Most microbiome-based studies in both chickens and turkeys have focused on the microbiome related to carriage of pathogens (11–13). Because of a primary emphasis on pathogens in the more distal portions of the intestinal tract, fewer studies have examined the ileum microbiome. Pioneering work by Lu et al. examined the ileal and cecal bacterial communities of the chicken during bird development (14). They found that the broiler ileum was dominated by Lactobacillaceae, whereas the cecum was dominated by Clostridiaceae.

A number of studies have sought to examine the effects of antibiotic growth promoters (AGPs) on the intestinal microbiome. For example, virginiamycin and other AGPs applied in broilers were shown to exert the greatest modulatory effect on the proximal small intestinal microbiome correlating with increased average daily weight gain, as compared to the distal intestine and ceca (9, 15). Several AGPs [avilamycin, bacitracin methylene disalicylate (BMD), and enramycin] applied to broilers housed in floor pens resulted in improvements in growth performance, grossly correlated with changes to the intestinal microbiota (16). An interesting result validated through multiple studies is that AGP treatment decreased bacterial diversity in the avian ileum and decreased *Lactobacillus* populations (17–19). AGPs also appear to decrease bird-to-bird variations in weight and performance (20).

Penicillin G procaine has been shown to enhance weight gain and feed efficiency in commercial poultry (2). However, the underlying mechanisms by which administration of penicillin in feed is effective have not been fully examined. The purpose of this study was to define the baseline correlations between the bacterial populations inhabiting the turkey cecum, ileum, and surrounding litter environment and to assess the impact of penicillin in feed on the ileum bacterial microbiome of turkeys during the early brood period when the turkey gastrointestinal microbiome is most dynamic (10).

MATERIALS AND METHODS

Study Design

All studies were performed on commercial turkeys; therefore, ethical standards for commercial turkey production were followed by the company performing the study. Animals were euthanized using methods approved by the American Veterinary Medical Association. Two trials were performed at a commercial turkey research facility in Willmar, Minnesota. The barn was divided into 24 pens, with 16 pens on one half of the barn each housing 1,500 turkey poults, and 8 pens on the other half of the barn each housing 3,000 birds. Feed was mixed and supplied using a Feedlogic robot (Feedlogic Corporation, Willmar, MN, USA). In the first trial, Hybrid Converter female poults (Willmar Poultry Company, Willmar, MN, USA) were placed at day-of-hatch into a pen housing 3,000 birds. At days 7, 14, 21, 28, 35, 42, 56, 70, and 84, five birds were randomly selected and euthanized. For this trial, birds were moved to a commercial grow-out facility at 5 weeks and were separated from other commercial birds by fencing within the grow-out barn. They were subsequently raised under standard commercial turkey management practices. The following measurements were taken from each bird sampled: total body weight, intestinal weight, intestinal length, and cecal score. Cecal score was recorded throughout the study by a single person blinded to the experimental groups. The scoring system ranged from 0 to 3, based upon consistency, color, and gas present in the cecal contents. A score of 0 indicated pasty and dark brown cecal content; a score of 1 indicated changes in consistency toward watery but still dark brown content; a score of 2 indicated changes in color and consistency of the cecal contents toward watery and yellow color; and a score of 3 indicated watery, gassy, and yellow-colored cecal content. Both ceca and the ileum from euthanized poults were aseptically collected intact, homogenized, and frozen at −20°C for future processing. Grab litter samples of representative bedding from each group were aseptically collected in whirl-pak bags at the same time points. Each litter sample collected was composed of a pool of five samples collected randomly from dry areas in the barn not including fecal or cecal droppings.

In the second trial, four pens were used, including two replicates each of control and treatment groups. Birds were immediately placed on standard feed containing 50 g/ton of BMD for control birds, and 50 g/ton BMD plus 50 g/ton penicillin G procaine for treatment birds. At days 7, 14, and 21, five birds per pen were randomly selected and euthanized. The following measurements were taken: total body weight, intestinal weight, intestinal length, and cecal score. Ilea from euthanized poults were aseptically collected intact, homogenized, and frozen at −20°C for future processing.

Sample Processing and Sequencing

DNA was extracted using a bead-beating procedure and the QIAmp® DNA Stool Kit (Qiagen, Valencia, CA, USA) as previously described (21). PCR was used to amplify the V3 hypervariable region of the 16S rRNA gene using primers containing Illumina barcoding and sequencing primers, as well as sample-specific barcodes on the reverse primers, as previously described (22). The PCR conditions used were an initial denaturation step at 95°C for 2 min, followed by 25 cycles of 95°C for 30 s, 60°C for 30 s, and 72°C for 30 s, with a final extension at 72°C for 7 min. The PCR product was excised from a 1.5% gel and purified using the QIAquick Gel Extraction Kit following manufacturer's instructions (Qiagen). Sample DNA quality and quantity were assessed on a Bioanalyzer 2100 (Agilent, Palo Alto, CA, USA) using a DNA-1000 lab chip. Sequencing was performed at the University of Minnesota Genomics Center using Illumina MiSeq paired-end 2 × 250 bp technology.

Data Analyses

Following sequencing, sorting by barcode was performed to generate fastq files for each sample. Paired-end reads were assembled and quality screened using Pandaseq, using a threshold quality cut-off value of 0.6 and eliminating any assembled reads with ambiguous base calls (23). Proximal and distal primers were trimmed from the sequence reads. Random subsets of 20,000 high-quality reads per sample for Trial #1 and 40,000 reads per sample for Trial #2 were selected using the sub.sample approach in Mothur (24). In total, 45 cecum samples, 45 ileum samples, and 16 pooled litter samples were analyzed from Trial #1 (2.12 million reads), and 30 ileum samples were analyzed from Trial #2 (1.2 million reads). A *de novo* operational taxonomic unit (OTU) picking approach was used in QIIME (25) using uclust (26) independently for each dataset (Trial #1 and Trial #2). OTUs containing <25 sequences were removed to eliminate possible spurious OTUs due to sequencing error. Potential chimeras were removed using ChimeraSlayer (27). QIIME was used for assessments of alpha diversity, beta diversity using Unifrac (28), and phylogenetic classifications using the RDP database (29). Differential abundances of OTUs and other phylogenetic classifications were identified using METASTATS (30). Construction of heatmaps was performed using the R statistical software (31). Statistical analyses for differences in community structure were performed using distance matrices analyzed via the AMOVA command in Mothur (24). A paired two-sample *t*-test was used to statistically compare total body weights, intestinal weights, intestinal lengths, and cecal scores at each time point during trial #2.

The data from this project is freely available at the Data Repository for the University of Minnesota (DRUM) at the following link: http://hdl.handle.net/11299/174930.

RESULTS

Trial #1: Relationships Between Cecum, Ileum, and Litter Bacterial Microbiomes During Flock Succession

In Trial #1, 38,861 OTUs were identified using open reference OTU picking. Our goal was to assess the dominant bacterial populations and avoid spurious OTU calling due to sequencing error. After removing OTUs with <25 total sequencing reads, 1,101 OTUs remained in the dataset. Using the greengenes database, OTUs were classified at the bacterial class level (**Figure 1**). In cecal samples, Clostridia was the dominant class (>70% of the population) throughout trial 1 with lower levels of Bacteroidia (5–20% of the population) appearing at 28 days and beyond. Levels of Gammaproteobacteria remained low throughout, typically <1% of the total population. In contrast, Bacilli was the dominant bacterial class in ileum samples throughout trial 1 (50–90% of the population), with levels of Clostridia increasing (0–75% of the population) throughout the study. Gammaproteobacteria were high (up to 50% of the population) in ileum samples at day 7, then decreased substantially in the subsequent weeks. Actinobacteria also increased in abundance in ileum samples (5–30% of the population) at day 28 and beyond. Litter samples were distinct from both ceca and ileum in terms of bacterial class composition, but more closely represented ileum samples than ceca samples. Notably, Gammaproteobacteria and Actinobacteria were of substantially higher relative abundance in litter samples at day 7 and days 21–56, respectively.

Using an OTU-based approach, bacterial species richness was highest in ceca samples throughout the study, followed by litter and ileum samples (**Figure 2**). Species richness increased in samples through 35 days, when the birds were moved to a commercial grow-out barn. At day 42, following movement to the grow-out barn and change in feed to reduced protein composition, bacterial species richness decreased in the ceca and litter samples but remained the same in ileum samples. At day 56, bacterial species richness in these samples increased to pre-movement levels or greater. Ileum and ceca samples continued to increase in species richness through day 84. Using a non-parametric two-sample *t*-test with Bonferroni correction, alpha diversity measurements were significantly different ($P = 0.003$) comparing ileum versus cecum samples ($P = 0.003$) and litter versus cecum samples ($P = 0.003$), but not ileum versus litter samples.

Community-level similarities in the bacterial microbiome of samples were compared using principal coordinates analysis (PCoA; **Figure 3**). Samples were stratified primarily by age of flock, and also separated by sample type. Using AMOVA based upon distance matrix, bacterial communities from all three sample types were distinct ($P < 0.001$). Upon visualization of the PCoA plots, litter and ileum samples had some overlap, while both of these sample types were clearly distinct from cecal samples. However, all sample types shifted similarly over time on the plot, indicating that bird age has a predominant impact on the barn bacterial microbiome irrespective of sample type.

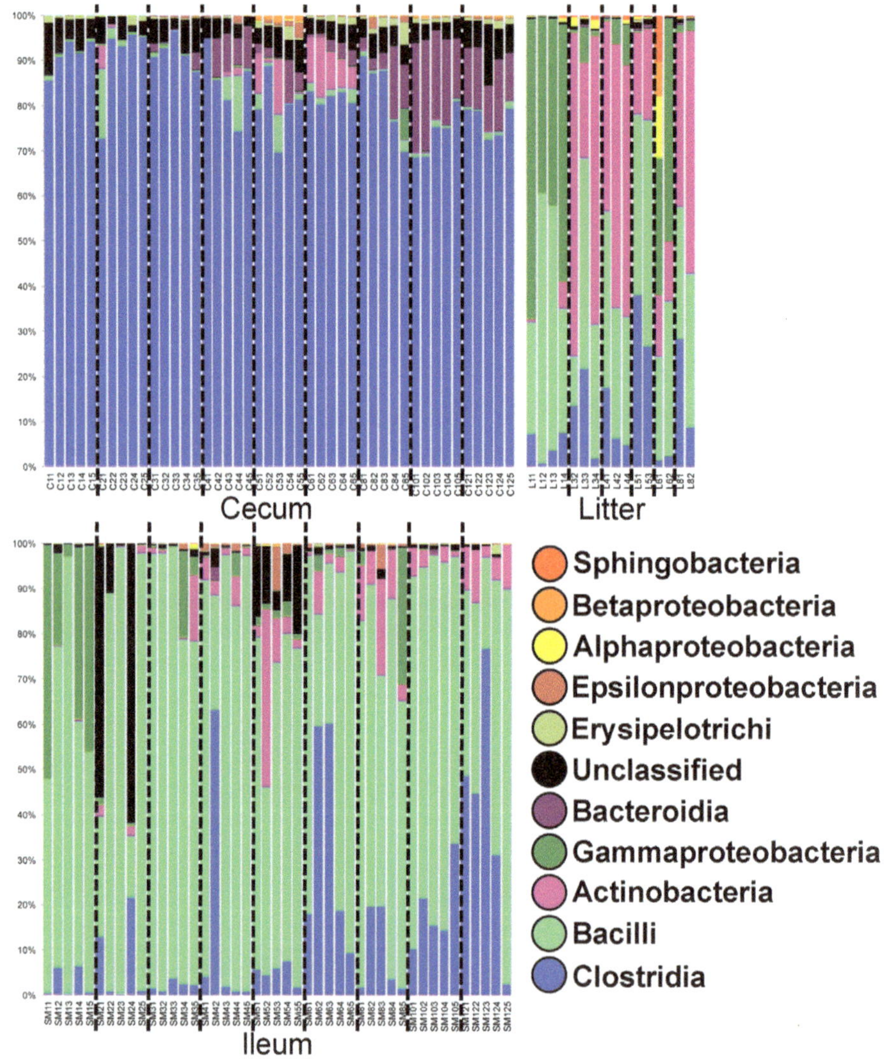

FIGURE 1 | Class-level taxonomic compositions of bacterial microbiome samples in Trial #1. For each sample type (ileum = SM, litter = L, and cecum = C) individual samples are depicted by age (weeks 1–12) followed by bird number (1–5). Black dashed lines divide samples by age.

Samples were also analyzed at the OTU level for specific subsets of OTUs representing sample types and age (Figure S1 in Supplementary Material; **Figure 4**). It was clear from this analysis that there were shared subsets of OTUs present across all samples, unique subsets that were defining of a particular sample type(s), and OTUs that were dependent on flock age. For example, numerous OTUs were identified belonging to the phylum Firmicutes and class Clostridia that were dominant in cecal samples, and present in ileum and litter samples but at much lower abundance. Similarly, OTUs belonging to phylum Firmicutes and class Bacilli were dominant in ileum and litter samples but present in cecal samples at much lower abundance. OTUs classified at the genus level such as *Brachybacterium*, *Brevibacterium*, *Staphylococcus*, *Corynebacterium*, *Jeotgalicoccus*, and *Weissella* were found in ileum and litter samples, but were absent from cecal samples. An OTU that we had previously identified as Candidatus division Arthromitus (10) was identified in ileum samples but not found in litter or cecal samples. Finally, some OTUs displayed a temporal trend and were found more prominently in later-aged samples, such as those classified as *Lactobacillus aviarius*, *Lactobacillus johnsonii*, Clostridium group XI, *Megamonas*, and *Lactobacillus ingluviei*. OTU-based clustering of the sample confirmed what was observed with PCoA-based analysis, with cecum samples clearly separating from ileum/litter samples which contained considerable overlap in bacterial microbiome composition (Figure S2 in Supplementary Material).

Trial #2: Effects of Low-Dose Penicillin Treatment on the Ileum Bacterial Microbiome

The effect of low-dose penicillin (50 g/ton) in feed on commercial turkey poults was examined in a second trial. Total bird weights were significantly higher at days 14 and 21 in the penicillin-treated

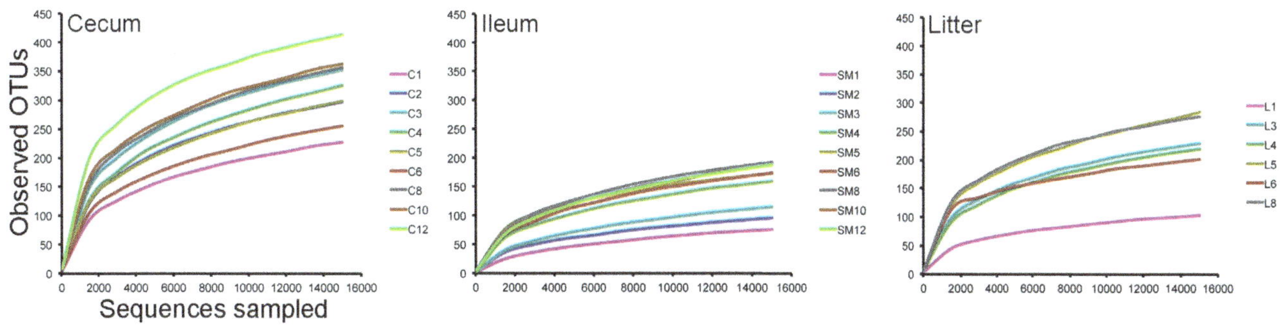

FIGURE 2 | Rarefaction curves of cecum, ileum, and litter samples. Legends refer to sample type (C = cecum, SM = ileum, L = litter) and weeks of age (1–12) for each sample type.

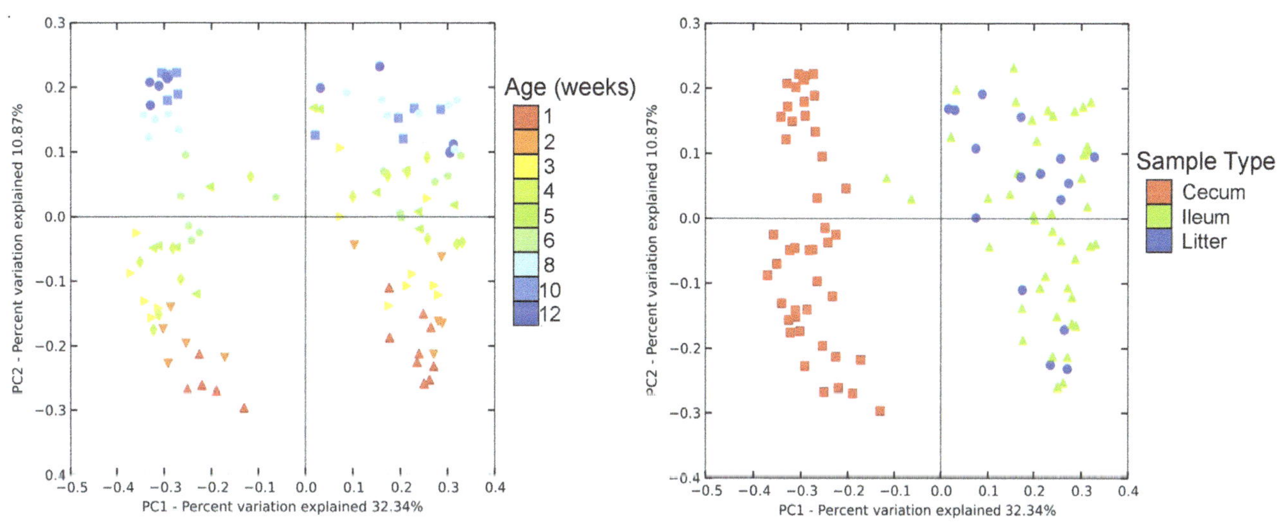

FIGURE 3 | Principal coordinates analysis (PCoA) of individual samples from turkey cecum, ileum, and litter within a single flock. Left image depicts PCoA by flock age, and right image depicts PCoA by sample type.

groups compared to control groups (**Table 1**; $P < 0.05$). Intestinal weights and lengths were also significantly higher in penicillin-treated groups at day 21 ($P < 0.05$), but cecal score was unaffected (**Table 2**).

Analysis of the ileum bacterial microbiome was performed on five individual birds per treatment group and time point to determine if there were shifts in the microbiome associated with penicillin treatment. In total, 7,857 OTUs were identified from these samples using open reference OTU picking. After removing OTUs with <25 total sequencing reads, 786 OTUs remained in the dataset. OTUs were examined by treatment group and flock age (**Figure 5**), and hierarchical clustering suggested that penicillin treatment had effects on the ileum bacterial microbiome at weeks 2 and 3. AMOVA also revealed significantly different community structures in the control versus penicillin-treated groups at days 14 ($P = 0.003$) and 21 ($P < 0.001$). Using METASTATS comparison, OTUs that were of significantly higher abundance ($P < 0.05$) at days 14 and 21 in penicillin-treated groups included those classified as *L. aviarius*, *L. johnsonii*, *Streptococcus* sp., and several other *Lactobacillus* spp. that were unclassified beyond genus level (Data Sheet S1 in Supplementary Material). A PCoA plot confirmed bacterial community differences between control and treatment groups, with day 14 and day 21 samples shifted on the plot in the penicillin-treated groups (**Figure 6**). Shannon diversity and species richness were also assessed, and at days 7 and 14, the penicillin-treated groups were significantly increased compared to the control groups ($P < 0.05$) (Figure S3 in Supplementary Material).

DISCUSSION

Recent bans on the use of AGPs in the European Union (EU) broiler industry have been associated with numerous production-associated problems, including decreased feed

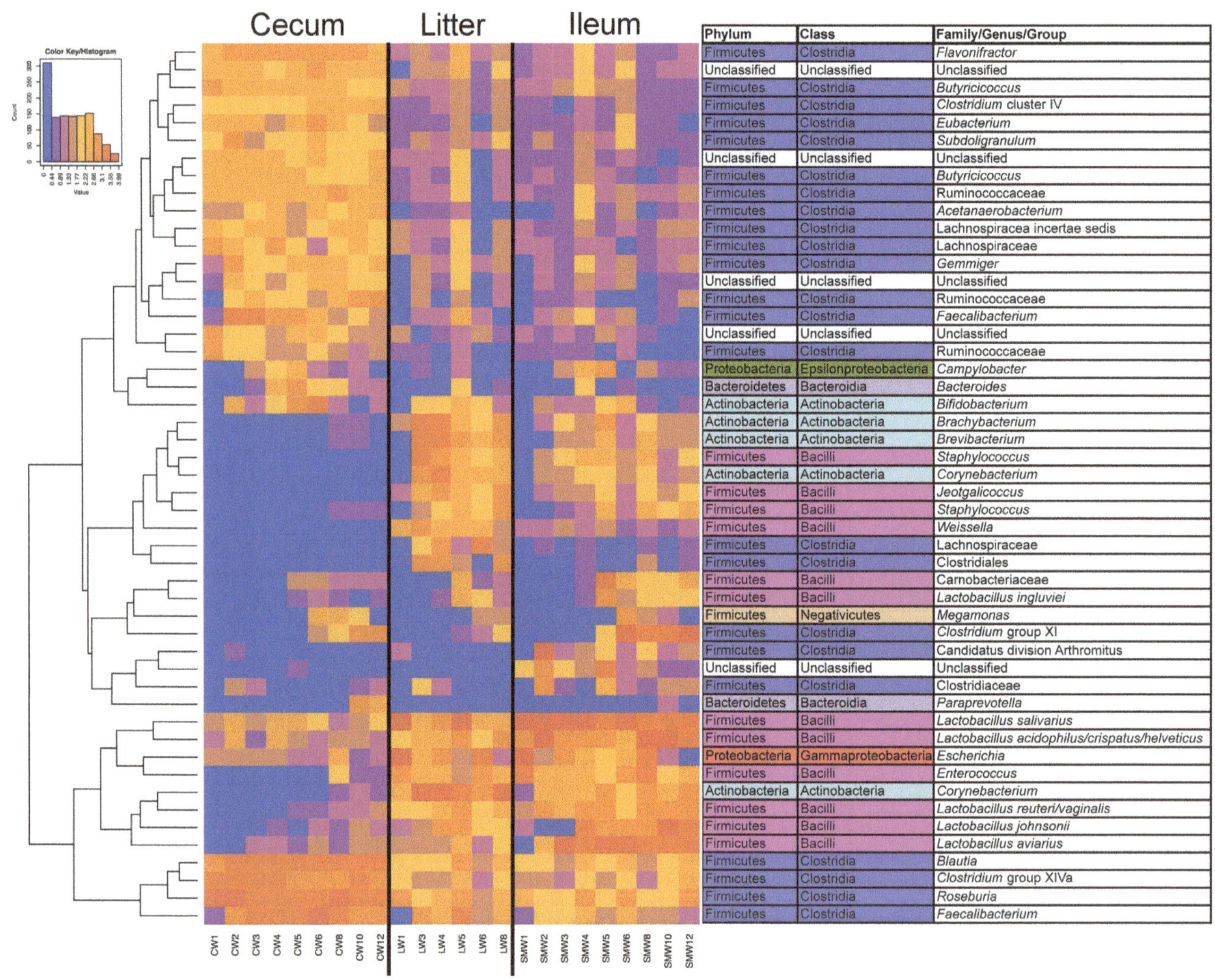

FIGURE 4 | Heatmap depicting abundance of the top 50 OTUs by overall abundance across samples, averaged by age/sample. Heatmap was constructed using normalized $\log_{10}$ abundance of each OTU in each sample type. To the right of the heatmap is a table depicting classification of each OTU using RDP database assignment or best-hit classification where appropriate. "W" depicts the age of sample in weeks.

TABLE 1 | Total body weights of turkeys treated with and without 50 g/ton of penicillin in feed.

	Day 7 weight (g)		Day 14 weight (g)		Day 21 weight (g)	
	Control	Penicillin	Control	Penicillin	Control	Penicillin
Average weight replicate 1	148.4	156.4	338	390.8[a]	665.8	779.8[a]
Average weight replicate 2	141.6	152.4	302.6	378.4[a]	664.4	736.8[a]
Standard deviation overall	21.6	18.0	54.1	44.5	111.2	59.4

[a]*Significantly different from control group ($P < 0.05$) using Student's t-test.*

efficiency, watery feces, and disease, among other conditions (32). Considering this, and that supplementation of antibiotics in poultry feed is a highly controversial issue (33), it is apparent that alternatives with similar modes of action are greatly needed. In order to identify these alternatives, we need to also understand the mechanisms by which antibiotic usage results in accelerated weight gain.

The purpose of Trial 1 was to examine the relationship between bacterial populations in the ileum, cecum, and litter within one flock over time. Age was a key factor in population shifts across all sample types, which has also been previously observed in turkey cecum and ileum studies (10, 21). Several OTUs were found predominantly in later time points across samples, including several classified *Lactobacillus* spp (*L. aviarius*, *L. johnsonii*, and

TABLE 2 | Intestinal measurements and cecal scores of turkeys with and without 50 g/ton of penicillin in feed.

		Cecal score	Intestinal length (cm)	Intestinal weight (g)
Day 7	Control	1.5 ± 0.8	93.0 ± 6.4	18.2 ± 2.2
	Penicillin	1.5 ± 0.4	95.1 ± 6.4	16.5 ± 2.1
Day 14	Control	2.4 ± 0.5	122.3 ± 9.9	35.2 ± 5.5
	Penicillin	2.0 ± 0.7	127.4 ± 6.2	37.1 ± 3.7
Day 21	Control	1.6 ± 0.6	148.1 ± 7.4	52.0 ± 6.4
	Penicillin	1.8 ± 0.5	158.8 ± 10.8[a]	65.9 ± 11.9[a]

[a]*Significantly different from control group ($P < 0.05$) using Student's t-test.*

L. ingluviei), which have been previously identified as key marker species of turkey ileum microbiome succession (10). In addition, *Clostridium* group XI was another OTU increasing in abundance with age of the flock; this diverse group includes *Eubacterium* and *Peptostreptococcus* spp, as well as *Clostridium bartlettii* (34), which may be another indicator of gut microbiome succession (10), in part due to the high ability of this species to ferment aromatic amino acids in the gut (35).

Sample type appeared to be another dominant factor affecting bacterial populations, with clear distinctions between the ileum and cecum populations; the litter samples were also distinct, but

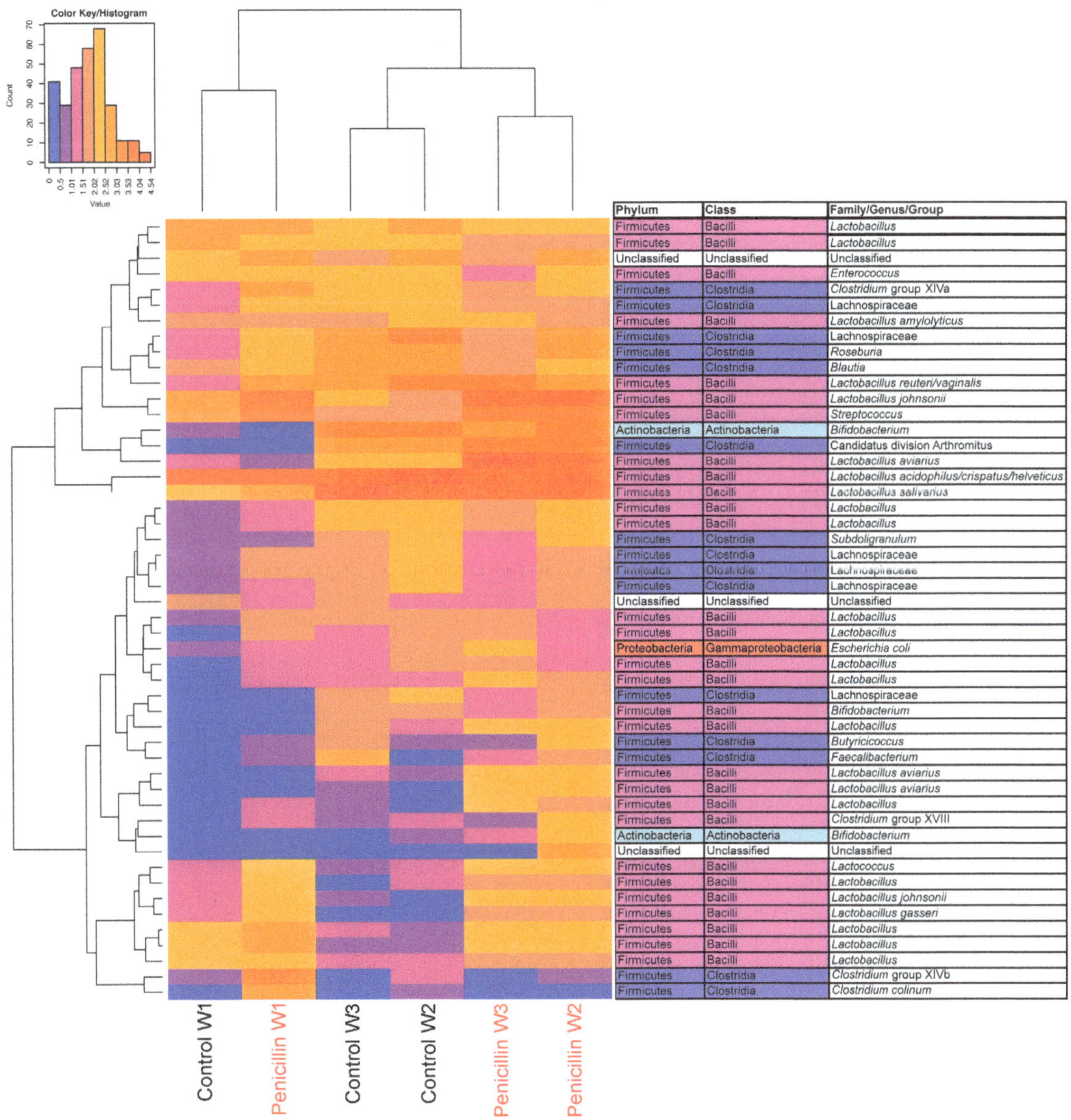

FIGURE 5 | Heatmap depicting abundance of the top 50 OTUs by overall abundance across samples, averaged by age/sample. Heatmap was constructed using normalized log_{10} abundance of each OTU in each sample type. To the right of the heatmap is a table depicting classification of each OTU using RDP database assignment or best-hit classification where appropriate. "W" depicts the age of sample in weeks. Control = birds receiving standard feed with BMD, penicillin = birds receiving BMD plus penicillin in feed.

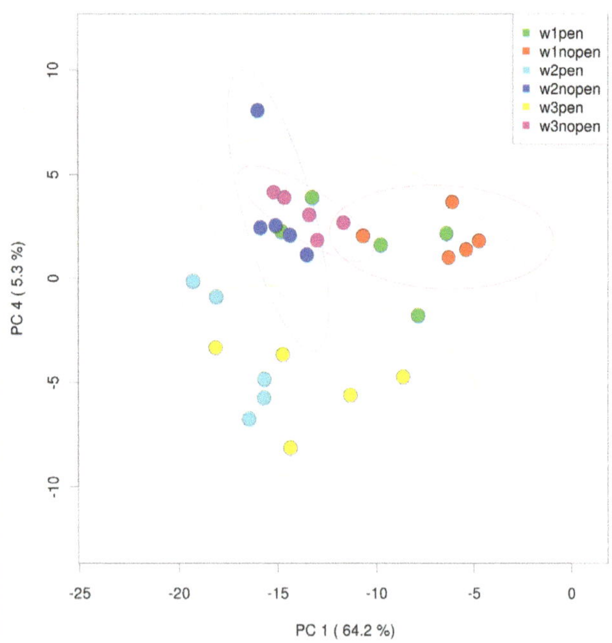

FIGURE 6 | Principal coordinates analysis (PCoA) of individual ileum samples from penicillin-treated versus control groups. "W" = flock age in weeks; "pen" = penicillin-treated samples; "nopen" = control samples.

more closely represented the ileum. The differences between the cecum samples and ileum and litter samples were largely within the Firmicutes phylum; more specifically, Clostridia OTUs were enriched in the cecal samples, whereas Bacilli were more abundant in the ileum and litter. Several identified OTUs were present only in ileum and litter samples, including *Brachybacterium*, which was first detected in poultry litter (36), and *Brevibacterium*, a soil bacterium that has been used as an indicator organism for poultry waste contamination in the environment (37). Other OTUs identified only in the ileum and litter were *Staphylococcus*, *Corynebacterium*, *Jeotgalicoccus*, the latter of which is a lactic acid bacterium also found in the air in poultry houses (38), and *Weissella*, a genus reported in high abundance in healthy birds (39). A recently published study found that cecal content populations reflect cecal drop, whereas fecal drop populations were dissimilar to cecal populations, further suggesting that ileum populations would be more closely related to litter than to cecal community structure (40). However, another study found that the fecal microbiome represents a large portion of the cecal diversity, though it was not a good quantitative measure (41). The birds in the present study were placed on clean litter for the brood period (first 5 weeks), suggesting that the ileum microbiome influenced the litter microbiome; however, before week 6 the birds were moved into a commercial finisher barn setting, in which the bedding was mostly reused with just a thin layer of clean litter, which could have resulted in the litter microbiome influencing ileum populations from weeks 6 to 12. The reasons for litter more closely reflecting ileum are likely due to less frequent cecal discharge and a litter growth environment that would better support facultative anaerobes compared to strict anaerobes.

One OTU that was found only in the ileum samples was classified as Candidatus division Arthromitus, a segmented filamentous bacteria (SFB) previously reported to play a potential role in gut health in turkeys and other animals (10, 42). Little is known about this bacterium, as it has only recently been sequenced (43) and grown *in vitro* (44). SFBs are thought to be host-specific as they have reduced genomes and rely heavily on host metabolic functions, and very little is known about the turkey-specific strains; however, these bacteria have been reported to play a role in early innate immune system development in mice as well (45). Overall, while temporal succession of bacterial populations was observed in this flock similar to previous studies (10), differences in sample type were more prominent. In addition, our results corroborate findings that poultry fecal droppings or litter samples are a better predictor of ileal rather than cecal bacterial composition (40).

It is a well-known fact that antibiotics are commonly used as a feed additive in poultry operations as a way to enhance the growth of birds to reach market weights faster (46). In previous studies, supplementation of subtherapeutic levels of several antibiotics, such as penicillin, to poultry broiler feeds have been associated with increases in weight gain (9). Through our study, we have also shown that antibiotic usage, specifically penicillin combined with BMD, results in significantly increased weight gain in turkey broilers up to at least 3 weeks. A limitation of the study was that BMD was used in the control groups, thus the sole effects of penicillin on the microbiome were not identified in this study. However, the scenario used in these experiments reflects commonly applied practices in the turkey industry, so it is more relevant as a real-life application.

While limited information currently exists, hypotheses aimed at explaining mode of action of AGPs have been proposed, including shifts in microbiome composition in gastrointestinal tract act to improve feed efficiency (32). In our study, the relative increase in weight gain in penicillin-supplemented broilers as compared to control groups can be temporally correlated with shifts in microbiome composition. Given our findings, we believe mining the microbiome is a means for finding potential replacements for AGPs, such as by identifying specific bacterial taxa responsible for improving feed efficiency, which can be used as probiotics.

Of the probiotics that have been investigated as growth promoters in poultry, many have included *Lactobacillus* spp. (47). In our study, relative abundances of *Lactobacillus* spp., including *L. johnsonii* and *L. aviarius*, were higher in penicillin-supplemented groups as compared to control groups. In terms of growth promotion, *Lactobacillus* spp. have been associated with both beneficial and detrimental effects. One mechanism whereby lactobacilli have been shown to decrease weight gain in a pig model is through the production of bile salt hydrolase (BSH) (48). On the contrary, *Lactobacillus* spp. has been demonstrated in broiler chicks to antagonize pathogenic bacteria, thus resulting in weight gain (47). *Lactobacillus* spp., specifically *L. johnsonii*, has been shown to possess antibacterial activity against pathogenic bacteria (49), and Zulkifli et al. showed that feeding lactobacilli cultures to broiler chicks resulted in increased weight gain (50), comparable to feeding oxytetracycline. It seems plausible that supplementing poultry feeds with appropriate lactobacilli cultures could serve as an alternative method for improving feed efficiency in poultry flocks.

Few studies have investigated the ileum bacterial community structure focusing on commercial turkeys. Our data suggest that low-dose penicillin treatment has a discernable impact on ileum bacterial community structure. The initial effects during the first week of age increase bacterial diversity in the ileum, and subsequent effects apparently drive the ileal microbiome composition toward a state correlating with significant enhancements of body weight (10). Some important factors remain to be examined, such as the effects of AGP treatment on total microbial biomass and on the turkey immune system. Since penicillin treatment modulates the turkey ileal microbiome in a fashion similar to that previously observed between commercial turkey flocks with differing weight outcomes, modulating the ileal microbiome similarly using antibiotic-free approaches may provide an alternative approach by which to enhance performance and prevent disease in the commercial bird.

AUTHOR CONTRIBUTIONS

TJ and BM conceived the study. JD and BM performed the experiments. JC, HH, DK, and TJ analyzed the data. TJ, JC, JD, and SH wrote the manuscript.

ACKNOWLEDGMENTS

The authors are grateful to Willmar Poultry Company for providing animal resources for this study. Bioinformatics were supported using tools available from the Minnesota Supercomputing Institute.

FUNDING

Funding was provided by the Minnesota Turkey Research and Promotion Council (award 2013-01), University of Minnesota MNDrive Initiative, University of Minnesota Rapid Agricultural Response Funds, and the National Institutes of Health PharmacoNeuroImmunology Fellowship (NIH/NIDA T32 DA007097-32) awarded to JC.

REFERENCES

1. National Agricultural Statistics Service. *Turkeys Raised. United States Department of Agriculture Economics, Statistics and Market Information System.* (2012). Available at: https://usda.mannlib.cornell.edu/MannUsda/viewDocumentInfo.do?documentID=1498
2. Feighner SD, Dashkevicz MP. Subtherapeutic levels of antibiotics in poultry feeds and their effects on weight gain, feed efficiency, and bacterial cholyltaurine hydrolase activity. *Appl Environ Microbiol* (1987) **53**:331–6.
3. Calvert A. *Light Turkey Syndrome: Field Study and Inoculation Trial.* M S thesis, Department of Animal Science, University of Minnesota, Saint Paul, MN, USA (2012).
4. Mor SK, Sharafeldin TA, Abin M, Kromm M, Porter RE, Goyal SM, et al. The occurrence of enteric viruses in light Turkey syndrome. *Avian Pathol* (2013) **42**:497–501. doi:10.1080/03079457.2013.832145
5. Sekelja M, Rud I, Knutsen SH, Denstadli V, Westereng B, Naes T, et al. Abrupt temporal fluctuations in the chicken fecal microbiota are explained by its gastrointestinal origin. *Appl Environ Microbiol* (2012) **78**:2941–8. doi:10.1128/AEM.05391-11
6. Apajalahti J, Kettunen A, Graham H. Characteristics of the gastrointestinal microbial communities with special reference to the chicken. *World Poult Sci J* (2004) **60**:223–32. doi:10.1079/WPS20040017
7. Lan PT, Hayashi H, Sakamoto M, Benno Y. Phylogenetic analysis of cecal microbiota in chicken by the use of 16S rDNA clone libraries. *Microbiol Immunol* (2002) **46**:371–82. doi:10.1111/j.1348-0421.2002.tb02709.x
8. Zhu XY, Zhong T, Pandya Y, Joerger RD. 16S rRNA-based analysis of microbiota from the cecum of broiler chickens. *Appl Environ Microbiol* (2002) **68**:124–37. doi:10.1128/AEM.68.1.124-137.2002
9. Dumonceaux TJ, Hill JE, Hemmingsen SM, Van Kessel AG. Characterization of intestinal microbiota and response to dietary virginiamycin supplementation in the broiler chicken. *Appl Environ Microbiol* (2006) **72**:2815–23. doi:10.1128/AEM.72.4.2815-2823.2006
10. Danzeisen JL, Calvert AJ, Noll SL, McComb B, Sherwood JS, Logue CM, et al. Succession of the turkey gastrointestinal bacterial microbiome related to weight gain. *PeerJ* (2013) **1**:e237. doi:10.7717/peerj.237
11. Scupham AJ. Campylobacter colonization of the Turkey intestine in the context of microbial community development. *Appl Environ Microbiol* (2009) **75**:3564–71. doi:10.1128/AEM.01409-08
12. Juricova H, Videnska P, Lukac M, Faldynova M, Babak V, Havlickova H, et al. Influence of *Salmonella enterica* serovar enteritidis infection on the development of the cecum microbiota in newly hatched chicks. *Appl Environ Microbiol* (2013) **79**:745–7. doi:10.1128/AEM.02628-12
13. Videnska P, Sisak F, Havlickova H, Faldynova M, Rychlik I. Influence of *Salmonella enterica* serovar enteritidis infection on the composition of chicken cecal microbiota. *BMC Vet Res* (2013) **9**:140. doi:10.1186/1746-6148-9-140
14. Lu J, Idris U, Harmon B, Hofacre C, Maurer JJ, Lee MD. Diversity and succession of the intestinal bacterial community of the maturing broiler chicken. *Appl Environ Microbiol* (2003) **69**:6816–24. doi:10.1128/AEM.69.11.6816-6824.2003
15. Wise MG, Siragusa GR. Quantitative analysis of the intestinal bacterial community in one- to three-week-old commercially reared broiler chickens fed conventional or antibiotic-free vegetable-based diets. *J Appl Microbiol* (2007) **102**:1138–49. doi:10.1111/j.1365-2672.2006.03153.x
16. Pedroso AA, Menten JF, Lambais MR, Racanicci AM, Longo FA, Sorbara JO. Intestinal bacterial community and growth performance of chickens fed diets containing antibiotics. *Poult Sci* (2006) **85**:747–52. doi:10.1093/ps/85.4.747
17. Lu J, Hofacre C, Smith F, Lee MD. Effects of feed additives on the development on the ileal bacterial community of the broiler chicken. *Animal* (2008) **2**:669–76. doi:10.1017/S1751731108001894
18. Thompson K, Burkholder K, Patterson J, Applegate TJ. Microbial ecology shifts in the ileum of broilers during feed withdrawal and dietary manipulations. *Poult Sci* (2008) **87**:1624–32. doi:10.3382/ps.2007-00324
19. Lin J, Hunkapiller AA, Layton AC, Chang YJ, Robbins KR. Response of intestinal microbiota to antibiotic growth promoters in chickens. *Foodborne Pathog Dis* (2013) **10**:331–7. doi:10.1089/fpd.2012.1348
20. Torok VA, Allison GE, Percy NJ, Ophel-Keller K, Hughes RJ. Influence of antimicrobial feed additives on broiler commensal posthatch gut microbiota development and performance. *Appl Environ Microbiol* (2011) **77**:3380–90. doi:10.1128/AEM.02300-10
21. Danzeisen JL, Kim HB, Isaacson RE, Tu ZJ, Johnson TJ. Modulations of the chicken cecal microbiome and metagenome in response to anticoccidial and growth promoter treatment. *PLoS One* (2011) **6**:e27949. doi:10.1371/journal.pone.0027949
22. Bartram AK, Lynch MD, Stearns JC, Moreno-Hagelsieb G, Neufeld JD. Generation of multimillion-sequence 16S rRNA gene libraries from complex microbial communities by assembling paired-end illumina reads. *Appl Environ Microbiol* (2011) **77**:3846–52. doi:10.1128/AEM.02772-10
23. Masella AP, Bartram AK, Truszkowski JM, Brown DG, Neufeld JD. PANDAseq: paired-end assembler for illumina sequences. *BMC Bioinformatics* (2012) **13**:31. doi:10.1186/1471-2105-13-31
24. Schloss PD, Westcott SL, Ryabin T, Hall JR, Hartmann M, Hollister EB, et al. Introducing mothur: open-source, platform-independent,

community-supported software for describing and comparing microbial communities. *Appl Environ Microbiol* (2009) **75**:7537–41. doi:10.1128/AEM.01541-09
25. Caporaso JG, Kuczynski J, Stombaugh J, Bittinger K, Bushman FD, Costello EK, et al. QIIME allows analysis of high-throughput community sequencing data. *Nat Methods* (2010) **7**:335–6. doi:10.1038/nmeth.f.303
26. Edgar RC. Search and clustering orders of magnitude faster than BLAST. *Bioinformatics* (2010) **26**:2460–1. doi:10.1093/bioinformatics/btq461
27. Haas BJ, Gevers D, Earl AM, Feldgarden M, Ward DV, Giannoukos G, et al. Chimeric 16S rRNA sequence formation and detection in Sanger and 454-pyrosequenced PCR amplicons. *Genome Res* (2011) **21**:494–504. doi:10.1101/gr.112730.110
28. Lozupone C, Knight R. UniFrac: a new phylogenetic method for comparing microbial communities. *Appl Environ Microbiol* (2005) **71**:8228–35. doi:10.1128/AEM.71.12.8228-8235.2005
29. Cole JR, Wang Q, Cardenas E, Fish J, Chai B, Farris RJ, et al. The ribosomal database project: improved alignments and new tools for rRNA analysis. *Nucleic Acids Res* (2009) **37**:D141–5. doi:10.1093/nar/gkn879
30. White JR, Nagarajan N, Pop M. Statistical methods for detecting differentially abundant features in clinical metagenomic samples. *PLoS Comput Biol* (2009) **5**:e1000352. doi:10.1371/journal.pcbi.1000352
31. Dean CB, Nielsen JD. Generalized linear mixed models: a review and some extensions. *Lifetime Data Anal* (2007) **13**:497–512. doi:10.1007/s10985-007-9065-x
32. Huyghebaert G, Ducatelle R, Van Immerseel F. An update on alternatives to antimicrobial growth promoters for broilers. *Vet J* (2011) **187**:182–8. doi:10.1016/j.tvjl.2010.03.003
33. Singer RS, Hofacre CL. Potential impacts of antibiotic use in poultry production. *Avian Dis* (2006) **50**:161–72. doi:10.1637/7569-033106R.1
34. Song YL, Liu CX, McTeague M, Summanen P, Finegold SM. *Clostridium bartlettii* sp. nov., isolated from human faeces. *Anaerobe* (2004) **10**:179–84. doi:10.1016/j.anaerobe.2004.04.004
35. Russell WR, Duncan SH, Scobbie L, Duncan G, Cantlay L, Calder AG, et al. Major phenylpropanoid-derived metabolites in the human gut can arise from microbial fermentation of protein. *Mol Nutr Food Res* (2013) **57**:523–35. doi:10.1002/mnfr.201200594
36. Lapidus A, Pukall R, Labuttii K, Copeland A, Del Rio TG, Nolan M, et al. Complete genome sequence of *Brachybacterium faecium* type strain (Schefferle 6-10). *Stand Genomic Sci* (2009) **1**:3–11. doi:10.4056/sigs.492
37. Ryu H, Elk M, Khan IU, Harwood VJ, Molina M, Edge TA, et al. Comparison of two poultry litter qPCR assays targeting the 16S rRNA gene of *Brevibacterium* sp. *Water Res* (2014) **48**:613–21. doi:10.1016/j.watres.2013.10.015
38. Martin E, Klug K, Frischmann A, Busse HJ, Kampfer P, Jackel U. *Jeotgalicoccus coquinae* sp. nov. and *Jeotgalicoccus aerolatus* sp. nov., isolated from poultry houses. *Int J Syst Evol Microbiol* (2011) **61**:237–41. doi:10.1099/ijs.0.021675-0
39. Stanley D, Keyburn AL, Denman SE, Moore RJ. Changes in the caecal microflora of chickens following *Clostridium perfringens* challenge to induce necrotic enteritis. *Vet Microbiol* (2012) **159**:155–62. doi:10.1016/j.vetmic.2012.03.032
40. Pauwels J, Taminiau B, Janssens GP, De Beenhouwer M, Delhalle L, Daube G, et al. Cecal drop reflects the chickens' cecal microbiome, fecal drop does not. *J Microbiol Methods* (2015) **117**:164–70. doi:10.1016/j.mimet.2015.08.006
41. Stanley D, Geier MS, Chen H, Hughes RJ, Moore RJ. Comparison of fecal and cecal microbiotas reveals qualitative similarities but quantitative differences. *BMC Microbiol* (2015) **15**:51. doi:10.1186/s12866-015-0388-6
42. Prakash T, Oshima K, Morita H, Fukuda S, Imaoka A, Kumar N, et al. Complete genome sequences of rat and mouse segmented filamentous bacteria, a potent inducer of Th17 cell differentiation. *Cell Host Microbe* (2011) **10**:273–84. doi:10.1016/j.chom.2011.08.007
43. Bolotin A, De Wouters T, Schnupf P, Bouchier C, Loux V, Rhimi M, et al. Genome sequence of "*Candidatus Arthromitus*" sp. strain SFB-mouse-NL, a commensal bacterium with a key role in postnatal maturation of gut immune functions. *Genome Announc* (2014) **2**:e705–14. doi:10.1128/genomeA.00705-14
44. Schnupf P, Gaboriau-Routhiau V, Gros M, Friedman R, Moya-Nilges M, Nigro G, et al. Growth and host interaction of mouse segmented filamentous bacteria in vitro. *Nature* (2015) **520**:99–103. doi:10.1038/nature14027
45. Ivanov II, Atarashi K, Manel N, Brodie EL, Shima T, Karaoz U, et al. Induction of intestinal Th17 cells by segmented filamentous bacteria. *Cell* (2009) **139**:485–98. doi:10.1016/j.cell.2009.09.033
46. Jones FT, Ricke SC. Observations on the history of the development of antimicrobials and their use in poultry feeds. *Poult Sci* (2003) **82**:613–7. doi:10.1093/ps/82.4.613
47. Jin LZ, Ho YW, Abdullah N, Jalaludin S. Probiotics in poultry: modes of action. *Worlds Poult Sci J* (1997) **53**:351–8. doi:10.1079/WPS19970028
48. Collier CT, Smiricky-Tjardes MR, Albin DM, Wubben JE, Gabert VM, Deplancke B, et al. Molecular ecological analysis of porcine ileal microbiota responses to antimicrobial growth promoters. *J Anim Sci* (2003) **81**:3035–45. doi:2003.81123035x
49. Makras L, Triantafyllou V, Fayol-Messaoudi D, Adriany T, Zoumpopoulou G, Tsakalidou E, et al. Kinetic analysis of the antibacterial activity of probiotic lactobacilli towards *Salmonella enterica* serovar typhimurium reveals a role for lactic acid and other inhibitory compounds. *Res Microbiol* (2006) **157**:241–7. doi:10.1016/j.resmic.2005.09.002
50. Zulkifli I, Abdulllah N, Azrin NM, Ho YW. Growth performance and immune response of two commercial broiler strains fed diets containing *Lactobacillus* cultures and oxytetracycline under heat stress conditions. *Br Poult Sci* (2000) **41**:593–7. doi:10.1080/713654979

Conflict of Interest Statement: Dr. Brian McComb was an employee at Willmar Poultry Company at the time of this study. The remaining authors have no conflict of interest to declare.

10

Oxidant/antioxidant balance in animal nutrition and health: the role of protein oxidation

Pietro Celi[1,2] and Gianfranco Gabai[3]*

[1] DSM Nutritional Products, Animal Nutrition and Health, Columbia, MD, USA, [2] Faculty of Veterinary and Agricultural Sciences, The University of Melbourne, Parkville, VIC, Australia, [3] Department of Comparative Biomedicine and Food Science, University of Padova, Legnaro, Italy

This review examines the role that oxidative stress (OS), and protein oxidation in particular, plays in nutrition, metabolism, and health of farm animals. The route by which redox homeostasis is involved in some important physiological functions and the implications of the impairment of oxidative status on animal health and diseases is also examined. Proteins have various and, at the same time, unique biological functions and their oxidation can result in structural changes and various functional modifications. Protein oxidation seems to be involved in pathological conditions, such as respiratory diseases and parasitic infection; however, some studies also suggest that protein oxidation plays a crucial role in the regulation of important physiological functions, such as reproduction, nutrition, metabolism, lactation, gut health, and neonatal physiology. As the characterization of the mechanisms by which OS may influence metabolism and health is attracting considerable scientific interest, the aim of this review is to present veterinary scientists and clinicians with various aspects of oxidative damage to proteins.

Keywords: protein oxidation, biomarkers, oxidative stress, inflammation, animal welfare

Edited by:
Stephen Brent Smith, Texas A&M University, USA

Reviewed by:
Sung Woo Kim, North Carolina State University, USA
Sungkwonk Park, Sejong University, South Korea

****Correspondence:***
Pietro Celi
pietro.celi@dsm.com

INTRODUCTION

In aerobic organisms, mitochondrial and cytochrome P450 metabolism, inflammation processes (e.g., phagocyte respiratory burst) and several environmental factors are endogenous sources of reactive oxygen species (ROS) (1). In low concentrations, ROS are involved in numerous physiological events (2, 3), but they can be detrimental for living cells if they are present in excessive amounts (4) that cannot be overridden by the body antioxidants. The imbalance between pro-oxidants and antioxidants lead to oxidative stress (OS), eventually resulting in damages of macromolecules.

The role of OS in farm animals' health and disease has been reviewed elsewhere (5–7). The most investigated causes of OS in veterinary medicine are metabolic and inflammatory events, and environmental factors (heat stress and nutrition) (**Figure 1**). In dairy cows, conditions, such as high body condition score at calving (8), high milk yield (9), negative energy balance (10) and diet (11), and suppressed dry period (12) are all factors contributing to increased OS. Several observations suggest that excessive lipid mobilization plays a pivotal role as a link between altered energy metabolism, OS and decrease immune system efficiency (13, 14). Indeed, the adipose tissue secretes a great number of substances involved in the modulation of the immune response (5, 15), and during excessive adipose tissue mobilization, adipose tissue produces proinflammatory cytokines, while the production

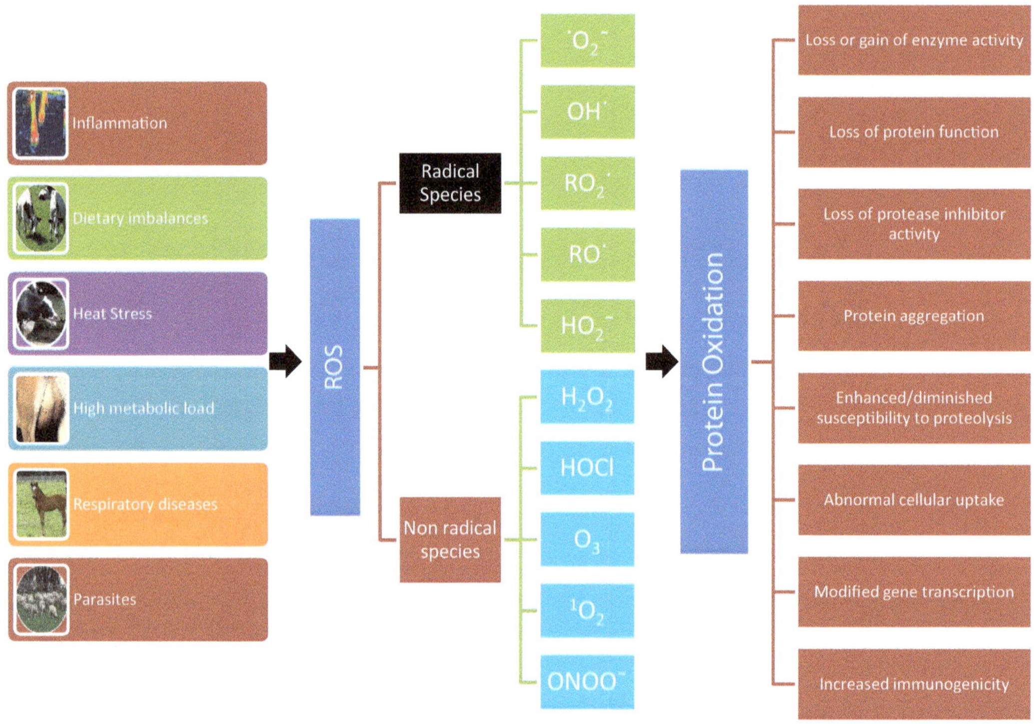

FIGURE 1 | Consequences of protein oxidation. A number of conditions (inflammation, dietary imbalances, heat stress, high metabolic load, respiratory diseases, and parasites) can lead to the formation of reactive oxygen metabolites (ROS). ROS leading to protein oxidation that includes radical species, such as superoxide ($^{\cdot}O_2^-$), hydroxyl (OH•), peroxyl ($RO_2^{\cdot}$), alkoxyl (RO•), hydroperoxyl (HO_2^-), and non-radical species, such as hydrogen peroxide (H_2O_2), hypochlorous acid (HOCl), ozone (O_3), singlet oxygen ($^1O_2$), and peroxynitrite ($ONOO^-$). The oxidation of protein can result in loss or gain of enzyme activity, loss of protein function and of protease inhibitor activity, protein aggregation, enhanced/diminished susceptibility to proteolysis, abnormal cellular uptake, modified gene transcription, and increased immunogenicity.

of adiponectin is reduced (16). In addition, changes in bovine NEFA concentrations and composition may alter the response of monocyte and neutrophil (17).

Activated phagocytes and neutrophils represent another source of OS, which contribute to OS by generating hydrogen peroxide and superoxide via a respiratory burst, and the release of the enzyme myeloperoxidase (MPO), which catalyzes the reaction of hydrogen peroxide with physiological concentrations of chlorine ions and gives rise to the potent oxidant hypochlorous acid. Hypochlorous acid plays an important role in killing invading pathogens; however, excessive or misplaced generation of this oxidant can cause tissue damage, and it is believed to be involved in a number of human and animal diseases (18).

Oxidative stress can virtually damage all biological molecules (DNA, RNA, cholesterol, lipids, carbohydrates, and proteins). In turn, the oxidation of these macromolecules produces various endproducts that can be measured to assess OS *in vivo*. Proteins are the molecules most susceptible to oxidative damage in cells because they are often catalysts rather than stoichiometric mediators; hence, the effect of damage to one molecule is greater than stoichiometric (19). Proteins have various and unique biological functions, and their oxidation can result in structural changes and consequently in various modifications in their functions (**Figure 1**) (20–22).

TABLE 1 | Approximate constitution of various biological materials and number of papers published in PubMed related to protein, DNA, and lipid oxidation [adapted from Ref. (23)].

	Protein	DNA	Total lipid	Cholesterol
Organ level (liver, g/kg wet weight)	146	2.6	49	3.9
Cellular level (g/10^{12} leukocytes)	100	6.9	15.6	2
Plasma (g/L)	73		0.5	1.5–2.5
Papers (PubMed)	106,508	19,561	55,287	7,394

The study of the physiopathology of protein oxidation has attracted considerable interest in human medicine (**Table 1**), but similar studies in veterinary medicine are still scarce. Therefore, the aim of this review is to present veterinary scientists and clinicians with various aspects of oxidative damage to proteins, with emphasis on using oxidized proteins as markers of OS in veterinary medicine. We will also discuss the involvement of protein oxidation in pathological conditions relevant to farm animals. In this regard, we have used the modern dairy cow as it has been the objective of the majority of studies conducted in this field; examples of other species have been given when available. Besides oxygen, nitrogen also plays an important role in damaging biological molecules via "reactive nitrogen species." However, this review will not deal with this family of reactive species.

PROTEIN OXIDATION

It has been estimated that proteins can scavenge up to 75% of free radicals, such as hydroxyl (24). On the basis of this evidence and considering that oxidized proteins have considerably long half-lives, it is reasonable to assume that proteins are likely to accumulate "evidence" of oxidative insult making those suitable markers of oxidative damage (23, 25).

Protein oxidation is defined as the covalent modification of a protein induced either directly by ROS or indirectly by reaction with secondary by-products of OS (22). Oxidative damage to proteins can affect their functions as receptors, enzymes, transport, or structural proteins, etc.; moreover, oxidized proteins can generate new antigens and provoke immune response (26).

Reactive species leading to protein oxidation are outlined in **Figure 1** and include radical and non-radical species (21, 25). Other agents that lead to protein oxidation include reagents, such as xenobiotics, such as paraquat, CCl_4, and acetaminophen, cigarette smoke, reduced transition metals, such as Fe^{2+} or Cu^+, γ-irradiation in the presence of O_2, activated neutrophils, ultraviolet light, ozone, oxidoreductase enzymes, and by-products of lipid and free amino acid oxidation (21, 25). For example, pigs exposed to whole body γ-irradiation showed a significant increase in protein carbonyls (27). As a consequence of the large variety of agents that cause protein oxidation and because all of the amino acyl side chains can become oxidatively modified, there are numerous different types of protein oxidative modification (22).

Reactions of ROS with proteins and peptides can induce alterations to both the backbone and side chains (25). The use of backbone fragmentation as a marker of protein oxidation *in vivo* is very limited because of the quantity of other proteins present and the potential role of proteases that can bias the results (28). Nevertheless, the use of protein fragmentation as a potential source of biomarkers is very attractive in veterinary science, and mastitis detection seems a promising field of investigation. During mastitis infection, pathogenic bacteria elude the defense mechanisms of the mammary gland, start multiplying and liberate enzymes and toxins. Circulating polymorphonuclear neutrophils (PMNs) are attracted to the site of infection and release oxidants and proteases to destroy the invading pathogens (29). Enzymes and oxidants secreted by both bacteria and PMNs result in the damage of the mammary cells and milk components, milk proteins in particular. Interestingly, the peptidome resulting from the fragmentation of milk proteins in diseased animals shows peculiar differences from that observed in healthy animals, and it may be possible to obtain a panel of protein fragments, which can be used for differential diagnosis of causative bacteria of mammary infection (29).

Products of protein side chain oxidation, on the other hand, are relatively stable and there are several assays available for their detection (30). The most frequently used biomarker of protein oxidation is the carbonyl assay, which measures protein carbonyl groups (26, 30). Protein carbonylation occurs when ROS attack the amino acid side chains of proline, arginine, lysine, and threonine in presence of transition metals (Fe^{2+}, Cu^+, etc.). This process can be defined as "primary protein carbonylation," and refers to the formation of reactive ketones or aldehydes that can react with 2,4-dinitrophenylhydrazine (DNPH) (31). Alternatively, reactive carbonyl compounds, such as carbohydrates and lipids having reactive carbonyl groups produced during glycoxidation and lipoperoxidation, can bind to amino acid side chains (mainly on lysine, cysteine, and histidine residues) generating the so-called "secondary protein carbonylation" (31, 32).

Protein carbonylation is the most frequent irreversible transformation and also the one most often studied (30), and accumulation of protein carbonyls has been observed in several human diseases (21, 33, 34). In general, the accumulation of oxidized proteins depends on the rate of their clearance. Degradation of oxidized proteins is influenced by the presence and the activity of specific proteases and the extent of their chemical modification, with mildly oxidized proteins highly prone to degradation, while extremely oxidized proteins (i.e., carbonylated) can form cross-links and aggregates, which are poor substrates for proteolysis (35). Therefore, these molecules are chemically stable, which is advantageous for both their detection and storage, with several assays being available for their detection.

Carbonyls have no specific UV or visible spectrophotometric absorbance/fluorescence properties; therefore, it is not possible to detect them directly. Products of both primary and secondary carbonylation react with chemical probes, such as DNPH, which allows the determination of total protein carbonyl groups. Once a protein carbonyl reacts with DNPH, a 2,4-dinitrophenylhydrazone (DNP)-protein adduct is formed, and total carbonyl groups in a mixture of proteins can be detected and quantified spectrophotometrically due to the characteristic absorption spectrum of DNP with a maximum at 365–375 nm. Moreover, as several antibodies against DNP are commercially available, carbonyl groups can be detected also by immunoassays, such as ELISA and Western blot (36).

Proteins can be oxidized in more than 35 ways, and many of these modifications involve some form of carbonylation (37), thus the carbonyl assay applied to tissues or body fluids measures the average protein modifications (26). However, total carbonyl determination does not provide accurate information on the source of the OS insult, as in most cases, the carbonylated protein(s) cannot be identified. Moreover, an inaccurate estimation of carbonyl groups can occur when they are measured spectrophotometrically using DNPH as the chemical probe, because some proteins (e.g., hemoglobin, cytochrome c) have absorbance wavelengths similar to DNPH (38).

In the last decade, the development of mass spectrometry (MS) methods, coupled with suitable protein fractionation strategies, have been developed. Comprehensive reviews of MS methods and enrichment strategies to study post-translational protein modifications have been recently published (36, 39). Here, it is worth remembering that combining the derivatization of carbonyl groups with reagents, such as DNPH with proteomic techniques, leads to the identifications of specific carbonylated proteins in several diseases in humans, animal models, and cell models (31, 36, 37). Indeed, proteomic approaches suggest that not all the proteins in a given proteome are subjected to the same oxidative attack, and carbonyl accumulation during OS, disease, or aging is a selective process (40).

Proteins rich in cysteine and methionine residues, both of which contain susceptible sulfur atoms, are particularly prone to OS damage. In the case of cysteine, oxidation leads to the formation of disulfide bonds, mixed disulfides, and thiyl radicals, while methionine sulfoxide is the major product of methionine oxidation (22, 28). The oxidation of cysteine and methionine is reversible as cells are equipped with systems, such as methonine sulfoxide reductase, glutathione, and thioredoxin redox system, capable of reversing the oxidation. It seems that the reversible oxidation/reduction of methionine may prevent the formation of more damaging forms of protein oxidative modification, namely protein carbonyl formation (22). Oxidation of cysteine and methionine can also result in the reversible formation of disulfides bonds between thiol groups (41). Detection of reversible oxidative modifications, however, cannot be considered as useful biomarkers of protein oxidation.

Hypochlorous acid-induced products are another major group of protein oxidation products. Primary products are chloro- and di-tyrosyl residues, amino acyl aldehyde adducts, and chloramines. They represent unique products of MPO activity, reflecting neutrophil and monocyte activity and therefore they can serve as indicators of OS markers generated during the inflammatory response (22). The availability of biomarkers for HOCl is important for investigating the pathological role of MPO and its products.

Dityrosine is a fluorescent molecule that represents one of the normal post-translational modifications of proteins, which implies a protein-protein cross-linking through tyrosine-tyrosine binding. In addition, dityrosine can be found as the product of oxidative or nitrative stress under a number of disease conditions, such as in the atherosclerotic plaque, Alzheimer's brain tissue, human blood plasma, and urine of humans and animals (42, 43). The ionized form of dityrosine have maximum absorption at 315 nm (44) and it is characterized by an intense fluorescence at 420 nm measurable upon excitation at either 315 nm (alkaline solution) or 284 nm (acidic solution) (43). Dityrosine is widely used as an important biomarker of oxidative modified proteins as it is a stable product and it is released by proteolysis of proteins modified by OS. Moreover, free dityrosine cannot be incorporated into proteins synthesized "*de novo*," thus suggesting that the levels of dityrosine reflect the oxidative damage of proteins (43).

Analytical methods to detect and measure dityrosine have been extensively reviewed elsewhere (42–44). The simplest way to monitor dityrosine formation "*in vitro*" is measuring the absorbance at 315 nm in a pure protein solution (45); however, spectrophotometric measurement of dityrosine cannot be used in a complex matrix, such as serum/plasma, as many chromophores absorb in the same wavelength interval. Dityrosine residues quantification can be performed in plasma samples by a fluorimetric method, after the sample is denaturated by dilution in PBS with 6 M urea (46, 47). The fluorescence emission is read near 410 nm after excitation at 325 nm, and the assay is calibrated using authentic synthesized dityrosine (48).

Dityrosine in tissues can be visualized by immunohistochemical staining using one of the commercially available antibodies. The availability of antibodies specific for dityrosine enabled also the development of immunoassays and Western blot analysis of solubilized protein extracts (43). However, the quantitative determination of dityrosine released by oxidized proteins usually employs the combinations of chromatographic techniques (42–44). Recently, quantitative measurement of dityrosine can be performed by MS, and the molecule has been detected in biological matrices of veterinary interest, such as bovine milk protein (49), cat urine (50), and rat plasma (51).

Dityrosine is a product of MPO and activated bovine neutrophils can produce a significant amount of dityrosine from bovine serum albumin (45). When proteins containing tyrosyl residues are exposed to HOCl, other compounds, such as 3-chlorotyrosin and 3,5-dichlorotyrosine are formed, but sensitive and complex procedures are required to detect tyrosine chlorination after exposure to physiological amounts of HOCl (18).

Advanced oxidation protein products (AOPP) can be defined as synthetic markers of protein oxidation. Spectral characteristics of AOPP correspond to chromophores induced by chlorinated oxidants, such as 3-chlorotyrosin and 3,5-dichlorotyrosine (52). Moreover, AOPP contain abundant dityrosine and disulfide bridges, which allow cross-linking, and carbonyl groups (46, 53). AOPP increase as a result of neutrophil activation during infections as they represent useful markers of MPO/HOCl protein oxidation. Conversely, although protein carbonyls can arise through the breakdown of chloramines, they cannot be taken as being specific biomarkers for HOCl (18) as a variety of other oxidation mechanisms can lead to their formation (25).

When measuring AOPP in plasma by the original method developed by Witko-Sarsat et al. (46), it should be considered that AOPP comprises several chromophores (46, 52, 53). In humans, fibrinogen (54) and serum albumin (46) modifications, and dityrosine cross-links are the major contributors to AOPP formation. Indeed, AOPP measurement can be used to estimate the dityrosine content in a biological matrix (54). The original assay (46), however, could lead to an overestimation of AOPP, particularly due to the influence of plasma turbidity induced by triglycerides (55). For this reason, a modified AOPP assay, which included a sample preparation procedure to precipitate plasma lipoproteins, has been developed (56). More recently, a method using citric acid to solubilize plasma lipids was developed in order to overcome the reported overestimation of AOPP levels (57). This method should allow a more accurate measure of chromophore absorption at 340 nm. However, AOPP analysis based on absorbance of light at 340 nm is not a selective way to measure oxidized proteins, and we consider of the utmost importance to test the potential interference of lipids or other substances when applying the AOPP assay to a new animal species or to a different biological fluid.

DISEASES AND PROTEIN OXIDATION IN FARM ANIMALS

Protein Oxidation and Female Reproduction

It is apparent that OS plays a crucial role in the cause and progression of a number of reproductive events, such as fertilization and early embryo development (58), and indeed it seems that OS is involved in the regulation of the female reproductive system at different levels (7, 59). For example, it has been shown that OS is associated with embryonic losses in dairy cows (60, 61) and that OS is involved in the pathogenesis of follicular cysts and repeat breeder syndrome in dairy cows (62–64).

It has been observed that the plasma profiles of the AOPP/albumin ratio provide a more sensitive indicator of OS (60, 61). This observation supports the proposed development and validation of a protein oxidation index. Considering that in dairy cows, pathogens are often introduced in the uterus during the artificial insemination procedure, it could be argued that they could generate an inflammatory reaction leading to OS and AOPP generation. Indeed, the development of subclinical endometritis seems to be a common event in dairy cows after artificial insemination (65), therefore the increase in plasma AOPP in cows that experience embryonic mortality might be indicative of subclinical uterine infection. It is important to consider that when uterine physical defenses are breached, the next line of defense is represented by neutrophils and macrophages triggering an inflammation process: the resulting activated leukocyte and vasoactive substances released during inflammation can increase blood vessel permeability resulting in plasma protein leaking into the endometrial surface (66, 67). We, therefore, propose that the assessment of OS and protein oxidation in particular, might improve our understanding of the role of OS and protein oxidation in the pathophysiology of reproductive wastage.

As consequence of the rapid fetal growth during the last trimester of pregnancy and the production of large amounts of colostrum and milk at the beginning of lactation, both maternal and fetal metabolism is increased in consequence of augmented mitochondrial activity in maternal tissues and the conceptus (68). This results in an increase in the production of ROS, particularly in dairy cows during late gestation (69) and early lactation (10). Considering that the activity of monocytes and macrophages is increased during pregnancy, and that the concentration of several markers of OS is concomitantly increased, it could be argued that pregnancy is characterized by a proinflammatory state (70). The observation of a positive correlation between AOPP and C-reactive protein during pregnancy brings further support to the association between inflammation and OS during pregnancy (71).

Studies in sows have reported a close relationship between protein oxidation and reproductive performance, with negative correlations between plasma protein carbonyl and litter size and litter weights (72). It is possible that the observed increase in protein oxidation and consequent increase in functional modification of proteins, protein turnover, and cell death, as discussed above, might be responsible for the observed decrease in litter size in sows in high social rank treatment (72).

One possible approach to reduce OS during late gestation is given by antioxidant supplementation. Studies in pigs have been able to demonstrate that silymarin supplementation of gilts' diets decreased liver and circulating protein carbonyl (73). Conversely, the administration of polyphenols rich foods (dried tomatoes, dried apples, dried green tea leaves, and raw soy grains) in pregnant ewes resulted in an increase in protein carbonyls and a decrease in lipid peroxidation and non-protein thiols (74). Considering the complexity of numerous interactions between antioxidants and body systems (genome, proteome, and metabolome), it is conceivable that a thorough analysis of antioxidants–animal interactions is necessary to achieve a deeper understanding of the effects of antioxidant supplementation in animal diets. The use of plants and plant rich in antioxidants is a new goal in animal nutrition (75–77), which needs to be explored.

Protein Oxidation, Nutrition, and Gut Health

In dairy cattle, prolonged concentrate feeding increased lipid peroxidation, and decreased α-tocopherol and ferric reducing ability of plasma (78). An increase in OS has also been observed when high levels of starch have been fed to dairy cows (11). It has been demonstrated that an increase in dietary concentrate content and a reduction in dietary NDF content are associated with an increase in ruminal endotoxin (79), which may stimulate the production of proinflammatory cytokines, ROS, and bioactive lipids (80). When ruminal endotoxin and plasma OS biomarker concentrations were evaluated in dairy heifers fed with grain, fructose, and histidine, and their combinations under subacute ruminal acidosis (SARA) challenge conditions, no effects of dietary treatments were observed on OS biomarkers (81). Considering the observed decreases in ruminal pH, increases in total VFA, and marked increases in lactic acid in fructose-fed heifers (82), changes in OS biomarkers were expected; however, the lack of OS response including protein oxidation (AOPP) to the dietary treatments could be ascribed to the lack of treatment effects on ruminal endotoxin (81), which is consistent with the hypothesis that AOPP increase early during the inflammatory pathway, when PMN cells are recruited and activated. The absence of effects on AOPP may also be indicative of the acute, as opposed to the chronic challenge of the study. In support of this hypothesis are the observations made in growing lambs that were fed a pelleted diet for 8 weeks, where a significant increase in concentrate intake was paralleled by an increase in AOPP concentration in lambs supplemented with Yerba Mate (83). Considering that high level of feed intake are negatively associated with rumen buffering capacity (84), it is likely that the higher levels of concentrate intake in the Yerba Mate supplemented lambs might have caused a transient state of SARA and that the observed higher levels of AOPP may reflect subclinical inflammatory events. Further research is needed to explore the relationships between abruptly feeding rapidly fermentable carbohydrates, endotoxin, and OS and to determine thresholds for OS induced changes in metabolism. In this context, plasma concentration of AOPP may be indicative of an early inflammatory event. Considering that AOPP are very easy to measure, it seems worthwhile exploring the possible applications of using this biomarker by veterinary scientists and clinicians.

In horses, the ingestion of excessive amount of rapidly fermentable carbohydrates, for example, an overload of starch from cereal grains or sugar and fructans from pasture or the feeding of black walnut extract can reproducibly induce laminitis (85), a condition that has been associated with OS (6). Rapidly fermented carbohydrates induce lactic acid production, increase hindgut mucosal permeability and therefore endotoxins [lipopolysaccharides (LPS)], exotoxins (protease), and amines are released by the disturbed gut microflora leading to the activation of neutrophils, release of cytokines and other inflammatory and OS mediators, which ultimately lead to the activation of matrix metalloproteinase which results in laminitis (85). Evidence of OS has been reported in the pathophysiology of black walnut extract induced laminitis (86), and it has been thought that both lipid and protein oxidation might be more prominent in the carbohydrates overload model (87). However, while the results of Burns et al. (87) study did not show an increase in laminar protein carbonyl content in either the black walnut extract and carbohydrates overload induced laminitis, it could be argued that the sampling window adopted in that study was not able to capture the formation of these products or that some antioxidant mechanism might have been upregulated in these models (87), conferring some degree of protection of the laminar tissue. Finally, it has been reported that synovial fluid protein carbonyl content is increased in equine joints under degenerative process (88, 89). While the increase in protein oxidation could have been the consequence of a post traumatic inflammatory response, further studies are required to determine the overall contribution of OS to the pathophysiology of these diseases.

An increase in AOPP concentration has also been observed in dairy cows when they are fed maize silage (77, 90) and in growing dairy calves (91). Silage is characterized by low antioxidant content (92), and when its level in the diet is increased it could lead to OS. In addition, as the antioxidant capacity of rumen bacteria is less developed than that of aerobe microbes, the lower antioxidant content of the silage might also expose ruminal bacteria to OS, impairing their activity, growth, and finally decreasing ruminant production. Indeed, a negative correlation between AOPP concentration and milk yield has been observed in dairy cows (90). Interestingly, an increase in AOPP concentration has also been observed in obese ponies subjected to high level of energy restriction (93). This observation seems to be ascribable to the high level of lipomobilization as reflected by the increase in triglycerides and NEFA concentrations, which are then prone to oxidation. This observation further supports the link between energy balance, metabolism and oxidant-antioxidant balance (7, 8, 10). Finally, supplementing pigs' diet L-methionine (L-Met) resulted in a reduction of MDA and protein carbonyl levels in duodenal mucosal samples, indicating a decrease in OS in the mucosa of the duodenum (94). It seems that this observation is due to the greater efficiency of L-Met, compared to DL-Met, in enhancing GSH synthesis in the intestinal mucosa. L-Met is also known to be a potent ROS scavenger (95); free L-Met and L-Met residues in protein act as endogenous antioxidants in cells, namely duodenal mucosal cells in Shen et al.'s (94) study.

Oxidative stress can be induced by dietary manipulation in poultry, for example, oxidized feeds can induce protein oxidation in birds (96). Indeed, feeding diets with oxidized oil (97) or animal-vegetable fat (98) increased plasma protein carbonyl content. Dietary antioxidant supplementation with organic selenium and minerals (97) or with saponins isolated from ginseng stems and leaves (99) is able to reduce OS in poultry by eliminating or decreasing the production of protein carbonyls. Therefore, we propose to include AOPP and protein carbonyl in the panel of biomarkers to study the relationships between OS, nutrition, metabolism, and gut health in veterinary medicine.

Protein Oxidation and Mammary Gland Function

To the best of our knowledge, no thorough studies were undertaken to measure markers of protein oxidation in the periparturient cow, where a state of OS can be observed in response to the copious milk yield and mammary gland remodeling. At least three sources of OS can be identified: the shift in cellular metabolism during the transition period, the contribution of immune cells (PMN and phagocytes), and the intensive mammary epithelial cell replacement occurring after termination of milking. In a preliminary study, we observed that plasmatic AOPP significantly decreased and plasmatic carbonyl groups significantly increased in cows around parturition, suggesting that different radicals can produce different alteration in the protein structure and a panel of parameters may better characterize the OS status (100). However, further work is required to investigate the relationships between protein oxidation and mammary gland function.

Between two consecutive milking bouts most of milk produced resides within mammary alveoli and ducts for a significant time, exposing milk proteins to the action of oxidizing enzymes, such as MPO, lactoperoxidase, and xanthine oxidase, present in the surrounding mammary and immune cells (101). Thus, OS biomarkers in colostrum and milk may reflect the oxidative status within the mammary gland; and, perhaps, oxidized protein products in milk and whey can be non-invasive tools for investigating the oxidative status of the dairy cow. We are currently undertaking a series of experiments to investigate if biomarkers of oxidized protein can be measured in colostrum and milk, and to characterize differences in oxidized protein products potentially related to HOCl and SCC. Preliminary results suggested that exposure of milk to increasing HOCl concentrations (HOCl/protein ratio from 0.3 to 3 μmol/mg) induces a 20–30% increase in AOPP concentrations and a three to sixfold increase in carbonyl group concentrations (102). In addition, a significant correlation has been observed between milk AOPP and somatic cell count (100), further supporting the involvement of OS in mammary gland function. A deeper characterization of the role of protein oxidation during lactation might allow the development of targeted antioxidant supplementation that might optimize mammary gland health by favoring tissue repair and cell turnover and prevent diseases like mastitis.

Protein Oxidation and Respiratory Diseases

The respiratory system is a major site of OS insult and it seems that pulmonary OS is crucial for the progression of respiratory disease especially in horses (103). It has been reported that AOPP concentration was numerically but not significantly elevated in foals affected by *Rhodococcus equi* (104). A possible explanation for the non-significant difference in AOPP in Crowley's study is that neutrophil counts did not differ between healthy and affected foals. Considering that higher neutrophil counts have been observed in foals with manifest clinical signs of *R. equi* pneumonia (105), it is possible to speculate that AOPP concentrations may differ beyond the subclinical state. Indeed, the observations that AOPP values were greatly elevated in a foal showing overt evident of upper respiratory tract disease associated with a heavy nasal culture of *Streptococcus equi* suggest that this might be the case (106). In Crowley's study, the AOPP/albumin ratio was significantly higher in *R. equi* affected foals compared to their healthy counterparts. This observation brings further evidence that AOPP/albumin ratio seems to be a more sensitive biomarker of OS suggesting that a more integrated approach to OS research and its role in the inflammatory events is required (107).

Lungs are quite susceptible to LPS, a major component of the outer membrane of gram-negative bacteria. Studies in piglets have shown that ampelopsin, a flavonoid with known antioxidant activity, is able to reduce the lung protein carbonyl content in LPS-challenged piglets (108). Recently in a study designed to evaluate OS responses in fetal lambs exposed to intra-amniotic endotoxin, a significant increase in protein carbonyls was observed in their bronchoalveolar lavage fluid (BALF) and in their plasma (109). Therefore, the investigation of proteins oxidation could represent a novel tool to study the role of OS in the etiopathogenesis of respiratory diseases in veterinary medicine.

Protein Oxidation and Parasitic Infection

Microorganisms, like bacteria, viruses, and parasites, can increase ROS production inducing OS (6). Parasitic diseases induce inflammation resulting in an influx of eosinophils, which seems to be responsible for tissue damage, possibly via their potent ROS production and therefore exposing farm animals to OS (7). Gastrointestinal nematode infections are quite prevalent in grazing animals and it has been observed that the selenium status of sheep may influence the acquired immunity to parasitic infestation (110). For example, during *Strongyloides papillosus* infections, it has been observed that OS damage seems to be related to the severity of the parasitic infection, and that sheep were exposed to OS even after they were treated with albendazole (111). The observed decrease in albumin and total thiol groups, which was accompanied by an increase in urea and protein carbonyl groups in the study of Dimitrijević et al. (111), clearly indicates that protein oxidation plays an important role in the etiopathogenesis of parasitic infections. Of particular interest is the observation that the changes in protein oxidation markers were correlated with the intensity of parasitic infection, which not only brings further proof of an impaired oxidant/antioxidant balance, but it also suggests that changes in protein oxidation markers may reflect the extent of damage induced by parasites and potentially different stages of the parasitic infection.

Theileriosis is another parasitic disease caused by a small protozoan that infects both red and white blood cells. In cattle, *Theileria annulata* infection induces high levels of proinflammatory cytokines (112) and OS damage of erythrocytes' skeletal membrane protein resulting in an increase in protein carbonyls (113). The observation that *T. annulata* infection in calves is associated with higher levels of protein oxidation than lipid oxidation suggests that protein carbonyls might be more reliable markers of OS damage during parasitic infection. Therefore, protein oxidation biomarkers could be used as monitoring tools aiding in diagnostic, prognosis, and anthelmintic therapeutic decision-making processes.

Protein Oxidation and Husbandry Practices

Oxidative stress biomarkers have been proposed as new and reliable indicators of animal welfare since stress of any origin can deplete the body's antioxidant resources (114). For example, an increase in plasma protein oxidation has been reported in pigs housed at high densities (115). Observations made in cattle kept in good or harsh conditions by the same research group have revealed that protein oxidation was highest in cattle living in hard conditions (116). While these observations could be due to several factors (nutrition, environmental conditions), they also suggest that animals might adopt different behavioral strategies in order to cope with stress (115). This observation highlights the need of a multidisciplinary approach to the characterization of OS-related diseases as both nutrition, metabolism, behavior and their interactions with potential pathogens might contribute to the exacerbation of OS.

Protein Oxidation and Neonatal Physiology

There is much interest in the mechanisms by which OS may influence postnatal growth, metabolism, and health in neonatal animals (117). At birth, the passage from the intrauterine hypoxic environment to the relatively hyperoxic external environment induces an abrupt exposure of mammalian neonates to environmental oxygen. In response to the changes in extracellular environmental conditions, the cells of new-born animals generate large amount of reactive ROS leading to neonatal OS (117).

In a study designed to evaluate the oxidant/antioxidant balance in dairy calves from birth to weaning, it has been reported that antioxidative defenses increased with time in new-born calves and this process seemed to be related to protein oxidation (118). In particular, it was observed that plasma AOPP concentration and the AOPP/albumin ratio progressively decreased from birth to weaning, while the opposite trend was observed for albumin and thiol groups. Albumin not only is the predominant oxidized protein contributing to AOPP formation but also constitutes the largest pool of circulating thiols; indeed, a positive correlation between albumin and thiol groups has been reported (119). A negative correlation between plasma albumin and thiol groups concentration, and AOPP concentrations and with the AOPP/albumin ratio was also observed in Ranade et al. (118) study, bringing further supports to the role of albumin as the predominant plasma protein contributing to AOPP formation.

It has been reported that protein carbonyls concentration in the serum of fetal and neonatal pigs were quite similar, suggesting that the oxidative mechanisms that regulate the production and degradation of circulating protein carbonyls are similar *in utero* and during early post-uterine life (119). In their study, Caperna et al. (119) also compared protein carbonyls between normal and low birth-weight piglets finding no differences. While this observation needs to be further explored, an interesting finding from this study was that two potential specific upregulated carbonylated markers were observed in low birth-weight piglets at birth (119). In a study aimed at investigating OS and the development of an antioxidant system after early weaning in piglets, it has been observed that plasma protein carbonyl levels were increased from day 1 to day 5 after early weaning (120). While weaning can alter the oxidant/antioxidant balance in piglets, this balance seems to be restored with the development of an antioxidant system via feedback regulation (120). Although additional studies are needed to isolate and identify them, these findings suggest that the study protein oxidation markers might increase our knowledge of redox homeostasis during the neonatal period, allowing the development of specific antioxidant interventions.

Protein Oxidation and Environmental Conditions

Heat stress has been implicated in the generation of OS either through excessive ROS production or decreased antioxidant defenses (121–123). Heat stress increases AOPP concentration in sheep and pigs and supra-physiological doses of Vitamin E and selenium are able to reduce the oxidation of plasma protein (124, 125). The lower AOPP concentration in heat stressed lambs fed supra-physiological doses of Vitamin E and selenium is indicative of protective role of these two antioxidants against the OS damage of proteins induced by heat stress and reinforces the need for higher levels of antioxidants than the current recommended levels under stressful conditions. Studies in broiler chickens have also demonstrated that high temperatures induce both lipid and protein oxidation (126); however, in another study aimed at assessing the effect of acute and chronic heat stress in broiler breeders, no changes in both lipid and protein oxidation were observed (127). While this apparent inconsistency could be ascribed to the different temperature regimes adopted in the two studies, it seems that acute heat stress might induce OS by disrupting the respiratory chain complex (126). Interestingly, low ambient temperature conditions increase the amount of protein carbonyls in liver and lung of broiler chickens; however, vitamin C dietary supplementation was not able to reverse this effect (128). Cold can be considered as a stressor and therefore lower temperature can induce OS.

The increase in protein oxidation following heat stress is of particular interest as it may have important implications on protein accretion and oxidative stability in lamb muscles, which is very important from meat quality perspectives for both ruminants and poultry (4, 96). The increase in AOPP during heat stress was accompanied by an increased expression of TNF-α in skeletal muscle in non-supplemented sheep (123), that further suggests a strong association between protein oxidation and mediators of proinflammatory responses (107, 129), and indicating that heat stress leads to undesired proinflammatory responses that may compromise animal performance (4). Maintaining animal performance during hot and humid weather requires continued advances in nutritional strategies to enhance animal resilience to heat stress. Therefore, the manipulation of dietary micronutrients and antioxidants has the potential to prevent the effects of oxidative damage (4, 130). Considering the capacity for interactions of antioxidants with other dietary substrates and environmental conditions, such as heat stress (131), it is possible that a more sophisticated understandings of the mechanisms responsible for the impairment of redox homeostasis induced by heat stress may help to generate mitigation strategies (132) and to develop potential nutritional interventions to alleviate the negative consequences of heat stress (133).

CONCLUSION

For a better understanding of the role of OS and protein oxidation in veterinary medicine, future studies should identify a panel of biomarker of protein oxidation to be used in veterinary medicine. While an OS biomarker should meet a number of criteria (**Table 2**), it is clear then that each biomarker of protein oxidation has its benefits and shortcomings. The biomarkers that have been used so far, while it could be argued that some of them could be considered too generic, they have been useful in the characterization of pathophysiology of protein oxidation. In our opinion, the translation of the current knowledge into practical applications for veterinary scientists and clinicians needs to be made a priority by the scientific community as this would allow to achieve a better insight in the evaluation and in the progression of several conditions and associated therapeutic interventions. Future studies should be combined with a proteomic analysis approach so that we can identify the specific sites of oxidation damage on particular proteins allowing us to refine the panel of protein oxidation biomarkers to be used in the characterization of OS induced conditions that lead to decreased welfare and productive performances.

This review has highlighted how considerable evidence on the involvement of OS and protein oxidation in a number of diseased and conditions of farm animals has been obtained in the past

TABLE 2 | Key criteria of the validation process of a suitable biomarker of protein oxidation.

Selection of biomarker of protein oxidation
Directly implicated in the onset and progression of disease
Development and validation of method for measuring the biomarker
Verification of potential for pitfalls and artifacts
Verification of biomarker in suitable animal models
Identification of modifying factor of the biomarker (nutrition, physiological status, and photoperiod)
Establishment of reference intervals and values
Adaptation of the method to field condition (sensitivity, simplicity, and throughput)

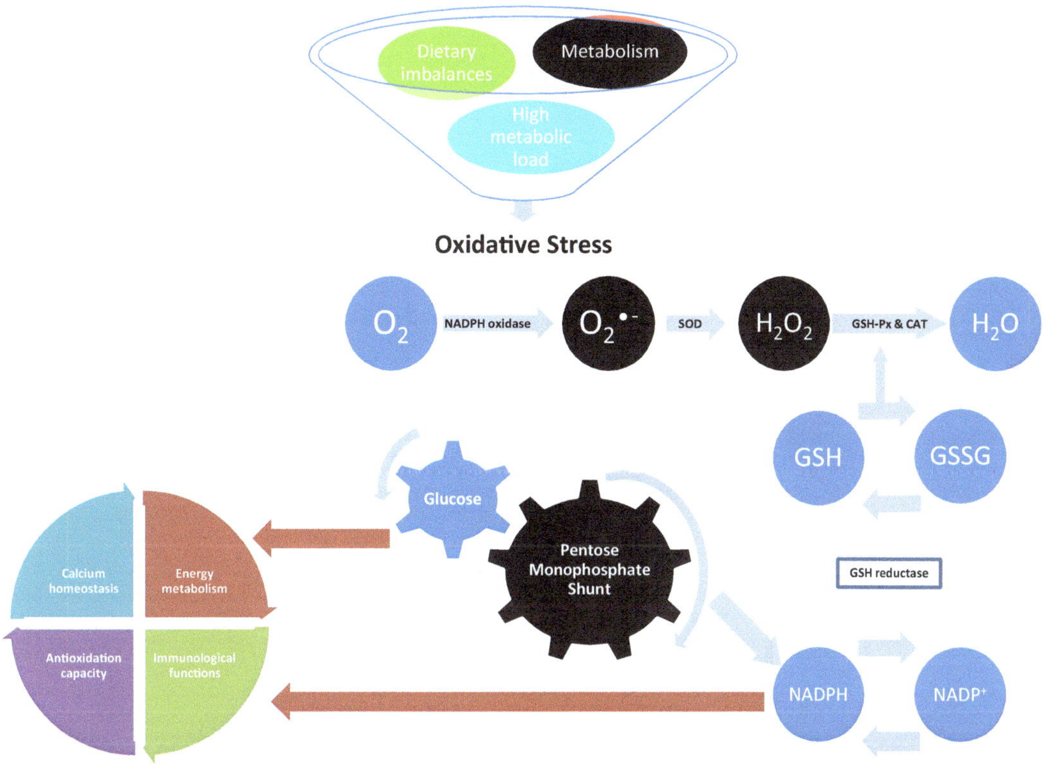

FIGURE 2 | Effect of oxidative stress on NADPH-dependent metabolic pathways. Superoxide (O_2^{-}) is generated during normal metabolism by the activity of the NADPH oxidase. Dietary imbalances and high metabolic load also stimulate the activity of the NADPH oxidase leading to oxidative stress if not removed by the antioxidant system. In normal conditions, O_2^{-} is converted in hydrogen peroxide (H_2O_2) by superoxide dismutase (SOD); H_2O_2 is then converted in water (H_2O) by the activity of glutathione peroxidase (GSH-Px) and catalase (CAT). Reduction of peroxides is accompanied by oxidation of reduced glutathione (GSH), which can be regenerated from glutathione disulfide (GSSG) by reducing equivalents from NADPH, which is generated by the pentose monophosphate shunt. The resulting destruction of GSH increases consumption of reducing equivalents, diverting glucose from important physiological pathways and competing with NADPH-dependent metabolic pathways, such as energy metabolism, immunological functions, antioxidation capacity, and calcium homeostasis.

few years. These studies span from important physiological functions, such as reproduction, nutrition, metabolism, lactation, gut health, and neonatal physiology, to respiratory diseases and parasitic infection. Despite this body of evidence, there are several questions that need to be explored about the role that OS and protein oxidation play in animal health. Animal health and welfare is crucial for a sustainable production system, and the characterization of the mechanisms by which OS may influence metabolism and health is now attracting international interest. The study of oxidant/antioxidant balance is contributing to the understanding of important pathways involved in regulation of cellular functions and metabolism. When ROS accumulates because of high metabolic rates, this may result in an impairment of the redox balance leading to OS (**Figure 2**). Therefore, as OS can negatively impact immune function and associated health disorders, future research should investigate the mechanisms involved in the maintenance of redox homeostasis especially during particular physiological conditions when animal metabolism is significantly increased, and homeostatic and homeorethic mechanisms are challenged.

REFERENCES

1. Höhn A, König J, Grune T. Protein oxidation in aging and the removal of oxidized proteins. *J Proteomics* (2013) **92**:132–159. doi:10.1016/j.jprot.2013.01.004
2. Miller JK, Brzezinska-Slebodzinska E, Madsen FC. Oxidative stress, antioxidants, and animal function. *J Dairy Sci* (1993) **76**(9):2812–2823. doi:10.3168/jds.S0022-0302(93)77620-1
3. Droge W. Free radicals in the physiological control of cell function. *Physiol Rev* (2002) **82**(1):47–95. doi:10.1152/physrev.00018.2001
4. Chauhan SS, Celi P, Ponnampalam EN, Leury BJ, Liu F, Dunshea FR. Antioxidant dynamics in the live animal and implications for ruminant health and product (meat/milk) quality: role of vitamin E and selenium. *Anim Prod Sci* (2014) **54**(10):1525–1536. doi:10.1071/AN14334
5. Sordillo LM, Aitken SL. Impact of oxidative stress on the health and immune function of dairy cattle. *Vet Immunol Immunopathol* (2009) **128**(1–3):104–109. doi:10.1016/j.vetimm.2008.10.305
6. Lykkesfeldt J, Svendsen O. Oxidants and antioxidants in disease: oxidative stress in farm animals. *Vet J* (2007) **173**(3):502–511. doi:10.1016/j.tvjl.2006.06.005
7. Celi P. Oxidative stress in ruminants. In: Mandelker L, Vajdovich P, editors. *Studies on Veterinary Medicine. Oxidative Stress in Applied Basic Research and Clinical Practice*. **5**. New York: Humana Press (2011). p. 191–231.

8. Bernabucci U, Ronchi B, Lacetera N, Nardone A. Influence of body condition score on relationships between metabolic status and oxidative stress in periparturient dairy cows. *J Dairy Sci* (2005) **88**(6):2017–2026. doi:10.3168/jds.S0022-0302(05)72878-2
9. Lohrke B, Viergutz T, Kanitz W, Gollnitz K, Becker F, Hurtienne A, et al. High milk yield in dairy cows associated with oxidant stress. *Online J Vet Res* (2004) **8**:70–78.
10. Pedernera M, Celi P, García SC, Salvin HE, Barchia I, Fulkerson WJ. Effect of diet, energy balance and milk production on oxidative stress in ea*rly-lactating* dairy cows grazing pasture. *Vet J* (2010) **186**(3):352–357. doi:10.1016/j.tvjl.2009.09.003
11. Gabai G, Testoni S, Piccinini R, Marinelli L, Stradaioli G. Oxidative stress in primiparous cows in relation to dietary starch and the progress of lactation. *Anim Sci* (2004) **79**:99–108.
12. Mantovani R, Sgorlon S, Marinelli L, Bailoni L, Bittante G, Gabai G. Oxidative stress indicators and metabolic adaptations in response to the omission of the dry period in dairy cows. *J Dairy Res* (2010) **77**(03):273–279. doi:10.1017/S0022029910000117
13. Sordillo LM, Raphael W. Significance of metabolic stress, lipid mobilization, and inflammation on transition cow disorders. *Vet Clin North Am* (2013) **29**(2):267–278. doi:10.1016/j.cvfa.2013.03.002
14. Sordillo LM, Mavangira V. The nexus between nutrient metabolism, oxidative stress and inflammation in transition cows. *Anim Prod Sci* (2014) **54**(9):1204–1214. doi:10.1071/AN14503
15. Contreras GA, Sordillo LM. Lipid mobilization and inflammatory responses during the transition period of dairy cows. *Comp Immunol Microbiol Infect Dis* (2011) **34**(3):281–289. doi:10.1016/j.cimid.2011.01.004
16. Kabara E, Sordillo LM, Holcombe S, Contreras GA. Adiponectin links adipose tissue function and monocyte inflammatory responses during bovine metabolic stress. *Comp Immunol Microbiol Infect Dis* (2014) **37**(1):49–58. doi:10.1016/j.cimid.2013.10.007
17. Raphael W, Sordillo L. Dietary polyunsaturated fatty acids and inflammation: the role of phospholipid biosynthesis. *Int J Mol Sci* (2013) **14**(10):21167–21188. doi:10.3390/ijms141021167
18. Winterbourn CC. Biological reactivity and biomarkers of the neutrophil oxidant, hypochlorous acid. *Toxicology* (2002) **181–182**:223–227. doi:10.1016/S0300-483X(02)00286-X
19. Dalle-Donne I, Scaloni A, Giustarini D, Cavarra E, Tell G, Lungarella G, et al. Proteins as biomarkers of oxidative/nitrosative stress in diseases: the contribution of redox proteomics. *Mass Spectrom Rev* (2005) **24**(1):55–99. doi:10.1002/mas.20006
20. Stadtman ER. Metal ion-catalyzed oxidation of proteins: biochemical mechanism and biological consequences. *Free Radic Biol Med* (1990) **9**(4):315–325. doi:10.1016/0891-5849(90)90006-5
21. Berlett BS, Stadtman ER. Protein oxidation in aging, disease, and oxidative stress. *J Biol Chem* (1997) **272**(33):20313–20316. doi:10.1074/jbc.272.33.20313
22. Shacter E. Quantification and significance of protein oxidation in biological samples. *Drug Metab Rev* (2000) **32**(3–4):307–326. doi:10.1081/DMR-100102336
23. Davies MJ. The oxidative environment and protein damage. *Biochimica et Biophys Acta* (2005) **1703**(2):93–109. doi:10.1016/j.bbapap.2004.08.007
24. Gebicki JM. Protein hydroperoxides as new reactive oxygen species. *Redox Rep* (1997) **3**:99–110.
25. Dean RT, Fu S, Stocker R, Davies MJ. Biochemistry and pathology of radical-mediated protein oxidation. *Biochem J* (1997) **324**(1):1–18. doi:10.1042/bj3240001
26. Halliwell B, Whiteman M. Measuring reactive species and oxidative damage in vivo and in cell culture: how should you do it and what do the results mean? *Br J Pharmacol* (2004) **142**(2):231–255. doi:10.1038/sj.bjp.0705776
27. Smutná M, Beňová K, Dvořák P, Nekvapil T, Kopřiva V, Maté D. Protein carbonyls and traditional biomarkers in pigs exposed to low-dose γ-radiation. *Res Vet Sci* (2013) **94**(2): 214–218. doi:10.1016/j.rvsc.2012.09.002
28. Davies MJ, Fu S, Wang H, Dean RT. Stable markers of oxidant damage to proteins and their application in the study of human disease. *Free Radic Biol Med* (1999) **27**(11–12):1151–1163. doi:10.1016/S0891-5849(99)00206-3
29. Mansor R, Mullen W, Albalat A, Zerefos P, Mischak H, Barrett DC, Biggs A, Eckersall PD. A peptidomic approach to biomarker discovery for bovine mastitis. *J Proteomics* (2013) **85**:89–98. doi:10.1016/j.jprot.2013.04.027
30. Dalle-Donne I, Rossi R, Giustarini D, Milzani A, Colombo R. Protein carbonyl groups as biomarkers of oxidative stress. *Clin Chim Acta* (2003) **329**(1–2):23–38. doi:10.1016/S0009-8981(03)00003-2
31. Suzuki YJ, Carini M, Butterfield DA. Protein carbonylation. *Antioxid Redox Signal* (2010) **12**(3):323–325. doi:10.1089/ars.2009.2887
32. Gillery P, Jaisson S. Usefulness of non-enzymatic post-translational modification derived products (PTMDPs) as biomarkers of chronic diseases. *J Proteomics* (2013) **92**:228–238. doi:10.1016/j.jprot.2013.02.015
33. Stadtman ER, Berlett BS. Reactive oxygen-mediated protein oxidation in aging and disease. *Chem Res Toxicol* (1997) **10**(5):485–494. doi:10.1021/tx960133r
34. Chevion M, Berenshtein E, Stadtman ER. Human studies related to protein oxidation: protein carbonyl content as a marker of damage. *Free Radic Res* (2000) **33**(Suppl):S99–S108.
35. Catalgol B, Grune T. Turnover of oxidatively modified proteins: the usage of in vitro and metabolic labeling. *Free Radic Biol Med* (2009) **46**(1):8–13. doi:10.1016/j.freeradbiomed.2008.09.024
36. Baraibar MA, Ladouce R, Friguet B. Proteomic quantification and identification of carbonylated proteins upon oxidative stress and during cellular aging. *J Proteomics* (2013) **92**:63–70. doi:10.1016/j.jprot.2013.05.008
37. Madian AG, Regnier FE. Proteomic identification of carbonylated proteins and their oxidation sites. *J Proteome Res* (2010) **9**(8):3766–3780. doi:10.1021/pr1002609
38. Yan LJ. Analysis of oxidative modifications of proteins. *Curr Protoc Protein Sci* (2013) **56**(14.4):14.4.1–14.4.28. doi:10.1002/0471140864.ps1404s56
39. Silva AMN, Rui V, Domingues MRM, Spickett CM, Domingues P. Post-translational modifications and mass spectrometry detection. *Free Radic Biol Med* (2013) **65**: 925–941. doi:10.1016/j.freeradbiomed.2013.08.184
40. Baraibar MA, Barbeito AG, Muhoberac BB, Vidal R. A mutant light-chain ferritin that causes neurodegeneration has enhanced propensity toward oxidative damage. *Free Radic Biol Med* (2012) **52**(9):1692–1697. doi:10.1016/j.freeradbiomed.2012.02.015
41. Eaton P. Protein thiol oxidation in health and disease: techniques for measuring disulfides and related modifications in complex protein mixtures. *Free Radical Biol Med* (2006) **40**(11):1889–1899. doi:10.1016/j.freeradbiomed.2005.12.037
42. Giulivi C, Traaseth NJ, Davies KJA. Tyrosine oxidation products: analysis and biological relevance. *Amino Acids* (2003) **25**(3–4):227–232. doi:10.1007/s00726-003-0013-0
43. DiMarco T, Giulivi C. Current analytical methods for the detection of dityrosine, a biomarker of oxidative stress, in biological samples. *Mass Spectrom Rev* (2007) **26**(1):108–120. doi:10.1002/mas.20109
44. Malencik DA, Anderson SR. Dityrosine as a product of oxidative stress and fluorescent probe. *Amino Acids* (2003) **25**(3–3): 233–247. doi:10.1007/s00726-003-0014-z
45. Bordignon M, Da Dalt L, Marinelli L, Gabai G. Advanced oxidation protein products are generated by bovine neutrophils and inhibit free radical production in vitro. *Vet J* (2014) **199**(1):162–168. doi:10.1016/j.tvjl.2013.10.028
46. Witko-Sarsat V, Friedlander M, Capeillère-Blandin C, Nguyen-Khoa T, Nguyen AT, Zingraff J, et al. Advanced oxidation protein products as a novel marker of oxidative stress in uraemia. *Kidney Int* (1996) **49**:1304–1313. doi:10.1038/ki.1996.186
47. Capelliere-Blandin C, Delaveau T, Descamps-Latscha B. Structural modifications of human β_2 microglobulin treated with oxygen-derived radicals. *Biochem J* (1991) **277**(1):175–182. doi:10.1042/bj2770175
48. Malencik DA, Sprouse JD, Swanson CA, Anderson SR. Dityrosine: preparation, isolation and analysis. *Anal Biochem* (1996) **242**(2): 202–213. doi:10.1006/abio.1996.0454
49. Fenaille F, Parisod V, Vuichoud J, Tabet JC, Guy PA. Quantitative determination of dityrosine in milk powders by liquid chromatography coupled with tandem mass spectrometry using isotope dilution. *J Chromatogr A* (2004) **1052**(1–2): 77–84. doi:10.1016/j.chroma.2004.08.104
50. Marvin LF, Delatour T, Tavizzi I, Fay LB, Cupp G, Guy PA. Quantification of o,o'-dityrosine, o-nitrotyrosine and o-tyrosine in cat urine samples by LC/electrospray ionization-MS/MS using isotope dilution. *Anal Chem* (2003) **75**(2): 261–267. doi:10.1021/ac020309w
51. Yin J, Aviles P, Ly C, Lee W, Guillen MJ, Munt S, Cuevas C, Faircloth G. Quantitative analysis of variolin analog (PM01218) in mouse and rat plasma by high-performance liquid chromatography/electrospray ionization tandem

mass spectrometry. *J Chromatogr B* (2006) **832**(2): 268–273. doi:10.1016/j.jchromb.2006.01.027

52. Capeillère-Blandin C, Gausson V, Descamps-Latscha B, Witko-Sarsat V. Biochemical and spectrophotometric significance of advanced oxidized protein products. *Biochim Biophys Acta* (2004) **1689**(2):91–102. doi:10.1016/j.bbadis.2004.02.008
53. Kalousová M, Zima T, Tesar V, Dusilová-Sulková S, Skrha J. Advanced glycoxidation end products in chronic diseases – clinical chemistry and genetic background. *Mutat Res* (2005) **579**(1–2):37–46. doi:10.1016/j.mrfmmm.2005.03.024
54. Colombo G, Clerici M, Giustarini D, Portinaro N, Badalamenti S, Rossi R, Milzani A, Dalle-Donne I. A central role for intermolecular dityrosine cross-linking of fibrinogen in high molecular weight advanced oxidation protein product (AOPP) formation. *Biochim Biophys Acta* (2015) **1850**(1): 1–12. doi:10.1016/j.bbagen.2014.09.024
55. Valli A, Suliman ME, Meert N, Vanholder R, Lindholm B, Stenvinkel P, Watanabe M, Barany P, Alvestrand A, Anderstam B. Overestimation of advanced oxidation protein products in uremic plasma due to presence of triglycerides and other endogenous factors. *Clin Chim Acta* (2007) **379**(1–2): 87–94. doi:10.1016/j.cca.2006.12.026
56. Anderstam B, Bragfors-Helin A-C, Valli A, Stenvinkel P, Lindholm B, Suliman ME. Modification of the oxidative stress biomarker AOPP assay: application in uremic samples. *Clin Chim Acta* (2008) **393**(2): 114–118. doi:10.1016/j.cca.2008.03.029
57. Hanasand M, Omdal R, Norheim KB, Goransson LG, Brede C, Jonsson G. Improved detection of advanced oxidation protein products. *Clin Chim Acta* (2012) **413**(9–10): 901–906. doi:10.1016/j.cca.2012.01.038
58. Al-Gubory KH, Fowler PA, Garrel C. The roles of cellular reactive oxygen species, oxidative stress and antioxidants in pregnancy outcomes. *Int J Biochem Cell Biol* (2010) **42**(10):1634–1650. doi:10.1016/j.biocel.2010.06.001
59. Rizzo A, Roscino MT, Binetti F, Sciorsci RL. Roles of reactive oxygen species in female reproduction. *Reprod Domest Anim* (2012) **47**:344–352. doi:10.1111/j.1439-0531.2011.01891.x
60. Celi P, Merlo M, Barbato O, Gabai G. Relationship between oxidative stress and the success of artificial insemination in dairy cows in a pasture-based system. *Vet J* (2012) **193**(2):498–502. doi:10.1016/j.tvjl.2012.02.002
61. Celi P, Merlo M, Da Dalt L, Stefani A, Barbato O, Gabai G. Relationship between late embryonic mortality and the increase in plasma advanced oxidised protein products (AOPP) in dairy cows. *Reprod Fertil Dev* (2011) **23**(4):527–533. doi:10.1071/RD10268
62. Rizzo A, Minoia G, Trisolini C, Manca R, Sciorsci RL. Concentrations of free radicals and beta-endorphins in repeat breeder cows. *Anim Reprod Sci* (2007) **100**(3–4):257–263. doi:10.1016/j.anireprosci.2006.08.013
63. Rizzo A, Minoia G, Trisolini C, Mutinati M, Spedicato M, Jirillo F, et al. Reactive oxygen species (ROS): involvement in bovine follicular cysts etiopathogenesis. *Immunopharmacol Immunotoxicol* (2009) **31**(4):631–635. doi:10.3109/08923970902932962
64. Talukder S, Ingenhoff L, Kerrisk KL, Celi P. Plasma oxidative stress biomarkers and progesterone profiles in a dairy cow diagnosed with an ovarian follicular cyst. *Vet Q* (2014) **34**(2):113–117. doi:10.1080/01652176.2014.953264
65. Kaufmann TB, Drillich M, Tenhagen BA, Forderung D, Heuwieser W. Prevalence of bovine subclinical endometritis 4h after insemination and its effects on first service conception rate. *Theriogenology* (2009) **71**(2):385–391. doi:10.1016/j.theriogenology.2008.08.005
66. Bondurant RH. Inflammation in the bovine female reproductive tract. *J Anim Sci* (1999) **77** (Suppl. 2):101–110.
67. Singh J, Murray RD, Mshelia G, Woldehiwet Z. The immune status of the bovine uterus during the peripartum period. *Vet J* (2008) **175**(3):301–309. doi:10.1016/j.tvjl.2007.02.003
68. Aurousseau B, Gruffat D, Durand D. Gestation linked radical oxygen species fluxes and vitamins and trace mineral deficiencies in the ruminant. *Reprod Nutr Dev* (2006) **46**(6):601–620. doi:10.1051/rnd:2006045
69. Castillo C, Hernandez J, Bravo A, Lopez-Alonso M, Pereira V, Benedito JL. Oxidative status during late pregnancy and early lactation in dairy cows. *Vet J* (2005) **169**(2):286–292. doi:10.1016/j.tvjl.2004.02.001
70. Ness RB. The consequences for human reproduction of a robust inflammatory response. *Q Rev Biol* (2004) **79**(4):383–393. doi:10.1086/426089
71. Fialovà L, Malbohan I, Kalousova M, Soukupova J, Krofta L, Štipek S, et al. Oxidative stress and inflammation in pregnancy. *Scand J Clin Lab Invest* (2006) **66**:121–128. doi:10.1080/00365510500375230
72. Zhao Y, Flowers WL, Saraiva A, Yeum K-J, Kim SW. Effect of social ranks and gestation housing systems on oxidative stress status, reproductive performance, and immune status of sows. *J Anim Sci* (2013) **91**(12):5848–5858. doi:10.2527/jas.2013-6388
73. Farmer C, Lapointe J, Palin M-F. Effects of the plant extract silymarin on prolactin concentrations, mammary gland development, and oxidative stress in gestating gilts. *J Anim Sci* (2014) **92**(7):2922–2930. doi:10.2527/jas.2013-7118
74. Bubols GB, Zielinsky P, Piccoli AL, Nicoloso LH, Vian I, Moro AM, et al. Nitric oxide and reactive species are modulated in the polyphenol-induced ductus arteriosus constriction in pregnant sheep. *Prenat Diagn* (2014) **34**(13):1268–1276. doi:10.1002/pd.4463
75. Makkar HPS, Francis G, Becker K. Bioactivity of phytochemicals in some lesser-known plants and their effects and potential applications in livestock and aquaculture production systems. *Animal* (2007) **1**(09):1371–1391. doi:10.1017/S1751731107000298
76. Rochfort S, Parker AJ, Dunshea FR. Plant bioactives for ruminant health and productivity. *Phytochemistry* (2008) **69**(2):299–322. doi:10.1016/j.phytochem.2007.08.017
77. Celi P. Yerba Mate (*Ilex paraguariensis*) as strategic supplement for dairy cows. In: Makkar HPS, editor. *Enhancing Animal Welfare and Farmer Income Through Strategic Animal Feeding – Some Case Studies. Paper No. 175.* Rome, Italy: FAO Animal Production and Health (2013). p. 11–8.
78. Wullepit N, Raes K, Beerda B, Veerkamp RF, Fremaut D, De Smet S. Influence of management and genetic merit for milk yield on the oxidative status of plasma in heifers. *Livest Sci* (2009) **123**(2–3):276-282. doi:10.1016/j.livsci.2008.11.013
79. Zebeli Q, Metzler-Zebeli BU. Interplay between rumen digestive disorders and diet-induced inflammation in dairy cattle. *Res Vet Sci* (2012) **93**(3):1099–1108. doi:10.1016/j.rvsc.2012.02.004
80. Rietschel ET, Kirikae T, Schade FU, Mamat U, Schmidt G, Loppnow H, et al. Bacterial endotoxin: molecular relationsh+ips of structure to activity and function. *FASEB J* (1994) **8**(2):217–225.
81. Golder HM, Lean IJ, Rabiee AR, King R, Celi P. Effects of grain, fructose, and histidine feeding on endotoxin and oxidative stress measures in dairy heifers. *J Dairy Sci* (2013) **96**(12):7881–7891. doi:10.3168/jds.2013-7113
82. Golder HM, Celi P, Rabiee AR, Heuer C, Bramley E, Miller DW, et al. Effects of grain, fructose, and histidine on ruminal pH and fermentation products during an induced subacute acidosis protocol. *J Dairy Sci* (2012) **95**(4):1971–1982. doi:10.3168/jds.2011-4671
83. Po E, Horsburgh K, Raadsma HW, Celi P. Yerba Mate (*Ilex paraguarensis*) as a novel feed supplement for growing lambs. *Small Ruminant Res* (2012) **106**(2–3):131–136. doi:10.1016/j.smallrumres.2012.05.016
84. Robinson PH, Tamminga S, van Vuuren AM. Influence of declining level of feed intake and varying the proportion of starch in the concentrate on rumen fermentation in dairy cows. *Livest Prod Sci* (1986) **15**(2):173–189. doi:10.1016/0301-6226(86)90026-6
85. Harris P, Bailey SR, Elliott J, Longland A. Countermeasures for pasture-associated laminitis in ponies and horses. *J Nutr* (2006) **136**(7): 2114S–2121S.
86. Yin C, Pettigrew A, Loftus JP, Black SJ, Belkna JK. Tissue concentrations of 4-HNE in the black walnut extract model of laminitis: indication of oxidant stress in affected laminae. *Vet Immunol Immunopathol* (2009) **129** (3–4): 211–215. doi:10.1016/j.vetimm.2008.11.016
87. Burns TA, Westerman T, Nuovo GJ, Watts MR, Pettigrew A, Yin C, Belknap JK. Role of oxidative tissue injury in the pathophysiology of experimentally induced equine laminitis: a comparison of 2 models. *J Vet Intern Med* (2011), **25**(3): 540–548. doi:10.1111/j.1939-1676.2011.0706.x
88. Villasante A, Araneda OF, Behn C, Galleguillos M, Adarmes H. Antioxidant capacity and oxidative damage determination in synovial fluid of chronically damaged equine metacarpophalangeal joint. *Vet Res Commun* (2010) **34**(2): 133–141. doi:10.1007/s11259-009-9338-9
89. Dimock AN, Siciliano PD, McIlwraith CW. Evidence supporting an increased presence of reactive oxygen species in the diseased equine joint. *Equine Vet J* (2000) **32**(5):439–443. doi:10.2746/042516400777591129

90. Celi P, Raadsma HW. Effects of Yerba Mate (*Ilex paraguariensis*) supplementation on the productive performance of dairy cows during mid-lactation. *Anim Prod Sci* (2010) **50**(6):339–344. doi:10.1071/AN09170
91. Celi P, Robinson A. Effect of Yerba Mate (*Ilex paraguariensis*) supplementation on the performance of dairy calves. *Anim Prod Sci* (2010) **50**(6):376–381. doi:10.1071/AN09170
92. Ballet N, Robert JC, Williams PEV. Chapter 19: Vitamins in forages. In: Givens D.I. Owen E., Axford R.F.E., Omed H.M., editors. *Forage Evaluation in Ruminant Nutrition*. Oxon, UK: CABI Publishing (2000). p. 399–431.
93. Bruynsteen L, Janssens GPJ, Harris PA, Duchateau L, Valle E, Odetti P, et al. Changes in oxidative stress in response to different levels of energy restriction in obese ponies. *Br J Nutr* (2014) **112**(08):1402–1411. doi:doi:10.1017/S0007114514001974
94. Shen YB, Weaver AC, Kim SW. Effect of feed grade l-methionine on growth performance and gut health in nursery pigs compared with conventional dl-methionine. *J Anim Sci* (2014) **92**(12):5530–5539. doi:10.2527/jas.2014-7830
95. Levine RL, Mosoni L, Berlett BS, Stadtman ER. Methionine residues as endogenous antioxidants in proteins. *Proc Natl Acad Sci U S A* (1996) **93**(26):15036–15040. doi:10.1073/pnas.93.26.15036
96. Estévez M. Oxidative damage to poultry: from farm to fork. *Poult Sci* (2015) **94** (6): 1368–1378. doi:10.3382/ps/pev094
97. Delles RM, Xiong YL, True AD, Ao T, Dawson KA. Dietary antioxidant supplementation enhances lipid and protein oxidative stability of chicken broiler meat through promotion of antioxidant enzyme activity. *Poult Sci* (2014) **93**(6):1561–1570. doi:10.3382/ps.2013-03682
98. Zhang W, Xiao S, Lee EJ, Ahn DU. Consumption of oxidized oil increases oxidative stress in broilers and affects the quality of breast meat. *J Agric Food Chem* (2011) **59**(3):969–974. doi:10.1021/jf102918z
99. Yu J, Chen Y, Zhai L, Zhang L, Xu Y, Wang S, Hu S. Antioxidative effect of ginseng stem-leaf saponins on oxidative stress induced by cyclophosphamide in chickens. *Poult Sci* (2015) **94**(5):927–933. doi:10.3382/ps/pev055
100. Guzzo N, Bailoni L, Mantovani R, Da Dalt L, Gabai G. Oxidized protein biomarkers in the blood and milk of cows supplemented with flaxseed during the dry period. In: Knight C.H., editor. *2nd DairyCare Conference*; 2015 Mar 3-4. Cordoba, Spain: DairyCare COST Action FA1308 (2015). p. 60.
101. Silanikove N, Shapiro F, Shamay A, Leitner G. Role of xanthine oxidase, lactoperoxidase, and NO in the innate immune system of mammary secretion during active involution in dairy cows: manipulation with casein hydrolyzates. *Free Radic Biol Med* (2005) **38**(9):1139–1151. doi:10.1016/j.freeradbiomed.2004.12.011
102. Gabai G, Magro M, Baratella D, Miotto G, Da Dalt L, Vianello F, editors. Oxidized whey proteins as potential biomarkers of oxidative stress: preliminary studies of milk exposure to the myeloperoxidase product HOCl. *1st DairyCare Conference*; 2015 Aug 22–23. Copenhagen, Denmark: DairyCare COST Action FA1308 (2014) p. 42.
103. Kirschvink N, Moffarts BD, Lekeux P. The oxidant/antioxidant equilibrium in horses. *Vet J* (2008) **177**(2):178–191. doi:10.1016/j.tvjl.2007.07.033
104. Crowley J, Po E, Celi P, Muscatello G. Systemic and respiratory oxidative stress in the pathogenesis and diagnosis of *Rhodococcus equi* pneumonia. *Equine Vet J* (2013) **45**:20–25. doi:10.1111/evj.12166
105. Leclere M, Magdesian KG, Kass PH, Pusterla N, Rhodes DM. Comparison of the clinical, microbiological, radiological and haematological features of foals with pneumonia caused by *Rhodococcus equi* and other bacteria. *Vet J* (2011) **187**(1):109–112. doi:10.1016/j.tvjl.2009.10.025
106. Po E, Williams C, Muscatello G, Celi P. Assessment of oxidative stress biomarkers in exhaled breath condensate and blood of Thoroughbred foals. *Vet J* (2013) **196**(2):269–271. doi:10.1016/j.tvjl.2012.08.018
107. Celi P. Biomarkers of oxidative stress in ruminant medicine. *Immunopharmacol Immunotoxicol* (2011) **33**(2):233–240. doi:10.3109/08923973.2010.514917
108. Hou X, Zhang J, Ahmad H, Zhang H, Xu Z, Wang T. Evaluation of antioxidant activities of ampelopsin and its protective effect in lipopolysaccharide-induced oxidative stress piglets. *PLoS One* (2014) **9**(9):e108314. doi:10.1371/journal.pone.0108314
109. Cheah F-C, Jobe AH, Moss TJ, Newnham JP, Kallapur SG. Oxidative stress in fetal lambs exposed to intra-amniotic endotoxin in a chorioamnionitis model. *Pediatr Res* (2008) **63**(3):274–279. doi:10.1203/PDR.0b013e31815f653b
110. Celi P, Eppleston J, Armstrong A, Watt B. Selenium supplementation increases wool growth and reduce faecal egg counts of Merino weaners in a selenium deficient area. *Anim Prod Sci* (2010) **50**(7):688–692. doi:10.1071/AN09168
111. Dimitrijević B, Borozan S, Katić-Radivojević S, Stojanović S. Effects of infection intensity with *Strongyloides papillosus* and albendazole treatment on development of oxidative/nitrosative stress in sheep. *Vet Parasitol* (2012) **186**(3–4):364–375. doi:10.1016/j.vetpar.2011.11.017
112. Forsyth LMG, Minns FC, Kirvar E, Adamson RE, Hall FR, McOrist S, et al. Tissue damage in cattle infected with *Theileria annulata* accompanied by metastasis of cytokine-producing, schizont-infected mononuclear phagocytes. *J Comp Pathol* (1999) **120**(1):39–57. doi:10.1053/jcpa.1998.0256
113. Saleh MA, Mahran OM, Al-Salahy MB. Corpuscular oxidation in newborn crossbred calves naturally infected with *Theileria annulata*. *Vet Parasitol* (2011) **182**(2–4):193–200. doi:10.1016/j.vetpar.2011.05.011
114. Sconberg S, Nockels CF, Bennet DW, Bruyninclese W, Blancquaret AMB, Craig AM. Effect of shipping handling, adrenocortiocotropic hormone and epinephrine on L-tocopherol content of bovine blood. *Am J Vet Res* (1993) **54**:1287–1293.
115. Marco-Ramell A, Pato R, Peña R, Saco Y, Manteca X, Ruiz de la Torre JL, et al. Identification of serum stress biomarkers in pigs housed at different stocking densities. *Vet J* (2011) **190**(2):e66–e71. doi:10.1016/j.tvjl.2011.01.003
116. Marco-Ramell A, Arroyo L, Saco Y, García-Heredia A, Camps J, Fina M, et al. Proteomic analysis reveals oxidative stress response as the main adaptative physiological mechanism in cows under different production systems. *J Proteomics* (2012) **75**(14):4399–4411. doi:10.1016/j.jprot.2012.04.002
117. Mutinati M, Pantaleo M, Roncetti M, Piccinno M, Rizzo A, Sciorsci RL. Oxidative stress in neonatology. A review. *Reprod Domest Anim* (2014) **49**(1):7–16. doi:10.1111/rda.12230
118. Ranade R, Talukder S, Muscatello G, Celi P. Assessment of oxidative stress biomarkers in exhaled breath condensate and blood of dairy heifer calves from birth to weaning. *Vet J* (2014) **202**(3):583–587. doi:10.1016/j.tvjl.2014.10.025
119. Caperna TJ, Shannon AE, Blomberg LA, Garrett WM, Ramsay TG. Identification of protein carbonyls in serum of the fetal and neonatal pig. *Comp Biochem Physiol B Biochem Mol Biol* (2010) **156**(3):189–196. doi:10.1016/j.cbpb.2010.03.006
120. Yin J, Wu MM, Xiao H, Ren WK, Duan JL, Yang G, Li TJ, Yin YL. Development of an antioxidant system after early weaning in piglets. *J Anim Sci* (2014) **92**(2):612–619. doi:10.2527/jas.2013-6986
121. Bernabucci U, Ronchi B, Lacetera N, Nardone A. Markers of oxidative status in plasma and erythrocytes of transition dairy cows during hot season. *J Dairy Sci* (2002) **85**(9):2173–2179. doi:10.3168/jds.S0022-0302(02)74296-3
122. Di Trana A, Celi P, Claps S, Fedele V, Rubino R. The effect of hot season and nutrition on the oxidative status and metabolic profile in dairy goats during mid lactation. *Anim Sci* (2006) **82**:717–722. doi:10.1079/ASC200672
123. Chauhan SS, Celi P, Fahri FT, Leury BJ, Dunshea FR. Dietary antioxidants at supranutritional doses modulate skeletal muscle heat shock protein and inflammatory gene expression in sheep exposed to heat stress. *J Anim Sci* (2014) **92**(11):4897–4908. doi:10.2527/jas.2014-8047
124. Chauhan SS, Celi P, Leury BJ, Clarke IJ, Dunshea FR. Dietary antioxidants at supranutritional doses improve oxidative status and reduce the negative effects of heat stress in sheep. *J Anim Sci* (2014) **92**(8):3364–3374. doi:10.2527/jas.2014-7714
125. Liu F, Celi P, Chauhan S, Cottrell JJ, Abrasaldo A, Talukder S, et al., editors. Effects of heat stress and antioxidants (selenium or vitamin E) supplementation on oxidative status in growing pigs. *Proceedings of the American Society of Animal Science (ASAS) Midwest Section and the American Dairy Science Association® (ADSA®) Midwest Branch*; 2015 Mar 16–18; Des Moines, IA, USA (2015).
126. Tan GY, Yang L, Fu YQ, Feng JH, Zhang MH. Effects of different acute high ambient temperatures on function of hepatic mitochondrial respiration, antioxidative enzymes, and oxidative injury in broiler chickens. *Poult Sci* (2010) **89**(1):115–122. doi:10.3382/ps.2009-00318
127. Xie J, Tang L, Lu L, Zhang L, Lin X, Liu HC, Odle J, Luo X. Effects of acute and chronic heat stress on plasma metabolites, hormones and oxidant status in restrictedly fed broiler breeders. *Poult Sci* (2015) **94**(7):1635–1644. doi:10.3382/ps/pev105
128. Yang X, Luo YH, Zeng QF, Zhang KY, Ding XM, Bai SP, Wang JP. Effects of low ambient temperatures and dietary vitamin C supplement on growth

performance, blood parameters, and antioxidant capacity of 21-day-old broilers. *Poult Sci* (2014) **93**(4):898–905. doi:10.3382/ps.2013-03438
129. Celi P. The role of oxidative stress in small ruminants' health and production. *R Bras Zootec* (2010) **39**:348–363 doi:10.1590/S1516-35982010001300038
130. Lean IJ, DeGaris PJ, Celi P, McNeill DM, Rodney RM, Fraser DR. Influencing the future: interactions of skeleton, energy, protein and calcium during late gestation and early lactation. *Anim Prod Sci* (2014) **54**(9):1177–1189. doi:10.1071/AN14479
131. Dunshea FR, Leury BJ, Fahri F, DiGiacomo K, Hung A, Chauhan S, et al. Amelioration of thermal stress impacts in dairy cows. *Anim Prod Sci* (2013) **53**(9):965–975. doi:10.1071/AN12384
132. Baumgard LH, Rhoads RP. Ruminant Nutrition Symposium: ruminant production and metabolic responses to heat stress. *J Anim Sci* (2012) **90**(6):1855–1865. doi:10.2527/jas.2011-4675
133. Rhoads RP, Baumgard LH, Suagee JK, Sanders SR. Nutritional interventions to alleviate the negative consequences of heat stress. *Adv Nutr* (2013) **4**(3):267–276. doi:10.3945/an.112.003376

Conflict of Interest Statement: The authors declare that the research was conducted in the absence of any commercial or financial relationships that could be construed as a potential conflict of interest.

11

The effects of steroid implant and dietary soybean hulls on estrogenic activity of sera of steers grazing toxic endophyte-infected tall fescue pasture

Nancy W. Shappell[1]*, *Michael D. Flythe*[2] *and Glen E. Aiken*[2]

[1] *USDA-ARS Animal Metabolism-Agricultural Chemicals Research, Fargo, ND, USA,* [2] *USDA-ARS Forage-Animal Production Research Unit, Lexington, KY, USA*

Edited by:
Chang Bon Choi,
Yeungnam University, South Korea

Reviewed by:
Takeshi Ohkubo,
Ibaraki University, Japan
Sungkwonk Park,
Sejong University, South Korea

***Correspondence:**
Nancy W. Shappell,
Biosciences Research Laboratory,
USDA-ARS Animal Metabolism-Agricultural Chemicals Research,
1605 Albrecht Blvd., Fargo,
ND 58102, USA
nancy.shappell@ars.usda.gov

Soybean hulls (SBHs) have been fed to cattle pasturing on endophyte-infected tall fescue in attempts to increase rate of gain. Literature reports indicated some symptoms associated with fescue toxicosis were ameliorated by the use of steroidal implants containing estradiol (E2) and progesterone [implantation (IMP)], feeding SBHs, or the combination of the two. While the mechanism for amelioration was unclear, the SBHs were postulated as acting as a diluent of the toxic factors of the fescue. Alternatively, estradiol and phytoestrogens of SBHs might be acting through relaxation of the persistent vasoconstriction found in animals ingesting ergot alkaloids of endophyte-infected fescue. If so, estrogenic activity of serum of steers receiving SBHs, IMP, or a combination of the two should be elevated. Using the cellular proliferation assay of estrogenicity (E-Screen), estradiol equivalents (E_2Eqs) were determined on both SBHs and the serum of steers from a previously reported study. Range of SBHs was 5.0–8.5 ng Eqs g^{-1} DM (mean 6.5, $n = 4$ from different commercial sources of SBHs). At the rate fed, theoretically calculated blood E_2Eq could be physiologically relevant (~80 pg mL^{-1}, based on 2.3 kg SBHs d^{-1}, 300 kg steer, 5.7% blood volume, and 10% absorption). Serum E_2Eqs did increase in steers ($P \leq 0.05$) with steroidal implants or fed SBHs by 56 and 151% over control, respectively, and treatments were additive (211% increase). Serum prolactin was also greatest for the SBH + IMP group (188 ng mL^{-1}, $P < 0.05$), concentrations comparable to values reported for steers grazing endophyte-*free* fescue. Prolactin in the SBH group was higher than IMP or control groups (146 versus 76 and 60 ng mL^{-1}, respectively). Still unknown is if additional E_2Eqs from dietary phytoestrogens or exogenous sources of estradiol can further reduce symptoms of fescue toxicosis. The E-Screen assay was an effective tool in monitoring serum for estrogenic effects of dietary supplementation with SBHs or estrogenic implants.

Keywords: phytoestrogens, isoflavones, fescue toxicosis, prolactin, estrogenic activity

Introduction

Ergot alkaloids produced by a fungal endophyte [*Epichloë coenophiala* (Morgan-Jones & W. Gams) C.W. Bacon & Schardl] that infects tall fescue [*Lolium arundinaceum* (Schreb.) Darbysh] have a strong affinity for selected subclasses of α-adrenergic and serotonin receptors in the vasculature (1, 2). Ergot alkaloids consumed by grazing animals cause persistent constriction of blood flow to peripheral tissues, thereby disabling the animal's ability to regulate core body temperature, resulting in a condition referred to as fescue toxicosis. Various feeding regimens have been evaluated to mitigate the effects of fescue toxicosis on the rate of gain of steers (3–7). Soybean hulls (SBHs) are a high-fiber feed, the feeding of which has been effective in providing a higher plane of nutrition, resulting in a higher rate of gain, when fed to steers grazing toxic tall fescue pasture (6, 7). Feeding SBHs at a daily rate of 2.3 kg day^{-1} $steer^{-1}$ partially reversed the decreased serum prolactin concentrations and decreased the frequency of rough hair coats [Carter et al. (7)], both symptoms of fescue toxicosis (8). An estradiol–progesterone implant with no SBH treatment also reduced prevalence of rough hair, and a combination of the two treatments resulted in an additive effect on mitigating toxicosis. While the authors conjectured that SBHs diluted ergot alkaloids in steer diets, the phytoestrogens in SBHs could have been a contributing factor in the mitigation through positive effects on specific vasculature and overall circulation.

Though phytoestrogens (a subset known as isoflavones) have been linked to reproductive issues in cattle and sheep (9, 10), dietary isoflavones have also been demonstrated to benefit human health and well-being (11, 12). Various effects on the vasculature have been reported. For instance, isoflavones have been identified as an alternative to 17β-estradiol in ameliorating hot flashes in post-menopausal women, through relaxation of the vasculature by binding the estrogen receptors in the vascular endothelium, stimulating nitric oxide synthase (NOS), resulting in nitric oxide-mediated vasodilation (12–14). There also is evidence that genistein, considered the most estrogenic phytoestrogen in soybeans, exerts a vasodilatory effect as a β-adrenergic receptor agonist (15). Based on these findings, isoflavones may have the potential to induce relaxation of alkaloid-induced vasoconstriction, and perhaps mitigate other signs of toxicosis as described by Carter et al. (7) (rough hair coat, low prolactin concentrations, and poor thriftiness/performance).

Depending on species, variety, season and drying time, the amount of isoflavones found in legumes, such as soybeans, alfalfa, and clover, can vary (11, 16–18). While the estrogenic activity of soybean meal (SBM) (45% crude protein) was assessed using the *in vitro* cellular proliferation assay (E-Screen) and found to average 113 ng g^{-1} as fed (19), the estrogenic activity of SBHs has not been evaluated. Therefore, SBH samples collected from various suppliers, and serum samples collected from steers of the Carter et al. (7) study were analyzed by E-Screen to assess the estrogenicity of SBHs and determine if there is an association between serum prolactin and serum estrogenic activity.

Materials and Methods

Soybean Meal and Hulls

Samples of SBHs fed by Carter et al. (7) were no longer available for determination of estrogenic activity, therefore four samples from unrelated lots of SBHs were obtained from three feed suppliers representing three different years of harvest (**Table 1**, Woodford Feed Co., Versailles, KY, USA; Hallway Feed Co., Lexington, KY, USA, and North Dakota State University Feed Mill, Fargo, ND, USA). Sample size ranged from 120 to 750 g (as fed). Sample dry matter was determined in quintuplicate (dried at 100°C). Extractions were done as described for isoflavinoid analysis (20), with the exception of an additional hexane extraction step. Three subsamples of feed (1 g as fed) were extracted using sonication (47 kHz) and 25 mL of 60% acetonitrile at 37°C for 1 h, shaking samples every 10 min to resuspend feed and enhance sample/solvent contact. Particulates were removed by centrifugation (900 × *g*, 10 min). Supernatants were filtered through solvent-washed glass wool to remove remaining fines and volumes recorded. Acetonitrile was volatilized under N_2 at 37°C, and hexane (1:1, v:v) was added, vortexed for 1 min, then held at −20°C for ≥1 h. Phase separation was achieved by centrifugation as described above. The upper hexane layer was discarded, and the aqueous layer was subsequently diluted to ~90 mL with nanopure H_2O (npH_2O) after removing any pelleted material. Phytoestrogens were then concentrated by Oasis HLB solid phase extraction as described [Waters, Milford, MA, USA (21)], and the eluent taken to dryness and stored at −20°C for later analysis. On the day of assay, samples were resuspended in 400 μL of 5% dimethyl sulfoxide in npH_2O. Resuspended SBH samples were diluted (1:10,000–1:25,000) in cell culture medium described below to obtain cellular responses in the linear range of the E-Screen assay (~1×10^{-12} to 1×10^{-11} M).

Animal Treatment, Serum Collection

Estradiol equivalents were assayed on serum collected from steers used in a 2-year grazing experiment, evaluating the effect of combinations of steroid implantation (IMP) and SBH feeding on mitigation of fescue toxicosis (7). The experimental protocol was reviewed and accepted by Institution's Animal Care and Use Committee at the University of Kentucky (00996A2006). Treatments consisted of IMP (Synovex-S 200, 200 mg progesterone and 20 mg estradiol, Fort Dodge Animal Health, Fort Dodge,

TABLE 1 | Estrogenic equivalents of commercial soybean hull feedstuff by E-Screen assay.

Site of purchase/origin	Year of harvest	E_2Eqs^a ng E_2 Eqs g^{-1} DM	COV[b]
KY/na[c]	2011	8.5 ± 0.7	8%
ND/na	2013	5.0 ± 0.7	14%
KY/IN	2014	7.2 ± 0.3	5%
KY/IN	2014	5.3 ± 0.4	8%
	Mean	6.5 ± 1.6	25%

[a]*Mean ± SD of three replicate extractions, each dilution was tested on 4–6 wells of cells. Values do not reflect activity assayed in hexane phase, as ≤3% of SPE values.*
[b]*Coefficient of variation.*
[c]*Not available.*

IA, USA), SBHs (daily SBH feeding at 2.3 kg $steer^{-1}$ day^{-1}), SBH + IMP (combined feeding of SBHs and IMP), and Control (pasture-only). Steers were assigned to 12 3.0-ha pastures of toxic endophyte-infected tall fescue in a split-plot design. Main- and sub-plot treatments were ±SBH and ±IMP. Blood was collected from the jugular vein on 14 June and 5 July in 2007, and 24 June and 24 July in 2008. Blood was centrifuged for 15 min at 10,000 × *g* to obtain serum, which was stored frozen (−20°C) for prolactin analysis. Detailed descriptions of experimental design, sample preparation, and analyses (including prolactin) were provided by Carter et al. (7). Estrogenic activity (estradiol equivalents, E_2Eqs) was analyzed in serum from a subset of steers for which serum samples were available for all collection dates to provide an estimate of the bioavailability of isoflavones once they are absorbed into the animal's circulation.

Serum Extraction and E-Screen

Prior to E-Screen testing, serum samples required extraction to eliminate factors toxic to the MCF-7 cells as previously described (22). Sterile aliquots (typically 1 mL) of serum were diluted with acetonitrile (ACN, 1:2 v/v) in silanized glass conical centrifuge tubes. Serum weights were recorded, samples vortexed for 1 min, and centrifuged at 800 × *g* for 10 min (room temperature). The serum/ACN was removed from the pellet and transferred into a silanized glass vial, and residual liquid and pellet were weighed. The extracted serum was taken to dryness, and stored at −20°C until E-Screen analysis. Sample weights were used to calculate and adjust final estrogenic activity values for sample loss during extraction. Extracted serum samples were reconstituted in npH_20 at 1/5th the original serum volume. Samples were further diluted in cell culture medium (1:10 to up to 1:25 of the original serum) to obtain a proliferative response in the linear range of the E_2 standard curve. The limit of quantitation was ~0.2 pg mL^{-1} of E_2Eq in the original serum.

The MCF-7 BOS, estrogen-dependent cell line (derived from a human mammary epithelial carcinoma, provided by Drs. Ana Soto and Carlos Sonnenschein, Tufts University, Boston, MA, USA) was used to determine estrogenicity relative to 17β-estradiol as described by Shappell (21). Briefly, resuspended extracts were diluted in cell culture media. Twenty-four hours post-plating, steroid-containing medium (5% FBS) was removed and replaced with steroid-free medium (minus phenol red and containing 10% charcoal dextran-stripped FBS) containing diluted sample extracts of samples or 17β-E_2 (1×10^{-13} to 1×10^{-9} M). After 5 days of incubation, cells were fixed with trichloroacetic acid, stained for protein with sulforhodamine B (Sigma Chemicals, St. Louis, MO, USA), solubilized in buffer, and absorbance measured (490 nm). Estradiol equivalents were determined based on a regression analysis of the 17β-E_2 curve from the same experiment. Assay assessment, including range finding, was performed on serum samples from four steers on endophyte-infected tall fescue pasture, but not on trial. All extracts were tested over a wide range of dilutions, and those resulting in absorbance readings in the linear range of the E_2 standard curve were used for interpolation of the data. Evidence of toxicity was determined by evaluating cellular proliferation in the presence of the sample extract spiked with 17β-E_2 versus 17β-E_2 alone. The estrogen-dependence of cellular proliferation was confirmed by co-incubation with the E_2-receptor antagonist ICI 182,780 [Tocris, Ellisville, MO, USA (23)].

Statistical Analysis

Estradiol equivalents and prolactin concentrations were statistically analyzed using mixed models of SAS (24), with year, treatment, and blood collection month (June versus July) as fixed effects, and animal as a random effect. Mean separations were performed on least square means using the Tukey–Kramer adjustment of multiple comparisons of least square means. Estradiol equivalents data were transformed using the log function to stabilize the variances and analyzed as repeated measures using the AR(1) covariance structure.

Results

Soybean Hull Estrogenic Activity

Quantitation of E_2Eqs from extracts of SBHs yielded reproducible data. Coefficient of variation on triplicate extractions averaged 8.8%, with only one COV over 10% (14.2%). The hexane extractable phase contained ≤3% of the estrogenic activity from the SPE extraction. Estradiol equivalents of the SBH samples harvested in three different years and representing at least two different regions averaged 6.5 ± 1.65 ng g^{-1} dry matter or 5.8 ng g^{-1} wet weight (**Table 1**, overall COV 25%). As expected, the dry matter content of the processed SBHs were essentially identical (89 ± 1%). The estrogenic activity of SBH samples was more variable, though the range of values within a year was similar to the range across years.

Serum E_2Eqs

Range finding samples from the four steers on endophyte-infected tall fescue pasture, but not on trial yielded values similar to those from the control treatment group (4.9 ± 0.92 versus 6.1 ± 1.0 pg mL^{-1} E_2Eqs, respectively). Of the experimental treatments, all had mean serum estrogenicity greater ($P < 0.05$) than control steers (**Figure 1**). The smallest increase in E_2Eqs over control was found when feeding SBHs alone (9.6 ± 1.3 pg mL^{-1}), with the serum from IMP steers ranking next (15.3 ± 1.7 pg mL^{-1}). The highest mean serum E_2Eqs was of steers receiving the combined IMP and SBH treatment (19.0 ± 2.5 pg mL^{-1} and similar to IMP alone ($P = 0.44$). Serum E_2Eqs of IMP-SBH steers was greater ($P < 0.001$) than the SBH steers, indicating an additive effect of the two treatments.

Serum Prolactin

Unlike serum estrogenic activity, serum prolactin concentrations of IMP steers were not different from control concentrations (76.3 ± 7.6 IMP, versus 60.1 ± 12.9 ng mL^{-1} control, $P = 0.38$). SBH treatment alone resulted in elevated prolactin concentrations (145.5 ± 13.9 ng mL^{-1}, $P < 0.05$) with even greater prolactin concentrations when SBH and IMP treatments were combined (187.9 ± 17.3 ng mL^{-1}, $P < 0.05$) (**Figure 2**). There was a weak, but positive correlation between serum E_2Eqs and serum prolactin concentrations ($r = 0.29$; $P = 0.027$; $n = 59$).

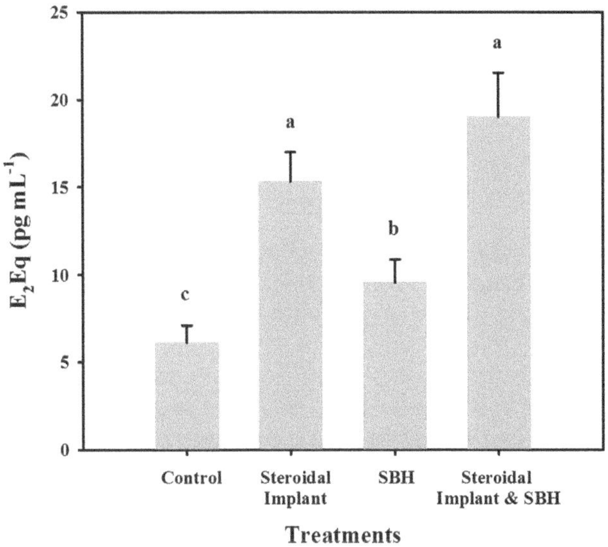

FIGURE 1 | Mean estrogenic equivalents (E_2Eqs) in steers grazing toxic endophyte-infected [*Epichloë coenophiala* (Morgan-Jones & W. Gams) C. W. Bacon & Schardl] tall fescue [*Lolium arundinaceum* (Schreb.) Darbysh] and treated (*n* = 4 steers per treatment groups) with or without an estradiol–progesterone ear implant and soybean hull (SBH) feeding combinations. Values are averages over 2 years, two sample dates per year (6/14 and 7/5/2007; 6/24 and 7/24/2008). Means with different letters are different ($P \leq 0.05$).

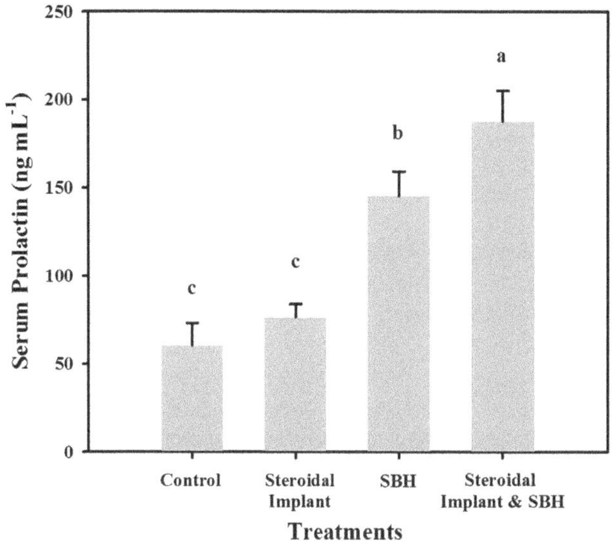

FIGURE 2 | Mean serum prolactin levels in steers grazing toxic endophyte-infected [*Epichloë coenophiala* (Morgan-Jones & W. Gams) C. W. Bacon & Schardl] tall fescue [*Lolium arundinaceum* (Schreb.) Darbysh] and treated (*n* = 4 steers per treatment groups) with or without an estradiol–progesterone ear implant and soybean hull (SBH) feeding combinations. Values are averages over 2 years, two sample dates per year (6/14 and 7/5/2007; 6/24 and 7/24/2008). Means with different letters are different ($P \leq 0.05$).

Discussion

Estrogenic Activity of SBHs

While soybeans and SBM have been evaluated for phytoestrogens and estrogenic activity, SBHs as an alternative feedstuff had not. The hulls are a co-product of milling meal that is derived from the fibrous, inert, soybean seed coat and are greater than 86% cellulose, hemicellulose, and lignin (25), with the remainder being primarily protein and minerals. Variability of E_2Eqs (5.0–8.5 ng g^{-1}) reported herein for SBHs from different suppliers was less than that reported for soybean *meal* using the yeast-based human α-estrogen receptor *in vitro* assay [YES (26)]. Meal from lots manufactured 1 month apart varied threefold in E_2Eqs by YES assay, while SBHs analyzed here varied by <2-fold. For context, based on data from our laboratory, the estrogenic activity of SBHs could be expected to range from 4 to 20% of SBM. These estimates are based on E-Screen analysis of SBM in our laboratory yielding 127 E_2Eqs ng g^{-1} dry matter (19), and are similar to analysis by YES assay [29–100 E_2Eqs]. The measured quantities of estrogenic activity of SBH are in line with the phytoestrogen content of hulls, reported to be 11–15% of whole soybeans or 15% of SBM from chemical analysis (27).

Physiological Context for Estrogenic Activity

A theoretical assessment of the potential for a physiological effect of SBH feeding of steers follows:

2,070 g DM SBHs per day (2,300 g as fed × 89% dry matter)
2,070 g SBHs DM × 6.5 E_2Eqs ng g^{-1} DM SBHs =
13.5 μg E_2Eqs per day per steer

For a 300 kg steer, blood volume estimates = 5.7% of body weight (28)

300 kg × 5.7% = 17.1 L or 17,100 mL blood volume

Of 13.5 μg E_2Eqs fed, if 10% are absorbed and bioavailable, then 1.35 μg E_2Eqs/17,100 mL blood = 79 pg mL^{-1} E_2Eqs in blood.

Obviously, this estimate has inherent assumptions requiring caution, if not skepticism. First, is the assumption of bolus delivery of phytoestrogens, second, no metabolism of phytoestrogens, either by steer or by their microflora, reducing the estrogenicity of the feedstuff. Though ingested phytoestrogens are found circulating in the serum of cattle (29), estimates of bioavailability were not reported. The peak blood concentrations (relative to time of consumption) resembled those in a study of women consuming phytoestrogen-rich diets (30). In women, the estimates of bioavailability for two phytoestrogens (genistein and daidzein) were 18–27% based on urinary recovery after 48 h. Similarly, oral bioavailability of genistein and daidzein in rats were 18 and 23%, respectively (31). Using a value of 10% bioavailability in the calculation above, though less than these reports, could still result in large overestimates due to ruminal metabolism (32). The estimate above also ignores any receptor-level competition between naturally circulating estrogens and the phytoestrogens. For context, the circulating concentration of estradiol for cows in estrus peak at ~10 pg mL^{-1} (28). Based on this calculation, it appears the dosage of estrogenic activity from SBHs, may be capable of eliciting an estrogenic response.

Supporting the potential for circulating E_2Eqs of steers consuming SBHs to be capable of exerting a physiological impact are the findings in rats receiving phytoestrogens. After 3 days of oral administration of ~75 mg kg body weight^{-1} day^{-1} of the phytoestrogens, genistein and daidzein (2:1 ratio), to 17 day old rats, an increase in wet uterine weight was observed (33). SBHs (as fed) were reported to contain 111 mg kg^{-1} of genistein and 200 mg kg^{-1} of daidzein (27). Using these values, the steers in our study received an estimated 250 and 460 mg kg body weight^{-1} day^{-1} of genistein and daidzein, respectively, substantially more than the above threshold for a uterine dose response in rats.

Serum E_2Eqs and Prolactin Response to Treatment

Historically little attention has been paid to the estrogenicity of various livestock feeds in comparison to estrogenicity of human foods. Exceptions include red clover and the associated infertility in sheep (34) or the effects of the estrogenic mycotoxin zearalenone-contaminated feed on heifers (35) and ewes (36). Soybeans have been used for livestock and poultry feed in the United States since the 1930s (37), and SBM is referred to as "the most important protein source used to feed farm animals" by the Feedipedia web site sponsored by the Institute for Agricultural Research, French Agricultural Center for International Development, French Association for Animal Production and the Food and Agriculture Organization of the United Nations (38). In contrast, their web site which provides many pages of information on SBM, mentions SBM's estrogenic properties in only one line – "soybean meal contains 1 g kg^{-1} of genistein, which has estrogenic properties." In contrast, a recent review in the International Journal of Endocrinology reports on the effect of phytoestrogens and specifically SBM on reproductive hormones in cows (29). SBHs, which contain only 5–20% of the estimated E_2Eqs of commonly fed SBM, nearly doubled the serum E_2Eq concentration of steer serum relative to control. These findings, at least conceptually, support the theoretical estimates of estrogenic activity made above, and are further supported by empirical findings of increased estrogenic activity of serum from SBH + IMP steers.

Estrogenic activity of serum from implanted steers was almost threefold that of control steers. These findings are in agreement with the plasma E_2 concentrations measured in steers with Synovex-S implants (20 mg estradiol). In two separate trials, Rumsey and Beaudry (39) found mean E_2 concentrations to be 4.4 and 34 times the non-implanted steers concentration, 60 days post-implantation ($n = 10$ steer per treatment per trial, using radioimmunoassay), with mean E_2 concentrations declining to near control concentrations by 106–120 days. Estrogenic activities in serum samples from steers in the current study are a mean of those collected at about 60 and 90 days post-implantation, and therefore could be expected to be lower than at 60 days.

While the findings of enhanced estrogenic activity with SBH feeding is novel, perhaps more unexpected is the trend for additivity of treatments (SBH + IMP) on E_2Eqs. The utility of the E-Screen assay can be fully realized here, because measurement of blood estrogens alone, either by immunoassay or by chemical analysis, would have failed to accurately reflect the full potential for systemic estrogenic activity. There have been some indications of additivity of *in vivo* responses to estrogenic chemicals in the literature, though often evidence of additivity occurs over a very limited range of concentrations [fish: (40, 41); frogs: (42); rats: (33)]. Lack of additive responses are most likely a reflection of the complexity of nature including differential rates of absorption, metabolism, receptor affinity, biofeedback, etc. The E-Screen assay has the unique potential to evaluate the effect of estrogenic modulators mid-experiment for an indication of an *overall* change in estrogenic activity of the animal's serum, not a specific hormonal response. Results from such monitoring could lead investigators to end experiments earlier than anticipated, or extend them.

One of the few measurable parameters indicative of fescue toxicosis is a decreased serum prolactin concentration (8). The control steers grazing endophyte-infected fescue had serum prolactin concentrations similar to bulls fed endophyte-infected fescue seed [~30 ng mL^{-1} (43)], indicating toxicity. While implants caused no significant increase in serum prolactin, SBHs did elevate prolactin, and the combination of SBH + IMP resulted in prolactin concentrations similar to those of bulls fed endophyte-free fescue seed [~250 ng mL^{-1} (43)]. In other words, the ~3-fold decrease in prolactin concentrations measured with consumption of endophyte-infected fescue, was reversed in SBH + IMP steers. The lack of elevation in serum prolactin in the IMP steers is puzzling, but could reflect suppression by progesterone contained in the implants. The literature has no reports of progesterone effects on prolactin in steers. Implants of estradiol alone are not widely used, but it would be of interest to compare serum prolactin in steers implanted with E2 versus E2 plus progesterone. These results appear to indicate that phytoestrogens of SBHs could be acting as surrogates for estradiol, overcoming any potential suppression by progesterone in the implant.

While the actions of prolactin on angiogenesis and the vasculature are complicated [review in Ref. (44)] and its causative role in fescue toxicosis is unclear, E_2 binding to E_2-α receptors in the plasma membrane of pituitary cells increased prolactin release (45). Estradiol also increased angiogenesis in the pituitary (46), another possible connection for an additive effect of the treatments, with phytoestrogens from SBHs. While elevated serum E_2 from implants might be relatively quickly metabolized by endogenous enzymes, the clearance rates of phytoestrogen might be slower, resulting in a more sustained physiological response.

Though Carter et al. (7) suggested that SBHs were acting merely through a passive role, diluting the ergot alkaloids, and thereby mitigating their adverse effects, we propose a more active role for SBHs. Both steers with implants or fed SBHs had a reduced percentage of rough hair coat (7). If a decrease in hair coat shedding (another indicator of fescue toxicosis) is a result of decreased blood flow to the hair follicle caused by the ergot alkaloids, then perhaps E_2 or phytoestrogens/isoflavones can ameliorate the effect by increasing follicular blood flow. Though several reports have found a lack of specific arterial responsiveness to isoflavones [brachial artery (12, 13)], a more global vascular effect was seen, including reduced peak flow velocity and lower peripheral flow resistance. Nestel et al. (47) noted that soy isoflavones increased vascular blood flow in menopausal and perimenopausal women. In addition, using biopsies of subcutaneous fat from men, the phytoestrogen genistein increased relaxation of small arteries, as determined by myograph (14). It is well accepted that arteries often have individual or tissue-specific responses to chemical stimuli, and that global measures, such as blood pressure and velocity, are not necessarily indicated by the responses of individual arteries (48). Though specific direct evidence may be hard to find, isoflavones of SBHs could be ameliorating coat effects via interaction with the vasculature nourishing the hair coat.

Mechanistically, vasorelaxation can be caused by nitric oxide (NO), which is generated by binding and activation of estrogenic receptors by E_2 or isoflavones (15). While NO was not measured in the current study, Schreihofer et al. (49) measured increased vasorelaxation in ovariectomized rats fed high-soy diets or treated with E_2. The increase was associated with a decrease in caveolin-1 activity, an enzyme that inhibits NO-induced vasorelaxation. Similar mechanisms could be expected to occur with SBH feeding of steers.

There is a tendency to focus on "the most estrogenic compounds" in SBHs and consider them the "players," although it is well known that isoflavones undergo degradation by bacteria in the gut/rumen (32, 50). And while some catabolites or conjugates of phytoestrogens are less active, some are more active, depending on the tissue or assay type. For instance, equol, the ruminal catabolite of daidzein (found in SBHs) has greater vasodilatory effects on the basilar artery of rats than its precursor daidzein (51), though they are equipotent on the carotid artery. Equol has been found not only in ruminal digesta of animals fed legumes, but bioavailability was confirmed by its presence in the kidneys and blood (9, 52). Assay and tissue specificity was also a factor in assignment of a "relative potency factor," as genistein evaluated by E-Screen (breast tissue origin) was ~6 times as potent as daidzein in eliciting MCF-7 cell proliferation (53), with daidzein and equol ~ equivalent, yet the two had different potencies based on E_2-receptor affinities and transcriptional efficiencies (54).

Conclusion

The estradiol–progesterone implant and SBH treatments enhanced E_2Eqs in sera of steers, with an additive effect when combined. It cannot be concluded that the increases in estrogenicity directly caused the mitigation of fescue toxicosis reported by Carter et al. (7) for these steers. But based on research with human subjects, exogenous sources of estradiol and isoflavones may relieve the ergot alkaloid-induced vasoconstriction that persists in livestock grazing toxic endophyte-infected tall fescue. Still unknown is the threshold at which estradiol and or isoflavones can alleviate or mitigate toxicosis. The E-Screen assay was shown to be an effective tool in monitoring serum for estrogenic effects of dietary supplementation with isoflavones or estrogenic implants, though threshold concentrations of estrogenic activity that result in vasculature responses have yet to be established.

Acknowledgments

Excellent technical assistance was provided by Mr. Lloyd Billey and Ms. DeeAnne Ellig. Mention of trade names or commercial products in the article is solely for the purpose of providing specific information and does not imply recommendation or endorsement by the USDA. The USDA is an equal opportunity provider and employer.

References

1. Oliver JW. Pathophysiologic response to endophyte toxins. In: Roberts CA, West CP, Spiers DE, editors. *Neotyphodium in Cool Season Grasses*. Ames, IA: Blackwell Publishing (2005). p. 291–301.
2. Strickland JR, Looper ML, Matthews JC, Rosenkrans CF Jr, Flythe MD, Brown KR. Board-invited review: St. Anthony's fire in livestock: causes, mechanisms, and potential solutions. *J Anim Sci* (2011) **89**:1603–26. doi:10.2527/jas.2010-3478
3. Goetsch, AL, Jones AL, Beers KW, Stokes SR, Piper EL. Effects of offering different amounts and types of supplemental feeds to growing dairy steers fed endphyte-infected fescue hay ad libitum on intake, digestion, passage rate and serum prolactin concentrations. *J Anim Sci* (1987) **64**:1769–78. doi:10.2134/jas1987.6461769x
4. Stokes, SR, Goetsch, AL, Nejad HH, Murphy GA, Jones L., Mashburn SK, et al. Effects of supplemental Bermuda grass hay or corn on intake, digestion and performance of cattle consuming endophyte-infected fescue. *J Anim Sci* (1988) **66**:204–12. doi:10.2134/jas1988.661204x
5. Aiken GE, Ball DM, Piper EL, West CP. Performance of steers fed a broiler litter-corn mixture on endophyte-infested and non-infested tall fescue. *Prof Anim Sci* (1998) **14**:51–5.
6. Aiken GE, McClanahan LK, Schrick FN. Steer responses to feeding soybean hulls on toxic tall fescue pasture. *Prof Anim Sci* (2008) **24**(5):399–403. doi:10.2527/jas.2009-2536
7. Carter JM, Aiken GE, Dougherty CT, Schrick FN. Steer responses to feeding soybean hulls and steroid hormone implantation on toxic tall fescue pasture. *J Anim Sci* (2010) **88**:3759–66. doi:10.2527/jas.2009-2536
8. Sleper DA, West CP. Tall fescue. In: Moser LE, Buxton DR, Casler MD, editors. *Cool Season Forage Grasses*. Madison, WI: American Society of Agronomy (1996). p. 471–502.
9. Lundh TJ-O, Pettersson HI, Martinsson KA. Comparative levels of free and conjugated plant estrogens in blood plasma of sheep and cattle fed estrogenic silage. *J Agric Food Chem* (1990) **38**:1530–4. doi:10.1021/jf00097a022
10. Adams NR. Detection of the effects of phytoestrogens on sheep and cattle. *J Anim Sci* (1995) **73**:1509–15.
11. Coward L, Barnes NC, Setchell KDR, Barnes S. Genistein, daidzein, and their β-glucoside conjugates: antitumor isoflavones in soybean foods from American and Asian diets. *J Agric Food Chem* (1993) **41**:1961–7. doi:10.1021/jf00035a027
12. Steinberg FM, Gutherie NL, Villablanca AC, Kumar K, Murray MJ. Soy protein with isoflavones has favorable effects on endothelial function that are independent of lipid and antioxidant effects in healthy postmenopausal women. *Am J Clin Nutr* (2003) **78**:123–30.
13. Teede HJ, McGrath BP, DeSilva L, Cehun M, Fassoulakis A, Nestel PJ. Isoflavones reduce arterial stiffness: a placebo-controlled study in men and postmenopausal women. *Arterioscler Thromb Vasc Biol* (2003) **23**:1066–71. doi:10.1161/01.ATV.0000072967.97296.4A
14. Cruz MN, Leonid L, Logman H, Poston L, Agewall S, Kublickiene K. Genistein, daidzein, and their β-glycoside conjugates: antitumor isoflavones in soybean foods from American and Asian diets. *Am J Physiol* (2006) **290**:H1969–75. doi:10.1152/ajpheart.01065.2005
15. Grossini E, Molinari C, Mary D, Uberti F, Caimmi P, Surico N, et al. Intracoronary genistein acutely increases coronary blood flow in anesthetized pigs through β-adrenergic mediated nitric oxide release and estrogenic receptors. *Endocrinology* (2008) **149**:2678–87. doi:10.1210/en.2007-1361
16. Livingston AL. Forage plant estrogens. *J Toxicol Environ Health* (1978) **4**:301–24. doi:10.1080/15287397809529663
17. Flythe M, Kagan I. Antimicrobial effect of red clover (*Trifolium pretense*) phenolic extract on the ruminal hyper ammonia-producing bacterium, *Clostridium sticklandii*. *Curr Microbiol* (2010) **61**:125–31. doi:10.1007/s00284-010-9586-5
18. Booth NL, Overk CA, Yao P, Totura S, Deng Y, Hedayat AS, et al. Seasonal variation of red clover (*Trifolium pretense* L., *Fabaceae*) isoflavones and estrogenic activity. *J Agric Food Chem* (2006) **54**:1277–82. doi:10.1021/jf052927u

19. Magolski JD, Shappell NW, Vonnahme KA, Anderson GM, Newman DJ, Berg EP. Consumption of ground beef obtained from cattle that had received steroidal growth promotants does not trigger early onset of estrus in prepubertal pigs. *J Nutr* (2014) **144**:1718–24. doi:10.3945/jn.114.198127
20. Bajer T, Adam M, Galla L, Ventura K. Comparison of various extraction techniques for isolation and determination of isoflavonoids in plants. *J Sep Sci* (2007) **30**:122–7. doi:10.1002/jssc.200600306
21. Shappell NW. Estrogenic activity in the environment: municipal wastewater effluent, river, ponds, and wetlands. *J Environ Qual* (2006) **35**:122–32. doi:10.2134/jeq2004.0464
22. Hiablie S, Church CD, Elliott HA, Shappell NW, Schoenfuss HL, Dreschsel P, et al. Serum estrogenicity and biological responses in African catfish raised in wastewater ponds in Ghana. *Sci Total Environ* (2013) **463-464**:1182–91. doi:10.1016/j.scitotenv.2013.06.032
23. Rassmussen TH, Nielsen JB. Critical parameters in the MCF-7 cell proliferation bioassay (E-Screen). *Biomarkers* (2002) **7**:322–36. doi:10.1080/13547500210132907
24. Littell RC, Milliken GA, Stroup WW, Wolfinger RD. *SAS System for Mixed Models*. Cary, NC: SAS Institute Inc. (1996).
25. Alemdar A, Sain M. Isolation and characterization of nanofibers from agricultural residues – wheat, straw, and soy hulls. *Bioresour Technol* (2008) **99**:1664–71. doi:10.1016/j.biortech.2007.04.029
26. Kato H, Iwata T, Katsu Y, Watanabe H, Ohta Y, Iguchi T. Evaluation of estrogenic activity in diets for experimental animals using *in vitro* assay. *J Agric Food Chem* (2004) **52**:1410–4. doi:10.1021/jf034896d
27. Wang H-J, Murphy PA. Mass balance study of isoflavones during soybean processing. *J Agric Food Chem* (1996) **44**:2377–83. doi:10.1021/jf950535p
28. Reece WO. *Dukes' Physiology of Domestic Animals*. 12th ed. Ithaca, NY: Cornell University Press (2004).
29. Woclawek-Potocka I, Piskula MK, Bah MM, Siemieniuch MJ, Korzekwa A, Brzezicka E, et al. Concentrations of isoflavones and their metabolites in the blood of pregnant and non-pregnant heifers fed soy bean. *J Reprod Dev* (2008) **54**:358–63. doi:10.1262/jrd.20013
30. Xu X, Wang HJ, Murphy PA, Hendrich S. Neither background diet nor type of soy food affects short-term isoflavone bioavailability in women. *J Nutr* (2000) **130**:798–801.
31. Mallis LM, Sarkahian AB, Harris HA, Zhang MY, McConnell OJ. Determination of rat oral bioavailability of soy-derived phytoestrogens using an automated on-column extraction procedure and electrospray tandem mass spectrometry. *J Chromatogr B Analyt Technol Biomed Life Sci* (2003) **796**:71–86. doi:10.1016/j.jchromb.2003.08.003
32. Nilsson A, Hill JL, Davies HL. An in vitro study of formononetin and biochanin A metabolism in rumen fluid from sheep. *Biochim Biophys Acta* (1967) **148**:92–8. doi:10.1016/0304-4165(67)90282-6
33. Charles GD, Gennings C, Tornesi B, Lynn Kan H, Zacharewski TR, Bhaskar Gollapudi B, et al. Analysis of the interaction of phytoestrogens and synthetic chemicals: an in vitro/in vivo comparison. *Toxicol Appl Pharmacol* (2007) **218**:280–8. doi:10.1016/j.taap.2006.11.029
34. Bennetts HW, Underwood EJ, Shier FL. A breeding problem of sheep in the south-west division of Western Australia. *J Agric West Aust* (1946) **23**:1–12.
35. Weaver GA, Kurtz HJ, Behrens JC, Robison TS, Seguin BE, Bates FY, et al. Effect of zearalenone on dairy cows. *Am J Vet Res* (1986) **47**:1826–8.
36. Smith JF, di Menna ME, McGowan LT. Reproductive performance of Coopworth ewes following oral doses of zearalenone before and after mating. *J Reprod Fertil* (1990) **89**:99–106. doi:10.1530/jrf.0.0890099
37. Aherne FX, Kennelly JJ. Oilseed meals for livestock feeding. In: Cole DJA, Haresign W, editors. *Recent Developments in Pig Nutrition*. Boston, MA: Butterworths (1985). p. 278–316.
38. Heuzé V, Tran G, Kaushik S. Soybean meal. *Feedipedia, a Programme by INRA, CIRAD, AFZ and FAO*. (Vol. **15**) (2015). 44 p. Available from: http://www.feedipedia.org/node/674
39. Rumsey TS, Beaudry N. Plasma estrogen concentrations in non-implanted and Synovex-S implanted feedlot steers. *Bull Environ Contam Toxicol* (1979) **23**:405–11. doi:10.1007/BF01769979
40. Brian JV, Harris CA, Scholze M, Backhaus T, Booy P, Lamoree M, et al. Accurate prediction of the response of freshwater fish to a mixture of estrogenic chemicals. *Environ Health Perspect* (2005) **113**:721–8. doi:10.1289/ehp.7598
41. Zhang H, Kong FX, Wang SH, Yu Y, Zhang M. Vitellogenin induction by a mixture of steroidal estrogens in freshwater fishes and relevant risk assessment. *Environ Toxicol* (2009) **24**:484–91. doi:10.1002/tox.20453
42. Palmer BD, Huth LK, Pieto DL, Selcer KW. Vitellogenin as a biomarker for xenobiotic estrogens in an amphibian model system. *Environ Toxicol Chem* (1998) **17**:30–6. doi:10.1002/etc.5620170105
43. Stowe HM, Miller M, Burns MG, Calcatera SM, Andrae JG, Aiken GE, et al. Effects of fescue toxicosis on bull growth, semen characteristics, and breeding soundness evaluation. *J Anim Sci* (2013) **91**:3686–92. doi:10.2527/jas.2012-6078
44. Clapp C, de la Escalera LM, de la Escalera GM. Prolactin and blood vessels: a comparative endocrinology perspective. *Gen Comp Endocrinol* (2012) **176**:336–40. doi:10.1016/j.ygcen.2011.12.033
45. Norfleet AM, Clarke CH, Gametchu B, Watson CS. Antibodies to the estrogen receptor-α modulate rapid prolactin release from rat pituitary tumor cells through plasma membrane estrogen receptors. *FASEB J* (2000) **14**:157–65. doi:10.106/fj.1530-6860
46. Lombardero M, Quintanar-Stephano A, Vidal S, Horvath E, Kovacs K, Lloyd RV, et al. Effect of estrogen on the blood supply of pituitary autografts in rats. *J Anat* (2009) **214**:235–44. doi:10.1111/j.1469-7580.2008.01037.x
47. Nestel PJ, Yamashita T, Sasahara T, Pomeroy S, Dart A, Komesaroff P, et al. Soy isoflavones improve systemic arterial compliance but not plasma lipids in menopausal and perimenopausal women. *Arterioscler Thromb Vasc Biol* (1997) **17**:3392–8. doi:10.1161/01.ATV.17.12.3392
48. Aiken GE, Kirch BH, Strickland JR, Bush LP, Looper ML, Schrick FN. Hemodynamic responses of the caudal artery to toxic tall fescue in beef heifers. *J Anim Sci* (2007) **85**:2337–45. doi:10.2527/jas.2006-821
49. Schreihofer DA, Deutsch C, Lovekamp-Swan T, Sullivan JC, Dorrance AM. Effect of high soy diet on the cerebrovasculature and endothelial nitric synthase in the ovariectomized rat. *Vascul Pharmacol* (2010) **52**:236–42. doi:10.1016/j.vph.2010.02.003
50. Matthies A, Loh G, Blaut M, Braune A. Daidzein and genistein are converted to equol and 5-hydroxy-equol by human intestinal *Slackia isoflavoniconvertens* in gnotobiotic rats. *J Nutr* (2012) **142**:40–6. doi:10.3945/jn.111.148247
51. Jackman KA, Woodman OL, Chrissobolis S, Sobey CG. Vasorelaxant and antioxidant activity of the isoflavone metabolite equol in carotid and cerebral arteries. *Brain Res* (2007) **1141**:99–107. doi:10.1016/j.brainres.2007.01.007
52. Dickinson JM, Smith GR, Randel RD, Pemberton IJ. In vitro metabolism of formononetin and biochanin a in bovine rumen fluid. *J Anim Sci* (1988) **66**:1969–73.
53. Shappell NW, Mostrom MS, Lenneman EM. E-Screen evaluation of sugar beet feedstuffs in a case of reduced embryo transfer efficiencies in cattle: the role of phytoestrogens and zearalenone. *In Vitro Cell Dev Biol Anim* (2012) **48**:216–28. doi:10.1007/s11626-012-9489-9
54. Schmitt E, Dekant W, Stopper H. Assaying the estrogenicity of phytoestrogens in cells of different estrogen sensitive tissues. *Toxicol In Vitro* (2001) **15**:433–9. doi:10.1016/S0887-2333(01)00048-0

Conflict of Interest Statement: The authors declare that the research was conducted in the absence of any commercial or financial relationships that could be construed as a potential conflict of interest.

12

Summer-Long Grazing of High vs. Low Endophyte (*Neotyphodium coenophialum*)-Infected Tall Fescue by Growing Beef Steers Results in Distinct Temporal Blood Analyte Response Patterns, with Poor Correlation to Serum Prolactin Levels

Joshua J. Jackson, Merlin D. Lindemann, James A. Boling and James C. Matthews*

Department of Animal and Food Sciences, University of Kentucky, Lexington, KY, USA

Edited by:
Glen Eris Aiken,
USDA Agricultural Research Service, USA

Reviewed by:
Marcello Mele,
University of Pisa, Italy
Kristy DiGiacomo,
The University of Melbourne, Australia

****Correspondence:***
James C. Matthews
jmatthew@uky.edu

Previously, we reported the effects of fescue toxicosis on developing Angus-cross steer growth, carcass, hepatic mRNA, and protein expression profiles of selected serum proteins, and blood clinical and chemical profiles, after summer-long grazing (85 days) of high endophyte (HE)- vs. low endophyte (LE)-infected fescue pastures. We now report the temporal development of acute, intermediate, and chronic responses of biochemical and clinical blood analytes determined at specified time intervals (period 1, day 0–36; period 2, day 37–58; and period 3, day 59–85). Throughout the trial, the alkaloid concentrations of the HE forage was consistently 19–25 times greater ($P \leq 0.002$) than the concentration in the LE forage, and HE vs. LE steers had continuously lower ($P \leq 0.049$) serum prolactin (85%), cholesterol (27%), and albumin (5%), but greater red blood cells (7%). The HE steers had decreased ($P = 0.003$) ADG only during period 1 (−0.05 vs. 0.4 kg/day). For period 1, HE steers had reduced ($P \leq 0.090$) numbers of eosinophils (55%) and lymphocytes (18%), serum triglyceride (27%), and an albumin/globulin ratio (9%), but an increased bilirubin concentration (20%). During period 2, serum LDH activities were 18% lower ($P = 0.022$) for HE vs. LE steers. During period 3, serum levels of ALP (32%), ALT (16%), AST (15%), creatine kinase (35%), glucose (10%), and LDH (23%) were lower ($P \leq 0.040$) for HE steers. Correlation analysis of serum prolactin and other blood analytes revealed that triglycerides ($P = 0.042$) and creatinine ($P = 0.021$) were moderately correlated ($r \leq 0.433$) with HE serum prolactin. In conclusion, three HE-induced blood analyte response patterns were identified: continually altered, initially altered, and subsequently "recovered," or altered only after long-term exposure. Blood

---

Abbreviations: ADG, average daily gain; ALP, alkaline phosphatase: ALT, alanine transaminase; AST, aspartate transaminase; BW, body weight; HE, high toxic endophyte-infected tall fescue; LE, low toxic endophyte tall fescue-mixed grass; LDH, lactate dehydrogenase; RBC, red blood cell.

analytes affected by length of grazing HE vs. LE forages were either not or poorly correlated with serum prolactin. These data reveal important, temporal, data about how young cattle respond to the challenge of consuming HE pasture.

Keywords: *Neotyphodium coenophialum*, ergot alkaloids, blood metabolites, blood cells, cattle

INTRODUCTION

Tall fescue (*Lolium arundinaceum*) is a forage grass that is commonly used by many livestock producers in the southeastern United States. The hardiness of the grass is primarily due to the fact that the majority of the fescue in the southeast is infected with the endophytic fungus, *Neotyphodium coenophialum*. Unfortunately, cattle consuming endophytic fescue manifest clinical symptoms of fescue toxicosis ("summer slump"), such as decreased body weight (BW) gain (1–3), reduced feed intake (4, 5), lowered milk production (6), retained winter hair coat during the summer (7), increased body temperature (6), and increased respiration rate (4).

The consumption of endophyte-infected tall fescue also is known to alter the blood parameter profiles of cattle and other livestock, with decreased plasma prolactin being the most commonly observed indicator of fescue toxicosis (8). Previously, we reported (9) the effects of fescue toxicosis on developing Angus-cross steer growth, carcass, hepatic mRNA, and protein expression profiles of selected serum proteins, and blood clinical and chemical profiles that were induced by whole-summer-long grazing of forages containing either high or low amounts of endophyte-infected tall fescue. Therefore, the primary objectives of the current research were to (a) characterize the temporal changes in blood clinical and chemical profiles of steers grazing forages containing either high or low amounts of endophyte-infected tall fescue over the course of the summer and then (b) evaluate the potential relationships between serum prolactin and measured blood analytes.

MATERIALS AND METHODS

Animals and Experimental Periods

All experimental procedures were approved by the University of Kentucky Institutional Animal Care and Use Committee (protocol no. 01012A2006). Nineteen predominately Angus crossbred beef steers were randomly allotted (day 0) to graze low-toxic endophyte tall fescue-mixed grass (LE, $n = 9$, 5.7 ha; BW = 266 ± 10.9 kg) or a high-toxic endophyte-infected tall fescue (HE, $n = 10$, 5.7 ha; BW = 267 ± 14.5 kg) for 85 days. Pastures were within 500 m of each other and are part of the University of Kentucky Agricultural Research Center, located in Woodford County, KY, USA. All steers had *ad libitum* access to fresh water and mineral supplement (Ca min. 13.0 – max. 15.0%; *P* 6.2%; NaCl min. 17.0 – max. 19.5%; Mg 3.0%; S 1.0%; K 0.8%; Zn 2300 μg/g; Mn 2200 μg/g; Cu 1450 μg/g; I 45 μg/g; Co 15 μg/g; Se 29 μg/g; Vit. A 661 IU/g; Vit. E 0.276 IU/g; as-fed). Shrunk (denied access to feed and water for 14 h) BW were determined on day 0 and 86 to determine overall experiment average daily gain (ADG). Full BW were taken on day 36 and 57 and shrunk BW calculated based on the mean percentage shrink of 4.04% from weight measurements taken on day 0 and 85. Experimental periods were as per weigh days: period 1 = day 0–36, period 2 = day 37–58, and period 3 = day 59–85.

Pasture Sampling and Analysis

On day 37, 59, and 88 of the study, leaf blades suitable for grazing were detached from each fescue plant in pasture for ergot alkaloid (ergovaline, ergovalinine, lysergic acid, and isolysergic acid) determination, and proximate analysis (9). Briefly, samples were obtained systematically from approximately 30 sites in each pasture, using a knife to cut the forage at approximately 2 cm above soil level. Samples were immediately placed into individual plastic bags, and then stored on ice during transportation to our laboratory. All samples were frozen and stored at −20°C. Analysis of ergot alkaloids was performed, as previously described (10), and isolysergic acid was quantified with a lysergic acid standard. Proximate analysis and mineral content were determined by a commercial laboratory (Dairy One Forage Lab, Ithaca, NY, USA).

Blood Collection and Analyses

Jugular venous blood samples were collected by venipuncture on day 36, 58, and 85. For plasma, 16 mL of blood was collected in EDTA-containing (0.9375 mg/mL) blood collection tubes (Becton, Dickinson and Company, Franklin, Lakes, NJ, USA). For serum, 16 mL of blood was collected in serum blood collection tubes without an anticoagulant. For whole blood, 2 mL of blood was collected in EDTA-containing (2.7 mg/mL) blood collection tubes (Becton Dickerson). Plasma and sera were recovered by refrigerated centrifugation at 3 000 × *g* for 10 min at 4°C and stored at −80°C. Plasma samples were analyzed for ammonia-N by modifications of the L-Glu dehydrogenase enzyme assay (11) using a Konelab 20XTi analyzer (Thermo Electron Corp., Finland). Serum prolactin analysis (12) was conducted (Dr. F. N. Schrick Laboratory, Johnson Animal Research and Teaching Unit, University of Tennessee-Knoxville). All other serum enzymes and analytes, and blood cell types, were analyzed by the American Association for Veterinary Laboratory Diagnosticians approved – University of Kentucky Livestock Disease Diagnostic Center (Lexington, KY, USA). For serum analytes, activities of alkaline phosphatase (ALP), E.C. 3.1.3.1; alanine transaminase (ALT), E. C. 2.6.1.2; aspartate transaminase (AST), E. C. 2.6.1.1; γ-glutamyltransferase, E. C. 2.3.22; creatine kinase, E. C. 2.7.3.2; and lactate dehydrogenase (LDH), E. C. 1.1.1.27 were determined as per the manufacturer of the reagent kits (Alfa Wassermann, Diagnostic Technologies, West Caldwell) using a VET-EX Chemical Analyzer (Alfa-Wassermann), as were the other serum analytes. The concentration of red blood cells (RBCs), white blood cells, packed cell volume, and hemoglobin in whole blood was determined using a Hemavet HV 950S cell analyzer (Drew Scientific Inc., Miami Lakes, FL, USA). The whole blood concentration of neutrophils, lymphocytes, monocytes, and eosinophils were determined by manual identification and counting of cells (13).

Statistical Methods

Data are presented as least square means (±SEM). Individual steers were the experimental units. The effect of grazing HE vs. LE pastures on all measured experimental parameters was evaluated by ANOVA, using the MIXED procedure of SAS (v 8.01, SAS Inst. Inc., Cary, NC, USA). The statistical model used fescue toxicosis, the experimental period, and their interaction as fixed effects. Class variables were fescue toxicosis and steer, with steer included in the random statement. The Kenward–Roger adjustment was used to calculate the denominator df (14). Linear and quadratic non-orthogonal polynomial contrasts were used to characterize the effect of treatment over time using the imi procedure of SAS. Partial correlations between prolactin concentrations and serum analytes were determined by using ANOVA (PROC GLM) by using the MANOVA/PRINTE statement of SAS. For all data, significance was declared when $P \leq 0.05$ and tendency to differ was declared when $0.10 \geq P > 0.05$.

RESULTS

Nutrient Profiles of HE and LE Forages

Across-periods, the % compositions of DM, ADF, and crude fat did not differ ($P \geq 0.205$) between HE and LE pastures (**Table 1**). However, the HE forage contained less ($P \leq 0.001$) lignin (24%) and NDF (4.3%), and more ($P \leq 0.001$) TDN (3.8%), CP (7.6%), and ash (7.3%) than did LE.

Ergot Alkaloid Profiles of Forages

Across-period analysis of ergot alkaloid levels between the two forages revealed that the HE steers were exposed to 19 and 25 times more ($P \leq 0.002$) ergovaline/ergovalinine and lysergic acid/isolysergic acid, respectively, than LE steers (**Table 2**). No period or treatment by period interactions was observed for lysergic and isolysergic acids indicating that the differences in the concentration between HE and LE forages were similar throughout the trial. For ergovaline and ergovalinine, however, period ($P \leq 0.004$) and treatment by period ($P \leq 0.008$) were observed, perhaps reflecting the exceptionally low values for LE forages during period 1.

Steer Growth

Across-periods, BW tended to be lower ($P = 0.097$), and ADG was lower ($P = 0.014$), for HE vs. LE steers (**Table 3**). For BW, a period effect was found ($P \leq 0.001$) reflecting the greater growth of HE and LE steers during period 3. Similarly, the ADG for period 3 appeared greater for both groups of steers than for the other periods. Moreover, a treatment by period interaction was found ($P = 0.026$) for ADG. That is, although the ADG of LE and HE steers did not differ ($P \geq 0.595$) in periods 2 and 3, during period 1 LE steers achieved an ADG of 0.4 kg, whereas HE steers lost ($P = 0.003$) BW (0.05 kg/day). Overall, from day 0 to 85, the ADG of HE steers was 0.18 kg more ($P = 0.014$) than for LE steers.

Prolactin

Across all three periods, serum prolactin levels of HE steers ($P \leq 0.001$) were 15% that of LE steers (**Table 4**). Steers grazing HE forage had serum prolactin values that were 14, 19, and 10% that of LE steers in period 1, 2, and 3, respectively. The level of prolactin decreased in a quadratic manner ($P \leq 0.012$) over time for both LE and HE steers (**Table 5**), with the concentration of prolactin in the steers grazing LE pasture decreasing 58.3 ng/mL from periods 1 to 3 (**Table 4**). Steers grazing HE pasture exhibited a smaller decrease in prolactin (9.9 ng/mL) across-periods, likely due to the fact that HE steer prolactin levels had already been suppressed severely in period 1. A treatment by period interaction likely reflects this time-dependent differential decrease in serum prolactin values.

Biochemical and Clinical Blood Profiles

As shown in **Table 4**, the mean value across-periods for 9 of the biochemical and clinical blood profile measurements did not change ($P \geq 0.212$), whereas ALP, ALT, AST, ammonia, albumin, albumin:globulin ratio, creatine kinase, glucose, LDH, and cholesterol were influenced ($P < 0.10$) by grazing treatment. The trend across time for each biochemical and blood parameter was also determined for each treatment group (**Table 5**).

Serum ALP activity for HE steers tended ($P = 0.079$) to exhibit 26% less activity than LE steers (**Table 4**). In period 3, ALP was reduced ($P = 0.006$) by 32% for HE steers. Furthermore, there was a significant ($P < 0.001$) period interaction (**Table 4**), which showed quadratic trends ($P = 0.024$) (**Table 5**) for ALP for LE steers that decreased 13% from period 1 to 2 and increased 97% from period 2 to 3. For HE steers, there was also a quadratic trend ($P = 0.080$) (**Table 5**), which reduced ALP by 7.1% from periods 1 to 2 and increased 64% from periods 2 to 3. The period by treatment interaction ($P = 0.009$) most likely was due to the large increase in ALP by the LE steers from periods 2 to 3 (**Table 4**).

Across-periods, ALT activity was reduced ($P = 0.040$) by 9.5% in HE consuming steers compared to the LE consuming steers (**Table 4**). In period 3, ALT also was found to be depressed 16% ($P = 0.009$) in HE steers (**Table 4**). The period effect ($P = 0.001$) (**Table 5**) can be explained by the quadratic response to time ($P \leq 0.035$) (**Table 5**) for both treatments, with activity depressed during period 2 compared to periods 1 and 3. ALT activity for steers consuming LE pastures decreased by 24% from periods 1 to 2 and increased by 28% from periods 2 to 3, whereas ALT activity for HE consuming steers decreased by 17% from periods 1 to 2 and increased by 8.8% from period 2 to 3 (**Table 4**).

Across-periods, HE steer serum AST activity decreased ($P = 0.092$) 9.1% (**Table 4**). Within-periods, AST was decreased ($P = 0.014$) by 15% in HE vs. LE steers in period 3 and demonstrated no period or period by treatment interaction (**Table 4**). Across-periods, there was a linear decrease ($P = 0.031$) (**Table 5**) of 4.9% for HE steers across-periods but no trend for LE steers. For AST, the mean differed but there was no period or treatment by period interaction unlike prolactin and ALT, despite the fact that LE appeared to increase and HE to decrease (**Table 4**).

The serum albumin content of HE steers was 5% lower ($P \leq 0.009$) than LE steers across-periods (**Table 4**). Within-periods 1, 2, and 3, serum albumin of the HE steers was 4.6, 6.1,

TABLE 1 | Proximate analysis of low endophyte (LE) and high endophyte (HE) pasture samples[a].

Item (%)	Pasture treatment			*P*-value		
	LE	HE	SEM	TRT	Period	TRT by period
Across-periods						
DM	25.5	26.1	0.46	0.356	<0.001	0.273
CP	17.10	18.40	0.195	0.001	0.002	<0.001
TDN	58.56	60.78	0.377	0.001	0.001	0.093
ADF	32.12	31.83	0.370	0.591	0.782	0.069
NDF	60.41	57.82	0.387	0.001	0.008	0.004
Crude fat	3.46	3.61	0.082	0.205	0.006	0.179
Lignin	6.23	4.76	0.247	0.001	0.012	0.215
Ash	8.20	8.80	0.09	0.001	0.077	0.007
Within-periods						
DM						
Period 1	28.5	27.8	0.79	0.544		
Period 2	26.8	28.8	0.79	0.100		
Period 3	21.1	21.6	0.79	0.623		
CP						
Period 1	16.50	20.83	0.34	<0.001		
Period 2	16.70	17.93	0.34	0.024		
Period 3	18.10	16.43	0.34	0.004		
TDN						
Period 1	56.00	60.00	0.653	0.001		
Period 2	58.67	60.33	0.653	0.096		
Period 3	61.00	62.00	0.653	0.300		
ADF						
Period 1	32.87	30.93	0.641	0.054		
Period 2	32.40	32.07	0.641	0.720		
Period 3	31.10	32.50	0.641	0.149		
NDF						
Period 1	62.83	57.47	0.670	<0.001		
Period 2	60.87	58.17	0.670	0.015		
Period 3	57.53	57.83	0.670	0.757		
Crude fat						
Period 1	3.07	3.50	0.142	0.052		
Period 2	3.77	3.93	0.142	0.423		
Period 3	3.53	3.40	0.142	0.520		
Lignin						
Period 1	7.33	5.03	0.428	0.003		
Period 2	6.37	4.93	0.428	0.035		
Period 3	5.00	4.30	0.428	0.270		
Ash						
Period 1	7.9	9.1	0.16	0.001		
Period 2	8.4	9.1	0.16	0.008		
Period 3	8.4	8.3	0.16	0.864		

[a]Proximate analysis values are presented on a DM basis. Samples were obtained systematically from approximately 30 sites in each pasture, using a knife to cut the forage at approximately 2 cm above soil level. Data are presented as least square means (±SEM).

and 5.7% less ($P \leq 0.032$), respectively, than that of LE steers. The period effect could be explained by the fact that LE and HE steers decreased linearly ($P < 0.001$) (**Table 5**) in a parallel manner by 15 and 16%, respectively (**Table 4**). Additionally, the albumin:globulin ratio in HE steers was decreased ($P = 0.037$) by 8.5% across-periods when compared to LE steers (**Table 4**). In period 1, the albumin:globulin ratio was decreased by 9.5% in HE when compared to LE steers. The period effect ($P < 0.001$) was evident in that both treatment groups decreased over time with LE steers decreasing linearly ($P < 0.001$), whereas HE steers displayed a quadratic ($P = 0.071$) decrease across-periods (**Table 5**).

Across treatments, the creatine kinase activity that was 24% less ($P = 0.032$) in HE vs. LE steers (**Table 4**). In period 3, creatine kinase activity in HE steers was ($P = 0.001$) 35% less than that of LE steers. From periods 1 to 2, LE and HE steers decrease in a parallel manner. Nonetheless, from periods 2 to 3, LE increased by 75% while HE consuming steers creatine kinase activity increased by only 27%, likely reflecting the period and period by treatment interaction.

TABLE 2 | Alkaloid analysis of composited low endophyte (LE)- and high endophyte (HE)-infected forage samples[a].

Alkaloid (μg/g)	Pasture treatments			*P*-value		
	LE	HE	SEM	TRT	Period	TRT by period
Across-periods						
Ergovaline	0.018	0.276	0.016	<0.001	0.004	0.008
Ergovalinine	0.004	0.152	0.005	<0.001	<0.001	<0.001
Lysergic acid	0.002	0.064	0.011	0.002	0.731	0.908
Isolysergic acid	0.007	0.156	0.019	0.001	0.821	0.893
Within-periods						
Ergovaline						
Period 1	<0.001	0.260	0.028	<0.001		
Period 2	0.023	0.173	0.028	0.002		
Period 3	0.030	0.393	0.028	<0.001		
Ergovalinine						
Period 1	<0.001	0.087	0.008	<0.001		
Period 2	0.010	0.100	0.008	<0.001		
Period 3	0.003	0.270	0.008	<0.001		
Lysergic acid						
Period 1	<0.001	0.053	0.019	0.071		
Period 2	0.007	0.077	0.019	0.023		
Period 3	<0.001	0.063	0.019	0.037		
Isolysergic acid						
Period 1	<0.001	0.140	0.032	0.010		
Period 2	0.020	0.160	0.032	0.010		
Period 3	<0.001	0.167	0.032	0.032		

[a]Across- and within-periods proximate analysis values are presented on a DM basis. Samples were obtained systematically from approximately 30 sites in each pasture, using a knife to cut the forage at approximately 2 cm above soil level. Data are presented as least square means (±SEM).

Glucose concentrations were 8.5% lower ($P = 0.068$) in HE vs. LE steers across-periods (**Table 4**). In period 3, HE steers exhibited ($P = 0.040$) a 10% lower concentration of glucose. The period effect could be explained by a slight parallel decrease in serum glucose from periods 1 to 2 for LE and HE steers of 4.3 and 1.6% and increased from periods 2 to 3 by 18 and 11%, respectively. LE steers showed a quadratic response ($P = 0.036$), whereas HE steers demonstrated no linear or quadratic response (**Table 5**).

Across-periods, LDH activity was reduced ($P = 0.007$) 16% of HE steers vs. LE steers (**Table 4**), with LDH activity decreased ($P \leq 0.022$) by 18 and 23%, respectively, in periods 2 and 3. Similar to AST, the means that for LDH differed but there was no period or treatment by period interaction, even though the LE steer mean appeared to increase and HE steer mean decreased across-periods (**Table 5**).

There was no significant change ($P = 0.212$) in triglycerides across-periods between the two treatment groups (**Table 4**). Nonetheless, serum triglyceride concentration was reduced ($P = 0.017$) by 27% during period 1 in HE steers. A treatment by period interaction ($P = 0.003$) reflects a decreased triglyceride concentration from periods 1 to 2 for HE steers and increased concentrations from periods 2 to 3.

Across-periods, HE steers exhibited a 27% decrease ($P < 0.001$) in cholesterol as compared to LE steers (**Table 4**), with serum cholesterol concentrations that were 25, 29, and 29% less ($P < 0.001$) that of LE steers in periods 1, 2, and 3, respectively. The period effect ($P < 0.001$) can be explained by the fact that both treatments responded in a parallel quadratic manner ($P \leq 0.005$) (**Table 5**). From periods 1 to 2, there was a decrease of 13 and 17%; and from periods 2 to 3, there was an increase of 29 and 29% for LE and HE, respectively (**Table 4**), which was consistent with the lack of a treatment by period interaction ($P = 0.354$).

In contrast to other biochemical parameters, ammonia plasma concentrations tended ($P = 0.077$) to be increased in HE steers (**Table 4**). Across-periods, ammonia levels were 19% greater for HE steers. Within-periods 2 and 3, the ammonia concentration of HE steers was 34 and 38% greater ($P \leq 0.035$), respectively, than that of LE steers. The period effect ($P < 0.001$) could be explained by the fact that over time both treatment groups exhibited a decrease. The treatment by time interaction ($P = 0.052$) was apparent as LE steers exhibited a quadratic trend ($P = 0.096$) (**Table 5**), decreasing 32% from periods 1 to 2 and then 15% from periods 2 to 3. Nonetheless, the HE steers exhibited a linear ($P = 0.001$) decrease of 21% in plasma ammonia (**Table 5**).

Blood Cell Types

Across-periods, the amount of RBCs was increased ($P = 0.049$) 6.9% in HE vs. LE steers (**Table 6**). By contrast, other types of blood cells were not affected ($P \geq 0.228$). Within-periods, RBC concentrations of HE steers were increased ($P \leq 0.10$) by 6.3, 7.2, and 7.1% that of LE steers in periods 1, 2, and 3, respectively. The period effect ($P = 0.092$) was due to the fact that both LE and HE steers displayed a decrease in RBC during period 2.

Period affected blood cell abundance ($P \leq 0.044$) with the exception of eosinophils, which demonstrated a treatment by period interaction ($P = 0.087$) (**Table 6**). This interaction appears to reflect the linear ($P = 0.016$) (**Table 7**) decrease with time of LE

TABLE 3 | Body weight and ADG gain of steers grazing forages containing low endophyte (LE)- and high endophyte (HE)-infected forages for 85 days.

Item	*P*-value			
	TRT	Period	TRT by period	
Across-periods				
BW (kg)[a]	0.097	<0.001	0.861	
ADG (kg)	0.014	<0.001	0.026	
Within-periods				
Item	**Pasture treatment[b]**			
	LE	**HE**	**SEM**	***P*-value**
No. of steers	9	10		
BW (kg)[a]				
Day 36	280	265	6.1	0.091
Day 58	287	273	6.1	0.094
Day 85	314	301	6.1	0.132
ADG (kg)				
Period 1	0.40	−0.05	0.10	0.003
Period 2	0.26	0.27	0.10	0.971
Period 3	1.3	1.4	0.10	0.595
Overall	0.58	0.40	0.05	0.014

[a]*BW are calculated, or measured shrunk weights, as described in text.*
[b]*Steers LE (ergovaline and ergovalinine 0.02 μg; lysergic acids 0.01 μg) or HE (ergovaline and ergovalinine 0.52 μg; lysergic acids 0.22 μg) endophyte-infected tall fescue pastures.*

eosinophils, whereas HE steer eosinophils appeared to increase in period 3. Lymphocytes were decreased ($P = 0.090$) in HE steers by 18% in period 1, and monocytes were decreased ($P = 0.070$) by 45% in period 3. The LE steers show a linear ($P = 0.060$) (**Table 7**) decline across-period for lymphocytes and the means of the HE steers appears to parallel that of the LE steers. The decline across-periods reflects a significant ($P = 0.044$) period effect for lymphocytes, but the parallel pattern did not allow for a treatment by period interaction ($P = 0.240$). The LE steers displayed a quadratic ($P = 0.016$) (**Table 7**) response for monocytes across-period with period 2 being depressed the most. The HE steers exhibited a linear ($P \leq 0.001$) decline for monocytes across-periods. The overall decline in monocytes across time was enough to account for a period effect, but the differences in the trends of each treatment group was not enough to allow for a significant treatment by period interaction ($P = 0.243$) (**Table 6**).

Correlation of Serum Prolactin with Blood Analytes

Correlation analyses were performed to determine if a relationship existed between prolactin levels and serum and plasma (**Table 8**) and blood cell types (**Table 9**). Across treatments, the relative abundance of prolactin was weakly ($0.321 \geq r \geq 0.236$) correlated with ALT ($P = 0.022$), blood urea nitrogen ($P = 0.092$), triglycerides ($P = 0.021$), and hemoglobin ($P = 0.043$). Within treatments, correlation coefficients for ALT ($r = 0.424$), blood urea nitrogen ($r = 0.405$), and hemoglobin ($r = 0.536$) were significant ($P \leq 0.045$) and stronger only for LE steers, whereas the correlation coefficient for triglycerides ($r = 0.388$) was significant ($P = 0.042$) and stronger only for HE steers. Within treatment prolactin by analyte correlation analysis also revealed a significant ($P = 0.021$) moderately strong correlation ($r = 0.433$) between prolactin and creatinine in HE but not LE steers, whereas correlations between prolactin and blood urea nitrogen:creatinine ($r = 0.377$; $P = 0.064$) and packed cell volume ($r = 0.375$; $P = 0.065$) were identified in LE but not HE steers.

DISCUSSION

Trial-Long (Across All Periods) Responses

The primary objectives of this research were to characterize the temporal changes in blood clinical and chemical profiles of beef steers grazing forages containing either high or low amounts of endophyte-infected tall fescue over the course of the summer. Forage analysis revealed that the high alkaloid concentration in HE vs. LE pastures was maintained throughout the trial. Of the 19 blood analytes and 8 blood cell type HE vs. LE treatment responses measured across all 3 experimental periods of the trial (**Tables 4** and **6**), 6 were decreased ($P \leq 0.049$; prolactin, ALT, albumin, creatine kinase, LDH, cholesterol, RBC) in HE steers, whereas 3 (ALP, AST, glucose) tended ($0.10 \geq P > 0.05.$) to be decreased and 1 (ammonia) increased ($P \leq 0.077$). However, only prolactin, albumin, and cholesterol were consistently affected in each of the three periods. Decreased serum prolactin is the most consistently observed, and accepted, indicator of cattle suffering from fescue toxicosis (2, 8, 17, 18). The accompanying decreased serum cholesterol also is consistent with that found by others for cattle suffering from fescue toxicosis and is thought to be caused by elevated body temperatures (19–21). Although shown to be consistently decreased through all periods of the current trial, albumin response to the consumption of HE forages can vary. For example, a number of studies report lower levels of albumin in the serum of cattle consuming HE and suggest that this response could be due to the reduced dietary intake, decreased uptake by the gut of AA for the biosynthesis of albumin, damaged tissue, or increased catabolism of albumin (9, 22, 23). Alternatively, others report increased albumin levels in cattle grazing HE forages, potentially due to dehydration (18).

As just described, of the nine analytes and cell types measured that had across-period treatment effects, only three were consistently affected for each of the three periods. To more discretely determine when metabolic alterations were concomitant with grazing HE forages (rather than a total across-period treatment effect after a whole summer of grazing), serum enzymes, and blood constituents were measured and analyzed within the three time periods over the 85-day trial. This analysis was critical to identify potential treatment effects that may have been dependent on the length of grazing, thus potentially identifying metabolic adaptations to the length of HE forage consumption. Of the blood analytes and cell types evaluated (**Tables 4** and **5**), 9/19 analytes and 5/8 had period-specific changes, putatively indicating period-dependent shifts in metabolic capacity as detailed below.

Period 1

Although the cohort groups was relatively small ($n = 9–10$), the large reduction in ADG of HE steers occurred only during the

TABLE 4 | Serum and plasma analytes of steers grazing low endophyte (LE)- or high endophyte (HE)-infected forages[a].

Item[b]	Pasture treatment			P-value			Reference range
	LE	HE	SEM[c]	TRT	Period	TRT by period	
Across-periods							
Prolactin (ng/mL)	70.8	10.8	3.09	<0.001	<0.001	<0.001	–
ALP (U/L)	111.3	82.4	7.08	0.079	<0.001	0.009	100.0–500.0[d]
ALT (U/L)	30.4	27.5	0.96	0.040	<0.001	0.149	11–40[e]
AST (U/L)	68.1	61.9	2.53	0.092	0.495	0.106	0–160[e]
AST/ALT ratio	2.30	2.33	0.115	0.823	0.007	0.961	–
Ammonia[f] (mM)	0.059	0.070	0.005	0.077	<0.001	0.052	–
Blood urea nitrogen (mg/100 mL)	17.0	17.7	0.60	0.459	<0.001	0.680	5.0–27.0[d]
Albumin (g/100 mL)	3.68	3.48	0.034	0.009	<0.001	0.860	2.30–3.70[d]
Globulin (g/100 mL)	3.27	3.34	0.062	0.556	<0.001	0.719	3.0–3.5[d]
Albumin/globulin ratio	1.17	1.07	0.025	0.037	<0.001	0.731	0.8–1.00[d]
γ-Glutamyltransferase (U/L)	12.1	11.3	0.43	0.276	<0.001	0.735	2.0–20.0[d]
Total bilirubin (mg/100 mL)	0.2	0.2	0.01	0.453	0.166	0.166	0.0–0.5[d]
Total protein (g/100 mL)	6.95	6.82	0.067	0.318	<0.001	0.569	6.50–7.50[d]
Creatinine (mg/100 mL)	1.29	1.28	0.049	0.857	<0.001	0.578	1.00–2.00[d]
Blood urea nitrogen:creatinine	13.33	13.90	0.387	0.305	0.424	0.489	40–100[d]
Creatine kinase (U/L)	165.0	126.0	8.70	0.032	<0.001	0.010	100.0–650[d]
Glucose (mg/100 mL)	71	65	1.6	0.068	0.001	0.530	40–100[d]
LDH (U/L)	1037	870	34.1	0.007	0.322	0.224	692–1445[e]
Triglycerides (g/100 mL)	30	26	1.4	0.212	0.002	0.003	–
Cholesterol (mg/100 mL)	95	69	2.2	<0.001	<0.001	0.354	62–193[d]
Within-periods							
Prolactin (ng/mL)							
Period 1	94.3	13.5	3.94	<0.001			
Period 2	82.1	15.2	3.94	<0.001			
Period 3	36.0	3.6	3.94	<0.001			
ALP (U/L)							
Period 1	93.0	71.6	12.27	0.218			
Period 2	81.2	66.5	12.27	0.393			
Period 3	159.8	109.1	12.27	0.006			
ALT (U/L)							
Period 1	33.3	30.1	1.41	0.102			
Period 2	25.4	25.1	1.41	0.860			
Period 3	32.6	27.3	1.41	0.009			
AST (U/L)							
Period 1	66.8	63.7	2.94	0.454			
Period 2	66.3	61.3	2.94	0.225			
Period 3	71.2	60.6	2.94	0.014			
AST/ALT ratio							
Period 1	2.05	2.14	0.180	0.723			
Period 2	2.63	2.63	0.180	0.995			
Period 3	2.21	2.23	0.180	0.934			
Ammonia[e] (mM)							
Period 1	0.078	0.078	0.0055	0.940			
Period 2	0.053	0.071	0.0055	0.026			
Period 3	0.045	0.062	0.0055	0.035			
Blood urea nitrogen (mg/100 mL)							
Period 1	18.8	19.8	0.73	0.314			
Period 2	16.1	16.8	0.73	0.496			
Period 3	16.2	16.4	0.73	0.860			
Albumin (g/100 mL)							
Period 1	3.94	3.76	0.060	0.032			
Period 2	3.77	3.54	0.060	0.009			
Period 3	3.33	3.14	0.060	0.025			
Globulin (g/100 mL)							
Period 1	2.93	3.08	0.107	0.327			
Period 2	3.04	3.07	0.107	0.864			

(Continued)

TABLE 4 | Continued

Item[b]	Pasture treatment			P-value			Reference range
	LE	HE	SEM[c]	TRT	Period	TRT by period	
Period 3	3.83	3.86	0.107	0.858			
Albumin/globulin							
Period 1	1.37	1.24	0.043	0.039			
Period 2	1.24	1.15	0.043	0.119			
Period 3	0.90	0.83	0.043	0.245			
γ-Glutamyltransferase (U/L)							
Period 1	12.0	11.6	0.75	0.699			
Period 2	13.8	13.0	0.75	0.454			
Period 3	10.6	9.2	0.75	0.195			
Total bilirubin (mg/100 mL)							
Period 1	0.20	0.24	0.01	0.055			
Period 2	0.23	0.22	0.01	0.515			
Period 3	0.20	0.20	0.01	1.000			
Total protein (g/100 mL)							
Period 1	6.88	6.84	0.117	0.816			
Period 2	6.81	6.61	0.117	0.220			
Period 3	7.17	7.00	0.117	0.308			
Creatinine (mg/100 mL)							
Period 1	1.44	1.39	0.057	0.496			
Period 2	1.19	1.21	0.057	0.791			
Period 3	1.23	1.23	0.057	0.967			
Blood urea nitrogen:creatinine							
Period 1	13.17	14.24	0.494	0.126			
Period 2	13.60	14.00	0.494	0.554			
Period 3	13.23	13.45	0.494	0.750			
Creatine kinase (U/L)							
Period 1	144.0	119.3	15.06	0.242			
Period 2	127.7	113.8	15.06	0.509			
Period 3	223.4	144.8	15.06	0.001			
Glucose (mg/100 mL)							
Period 1	69	64	2.8	0.181			
Period 2	66	63	2.8	0.455			
Period 3	78	70	2.8	0.040			
LDH (U/L)							
Period 1	952	889	59.0	0.440			
Period 2	1095	901	59.0	0.022			
Period 3	1063	821	59.0	0.004			
Triglycerides (g/100 mL)							
Period 1	33	24	2.4	0.017			
Period 2	27	23	2.4	0.204			
Period 3	30	31	2.4	0.695			
Cholesterol (mg/100 mL)							
Period 1	95	71	3.75	<0.001			
Period 2	83	59	3.75	<0.001			
Period 3	107	76	3.75	<0.001			

[a]*Data are presented as least squares means (±SEM) of LE (n = 9) and HE (n = 10) treatments.*
[b]*ALP, alkaline phosphatase; ALT, alanine aminotransferase; AST, aspartate aminotransferase; LDH, lactate dehydrogenase.*
[c]*Most conservative error of the mean.*
[d]*Taken from the University of Kentucky Livestock Disease Diagnostic Laboratory (Lexington, KY, USA).*
[e]*Taken from Kaneko et al. (15).*
[f]*Plasma.*

first period. In the latter two periods, the growth response of the HE steers paralleled the LE steers. Thus, the HE steers showed an adjustment in rate of BW gain to the alkaloid challenge but without a compensatory growth response. Concomitantly, there was a decrease in blood concentrations of triglycerides, albumin/globulin ratio, eosinophils, and lymphocytes but an increase in bilirubin. It was only during the first period that the concentrations of both serum cholesterol (27%) and triglycerides (25%) were depressed. The initial more than sixfold (14% of LE steers) depression of the classic endophytic fescue identifier, prolactin, in

TABLE 5 | Linear vs. quadratic time effects on serum and plasma analytes of steers grazing low endophyte (LE)- or high endophyte (HE)-infected forages[a,b].

Item[b]	LE		HE	
	Linear	Quadratic	Linear	Quadratic
Prolactin	<0.001	0.010	0.001	0.012
ALP	0.002	0.024	0.009	0.080
ALT	0.863	<0.001	0.194	0.035
AST	0.204	0.432	0.031	0.383
AST/ALT ratio	0.341	<0.001	0.822	0.066
Ammonia	<0.001	0.0960	0.001	0.954
Blood urea nitrogen	<0.001	0.002	0.001	0.050
Albumin	<0.001	0.180	<0.001	0.425
Globulin	<0.001	0.033	<0.001	0.008
Albumin/globulin ratio	<0.001	0.112	<0.001	0.071
γ-Glutamyltransferase	0.110	0.008	0.023	0.013
Total bilirubin	0.907	0.057	0.069	0.912
Total protein	0.062	0.156	0.283	0.044
Creatinine	0.001	0.002	0.011	0.032
Blood urea nitrogen:creatinine	0.952	0.335	0.170	0.809
Creatine kinase	0.010	0.055	0.003	0.024
Glucose	0.031	0.036	0.141	0.255
LDH	0.343	0.337	0.151	0.308
Triglycerides	0.482	0.253	0.015	0.075
Cholesterol	0.056	0.005	0.124	0.001

[a]*Data are P-values associated with linear and quadratic non-orthogonal polynomial contrasts used to characterize the effect of treatment over time on concentrations of blood analytes.*
[b]*ALP, alkaline phosphatase; ALT, alanine aminotransferase; AST, aspartate aminotransferase; LDH, lactate dehydrogenase.*

HE steers is consistent with reduced triglyceride synthesis in the presence of ergot peptides (24) and with the overall correlation found between serum triglyceride and prolactin concentrations (**Table 8**). This evidence of altered lipid metabolism has been associated with reduced forage intake of high endophyte fescue (25, 26). Although we did not measure these parameters, DiMarco et al. (25) found steers that had been fasted, and then refed, recovered their initially depressed cholesterol levels. With regard to correlating prolactin and triglyceride levels, cattle consuming high levels of endophyte forages have been shown to possess more saturated fatty acids in subcutaneous and perinephric fat than those consuming low levels of endophyte (27, 28). In the current study, a decreased in ADG and triglycerides was found in the first period, whereas ADG and triglyceride levels had recovered by the second and third period. By contrast, consumption of alkaloids is thought to be the cause of the loss of stimulation for insulin receptors that are involved in lipid metabolism (24), consistent with the trial-long depressed cholesterol levels of HE steers.

The reduced serum albumin and the albumin/globulin ratio in HE steers vs. LE steers would signify that albumin synthesis within the liver was impaired. For the HE steers, the 20% increased bilirubin also observed in period 1 signifies that excretory function may have been partially curtailed. The 6.3% increase in RBC concentration for HE steers indicates that the senescence of erythrocytes would not be the major contributor to the increased bilirubin (23). Moreover, increased RBC in HE steers is inconsistent with the understanding that prolactin increases erythropoiesis (29), as prolactin is decreased in HE steers. The unaltered value of total protein and γ-glutamyltransferase would suggest that even though some protein synthesis and excretory function may have been abridged, liver function was not uniformly impaired. The unaltered ammonia, blood urea nitrogen, creatinine, blood urea nitrogen:creatinine ratio, and creatine kinase between treatment groups indicates that nitrogen metabolism, urea synthesis, renal glomerular filtration function, and skeletal muscles were not influenced during period 1.

Eosinophils (55.2%) and lymphocytes (17.6%) numbers were decreased in HE steers in period 1, suggesting that immune function may have been impaired (30–32). The reduced level of eosinophils in these young HE steers also has been found in mature beef steers grazing endophyte-infected tall fescue (18).

Period 2

In contrast to the severe reduction in BW gains of HE steers found during period 1, the ADG by HE steers (0.26 kg/day) did not differ from that of LE steers (0.27 kg/day). Although moderate, this rate of gain suggests that the HE steers seemed to have adjusted to the physiological challenge of consuming forages that contained about 20 times more ergot alkaloids than LE steers. However, despite an equal rate of BW gain, prolactin, albumin, and cholesterol levels remained suppressed, and RBC increased in HE steers during period 2. By contrast, the albumin:globulin ratio and bilirubin levels no longer differed, indicating that hepatic albumin synthesis was still impaired, but possibly not to the overall extent as in period 1. Between treatment groups, similar values for bilirubin, total protein, and γ-glutamyltransferase would implied that hepatic excretory capacity was not affected during this period and that liver damage did not occur.

Some aspects of energy metabolism also appeared to have been altered in period 2 as compared to period 1. Although HE steers no longer possessed reduced levels of triglycerides relative to LE steers, they continued to have lower serum cholesterol, levels that were below the clinical reference range (9, 15). This suggests that the HE steers may be utilizing their cholesterol to supplement the altered energy metabolism. In addition, the reduced LDH of HE steers during period 2 could be indicative of a reduction in the transformation of pyruvate to lactate or a reduced "shuttling" of lactate between skeletal muscles and the liver. In rats, the sub-chronic exposure of rats to environmental toxins caused hepatotoxicity and a decrease in the serum levels of LDH (33). The increased duration of exposure to the high concentration of ergot alkaloids may have led to the reduced LDH as well for the HE steers.

Also occurring during period 2, increased (34%) plasma ammonia in HE vs. LE steers suggests that ammonia capturing and recycling mechanisms were impaired in the HE steers (34–36). However, because blood urea nitrogen did not differ, urea synthesis likely was not altered in HE vs. LE steers. Moreover, the unaffected creatinine, blood urea nitrogen:creatinine ratio, and creatine kinase between treatment groups suggests that renal glomerular filtration function and skeletal muscle turnover also were similar in HE and LE steers during period 2.

TABLE 6 | Blood cell types of steers grazing low endophyte (LE)- or high endophyte (HE)-infected forages[a].

Item	Pasture treatment			*P*-value			Reference range
	LE	HE	SEM[b]	TRT	Period	TRT × period	
Across-periods							
RBC[c] (1 × 10⁶/μL)	8.43	9.01	0.134	0.049	0.092	0.974	5.0–10[e]
Hemoglobin (g/dL)	10.8	10.9	0.17	0.811	0.001	0.539	8.0–15[e]
Packed cell volume (%)	30.1	30.5	0.50	0.701	<0.001	0.783	24–46[e]
WBC[d] (1 × 10³/μL)	9.26	8.89	0.606	0.663	0.010	0.296	4.0–12.0[e]
Neutrophils (1 × 10³/μL)	3.13	3.18	0.331	0.917	0.004	0.900	0.06–4.00[f]
Lymphocytes (1 × 10³/μL)	5.65	5.23	0.373	0.430	0.044	0.240	2.5–7.5[f]
Monocytes (1 × 10³/μL)	0.43	0.35	0.046	0.228	<0.001	0.243	0.0–0.9[f]
Eosinophils (1 × 10³/μL)	0.22	0.17	0.046	0.373	0.183	0.087	0.0–2.4[f]
Within-periods							
RBC[c] (1 × 10⁶/μL)							
Period 1	8.57	9.11	0.231	0.100			
Period 2	8.24	8.83	0.231	0.077			
Period 3	8.49	9.09	0.231	0.067			
Hemoglobin (g/dL)							
Period 1	10.8	11.1	0.29	0.472			
Period 2	10.5	10.5	0.29	0.989			
Period 3	11.1	11.1	0.29	0.945			
Packed cell volume (%)							
Period 1	29.5	30.2	0.87	0.580			
Period 2	28.6	29.2	0.87	0.657			
Period 3	32.3	32.3	0.87	0.973			
WBC[d] (1 × 10³/μL)							
Period 1	10.43	9.12	0.743	0.209			
Period 2	8.11	8.19	0.743	0.942			
Period 3	9.23	9.35	0.743	0.904			
Neutrophils (1 × 10³/μL)							
Period 1	3.14	3.03	0.411	0.857			
Period 2	2.62	2.72	0.411	0.864			
Period 3	3.65	3.80	0.411	0.792			
Lymphocytes (1 × 10³/μL)							
Period 1	6.58	5.42	0.483	0.090			
Period 2	5.11	5.09	0.483	0.976			
Period 3	5.25	5.18	0.507	0.924			
Monocytes (1 × 10³/μL)							
Period 1	0.64	0.53	0.066	0.263			
Period 2	0.27	0.31	0.066	0.723			
Period 3	0.38	0.21	0.070	0.081			
Eosinophils (1 × 10³/μL)							
Period 1	0.38	0.17	0.087	0.056			
Period 2	0.18	0.13	0.077	0.625			
Period 3	0.11	0.21	0.065	0.245			

[a]*Data are presented as least squares means (±SEM) of LE (n = 9) and HE (n = 10) treatments.*
[b]*Most conservative error of the mean.*
[c]*Red blood cells.*
[d]*White blood cells.*
[e]*Taken from the University of Kentucky Livestock Disease Diagnostic Laboratory (Lexington, KY, USA).*
[f]*Taken from Duncan et al. (16).*

Period 3

In the final period, ADG of the steers consuming the HE forage was the same as for LE steers. However, for both groups of steers, the ADG achieved was about four times greater than during period 2 (1.4 vs. 0.27 and 1.3 vs. 0.26, respectively). Despite these treatments, similar and good rates of gain for grazing steers, prolactin, albumin, and cholesterol levels remained suppressed, and ammonia and RBC levels remained higher in HE vs. LE steers. The prolonged high endophyte exposure allowed for further adaption by the HE steers. During period 3, the activities of creatinine kinase, AST, ALT, ALP, LDH, glucose concentration, and number of monocytes decreased.

Unlike periods 1 or 2, creatinine kinase in period 3 was depressed by 35% for steers grazing the HE pasture. The decreased level of creatine kinase was presumably the result of suppressed expression in striated muscle and possibly cardiac tissue or reduced tissue mass (9). Also, unique to period 3 was the serum reductions of clinical markers (ALP, ALT, and AST) for impaired metabolism. A reduction in serum ALP, a common indicator of high endophyte exposure (7, 37, 38), is related to decreased bone and intestinal isoenzymes activities (39). The decreased ALP could also be the result of reduced intakes and absorption of nutrients vital for ALP function (18). The reduced serum ALT presumably represents reduced cytosolic ALT in hepatocytes (40, 41), whereas reduced AST typically is interpreted as increased mitochondrial turnover in hepatocytes (41–43) and striated muscles (44). The lack of change in the AST:ALT ratio and decreased content of both enzymes is indicative of a relative constant rate of tissue turnover with either decreased concentrations of AST and ALT in tissue or diminished tissue mass (9), again indicating a "healthy" but metabolically altered liver in HE vs. LE steers.

TABLE 7 | Linear vs. quadratic time effects on blood cell type of steers grazing low endophyte (LE)- or high endophyte (HE)-infected forages[a].

Item	LE		HE	
	Linear	Quadratic	Linear	Quadratic
RBC[b]	0.808	0.195	0.994	0.388
Hemoglobin	0.347	0.124	0.979	0.119
Packed cell volume	0.008	0.025	0.090	0.095
WBC[c]	0.224	0.029	0.617	0.059
Neutrophils	0.260	0.093	0.029	0.039
Lymphocytes	0.060	0.117	0.639	0.581
Monocytes	0.033	0.016	<0.001	0.161
Eosinophils	0.016	0.307	0.599	0.473

[a]*Data are P-values associated with linear and quadratic non-orthogonal polynomial contrasts used to characterize the effect of treatment over time on blood cell type.*
[b]*Red blood cells.*
[c]*White blood cells.*

During period 3, the concentration of RBC continued to be greater in HE vs. LE steers by 7.1%, whereas the monocytes were 44.7% lower in HE vs. LE steers. Monocytes are vital for immune response, wound healing, and tissue homeostasis (31, 45, 46). This decreased concentration of monocytes is similar to the report of Saker et al. (31) and could be due to the accumulated stress from the effects of grazing HE vs. LE pastures.

Serum Prolactin was Poorly Correlated with Blood Analytes

Prolactin is reported to affect many physiological processes besides lactation (47). Therefore, the second objective of this study is to evaluate the potential relationships between serum prolactin and measured blood analytes. In general, little evidence was found to indicate that HE-decreased serum prolactin concentrations were associated with other assessed blood analytes. This lack of correlation was unexpected given that prolactin is a multifunctional hormone known to exert metabolic effects on many tissues due to the ubiquitous expression of prolactin receptors (48). In this regard, it is interesting to note that prolactin levels were lowest for both LE and HE steers in period 3, the period of greatest ADG for both steer groups. However, the correlation between triglycerides and prolactin levels in HE steers could prove to be very important as an indicator of altered energy metabolism (48, 49).

CONCLUSION

In summary, growth, clinical, and biochemical parameters that changed in response to grazing HE vs. LE pastures can be

TABLE 8 | Correlation of serum and plasma analytes with serum prolactin of steers grazing low endophyte (LE)- or high endophyte (HE)-infected forages.

Item[d]	Overall[a]		LE[b]		HE[c]	
	Coefficient	*P*-value	Coefficient	*P*-value	Coefficient	*P*-value
ALP	0.176	0.212	0.155	0.4617	0.272	0.161
ALT	0.317	0.022	0.424	0.035	0.268	0.168
AST	0.161	0.256	0.154	0.462	0.202	0.302
AST/ALT ratio	−0.119	0.398	−0.144	0.492	−0.140	0.477
Ammonia	−0.146	0.301	−0.231	0.267	0.088	0.657
Blood urea nitrogen	0.236	0.092	0.405	0.045	0.204	0.297
Albumin	−0.111	0.434	−0.237	0.254	0.116	0.558
Globulin	0.092	0.517	0.214	0.305	−0.149	0.449
Albumin/globulin ratio	−0.159	0.262	−0.342	0.094	0.215	0.272
γ-Glutamyltransferase	0.100	0.479	0.240	0.247	−0.136	0.490
Total bilirubin	0.122	0.389	0.220	0.290	−0.024	0.904
Total protein	0.028	0.845	0.083	0.695	−0.074	0.709
Creatinine	0.110	0.438	−0.019	0.927	0.433	0.021
Blood urea nitrogen:creatinine	0.121	0.392	0.377	0.064	−0.237	0.226
Creatine kinase	0.023	0.870	0.014	0.948	0.109	0.614
Glucose	−0.057	0.689	−0.145	0.490	0.120	0.542
LDH	0.018	0.898	0.046	0.827	−0.120	0.542
Triglycerides	0.321	0.021	0.314	0.126	0.388	0.042
Cholesterol	0.046	0.748	0.054	0.799	0.019	0.923

[a]*(LE + HE) analytes vs. (LE + HE) prolactin.*
[b]*LE analytes vs. LE prolactin.*
[c]*HE analytes vs. HE prolactin.*
[d]*ALP, alkaline phosphatase; ALT, alanine aminotransferase; AST, aspartate aminotransferase; LDH, lactate dehydrogenase.*

TABLE 9 | Correlation of blood cell type with serum prolactin of steers grazing low endophyte (LE)- or high endophyte (HE)-infected forages.

Item	Overall[a]		LE[b]		HE[c]	
	Coefficient	*P*-value	Coefficient	*P*-value	Coefficient	*P*-value
RBC[d]	−0.144	0.307	−0.322	0.116	0.039	0.842
Hemoglobin	0.282	0.043	0.536	0.006	0.013	0.949
Packed cell volume	0.197	0.162	0.375	0.065	−0.005	0.982
WBC[e]	0.112	0.430	0.099	0.639	0.177	0.368
Neutrophils	0.193	0.170	0.277	0.180	0.127	0.519
Lymphocytes	−0.033	0.818	−0.103	0.633	0.151	0.445
Monocytes	0.062	0.669	0.055	0.799	0.094	0.643
Eosinophils	−0.078	0.649	−0.142	0.627	−0.051	0.816

[a]*(LE + HE) analytes vs. (LE + HE) prolactin.*
[b]*LE analytes vs. LE prolactin.*
[c]*HE analytes vs. HE prolactin.*
[d]*Red blood cells.*
[e]*White blood cells.*

divided into three groups: those that were continually altered (serum prolactin, albumin, cholesterol, and RBCs), those that were initially altered and then "recovered" (ADG, triglycerides, albumin/globulin ratio, bilirubin, lymphocytes, and eosinophils), and, subsequently, those that developed after long-term exposure (AST, ALT, ammonia, creatine kinase, LDH glucose, and monocytes). These findings suggest that the differences in blood analyte profiles may be indicative of whether and when grazing young steers are adjusting, metabolically, to consumption of HE pastures. However, mechanisms responsible for initial loss of BW gain of HE steers that occurred in period 1, and the subsequent parallel rates of gain to LE steers, but not compensatory growth, awaits discovery. Unexpectedly, with the exception of triglycerides and creatine, blood analytes were poorly correlated with serum prolactin levels.

AUTHOR CONTRIBUTIONS

JJ, JB, and JM were responsible for the design and acquisition of the data. All authors (JJ, ML, JB, and JM) were responsible for the analysis and interpretation of the data, drafting and/or critical revision of the intellectual content, and are accountable for the accuracy and integrity of this work.

FUNDING

This is publication No. 15-07-119 of the Kentucky Agricultural Experiment Station and is published with approval of the Director. This work is supported by the National Institute of Food and Agriculture, U.S. Department of Agriculture, Special Cooperative Agreement (JM) and Multistate project No. 1000591.

REFERENCES

1. Schmidt SP, Hoveland CS, Clark EM, Davis ND, Smith LA, Grimes HW, et al. Association of an endophytic fungus with fescue toxicity in steers fed Kentucky 31 tall fescue seed or hay. *J Anim Sci* (1982) **55**:1259–63.
2. Goetsch AL, Jones AL, Stokes SR, Beers KW, Piper EL. Intake, digestion, passage rate and serum prolactin in growing dairy steers fed endophyte-infected fescue with noninfected fescue, clover or wheat straw. *J Anim Sci* (1987) **64**:1759–68.
3. Chestnut AB, Fribourg HA, Mclaren JB, Keltner DG, Reddick BB, Carlisle RJ, et al. Effects of *Acremonium-coenophialum* infestation, bermudagrass, and nitrogen or clover on steers grazing tall fescue pastures. *J Prod Agric* (1991) **4**:208–13. doi:10.2134/jpa1991.0208
4. Hemken RW, Bull LS, Boling JA, Kane E, Bush LP, Buckner RC. Summer fescue toxicosis in lactating dairy cows and sheep fed experimental strains of ryegrass-tall fescue hybrids. *J Anim Sci* (1979) **49**:641–6.
5. Jackson JA Jr, Hemken RW, Boling JA, Harmon RJ, Buckner RC, Bush LP. Summer fescue toxicity in dairy steers fed tall fescue seed. *J Anim Sci* (1984) **58**:1057–61.
6. Strahan SR, Hemken RW, Jackson JA Jr, Buckner RC, Bush LP, Siegel MR. Performance of lactating dairy cows fed tall fescue forage. *J Dairy Sci* (1987) **70**:1228–34. doi:10.3168/jds.S0022-0302(87)80135-2
7. Boling JA, Bunting LD, Davenport GM, Van der Veen JL, Meekins KM, Bradley NW, et al. Physiological responses of cattle consuming tall fescue to environmental temperature and supplemental phenothiazine. *J Anim Sci* (1989) **67**:2377–85.
8. Strickland JR, Looper ML, Matthews JC, Rosenkrans CF, Flythe MD, Brown KR. Board-invited review: St. Anthony's fire in livestock: causes, mechanisms, and potential solutions. *J Anim Sci* (2011) **89**:1603–26. doi:10.2527/jas.2010-3478
9. Brown KR, Anderson GA, Son K, Rentfrow G, Bush LP, Klotz JL, et al. Growing steers grazing high versus low endophyte (*Neotyphodium coenophialum*)-infected tall fescue have reduced serum enzymes, increased hepatic glucogenic enzymes, and reduced liver and carcass mass. *J Anim Sci* (2009) **87**:748–60. doi:10.2527/jas.2008-1108
10. Yates SG, Powell RG. Analysis of ergopeptine alkaloids in endophyte-infected tall fescue. *J Agric Food Chem* (1988) **36**:337–40. doi:10.1021/jf00080a023
11. Da Fonseca-Wollheim F. The significance of the hydrogen ion concentration and the addition of ADP in the determination of ammonia with glutamate dehydrogenase. An improved enzymic determination of ammonia. *Clin Biochem* (1973) **11**:421–5.
12. Bernard JK, Chestnut AB, Erickson BH, Kelly FM. Effects of prepartum consumption of endophyte-infested tall fescue on serum prolactin and subsequent milk-production of Holstein cows. *J Dairy Sci* (1993) **76**:1928–33. doi:10.3168/jds.S0022-0302(93)77526-8
13. Feldman BF, Zinkl JG, Jain NC, Schalm OW. *Schalm's Veterinary Hematology*. Philadelphia, PA: Lippincott Williams & Wilkins (2000).
14. Kenward MG, Roger JH. Small sample inference for fixed effects from restricted maximum likelihood. *Biometrics* (1997) **53**:983–97. doi:10.2307/2533558
15. Kaneko JJ, Harvey JW, Bruss ML. *Clinical Biochemistry of Domestic Animals*. San Diego, CA: Academic Press (1997).

16. Duncan JR, Prasse KW, Mahaffey EA. *Veterinary Laboratory Medicine: Clinical Pathology*. Ames, IA: Iowa State University Press (1994).
17. Davenport GM, Boling JA, Rahe CH. Growth and endocrine responses of cattle to implantation of estradiol-17 beta during continuous or discontinuous grazing of high- and low-endophyte-infected tall fescue. *J Anim Sci* (1993) **71**:757–64.
18. Oliver JW. Physiological manifestations of endophyte toxicosis in ruminant and laboratory species. In: Bacon CW, Hill NS, editors. *Neotyphodium/Grass Interactions*. New York, NY: Plenum Press (1997). p. 311–46.
19. Noble RC, O'Kelly JC. Observations on changes in lipid composition and lecithin-cholesterol-acyltransferase reaction of bovine plasma induced by heat exposure. *Lipids* (1973) **8**:216–23. doi:10.1007/BF02544638
20. O'Kelly JC, Reich HP. Plasma lipid changes in cattle during chronic hyperthermia induced by heat exposure and by pyrogen. *Comp Biochem Physiol B* (1975) **51**:283–8.
21. Stuedemann JA, Hoveland CS. Fescue endophyte: history and impact on animal agriculture. *J Prod Agric* (1988) **1**:39–44. doi:10.2134/jpa1988.0039
22. Peters T. Serum albumin: recent progress in the understanding of its structure and biosynthesis. *Clin Chem* (1977) **23**:5–12.
23. Dufour DR, Lott JA, Nolte FS, Gretch DR, Koff RS, Seeff LB. Diagnosis and monitoring of hepatic injury. II. Recommendations for use of laboratory tests in screening, diagnosis, and monitoring. *Clin Chem* (2000) **46**:2050–68.
24. Cincotta AH, Meier AH. Reductions of body fat stores and total plasma cholesterol and triglyceride concentrations in several species by bromocriptine treatment. *Life Sci* (1989) **45**:2247–54. doi:10.1016/0024-3205(89)90066-0
25. DiMarco NM, Beitz DC, Whitehurst GB. Effect of fasting on free fatty acid, glycerol and cholesterol concentrations in blood plasma and lipoprotein lipase activity in adipose tissue of cattle. *J Anim Sci* (1981) **52**:75–82.
26. Realini CE, Duckett SK, Hill NS, Hoveland CS, Lyon BG, Sackmann JR, et al. Effect of endophyte type on carcass traits, meat quality, and fatty acid composition of beef cattle grazing tall fescue. *J Anim Sci* (2005) **83**:430–9.
27. Townsend WE, Snook ME, Stuedemann JA, Wilson RL. Effect of level of endophyte infection, nitrogen fertilization rate, grazing period, and paddock exchange on some chemical properties of four bovine tissues. *J Anim Sci* (1991) **69**:2871–82.
28. Stuedemann JA, Thompson AM. Management strategies and potential opportunities to reduce the effects of endophyte-infested tall fescue on animal performance. In: Hume DE, Latch G, Easton HS, editors. *Proc. Second Int. Symp. Acremonium/Grass Interactions*. Plenary Papers (1993). p. 103–14.
29. Jepson JH, Lowenstein L. Effect of prolactin on erythropoiesis in the mouse. *Blood* (1964) **24**:726–38.
30. Minton JE, Apple JK, Parsons KM, Blecha F. Stress-associated concentrations of plasma cortisol cannot account for reduced lymphocyte function and changes in serum enzymes in lambs exposed to restraint and isolation stress. *J Anim Sci* (1995) **73**:812–7.
31. Saker KE, Allen VG, Kalnitsky J, Thatcher CD, Swecker WS Jr, Fontenot JP. Monocyte immune cell response and copper status in beef steers that grazed endophyte-infected tall fescue. *J Anim Sci* (1998) **76**:2694–700.
32. Murray SE, Lallman HR, Heard AD, Rittenberg MB, Stenzel-Poore MP. A genetic model of stress displays decreased lymphocytes and impaired antibody responses without altered susceptibility to *Streptococcus pneumoniae*. *J Immunol* (2001) **167**:691–8. doi:10.4049/jimmunol.167.2.691
33. Wade MG, Foster WG, Younglai EV, McMahon A, Leingartner K, Yagminas A, et al. Effects of subchronic exposure to a complex mixture of persistent contaminants in male rats: systemic, immune, and reproductive effects. *Toxicol Sci* (2002) **67**:131–43. doi:10.1093/toxsci/67.1.131
34. Haussinger D. Regulation of hepatic ammonia metabolism: the intercellular glutamine cycle. *Adv Enzyme Regul* (1986) **25**:159–80. doi:10.1016/0065-2571(86)90013-0
35. Reynolds CK. Metabolism of nitrogenous compounds by ruminant liver. *J Nutr* (1992) **122**:850–4.
36. Lobley GE, Milano GD. Regulation of hepatic nitrogen metabolism in ruminants. *Proc Nutr Soc* (1997) **56**:547–63. doi:10.1079/PNS19970057
37. Bond J, Powell JB, Undersander DJ, Moe PW, Tyrrell HF, Oltjen RR. Forage composition and growth and physiological-characteristics of cattle grazing several varieties of tall fescue during summer conditions. *J Anim Sci* (1984) **59**:584–93.
38. Nihsen ME, Piper EL, West CP, Crawford RJ, Denard TM, Johnson ZB, et al. Growth rate and physiology of steers grazing tall fescue inoculated with novel endophytes. *J Anim Sci* (2004) **82**:878–83.
39. Schultze AE, Rohrbach BW, Fribourg HA, Waller JC, Oliver JW. Alterations in bovine serum biochemistry profiles associated with prolonged consumption of endophyte-infected tall fescue. *Vet Hum Toxicol* (1999) **41**:133–9.
40. Fleisher GA, Wakim KG. The fate of enzymes in body fluids-an experimental study. I. Disappearance rates of glutamic-pyruvic transaminase under various conditions. *J Lab Clin Med* (1963) **61**:76–85.
41. Tennant BC. Hepatic function. 5th ed. In: Kaneko J, editor. *Clinical Biochemistry of Domestic Animals*. San Diego, CA: Academic Press (1997). p. 337–8.
42. Cardinet GH, Littrell JF, Freedland RA. Comparative investigations of serum creatine phosphokinase and glutamic-oxaloacetic transaminase activities in equine paralytic myoglobinuria. *Res Vet Sci* (1967) **8**:219–26.
43. Harris P. Equine rhabodomyolysis syndrome. 4th ed. In: Robinson NE, editor. *Current Therapy in Equine Medicine*. Philadelphia, PA: W.B. Saunders Company (1997). p. 115–21.
44. Wakim KG, Fleisher GA. The fate of enzymes in body fluids – an experimental study. II. Disappearance rates of glutamic-oxalacetic transaminase I under various conditions. *J Lab Clin Med* (1963) **61**:86–97.
45. Schultze AB. Condition in dairy calves and level of circulating eosinophils. *J Dairy Sci* (1957) **40**:672–6. doi:10.3168/jds.S0022-0302(57)94537-X
46. Parihar A, Eubank TD, Doseff AI. Monocytes and macrophages regulate immunity through dynamic networks of survival and cell death. *J Innate Immun* (2010) **2**:204–15. doi:10.1159/000296507
47. Freeman ME, Kanyicska B, Lerant A, Nagy G. Prolactin: structure, function, and regulation of secretion. *Physiol Rev* (2000) **80**:1523–631.
48. Ben-Jonathan N, Hugo ER, Brandebourg TD, LaPensee CR. Focus on prolactin as a metabolic hormone. *Trends Endocrinol Metab* (2006) **17**:110–6. doi:10.1016/j.tem.2006.02.005
49. Carré N, Binart N. Prolactin and adipose tissue. *Biochimie* (2014) **97**:16–21. doi:10.1016/j.biochi.2013.09.023

Conflict of Interest Statement: The authors declare that the research was conducted in the absence of any commercial or financial relationships that could be construed as a potential conflict of interest.

13

Steering Endogenous Butyrate Production in the Intestinal Tract of Broilers as a Tool to Improve Gut Health

*Lonneke Onrust, Richard Ducatelle, Karolien Van Driessche, Celine De Maesschalck, Karen Vermeulen, Freddy Haesebrouck, Venessa Eeckhaut and Filip Van Immerseel**

Department of Pathology, Bacteriology and Avian Diseases, Ghent University, Merelbeke, Belgium

The ban on antimicrobial growth promoters and efforts to reduce therapeutic antibiotic usage has led to major problems of gastrointestinal dysbiosis in livestock production in Europe. Control of dysbiosis without the use of antibiotics requires a thorough understanding of the interaction between the microbiota and the host mucosa. The gut microbiota of the healthy chicken is highly diverse, producing various metabolic end products, including gases and fermentation acids. The distal gut knows an abundance of bacteria from within the *Firmicutes Clostridium* clusters IV and XIVa that produce butyric acid, which is one of the metabolites that are sensed by the host as a signal. The host responds by strengthening the epithelial barrier, reducing inflammation, and increasing the production of mucins and antimicrobial peptides. Stimulating the colonization and growth of butyrate-producing bacteria thus may help optimizing gut health. Various strategies are available to stimulate butyrate production in the distal gut. These include delivery of prebiotic substrates that are broken down by bacteria into smaller molecules which are then used by butyrate producers, a concept called cross-feeding. Xylo-oligosaccharides (XOS) are such compounds as they can be converted to lactate, which is further metabolized to butyrate. Probiotic lactic acid producers can be supplied to support the cross-feeding reactions. Direct feeding of butyrate-producing *Clostridium* cluster IV and XIVa strains are a future tool provided that large scale production of strictly anaerobic bacteria can be optimized. Current results of strategies that promote butyrate production in the gut are promising. Nevertheless, our current understanding of the intestinal ecosystem is still insufficient, and further research efforts are needed to fully exploit the capacity of these strategies.

Edited by:
Ryan Arsenault, University of Delaware, USA

Reviewed by:
Sherry Layton, Vetanco, Argentina
Brian B. Oakley, Western University of Health Sciences, USA

***Correspondence:**
Filip Van Immerseel
filip.vanimmerseel@ugent.be

Keywords: broiler, endogenous butyrate, performance, probiotics, prebiotics

INTRODUCTION

For many years, broiler intestinal health was supported by the widespread use of antimicrobial growth promoters (AGPs). These AGPs are antibiotic substances that were added to the feed at subtherapeutic levels, leading to improved animal performance. In the European Union, the use of AGPs was banned in 2006 while the Center for Veterinary Medicine of the US Food and Drug

Administration, in 2012, wrote a "Guidance for Industry" document recommending that antibiotics should only be used in case of specific diseases and not for growth promotion. The most important reason for these precautionary measures was the likelihood that AGPs may increase antimicrobial resistance in bacteria, in some cases followed by introduction of these bacteria in humans (1). Most likely intestinal health problems in the chicken have been masked partly by the routine use of AGPs. Since the ban of AGPs in Europe alternative strategies for control of intestinal health have become a focus of research. These research efforts have revealed the complexity of the intestinal ecosystem. The gut indeed is an organ that contains many different cell types and exerts many different functions (2). In addition, the composition of the gut microbiota is diverse and varies depending on different factors, including the feed composition. The interaction between the host and the beneficial microbes in the intestine is mutualistic, as the host provides an anaerobic shelter and nutrients for the bacteria, which in turn provide enzymes that help digesting polysaccharides and other complex molecules (3). Nonetheless, the intestinal tract also contains facultative pathogenic microorganisms, which may be harmful and even life-threatening to the host under certain conditions. The challenge for the intestinal immune system is thus to simultaneously create a firm barrier and a powerful defense against the pathogenic bacteria, while at the same time, foster the beneficial bacteria and create an open entrance for the nutrients. These apparently conflicting tasks are taken up by the intestinal mucosa forming the so-called intestinal barrier that receives signals from the intestinal bacteria (4). Microbial signals can originate from cell wall components, like lipopolysaccharides (LPS) and flagellin, DNA fragments, and metabolites such as short-chain fatty acids (SCFAs). Those signals can have proinflammatory or anti-inflammatory effects, depending on the signal (5). One important signal derived from the beneficial microbes is butyrate.

When considering signals derived from bacterial fermentation, butyric acid has been shown to be the main driving force toward an optimal gut health. The molecule exerts beneficial effects in the physiological concentration range (6, 7). Numerous butyrate products are available on the market in a wide range of formulations. However, another possibility to increase butyric acid in the gut is by stimulating the endogenous production of butyrate by the gut microbiota. This review focuses on the methods on how to increase the endogenous production of butyrate in the intestinal tract of broilers in order to improve gut health.

ROLE OF THE INTESTINAL BARRIER IN GUT HEALTH

The luminal side of the intestinal wall is lined with absorptive epithelial cells, needed for water and nutrient uptake, which form a semipermeable barrier between the outside world (the gut lumen) and the internal host tissues. This semipermeable barrier is not only formed by the cell membranes of the epithelial cells but also by tight junctions that connect neighboring epithelial cells (8). These connections are regulated at different levels (e.g., by cytokines). The permeability of the intestinal epithelial cell layer can be affected by epithelial cell death and also by luminal signals that increase the epithelial layer permeability by affecting the tight junctions and thus cause loss of integrity of this important barrier (4). This loss of integrity can have detrimental effects. First, it causes an efflux of host proteins ("leaky gut") into the lumen and can cause luminal molecules, including toxins, and microorganisms, to reach the basal side of the epithelial layer. Through coevolution, the host has developed the capacity to become tolerant to most bacteria present in the lumen at the apical side of the epithelial cells. However, bacterial components that closely interact with epithelial cells from the basolateral side do trigger an inflammatory response. This is mediated by the binding of pathogen-associated molecular patterns, such as LPS and flagellin, to the so-called Toll-like receptors that trigger the cascade of proinflammatory signals (9). It is evident that the loss of intestinal epithelial integrity and its consequences will have an effect on animal performance.

In addition to the absorptive epithelial cells, other cell types are present in the lining of the gut wall. These include mucin-producing goblet cells and antimicrobial peptide (AMP)-producing paneth cells in the crypts (10). Both cell types are very important in innate defenses. Enteroendocrine cells can also be found in the epithelial lining, secreting peptide hormones into the bloodstream. These peptide hormones have a variety of functions, including effects on epithelial cell proliferation, inflammation, and consequently intestinal barrier integrity. One of these hormones is glucagon-like peptide-2 (GLP-2), a hormone that is important in maintaining epithelial integrity (11). The enteroendocrine cells are activated by various luminal signals, including bacterial signals (see below).

Underneath the epithelial lining, many other cell types are present which together form the lamina propria of the intestinal mucosa. These cells include, among others, fibroblasts and endothelial cells. Immune cells are also present in the mucosa, both in organized lymphoid tissues and scattered between the other cells. All non-epithelial cell types are responsive to luminal triggers, whether transmitted by epithelial cell signals, including enteroendocrine cell hormones, or not, and thus can influence other cell types by themselves. Thus, intestinal barrier integrity, inflammation, and gut function are influenced by luminal signals, many of which are produced by the microbiota (12). The composition of the microbiota and the metabolites the bacteria produce are hence crucial for gut health.

EFFECTS OF BUTYRATE

One of the major terminal metabolites of intestinal bacteria is butyrate. The effects of butyrate on intestinal health have already been described in detail in many reports (6, 13). The main targets of butyrate are briefly described in the following paragraph. Supplementation of butyrate in the feed can beneficially influence growth performance and intestinal villus structure in broiler chickens (14). Presence of butyrate in the intestine plays a role in the control of pathogens such as *Salmonella* Enteritidis and *Clostridium perfringens*. Reduction of *Salmonella enterica* serovar Enteritidis colonization and shedding in chickens has been reported (15, 16), as well as a decrease of necrotic lesions induced by *C. perfringens* in the small intestine (17). In addition to the role of butyrate in growth performance and pathogen control, butyrate also has anti-inflammatory properties. One of the mechanisms is inhibition of nuclear factor-kappa B activation, resulting in decreased expression of proinflammatory cytokines (18, 19). As described above, the intestinal barrier plays an important role in maintaining intestinal health. Butyrate has an effect on several components of this barrier (13, 20), such as the tight junctions (21). Butyrate upregulates AMP-activated protein kinase, which regulates the assembly of tight junctions (22). The mucin-producing goblet cells in the small intestine and distal gastrointestinal tract are also influenced by the presence of butyrate (23, 24). Butyrate-induced expression of MUC2 genes results in secretion of mucin, a glycoprotein, which forms a protective layer on the enterocytes (23, 25). AMP-producing paneth cells in the crypts are another cell type influenced by butyrate. Expression of AMPs, such as cathelicidins and defensins, is upregulated upon supplementation of butyric acid (26, 27). Finally, it is assumed that butyrate affects enteroendocrine L-cells secreting GLP-2 (28). Beneficial effects of GLP-2 on general gut health, such as the stimulation of intestinal crypt cell proliferation and the reduction of apoptosis in the crypt compartment, have been described for several animal species (29, 30). Information about the function of GLP-2 in chickens is scarce. Honda et al. (31) reported suppressed feed intake after intracerebroventricular administration of GLP-2 in chickens, which suggests that GLP-2 plays a role in regulating appetite (31). Daily intraperitoneal injection of GLP-2 in healthy broiler chickens improves absorptive function of the small intestine and has a positive effect on growth performance (32). GLP-2 receptors are thought to be present in chicken proventriculus, duodenum, jejunum, ileum, cecum, and colon, as detected by PCR (33). L-cells containing GLP-2 are mainly found in the crypts of the distal ileum and the proximal jejunum (34). This information could prove useful in unraveling the functions of GLP-2 in birds and in finding out which physiological triggers lead to secretion of the hormone (35). In humans, it is reported that butyrate enhances GLP-2 secretion and increases GLP-2 plasma concentration (35, 36). However, studies in chickens are lacking, and further research is necessary to yield conclusive information about the effect of butyrate on the release of GLP-2 in chickens.

THE INTESTINAL MICROBIOTA WITH FOCUS ON ENDOGENOUS BUTYRATE PRODUCTION

The composition of the microbiota in the gut of chickens depends on the age and the gastrointestinal segment, i.e., there is both a temporal as well as a spatial variation (37). In general, the diversity of the microbiota increases with age. The composition of microbiota differs between the different segments of the chicken gut. In general, low numbers of bacteria are found in the proximal parts of the gut (stomach, duodenum, jejunum, $<10^3$ cfu/g content), while the numbers increase toward the distal ileum and ceca, the latter harboring more than 10^{10} bacteria/g of content. In addition, the diversity increases significantly toward the distal gut. While only a limited diversity can be observed in the small intestine, with lactobacilli often dominant, the ceca harbor a large number of different bacterial groups (38). The cecal ecosystem of healthy subjects is dominated by bacteria belonging to the phyla *Bacteroidetes* and *Firmicutes*, together comprising more than 80% of the microbiota. The former contains many polysaccharide-degrading bacterial species, while the latter contains a variety of bacterial families, of which the *Ruminococcaceae* (*Clostridium* cluster IV) and *Lachnospiraceae* (*Clostridium* cluster XIVa) families are capable of fermenting various substrates to butyrate. The bacterial community has the genetic potential to carry out an enormous number of physiological functions (37). They can play an important role in both immune and digestive functions. Commensal bacteria can exert anti-inflammatory properties by producing SCFA (see below). Moreover, the mucosal architecture, mucus composition, and production can be affected by the presence of the gastrointestinal bacteria (39). The number of microbial genes in the gut of a chicken exceeds the number of chicken genes. Together these form a so-called "hologenome" (40).

Butyrate-Producing Bacteria and Bacteria That Promote/Inhibit Butyrate Production

Butyrate-Producing Bacteria

While a large variety of bacteria can produce acetic acid, the most important butyric acid-producing bacteria belong to a limited number of families, including the *Ruminococcaceae* and *Lachnospiraceae* (41). These families contain strictly anaerobic bacteria that are highly abundant in the gut of healthy chickens, as well as mammals. Other *Clostridium* clusters, including clusters I and XVI, contain butyrate producers, but the level of butyrate produced is much lower in comparison with strains from cluster IV and XIVa (42, 43). Individual butyrate-producing strains isolated from chicken ceca have been characterized (44, 45). In 2011, a first study specifically investigated the diversity of butyrate-producing bacteria from chicken ceca. 16S rRNA gene sequence analysis of isolates revealed members of *Clostridium* clusters IV, XIVa, XIVb, and XVI (42). When butyrate-producing bacteria are present in a sufficiently high concentration, the epithelial barrier integrity will be stronger, the epithelial cells will proliferate more and thus the villi will be longer. Moreover, inflammatory reactions will be reduced, while the stimulation of regulatory T-lymphocytes will yield a state of tolerance toward non-harmful bacteria (46). Butyrate is mainly synthesized via the reductive acetyl-coenzyme A pathway (47). Via a four-step pathway, acetyl-CoA is converted to the intermediate butyryl-CoA and further to butyrate. The final step or actual butyrate formation in its synthesis is mostly catalyzed by butyryl-CoA:acetate CoA-transferase and is used by several families of the healthy gut microbiota, dominated by *Lachnospiraceae* and *Ruminococcaceae* (48, 49). Another, but less frequently used, enzyme in the final step is butyrate kinase that produces butyrate from butyrylphosphate that is derived after phosphorylation of butyryl-CoA (7). Recently, it has been hypothesized that a propionate CoA transferase related to the enzyme of *Clostridium propionicum* is responsible for butyrate formation in members of the family *Erysipelotrichaceae* (42). In addition, three other butyrate-producing pathways using amino acids as major substrates are known. These pathways, only present in 20% of potential butyrate producers, are the lysine, 4-aminobutyrate, and glutarate pathways (47).

Other Microorganisms That May Interact with Butyrate Production

The variety of metabolic functions of the intestinal microbiome encompasses degradation of complex substrates (polysaccharides, proteins, and fat), fermentation of substrates to yield acidic compounds, immunomodulation, communication with other bacteria, and much more. To break down complex substrates, the bacteria form a food web, with different species and strains involved in different steps of the substrate utilization process (50). In a simplified model, complex substrates such as polysaccharides, including arabinoxylans, pectins, and cellulose, are converted to oligosaccharides by specific bacterial populations such as lactobacilli and some *Bacteroides* species, among others. These oligosaccharides [e.g., arabinoxylan-oligosaccharides (AXOS)] are then used by other bacterial groups to produce lactic acid, hydrogen, and SCFAs such as acetic, propionic, and butyric acid (41). The system in which bacteria convert substrates to products that are converted by other bacteria is called cross-feeding. This is an important mechanism, clearly showing the need of a diverse bacterial community, in order to be able to degrade substrates (51, 52). In case of dysbiosis, an unfavorable shift in the composition of the microbiota occurs, leading to deficiencies in certain crucial steps in certain pathways, yielding changes in the bacterial metabolites produced in the gut (53). Bacteria that promote butyrate production through the production of intermediate metabolites, as well as bacteria that inhibit butyrate production by competition for substrates can be present in the gut. For example, the underlying mechanism by which lactic acid bacteria (LABs) can be beneficial can be explained by the effects of butyrate, considering that the lactic acid produced by these bacteria is then further consumed by *Clostridium* cluster XIV strains to produce butyrate (48). Lactic acid is toxic by itself when present in high concentrations and only has a benefit when it is converted (54). Sulfate-reducing bacteria (SRBs) compete for lactate with butyrate-producing bacteria from *Clostridium* cluster XIVa, with the outcome of this competition being a crucial factor for gut health. Apart from this, SRBs also have to compete for hydrogen with hydrogenotrophic acetogenic and methanogenic bacteria (55). They produce hydrogen sulfide as a terminal metabolite. Hydrogen sulfide, with proven cell death-inducing effects on intestinal epithelial cells, is a clearly toxic metabolite (56). One can thus conclude that a complex interaction between different bacterial populations for specific substrates exists, and the outcome of this interaction can drive the microbiota either to produce beneficial metabolites which promote gut health, or toward production of toxic metabolites.

TOOLS TO STIMULATE ENDOGENOUS BUTYRATE PRODUCTION

Probiotics

The term probiotics was first defined by FOA/WHO in 2001, and at the end of 2013, the definition was worded more grammatically correct as "live microorganisms that, when administered in adequate amounts, confer a health benefit on the host" (57). The majority of bacterial probiotics consist of LABs, mainly from the *Lactobacillus*, *Bifidobacterium*, *Enterococcus*, and *Streptococcus* genera (58, 59). As discussed above, lactic acid can be consumed by butyrate-producing bacteria to produce butyrate (48). Different types of products are currently available on the market. Beside single-strains, multi-strain products are available, as well as competitive exclusion (CE) products, which contain a freeze-dried mixture of gut content. The main purpose of CE products is replacing the natural route of microbiota succession, while probiotics enhance the functions of existing microbiota. Besides, only defined CE products can be registered for which the identities of the bacteria in the mixture are known to be safe for chickens and humans (60).

Reports of the effect of probiotics on animal performance have been published (61, 62), and studies on the beneficial effect on pathogen colonization and disease reduction are widely available (63–65). However, positive effects are not observed in all studies. One of the reasons for the inconsistency of observed beneficial effects may be that success depends partly on the conditions of the study, i.e., feed formulae and feed ingredients, management factors, and presence or absence of stress factors and challenge conditions. Indeed, unpublished data from our laboratory show that the efficacy of probiotics is highly dependent on the model used. However, based on the above described data, attempts could be made to develop probiotics that stimulate butyrate production in the intestinal tract, either directly or through cross-feeding.

Butyrate-Producing Bacteria as Probiotic Strains

Most butyrate-producing bacteria belong to the *Clostridium* clusters IV and XIVa (66, 67) and play an important role in maintaining a healthy gut primarily through production of butyrate (7). These bacteria are less abundant in the gut of people suffering from inflammatory bowel disease (IBD) as compared to healthy persons (68). More specifically, *Butyricicoccus pullicaecorum* and *Faecalibacterium prausnitzii*, species belonging to *Clostridium* cluster IV, have been shown to be less abundant in the gut of IBD patients (68, 69). Thus, oral administration of these strains as probiotics might counteract IBD inflammation. At the moment, no specific studies are available in literature that show beneficial effects of butyrate-producing bacteria from *Clostridium* clusters IV and XIVa as probiotic candidates in poultry. However, *Clostridium butyricum* from *Clostridium* cluster I, administered as a component of a tri-strain probiotic, significantly improved body weight gain and reduced feed conversion rate in broiler chickens (70). Similar results have been reported with supplementation of *C. butyricum* in the feed as single strain probiotic (71).

A major problem with the production of butyrate-producing bacteria as probiotic is the cultivation, as these microorganisms require strict anaerobic conditions (72). Another issue is that most poultry feed is pelleted, and probiotic strains are exposed to high temperatures during this process. Thus, ideally the probiotic strains should be heat-stable, for example, through spore formation (73). Unfortunately, most butyrate-producing bacteria seem to lack this characteristic.

Other Microorganisms as Probiotic Strains Increasing Butyrate Concentration

Instead of direct administration of butyrate-producing bacteria to the bird, attempts could be made to use strains that stimulate butyrate production by *Clostridium* cluster IV and XIVa strains. The *Clostridium* cluster XIVa strains consume lactic acid to produce butyric acid. Therefore, LABs could be useful probiotics for their property of indirect stimulation of butyrate production. This cross-feeding mechanism may explain the beneficial effects of lactobacilli and bifidobacteria (70, 74). Addition of lactobacilli in an *in vitro* fermentation system of cecal broiler content increases butyrate concentration (75). This suggests that lactobacilli, as probiotic bacteria, stimulate butyrate-producing bacteria in the chicken cecum. These effects are, however, hitherto not investigated *in vivo* in chickens.

Prebiotics

The definition of prebiotics as proposed by Gibson et al. (76) is "Selectively fermented ingredients that allow specific changes, both in the composition and/or activity of the gastrointestinal microflora that confer benefits upon host wellbeing and health" (76). Several prebiotics induce beneficial effects on broiler performance and pathogen control (77, 78). Most published studies involve oligosaccharides, such as fructo-oligosaccharides (FOS), galacto-oligosaccharides (GOS), arabinoxylo-oligosaccharides (AXOS), xylo-oligosaccharides (XOS), and raffinose family oligosaccharides (RFOs) (79). Prebiotics are complex molecules because of the chain length, the nature of the sugar bonds, and the nature of the side chains on the saccharides. These characteristics can affect their function as prebiotic (80). Prebiotics need to be converted into metabolites by the microbiota in the gut. Because they are saccharides, their end products will be SCFAs, lactate, and gases, and thus the beneficial effect can theoretically be evaluated or predicted by analyzing these metabolites.

Prebiotics Used By Butyrate-Producing Bacteria and Other Microorganisms

Prebiotics that stimulate colonization and activity of butyrate-producing *Clostridium* cluster IV and XIVa populations are considered to be beneficial. For example, our group showed that XOS supplementation to a broiler diet increases the number of lactobacilli and *Clostridium* cluster XIVa strains in the distal gut, thereby stimulating the cross-feeding between both groups, so that lactate is converted into butyrate (78). Different studies report improved growth performance and an increase of *Lactobacillus* and *Bifidobacterium* bacteria in the gut of broilers after administration of oligosaccharides (81–83). After supplementation of AXOS in the diet, a decrease of *Salmonella* Enteritidis and improved feed conversion rate is reported in poultry (44, 84). Contradictory results have been published with FOS supplementation in broilers. Several studies report a decrease of pathogen colonization, i.e., *Salmonella*, *C. perfringens*, and *Escherichia coli*, in the cecum of broilers (81, 85, 86), and an increase of *Bifidobacterium* spp. and *Lactobacillus* spp. (81). Other studies in broilers report no effect at all (87, 88). These discrepancies could be explained by differences in age, diet composition, and concentration of FOS in the diet. As discussed above, it can be hypothesized that the observed beneficial effects are at least partly due to the bacteria supporting the cross-feeding leading toward production of butyrate.

CONCLUSION

A large number of experimental and field trials in broilers have already been carried out, using a variety of feed additives. The most commonly measured outcome parameter is performance. Some studies were also done to determine the effect on pathogen colonization. The approach was mostly empirical and the products were therefore mainly developed without a clear understanding of the mode of action underlying the hoped-for beneficial effects. The only way to develop products with an enhanced activity as compared to the already existing products will be based on a thorough understanding of the intestinal ecosystem. Identification of the microbiota components that are crucial to gut health is ongoing and forms an essential part of the proper development of additives that support gut health (67). This needs to be done in both ways, i.e., identifying both the beneficial microbes as well as the harmful ones. Current knowledge indicates that butyrate-producing bacteria and their metabolite butyrate improve gut health in the physiological range (6). The amount of butyrate produced by the microbes in the lower intestinal tracts is impressive, considering that more than 50% of the microbiome is composed of butyrate producers (7). Deficiencies in butyrate production by the microbiota for whatever reason always seem to lead to inflammation in the intestinal tract (13). Providing a butyrate supplement in the feed only gives a partial answer to the problem, as the amount that can be added to the feed is limited. Thus, there is ample reason to try and stimulate endogenous butyrate production. This can be achieved by using feed additives, i.e., prebiotics that support the proliferation and the metabolic activities of the butyrate producers. Another possible strategy to stimulate endogenous butyrate production is by direct feeding of butyrate-producing bacteria. However, most probably a range of other metabolites exists with unknown mechanisms and influences on gut health. There is a need to investigate the specific effects of the different bacteria and metabolites that are found to play a role in gut health. Bacterial culturing is a crucial tool to foster our understanding of the intestinal ecosystem and essential in studying the effect of a specific species or strain on gut health parameters (2). Only a small minority of the microbial species residing in the gut has ever been cultured, and therefore isolation and characterization of new bacterial species from the gut will yield useful information (89).

Finally, the feed–microbiota–host interactions are extremely complex, but expertise on how to steer this interaction is growing rapidly. One way is to increase the abundance of butyrate-producing bacteria from *Clostridium* cluster IV and XIVa. In the future, many more health promoting as well as harmful bacterial groups and metabolites will doubtlessly be discovered. This will further contribute to optimizing gut health and animal performance.

REFERENCES

1. Butaye P, Devriese LA, Haesebrouck F. Antimicrobial growth promoters used in animal feed: effects of less well known antibiotics on gram-positive bacteria. *Clin Microbiol Rev* (2003) **16**(2):175–88. doi:10.1128/Cmr.16.2.175-188.2003
2. Walker AW, Duncan SH, Louis P, Flint HJ. Phylogeny, culturing, and metagenomics of the human gut microbiota. *Trends Microbiol* (2014) **22**(5):267–74. doi:10.1016/j.tim.2014.03.001
3. Backhed F, Ley RE, Sonnenburg JL, Peterson DA, Gordon JI. Host-bacterial mutualism in the human intestine. *Science* (2005) **307**(5717):1915–20. doi:10.1126/science.1104816
4. Hooper LV. Epithelial cell contributions to intestinal immunity. *Adv Immunol* (2015) **126**:129–72. doi:10.1016/bs.ai.2014.11.003
5. Hill DA, Artis D. Intestinal bacteria and the regulation of immune cell homeostasis. *Annu Rev Immunol* (2010) **28**:623–67. doi:10.1146/annurev-immunol-030409-101330
6. Guilloteau P, Martin L, Eeckhaut V, Ducatelle R, Zabielski R, Van Immerseel F. From the gut to the peripheral tissues: the multiple effects of butyrate. *Nutr Res Rev* (2010) **23**(2):366–84. doi:10.1017/S0954422410000247
7. Louis P, Flint HJ. Diversity, metabolism and microbial ecology of butyrate-producing bacteria from the human large intestine. *FEMS Microbiol Lett* (2009) **294**(1):1–8. doi:10.1111/j.1574-6968.2009.01514.x
8. Piche T. Tight junctions and IBS – the link between epithelial permeability, low-grade inflammation, and symptom generation? *Neurogastroenterol Motil* (2014) **26**(3):296–302. doi:10.1111/nmo.12315
9. Brown J, Wang H, Hajishengallis GN, Martin M. TLR-signaling networks: an integration of adaptor molecules, kinases, and cross-talk. *J Dent Res* (2011) **90**(4):417–27. doi:10.1177/0022034510381264
10. Muniz LR, Knosp C, Yeretssian G. Intestinal antimicrobial peptides during homeostasis, infection, and disease. *Front Immunol* (2012) **3**:310. doi:10.3389/fimmu.2012.00310
11. Baldassano S, Amato A. GLP-2: what do we know? What are we going to discover? *Regul Pept* (2014) **19**(4–195):6–10. doi:10.1016/j.regpep.2014.09.002
12. Havenaar R. Intestinal health functions of colonic microbial metabolites: a review. *Benef Microbes* (2011) **2**(2):103–14. doi:10.3920/BM2011.0003
13. Canani RB, Costanzo MD, Leone L, Pedata M, Meli R, Calignano A. Potential beneficial effects of butyrate in intestinal and extraintestinal diseases. *World J Gastroenterol* (2011) **17**(12):1519–28. doi:10.3748/wjg.v17.i12
14. Hu XF, Guo YM. Corticosterone administration alters small intestinal morphology and function of broiler chickens. *Asian Australas J Anim Sci* (2008) **21**(12):1773–8. doi:10.5713/ajas.2008.80167
15. Van Immerseel F, Boyen F, Gantois I, Timbermont L, Bohez L, Pasmans F, et al. Supplementation of coated butyric acid in the feed reduces colonization and shedding of *Salmonella* in poultry. *Poult Sci* (2005) **84**(12):1851–6. doi:10.1093/ps/84.12.1851
16. Fernandez-Rubio C, Ordonez C, Abad-Gonzalez J, Garcia-Gallego A, Honrubia MP, Mallo JJ, et al. Butyric acid-based feed additives help protect broiler chickens from *Salmonella* enteritidis infection. *Poult Sci* (2009) **88**(5):943–8. doi:10.3382/ps.2008-00484
17. Timbermont L, Lanckriet A, Dewulf J, Nollet N, Schwarzer K, Haesebrouck F, et al. Control of *Clostridium* perfringens-induced necrotic enteritis in broilers by target-released butyric acid, fatty acids and essential oils. *Avian Pathol* (2010) **39**(2):117–21. doi:10.1080/03079451003610586
18. Inan MS, Tolmacheva V, Wang QS, Rosenberg DW, Giardina C. Transcription factor NF-kappaB participates in regulation of epithelial cell turnover in the colon. *Am J Physiol Gastrointest Liver Physiol* (2000) **279**(6):G1282–91.
19. Place RF, Noonan EJ, Giardina C. HDAC inhibition prevents NF-kappa B activation by suppressing proteasome activity: down-regulation of proteasome subunit expression stabilizes I kappa B alpha. *Biochem Pharmacol* (2005) **70**(3):394–406. doi:10.1016/j.bcp.2005.04.030
20. Hamer HM, Jonkers D, Venema K, Vanhoutvin S, Troost FJ, Brummer RJ. Review article: the role of butyrate on colonic function. *Aliment Pharmacol Ther* (2008) **27**(2):104–19. doi:10.1111/j.1365-2036.2007.03562.x
21. Mitic LL, Van Itallie CM, Anderson JM. Molecular physiology and pathophysiology of tight junctions I. Tight junction structure and function: lessons from mutant animals and proteins. *Am J Physiol Gastrointest Liver Physiol* (2000) **279**(2):G250–4.
22. Peng L, Li ZR, Green RS, Holzman IR, Lin J. Butyrate enhances the intestinal barrier by facilitating tight junction assembly via activation of AMP-activated protein kinase in Caco-2 cell monolayers. *J Nutr* (2009) **139**(9):1619–25. doi:10.3945/jn.109.104638
23. Smirnov A, Perez R, Amit-Romach E, Sklan D, Uni Z. Mucin dynamics and microbial populations in chicken small intestine are changed by dietary probiotic and antibiotic growth promoter supplementation. *J Nutr* (2005) **135**(2):187–92.
24. Hatayama H, Iwashita J, Kuwajima A, Abe T. The short chain fatty acid, butyrate, stimulates MUC2 mucin production in the human colon cancer cell line, LS174T. *Biochem Biophys Res Commun* (2007) **356**(3):599–603. doi:10.1016/j.bbrc.2007.03.025
25. Willemsen LE, Koetsier MA, van Deventer SJ, van Tol EA. Short chain fatty acids stimulate epithelial mucin 2 expression through differential effects on prostaglandin E(1) and E(2) production by intestinal myofibroblasts. *Gut* (2003) **52**(10):1442–7. doi:10.1136/gut.52.10.1442
26. Goitsuka R, Chen CL, Benyon L, Asano Y, Kitamura D, Cooper MD. Chicken cathelicidin-B1, an antimicrobial guardian at the mucosal M cell gateway. *Proc Natl Acad Sci U S A* (2007) **104**(38):15063–8. doi:10.1073/pnas.0707037104
27. Sunkara LT, Achanta M, Schreiber NB, Bommineni YR, Dai G, Jiang W, et al. Butyrate enhances disease resistance of chickens by inducing antimicrobial host defense peptide gene expression. *PLoS One* (2011) **6**(11):e27225. doi:10.1371/journal.pone.0027225
28. Rowland KJ, Brubaker PL. The "cryptic" mechanism of action of glucagon-like peptide-2. *Am J Physiol Gastrointest Liver Physiol* (2011) **301**(1):G1–8. doi:10.1152/ajpgi.00039.2011
29. Drucker DJ. Glucagon-like peptides: regulators of cell proliferation, differentiation, and apoptosis. *Mol Endocrinol* (2003) **17**(2):161–71. doi:10.1210/me.2002-0306
30. Guan X, Karpen HE, Stephens J, Bukowski JT, Niu S, Zhang G, et al. GLP-2 receptor localizes to enteric neurons and endocrine cells expressing vasoactive peptides and mediates increased blood flow. *Gastroenterology* (2006) **130**(1):150–64. doi:10.1053/j.gastro.2005.11.005
31. Honda K, Saneyasu T, Yamaguchi T, Shimatani T, Aoki K, Nakanishi K, et al. Intracerebroventricular administration of novel glucagon-like peptide suppresses food intake in chicks. *Peptides* (2014) **52**:98–103. doi:10.1016/j.peptides.2013.12.008
32. Hu XF, Guo YM, Huang BY, Bun S, Zhang LB, Li JH, et al. The effect of glucagon-like peptide 2 injection on performance, small intestinal morphology, and nutrient transporter expression of stressed broiler chickens. *Poult Sci* (2010) **89**(9):1967–74. doi:10.3382/ps.2009-00547
33. Mo C, Zhong Y, Wang Y, Yan Z, Li J. Characterization of glucagon-like peptide 2 receptor (GLP2R) gene in chickens: functional analysis, tissue distribution, and developmental expression profile of GLP2R in embryonic intestine. *Domest Anim Endocrinol* (2014) **48**:1–6. doi:10.1016/j.domaniend.2014.01.002
34. Monir MM, Hiramatsu K, Nishimura K, Takemoto C, Watanabe T. Distribution of glucagon-like peptide (GLP)-2-immunoreactive cells in the chicken small intestine: antigen retrieval immunohistochemistry. *J Vet Med Sci* (2014) **76**(4):565–8. doi:10.1292/jvms.13-0513
35. Tappenden KA, Albin DM, Bartholome AL, Mangian HF. Glucagon-like peptide-2 and short-chain fatty acids: a new twist to an old story. *J Nutr* (2003) **133**(11):3717–20.
36. Mangian HF, Tappenden KA. Butyrate increases GLUT2 mRNA abundance by initiating transcription in Caco2-BBe cells. *JPEN J Parenter Enteral Nutr* (2009) **33**(6):607–17; discussion 17. doi:10.1177/0148607109336599
37. Stanley D, Hughes RJ, Moore RJ. Microbiota of the chicken gastrointestinal tract: influence on health, productivity and disease. *Appl Microbiol Biotechnol* (2014) **98**(10):4301–10. doi:10.1007/s00253-014-5646-2
38. Yeoman CJ, Chia N, Jeraldo P, Sipos M, Goldenfeld ND, White BA. The microbiome of the chicken gastrointestinal tract. *Anim Health Res Rev* (2012) **13**(1):89–99. doi:10.1017/S1466252312000138
39. Lan Y, Verstegen MWA, Tamminga S, Williams BA. The role of the commensal gut microbial community in broiler chickens. *Worlds Poult Sci J* (2005) **61**(1):95–104. doi:10.1079/WPS200445
40. Rosenberg E, Zilber-Rosenberg I. Symbiosis and development: the hologenome concept. *Birth Defects Res C Embryo Today* (2011) **93**(1):56–66. doi:10.1002/bdrc.20196

41. Pryde SE, Duncan SH, Hold GL, Stewart CS, Flint HJ. The microbiology of butyrate formation in the human colon. *FEMS Microbiol Lett* (2002) **217**(2):133–9. doi:10.1111/j.1574-6968.2002.tb11467.x
42. Eeckhaut V, Van Immerseel F, Croubels S, De Baere S, Haesebrouck F, Ducatelle R, et al. Butyrate production in phylogenetically diverse Firmicutes isolated from the chicken caecum. *Microb Biotechnol* (2011) **4**(4):503–12. doi:10.1111/j.1751-7915.2010.00244.x
43. De Maesschalck C, Van Immerseel F, Eeckhaut V, De Baere S, Cnockaert M, Croubels S, et al. *Faecalicoccus acidiformans* gen. nov., sp. nov., isolated from the chicken caecum, and reclassification of *Streptococcus pleomorphus* (Barnes et al. 1977), *Eubacterium* biforme (Eggerth 1935) and *Eubacterium cylindroides* (Cato et al. 1974) as *Faecalicoccus pleomorphus* comb. nov., *Holdemanella biformis* gen. nov., comb. nov. and *Faecalitalea cylindroides* gen. nov., comb. nov., respectively, within the family Erysipelotrichaceae. *Int J Syst Evol Microbiol* (2014) **64**(Pt 11):3877–84. doi:10.1099/ijs.0.064626-0
44. Eeckhaut V, Van Immerseel F, Teirlynck E, Pasmans F, Fievez V, Snauwaert C, et al. *Butyricicoccus pullicaecorum* gen. nov., sp. nov., an anaerobic, butyrate-producing bacterium isolated from the caecal content of a broiler chicken. *Int J Syst Evol Microbiol* (2008) **58**(Pt 12):2799–802. doi:10.1099/ijs.0.65730-0
45. Eeckhaut V, Van Immerseel F, Pasmans F, De Brandt E, Haesebrouck F, Ducatelle R, et al. *Anaerostipes butyraticus* sp. nov., an anaerobic, butyrate-producing bacterium from *Clostridium* cluster XIVa isolated from broiler chicken caecal content, and emended description of the genus Anaerostipes. *Int J Syst Evol Microbiol* (2010) **60**(Pt 5):1108–12. doi:10.1099/ijs.0.015289-0
46. Lopetuso LR, Scaldaferri F, Petito V, Gasbarrini A. Commensal Clostridia: leading players in the maintenance of gut homeostasis. *Gut Pathog* (2013) **5**(1):23. doi:10.1186/1757-4749-5-23
47. Vital M, Howe AC, Tiedje JM. Revealing the bacterial butyrate synthesis pathways by analyzing (Meta) genomic data. *MBio* (2014) **5**(2):e00889. doi:10.1128/mBio.00889-14
48. Duncan SH, Louis P, Flint HJ. Lactate-utilizing bacteria, isolated from human feces, that produce butyrate as a major fermentation product. *Appl Environ Microbiol* (2004) **70**(10):5810–7. doi:10.1128/AEM.70.10.5810-5817.2004
49. Louis P, Duncan SH, McCrae SI, Millar J, Jackson MS, Flint HJ. Restricted distribution of the butyrate kinase pathway among butyrate-producing bacteria from the human colon. *J Bacteriol* (2004) **186**(7):2099–106. doi:10.1128/Jb.186.7.2099-2106.2004
50. Flint HJ, Scott KP, Duncan SH, Louis P, Forano E. Microbial degradation of complex carbohydrates in the gut. *Gut Microbes* (2012) **3**(4):289–306. doi:10.4161/gmic.19897
51. Belenguer A, Duncan SH, Calder AG, Holtrop G, Louis P, Lobley GE, et al. Two routes of metabolic cross-feeding between *Bifidobacterium* adolescentis and butyrate-producing anaerobes from the human gut. *Appl Environ Microbiol* (2006) **72**(5):3593–9. doi:10.1128/AEM.72.5.3593-3599.2006
52. El Aidy S, Van den Abbeele P, Van de Wiele T, Louis P, Kleerebezem M. Intestinal colonization: how key microbial players become established in this dynamic process: microbial metabolic activities and the interplay between the host and microbes. *Bioessays* (2013) **35**(10):913–23. doi:10.1002/bies.201300073
53. Scott KP, Gratz SW, Sheridan PO, Flint HJ, Duncan SH. The influence of diet on the gut microbiota. *Pharmacol Res* (2013) **69**(1):52–60. doi:10.1016/j.phrs.2012.10.020
54. Hanstock TL, Mallet PE, Clayton EH. Increased plasma D-lactic acid associated with impaired memory in rats. *Physiol Behav* (2010) **101**(5):653–9. doi:10.1016/j.physbeh.2010.09.018
55. Marquet P, Duncan SH, Chassard C, Bernalier-Donadille A, Flint HJ. Lactate has the potential to promote hydrogen sulphide formation in the human colon. *FEMS Microbiol Lett* (2009) **299**(2):128–34. doi:10.1111/j.1574-6968.2009.01750.x
56. Carbonero F, Benefiel AC, Gaskins HR. Contributions of the microbial hydrogen economy to colonic homeostasis. *Nat Rev Gastroenterol Hepatol* (2012) **9**(9):504–18. doi:10.1038/nrgastro.2012.85
57. Hill C, Guarner F, Reid G, Gibson GR, Merenstein DJ, Pot B, et al. Expert consensus document. The international scientific association for probiotics and prebiotics consensus statement on the scope and appropriate use of the term probiotic. *Nat Rev Gastroenterol Hepatol* (2014) **11**(8):506–14. doi:10.1038/nrgastro.2014.66
58. Boesten RJ, de Vos WM. Interactomics in the human intestine: *Lactobacilli* and *Bifidobacteria* make a difference. *J Clin Gastroenterol* (2008) **42**(Suppl 3 Pt 2):S163–7. doi:10.1097/MCG.0b013e31817dbd62
59. Kleerebezem M, Vaughan EE. Probiotic and gut *Lactobacilli* and *Bifidobacteria*: molecular approaches to study diversity and activity. *Annu Rev Microbiol* (2009) **63**:269–90. doi:10.1146/annurev.micro.091208.073341
60. Wagner RD. Efficacy and food safety considerations of poultry competitive exclusion products. *Mol Nutr Food Res* (2006) **50**(11):1061–71. doi:10.1002/mnfr.200600058
61. Patterson JA, Burkholder KM. Application of prebiotics and probiotics in poultry production. *Poult Sci* (2003) **82**(4):627–31. doi:10.1093/ps/82.4.627
62. Kabir SML, Rahman MM, Rahman MB, Ahmed SU. The dynamics of probiotics on growth performance and immune response in broilers. *Int J Poult Sci* (2004) **3**:361–4. doi:10.3923/ijps.2004.361.364
63. Rantala M, Nurmi E. Prevention of growth of *Salmonella*-infantis in chicks by flora of alimentary-tract of chickens. *Br Poult Sci* (1973) **14**(6):627–30. doi:10.1080/00071667308416073
64. Fritts CA, Kersey JH, Motl MA, Kroger EC, Yan F, Si J, et al. *Bacillus subtilis* C-3102 (Calsporin) improves live performance and microbiological status of broiler chickens. *J Appl Poult Res* (2000) **9**(2):149–55. doi:10.1093/japr/9.2.149
65. Stern NJ, Cox NA, Bailey JS, Berrang ME, Musgrove MT. Comparison of mucosal competitive exclusion and competitive exclusion treatment to reduce *Salmonella* and *Campylobacter* spp. colonization in broiler chickens. *Poult Sci* (2001) **80**(2):156–60. doi:10.1093/ps/80.2.156
66. Gong J, Si W, Forster RJ, Huang R, Yu H, Yin Y, et al. 16S rRNA gene-based analysis of mucosa-associated bacterial community and phylogeny in the chicken gastrointestinal tracts: from crops to ceca. *FEMS Microbiol Ecol* (2007) **59**(1):147–57. doi:10.1111/j.1574-6941.2006.00193.x
67. Torok VA, Hughes RJ, Mikkelsen LL, Perez-Maldonado R, Balding K, MacAlpine R, et al. Identification and characterization of potential performance-related gut microbiotas in broiler chickens across various feeding trials. *Appl Environ Microbiol* (2011) **77**(17):5868–78. doi:10.1128/AEM.00165-11
68. Sokol H, Lay C, Seksik P, Tannock GW. Analysis of bacterial bowel communities of IBD patients: what has it revealed? *Inflamm Bowel Dis* (2008) **14**(6):858–67. doi:10.1002/ibd.20392
69. Eeckhaut V, Machiels K, Perrier C, Romero C, Maes S, Flahou B, et al. *Butyricicoccus pullicaecorum* in inflammatory bowel disease. *Gut* (2013) **62**(12):1745–52. doi:10.1136/gutjnl-2012-303611
70. Hossain MM, Begum M, Kim IH. Effect of *Bacillus subtilis*, *Clostridium butyricum* and *Lactobacillus acidophilus* endospores on growth performance, nutrient digestibility, meat quality, relative organ weight, microbial shedding and excreta noxious gas emission in broilers. *Vet Med* (2015) **60**(2):77–86. doi:10.17221/7981-VETMED
71. Yang CM, Cao GT, Ferket PR, Liu TT, Zhou L, Zhang L, et al. Effects of probiotic, *Clostridium butyricum*, on growth performance, immune function, and cecal microflora in broiler chickens. *Poult Sci* (2012) **91**(9):2121–9. doi:10.3382/ps.2011-02131
72. Van Immerseel F, Ducatelle R, De Vos M, Boon N, Van De Wiele T, Verbeke K, et al. Butyric acid-producing anaerobic bacteria as a novel probiotic treatment approach for inflammatory bowel disease. *J Med Microbiol* (2010) **59**(2):141–3. doi:10.1099/jmm.0.017541-0
73. Applegate TJ, Klose V, Steiner T, Ganner A, Schatzmayr G. Probiotics and phytogenics for poultry: myth or reality? *J Appl Poult Res* (2010) **19**(2):194–210. doi:10.3382/japr.2010-00168
74. Veiga P, Gallini CA, Beal C, Michaud M, Delaney ML, DuBois A, et al. *Bifidobacterium animalis* subsp. lactis fermented milk product reduces inflammation by altering a niche for colitogenic microbes. *Proc Natl Acad Sci U S A* (2010) **107**(42):18132–7. doi:10.1073/pnas.1011737107
75. Meimandipour A, Shuhaimi M, Hair-Bejo M, Azhar K, Kabeir BM, Rasti B, et al. In vitro fermentation of broiler cecal content: the role of *Lactobacilli* and pH value on the composition of microbiota and end products fermentation. *Lett Appl Microbiol* (2009) **49**(4):415–20. doi:10.1111/j.1472-765X.2009.02674.x
76. Gibson GR, Probert HM, Loo JV, Rastall RA, Roberfroid MB. Dietary modulation of the human colonic microbiota: updating the concept of prebiotics. *Nutr Res Rev* (2004) **17**(2):259–75. doi:10.1079/NRR200479
77. Kim YJ, Park WY, Choi IH. Effects of dietary alpha-tocopherol, selenium, and their different combinations on growth performance and meat quality of broiler chickens. *Poult Sci* (2010) **89**(3):603–8. doi:10.3382/ps.2009-00280
78. De Maesschalck C, Eeckhaut V, Maertens L, De Lange L, Marchal L, Nezer C, et al. Effects of xylo-oligosaccharides on broiler chicken performance and microbiota. *Appl Environ Microbiol* (2015) **81**(17):5880–8. doi:10.1128/AEM.01616-15

79. Ducatelle R, Eeckhaut V, Haesebrouck F, Van Immerseel F. A review on prebiotics and probiotics for the control of dysbiosis: present status and future perspectives. *Animal* (2015) **9**(1):43–8. doi:10.1017/S1751731114002584
80. Slavin J. Fiber and prebiotics: mechanisms and health benefits. *Nutrients* (2013) **5**(4):1417–35. doi:10.3390/nu5041417
81. Xu ZR, Hu CH, Xia MS, Zhan XA, Wang MQ. Effects of dietary fructooligosaccharide on digestive enzyme activities, intestinal microflora and morphology of male broilers. *Poult Sci* (2003) **82**(6):1030–6. doi:10.1093/ps/82.6.1030
82. Rebole A, Ortiz LT, Rodriguez ML, Alzueta C, Trevino J, Velasco S. Effects of inulin and enzyme complex, individually or in combination, on growth performance, intestinal microflora, cecal fermentation characteristics, and jejunal histomorphology in broiler chickens fed a wheat- and barley-based diet. *Poult Sci* (2010) **89**(2):276–86. doi:10.3382/ps.2009-00336
83. Nabizadeh A. The effect of inulin on broiler chicken intestinal microflora, gut morphology, and performance. *J Anim Feed Sci* (2012) **21**(4):725–34.
84. Courtin CM, Swennen K, Broekaert WF, Swennen Q, Buyse J, Decuypere E, et al. Effects of dietary inclusion of xylooligosaccharides, arabinoxylooligoscaccharides and soluble arabinoxylan on the microbial composition of caecal contents of chickens. *J Sci Food Agric* (2008) **88**(14):2517–22. doi:10.1002/jsfa.3373
85. YaC TC. Effect of adding chicory fructans in feed and fecal and intestinal microflora and excreta volatile ammonia. *Int J Poult Sci* (2003) **2**:188–94. doi:10.3923/ijps.2003.188.194
86. Cao BH, Karasawa Y, Guo YM. Effect of green tea polyphenols and fructo-oligosaccharides in semi-purified diets on broilers' performance and caecal microflora and their metabolites. *AsianAustralas J Anim Sci* (2005) **18**:85–9. doi:10.5713/ajas.2005.85
87. Fukata T, Sasai K, Miyamoto T, Baba E. Inhibitory effects of competitive exclusion and fructooligosaccharide, singly and in combination, on *Salmonella* colonization of chicks. *J Food Prot* (1999) **62**(3):229–33.
88. Rehman H, Hellweg P, Taras D, Zentek J. Effects of dietary inulin on the intestinal short chain fatty acids and microbial ecology in broiler chickens as revealed by denaturing gradient gel electrophoresis. *Poult Sci* (2008) **87**(4):783–9. doi:10.3382/ps.2007-00271
89. Lagier JC, Million M, Hugon P, Armougom F, Raoult D. Human gut microbiota: repertoire and variations. *Front Cell Infect Microbiol* (2012) **2**:136. doi:10.3389/fcimb.2012.00136

Conflict of Interest Statement: The authors declare that the research was conducted in the absence of any commercial or financial relationships that could be construed as a potential conflict of interest.

14

Long-Term Dynamics of *Coxiella burnetii* in Farmed Red Deer (*Cervus elaphus*)

*David González-Barrio[1], Isabel G. Fernández-de-Mera[1], José Antonio Ortiz[2], João Queirós[1,3,4] and Francisco Ruiz-Fons[1]**

[1] Health and Biotechnology (SaBio) Group, Spanish Wildlife Research Institute IREC (CSIC, Universidad de Castilla–La Mancha, Junta de Comunidades de Castilla–La Mancha), Ciudad Real, Spain, [2] Medianilla S. A., Benalup-Casas Viejas, Spain, [3] Centro de Investigacão em Biodiversidade e Recursos Genéticos (CIBIO), InBio Laboratório Associado, Universidade do Porto, Vairão, Portugal, [4] Departamento de Biologia, Faculdade de Ciências da Universidade do Porto, Porto, Portugal

Edited by:
Carl James Yeoman, Montana State University, USA

Reviewed by:
Eric Altermann, AgResearch Ltd, New Zealand
Stacey Gilk, Indiana University School of Medicine, USA

***Correspondence:**
Francisco Ruiz-Fons
josefrancisco.ruiz@uclm.es

Several aspects of the dynamics of *Coxiella burnetii* that are relevant for the implementation of control strategies in ruminant herds with endemic Q fever are unknown. We designed a longitudinal study to monitor the dynamics of exposure to *C. burnetii* in a red deer herd with endemic infection in order to allow the design of Q fever-specific control approaches. Other relevant aspects of the dynamics of *C. burnetii* – the effect of herd immune status, age, season, and early infection on exposure, the average half-life of antibodies, the presence and duration of maternal humoral immunity, and the age of first exposure – were analyzed. The dynamics of *C. burnetii* in deer herds seems to be modulated by host herd and host individual factors and by particular host life-history traits. Red deer females become exposed to *C. burnetii* at the beginning of their second year since maternal antibodies protect them after birth and during the main pathogen shedding season – at the end of spring-early summer. Infection pressure varies between years, probably associated with herd immunity effects, determining inter-annual variation in the risk of exposure. These results suggest that any strategy applied to control *C. burnetii* in deer herds should be designed to induce immunity in their first year of life immediately after losing maternal antibodies. The short average life of *C. burnetii* antibodies suggests that any protection based on humoral immunity would require re-vaccination every 6 months.

Keywords: control, epidemiology, Q fever, wildlife, zoonosis

INTRODUCTION

Coxiella burnetii is a worldwide-distributed Gram-negative intracellular bacterium that causes Q fever, a zoonotic disease shared by humans and animals. Infection with *C. burnetii* in humans is usually asymptomatic but it may trigger acute and chronic clinical manifestations. *C. burnetii* is also one of main pathogens causing reproductive losses in livestock (1) and reproductive failure in pets (2, 3) and wildlife (4–7). Clinical signs of Q fever in domestic ruminants are diverse; it has been associated with sporadic cases of abortion, premature delivery, stillbirth, and weak offspring in cattle, sheep, and goats, but epidemics with increased reproductive failure have been reported for sheep and goats mainly (8). Since *C. burnetii* infection does not always manifest clinically, the extent of *C. burnetii* infection in animals is probably underestimated.

Exposure to *C. burnetii* is increasingly reported in wildlife, e.g., (i) white-tailed deer – *Odocoileus virginianus* – in the eastern US (9); (ii) rats – *Rattus norvegicus* and *Rattus rattus* – in the UK (10) and the Netherlands (11); or (iii) European rabbits – *Oryctolagus cuniculus* – and Eurasian wild boar – *Sus scrofa* – in the Iberian Peninsula (12–14). Recently, González-Barrio et al. (15) found that *C. burnetii* circulates endemically in Iberian red deer populations. This study suggests that the red deer plays an important role in the maintenance of *C. burnetii* in Europe. Thus, the analysis of the dynamics of *C. burnetii* in red deer may be of interest to prevent Q fever transmission at the wildlife–livestock–human interface (16). Furthermore, the presence of *C. burnetii* in red deer may have implications for red deer itself and coexisting wild species (4, 7, 17, 18). Q fever may be an important cause of reproductive losses in red deer farming (7), an activity that is increasing worldwide (19). Therefore, deer producers could be interested in implementing Q fever prevention and control measures that would benefit from knowledge of the effect of deer farming particularities on *C. burnetii* dynamics.

Information on the dynamics of *C. burnetii* in endemic ruminant herds and on driving factors (host population, host individual, and environmental) is scarce. A trade-off between infection pressure and herd immunity may influence infection dynamics in *C. burnetii* endemic herds, which may modulate the efficiency of vaccination trials. Recently, it has been postulated that in endemic dairy cattle herds the immune status of the population drives exposure to *C. burnetii* (20). According to this postulate, high levels of protection in an endemic herd may lead to a reduction in environmental contamination with *C. burnetii*, therefore reducing transmission. However, as long as the immune status of the herd changes with time (i.e., herd immunity decreases due to culling of immune individuals) while *C. burnetii* persists in latently infected animals or in infected fomites (21), the circulation of *C. burnetii* reactivates and expands within the population. Currently, no long time series study has demonstrated that the immune status of a *C. burnetii* endemic ruminant population changes with time to support this postulate. Information from long time series would provide a significant boost to understand the epidemiology of Q fever and plan any prevention and/or control approach.

Apart from host population factors, host individual factors (e.g., age, maternal-derived immunity or acquired immunity, among others) may modulate the dynamics of *C. burnetii* (14). Currently, the presence, prevalence, and duration of maternal anti-*C. burnetii* antibodies and their effect in the outcome of natural exposure to *C. burnetii* are poorly understood. If vaccination of animals at early ages (before natural infection by *C. burnetii* takes place) is to be performed (22), knowledge on the exact timing for vaccination – i.e., the time at which maternal antibodies disappear and prior to exposure to *C. burnetii* – could be paramount to warrant protection. In dairy cattle, the transmission of colostral antibodies to calves borne from seropositive cows has been reported (23) but the duration of these antibodies was not monitored. Could early exposure to *C. burnetii* of individuals in endemic herds modulate infection with the individual's age? The effect of early exposure to *C. burnetii* on future protection against infection is also poorly known. In natural infections in domestic ruminant females, a non-immune animal is supposed to become infected and undergo a primary subclinical infection at early ages (24) that reactivates during the first pregnancy. Understanding the effect of natural early exposure to *C. burnetii* on future exposure would perhaps allow predicting the effect of vaccination at early ages on protection against *C. burnetii* infection. The likelihood of becoming infected by *C. burnetii* increases with age (25). Indeed, age-related *C. burnetii* serological patterns have been reported in domestic ruminants (26, 27) with highest seroprevalence in cows and sheep aged 3–5 years. Is this pattern similar in farmed red deer?

In this study, we aimed to answer different questions that are relevant to understand *C. burnetii* dynamics in endemic ruminant herds in the long time scale and that are, therefore, essential for the efficient planning and application of any Q fever control measure, such as vaccination. The following objectives were addressed in the study: (1) analysis of long-time variation in exposure to *C. burnetii*; (2) determination of the effect of herd immune status on the risk of exposure to *C. burnetii* of yearling females; (3) test of the effect of deer age on exposure and humoral response to *C. burnetii*; (4) study of the effect of deer life-history traits (i.e., concentrated calving) on exposure to *C. burnetii*; (5) investigation of the effect of natural exposure to *C. burnetii* at early ages over the future dynamics of exposure; (6) determination of the average half-life of antibodies against *C. burnetii*; (7) estimation of the presence, prevalence, and duration of maternal antibodies; and (8) determination of the age at which deer get exposed to *C. burnetii* for the first time in their life. To achieve our objectives, a *C. burnetii* endemic red deer herd was selected as model. Therefore, the present study provides a case report on the dynamics of *C. burnetii* in a red deer farm with a history of *C. burnetii* infection in humans and reproductive failure in deer.

MATERIALS AND METHODS

Study Farm and Management Schemes

The study was performed in a semi-extensive red deer farm located in the province of Cádiz (Southern Spain) that was found consistently positive to *C. burnetii* in consecutive studies (7, 28). The number of deer on the farm was approximately 500 females and 80 males along the study period, with only slight inter-annual variations in the number of reared animals. The deer are semi-extensively bred within large (6–8 has) enclosures separated by high-wire fencing in batches of approximately 60–80 females; males are kept in separate enclosures. The habitat in the deer enclosures consists on patches of natural Mediterranean scrubland – mainly composed by evergreen (*Quercus ilex*) and cork (*Quercus suber*) oak trees – with large areas of year-round irrigated prairies. Animals are bred in separate but contiguous batches according to sex and breeding status. Artificial feed is provided daily on the farm.

The deer are managed from two to four times per year at maximum to avoid excessive stress. Management is carried out for sanitary issues, weaning, reposition, and artificial insemination. Hinds give birth naturally – i.e., without human intervention – in hidden areas of scrubland patches within enclosures from the end of April to the beginning of May. Calves are weaned in August at 3.5 months of age and thereafter they are kept in male and female batches in separate enclosures. Ear tagging is performed at weaning for identification of individuals. Calves are managed again at 7 months of age for sanitary reasons. When animals are 13 months old, a selection of yearling females and males for farm reposition is performed and the rest of yearlings are sold. Reposition yearling females are inseminated at the age of 16 months when they join other hinds in existing batches of reproductive females. Selected yearling males are kept separate from stags in reproductive condition. Adult deer, both males and females, are managed for sanitary control in January and in August each year. Reproductive females (>16 months old) are annually managed for artificial insemination in September.

Reproductive hinds in the study farm are culled annually according to their reproductive fitness or health status. Average productive life of deer females in the farm is unknown; some hinds remain productive for 13–15 years but most are culled at 4–5 years of life.

Management schemes in the farm are scheduled to carry out batch, reproductive, and sanitary management issues without inducing excessive stress in the deer that, although farm-bred, still behave like wild animals. Therefore, animal sampling could only be performed according to the management schedule of the farm except for the monitoring of antibodies in the 2013 cohort (see details in the following section).

Survey Design

We designed a retrospective survey to search for the presence and the level of antibodies against *C. burnetii* in deer sera collected in the study farm for disease surveillance purposes. The retrospective survey was aimed at testing for variation in herd seroprevalence over time (Objective 1), the effect of herd immune status on the risk of exposure of yearling females (Objective 2), age-related variation in immune status of individual deer (Objective 3), seasonal variation in infection risk (Objective 4), influence of exposure at early ages on future exposure to *C. burnetii* (Objective 5) and the average half-life of *C. burnetii* antibodies (Objective 6). Blood samples were collected according to farm disease surveillance schemes and in the framework of Spanish and EU laws for notifiable disease surveillance. Therefore, no Animal Ethics Committee approval was required for the collection of blood samples from deer for the retrospective study.

To determine the inter-annual variation in exposure to *C. burnetii*, we carried out a selection of deer sera (yearling, 12–24 months old, and adult, >24 month-old females; $n = 1021$) collected in the farm along 12 consecutive years (2003–2014). Minimum annual sample size was estimated with WinEpi (http://winepi.net/sp/index.htm). The estimated sample size for each age-class – yearling and adult – with a 95% confidence level for a minimum seroprevalence of 5% with an accepted 10% error was 19; this minimum sample size was covered each year for each deer age-class. Selection of sera was carried out according to batch origin to obtain a balanced subset of samples that provides representative information of the real status of *C. burnetii* prevalence in the herd. For homogeneity of results, only sera collected in summer were selected to estimate inter-annual variation in the humoral immune status of deer in the farm.

To test for the rest of aforementioned objectives (2–6), we selected sera from reposition females belonging to three different cohorts – animals born in 2008, 2009, and 2010. Blood was collected from these females at least in four consecutive occasions (i.e., from 7 to 27 months old) and up to 13 consecutive occasions (i.e., from 7 to 78 months old). Deer were surveyed in summer and winter each year. Serum samples were obtained for the 2008 cohort at 7, 13, 20, 27, 32, 38, 44, 51, 56, 62, 67, 73, and 78 months of life. The same survey was carried out for the 2009 cohort but up to 67 months of life and the 2010 cohort could be surveyed up to the 56th month of life. Minimum sampling size at each survey time was estimated with WinEpi employing the same parameters described above. Although culling with age reduced the number of available samples with individuals' age, sampling size was above 19 for each month class except for individuals at 73 and 78 months of age ($n = 13$ in both cases).

Finally, to test for the presence, prevalence, and duration of maternal antibodies (Objective 7) and for the age at which deer get exposed to *C. burnetii* for their first time in life (Objective 8), serum samples from 21 calves born in 2013 were prospectively collected at 2, 3, 7, 13, 14, 19, and 20 months of life. This subset of the 2013 cohort was specifically surveyed to achieve these objectives since blood from calves in the farm is normally first collected at 7 months of age. The Research Ethics Commission of Castilla - La Mancha University Animal Ethics Committee (Spain) approved this research.

Since we initiated an experimental vaccination trial in the study herd in January 2012 with a *C. burnetii* phase I inactivated vaccine, animals that were included in this study for 2012, 2013, and 2014 were exclusively unvaccinated animals of the control group. The interpretation of the evolution of the immune status of the herd will be carried out in this study considering this potential confounding factor for 2012–2014 results.

Serological Analyses

Serology has been widely employed to test for the status of *C. burnetii* in ruminant populations (25, 28) and to understand its dynamics even though a proportion of infected individuals may not seroconvert (29). In a vaccination trial in the study, deer farm (the authors, unpublished) near the 90% of vaccinated seronegative deer seroconverted after a single dose of a *C. burnetii* inactivated phase I vaccine. This percentage was close to the 100% after a boosting dose 3 weeks later. Therefore, in contrast to domestic ruminants (e.g., sheep, 22), it is expected that a high percentage of infected red deer display detectable levels of anti-*C. burnetii* antibodies in ELISA. Therefore, ELISA was employed to study the dynamics of infection by *C. burnetii*.

Blood was collected from the jugular vein into sterile tubes and it was thereafter kept at 4°C and transported to the laboratory. Blood was centrifuged at 3,000 × *g* for 10 min and the serum obtained was preserved at −20°C until analyses were performed. The presence of specific antibodies against *C. burnetii* phase I and II antigens in deer sera was determined with a commercial indirect

ELISA test (LSIVet™ Ruminant Q Fever Serum/Milk ELISA Kit, Life Technologies, Carlsbad, CA, USA) with an in-house modification in the secondary antibody (Protein G–Horseradish peroxidase, Sigma-Aldrich, St. Louis, MO, USA) that had been validated for wild ungulates (15). ELISA results were expressed as the sample-to-positive control ratio (SP). For each sample, the SP was calculated according to the formula:

$$SP = \frac{(ODs - ODnc)}{(ODpc - ODnc)} \times 100$$

where "ODs" is the optical density of the sample at a dual wavelength 450–620 nm, "ODnc" is the optical density of the negative control, and "ODpc" is the optical density of the positive control. All SP values ≤40 were considered as negative, whereas SP values >40 were considered as positive. The SP ratio was considered as a proxy of the level of antibodies against *C. burnetii* as suggested by the manufacturer.

Statistical Analyses

Statistical analyses were carried out to test different hypotheses: (i) the immune status of the herd is negatively related to the incidence of infection by *C. burnetiii* in yearling females (Objective 2); (ii) the age of individuals is positively related to seroprevalence and antibody levels (Objective 3); (iii) there are seasonal variations in the rate of exposure to *C. burnetii* (Objective 4); and (iv) variations in the immune status at early ages modulates future exposure to *C. burnetii* (Objective 5).

To assess for the effect of herd immune status on the incidence of *C. burnetii* in yearling females, we performed Spearman correlations with the annual incidence (presence/absence of *C. burnetii* antibodies) in yearlings as response variable and three different explanatory variables that were tested separately: (i) seroprevalence in adult females in the same year (t); (ii) seroprevalence in adult females in the previous year (t−1); and (iii) average seroprevalence in adult females in years t, t−1, and t−2 (2 years before). Seroprevalence in adult females was employed as a proxy of herd seroprevalence because adult females constitute around the 75% of the herd. Spearman correlations were also employed to test the relationship between antibody levels and individuals' age.

Mann–Whitney *U* non-parametric tests for independent samples were employed to test for the alternative hypothesis of statistically significant differences in average antibody levels by season. Chi-square tests were employed for the same purpose with seroprevalence as response variable.

Finally, the influence of the immune status of individuals at early ages (7 months old; presence/absence of *C. burnetii* antibodies) on the evolution of the humoral immune response against *C. burnetii* infection along individual's age was tested by repeated measures ANOVA. Individual squared SP values were transformed into natural logarithms for normality and were employed as response variable. For this analysis, we used data obtained from the 2008, 2009, and 2010 deer cohorts.

IBM SPPS v22.0 (IBM, Armonk, NY, USA) was employed for statistical analyses. Exact Clopper–Pearson 95% confidence intervals (95%CI) were estimated for prevalence values using Quantitative Parasitology 3.0 software (http://www.zoologia.hu/qp/qp.html).

RESULTS

A total of 373 (inter-annual sampling size range: 19–92) and 648 (inter-annual sampling size range: 19–159) serum samples collected in summer from yearling and adult females, respectively, were selected for the cross sectional approach during 2003–2014. The inter-annual evolution of herd (yearling + adult) and age-class-specific seroprevalence from 2003 to 2014 is shown in **Figure 1**.

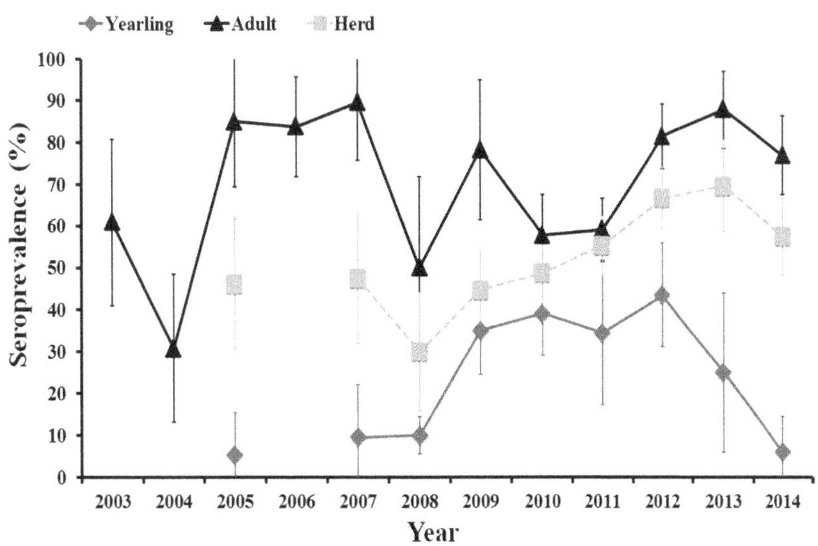

FIGURE 1 | Evolution of herd (yearling + adult) average and age-class-specific (yearling, 12–24 months old, and adult, >24 months old) seroprevalence (and associated 95% exact confidence intervals) from 2003 to 2014.

Average annual herd and age-specific seroprevalence values varied between years. There was no clear time scale pattern in inter-annual herd seroprevalence that remained above 30% and below 70% along the study period. Seroprevalence in adult females fluctuated between years with periods of 1–3 consecutive years of high values (above 70%) followed by periods of 1–2 consecutive years of medium values (from 30 to 60%). The high seroprevalence in unvaccinated females in 2012, 2013, and 2014, even though >70% of the herd had been vaccinated (the authors, unpublished), indicate a natural period of high herd humoral immunity similar to that observed in 2005–2007. A unimodal pattern was observed in yearlings. The observed age-related pattern of humoral immunity in individual deer shows that we can assimilate annual seroprevalence in yearlings to annual incidence ratio. Incidence in yearlings was low (5–10%) from 2005 to 2008 (although samples were not analyzed in 2006), it increased (35–43%) from 2008 to 2012, and it steeply decreased (25% in 2013 and 6% in 2014) from 2012 onward.

Incidence in yearlings remained low during the periods in which high seroprevalence was observed in adult females and increased during a period in which the seroprevalence in adult females was lower than in preceding years. Incidence was nonetheless not statistically influenced by seroprevalence in adult females at times t (survey year) and t−1 (previous year to survey), and by average seroprevalence in adult females in years t to t−2. However, trends in all three relationships were negative, that is increasing incidence in yearlings related to decreasing seroprevalence in adults in the same or in previous years.

One thousand four hundred and forty-five sera from 217 animals born in 2008 ($n = 97$), 2009 ($n = 92$), and 2010 ($n = 28$) were sequentially analyzed from 7 (calf) up to 78 (adult) months of life to estimate the evolution of antibodies against *C. burnetii* with age. Not every animal could be surveyed sequentially along the study period because of annual culling for health or productive reasons. On average, both seroprevalence and the level of antibodies in individual deer increased with age and this pattern was evidenced in animals from the three cohorts (**Figure 2**). Age (in months) and the level of antibodies were statistically significantly correlated (rho = 0.416, $p < 0.001$). This result confirms increasing levels of antibodies with deer age, but highest antibody levels were observed between 4 and 5 years of life.

The monitoring of individual deer sera by ELISA showed an evident seasonal pattern in antibody levels and seroprevalence. Both the level of antibodies and seroprevalence peaked in summer each year and decreased through winter (**Figure 2**). Seasonal differences were statistically significant: (i) Average SP in summer was 73.3 ± 2.5 in contrast to 37.8 ± 1.4 in winter ($Z = -12.89$, df = 1, $p < 0.001$) and (ii) 67.3% (95%CI: 62.8–71.7) of animals surveyed in summer had antibodies in contrast to 36.0% (95%CI: 32.6–39.5) in winter ($\chi^2 = 110.93$, df = 1, $p < 0.001$). This pattern was evident for any of the three cohorts surveyed (**Figure 2**).

Results from the repeated measures ANOVA showed that differences in the evolution of the level of antibodies in relation to the presence/absence of *C. burnetii* antibodies at 7 months of age were not statistically significant (**Figure 3**). Around the 82% of individuals in the 2008–2010 cohorts were seronegative at 7 months of age.

The evolution of the presence and level of antibodies in calves born in 2013 from 2–20 months of life are shown in **Figure 4**. High levels of antibodies were evidenced in calves at 2 months (June 2013), when 75% of them displayed an SP ratio > 40 (i.e., seropositive). Thereafter, both the level of antibodies and seroprevalence decreased sharply in 1 month (July 2013) and disappeared at 7 months (November 2013). Animals remained seronegative at 13 months of age (May 2014) and then became seropositive at 14 months (June 2014), 2 months after the calving season in the farm. This seroconversion was most probably caused by natural infection and affected 50% of the animals. The average level of antibodies derived from natural infection at 14 months was lower than that acquired from their mothers during lactation (at 2 months); in seropositive animals average SP ratio was 122.4 at 2 months ($n = 15$) in comparison to 77.8 in seropositive animals at 14 months of life ($n = 7$). Both seroprevalence and antibody level remained at similar values at 19 months (November 2014) but decreased thereafter notably a month later (December 2014). This observation and the seasonal pattern observed indicate that the expected average life of antibodies against *C. burnetii* could be around 6 months. These results show that deer become exposed to *C. burnetii* for the first time in life mainly at around 12–14 months of age.

DISCUSSION

Understanding the factors that drive the dynamics of endemic pathogens is paramount to design and efficiently apply any preventive or control measure. Vaccination with phase I inactivated *C. burnetii* vaccines – one of the main Q fever control tools in domestic ruminants (30) – is recommended for naïve or low-prevalence herds (31) but not for endemic herds (22, 32). However, the status of *C. burnetii* in an endemic host population may present inter-annual variation (20) with years in which the percentage of naïve individuals in the population is high, followed by years in which this percentage is low. Identification of time windows with high percentage of naïve individuals in a *C. burnetii* endemic population would allow the implementation of vaccination trials. During these time windows, the percentage of susceptible individuals that could be protected by vaccination would be enhanced. Determining the factors that modulate the dynamics of *C. burnetii* in endemic populations would allow predicting the occurrence of appropriate windows to implement vaccination. This study improves our understanding of the dynamics of *C. burnetii* in endemic ruminant herds and driving factors that could allow more efficient control approaches in the future.

Risks of Infection by *C. burnetii* Associated to Red Deer

Red deer may be a relevant reservoir of *C. burnetii* in Europe because of its increasing relevance as a game resource, its current demographic status and the status of *C. burnetii* in red deer populations. Deer farming is increasing (19) and likewise populations of free-roaming red deer currently display increasing demographic trends (33). Additionally, free-roaming deer populations are increasingly managed as extensively bred

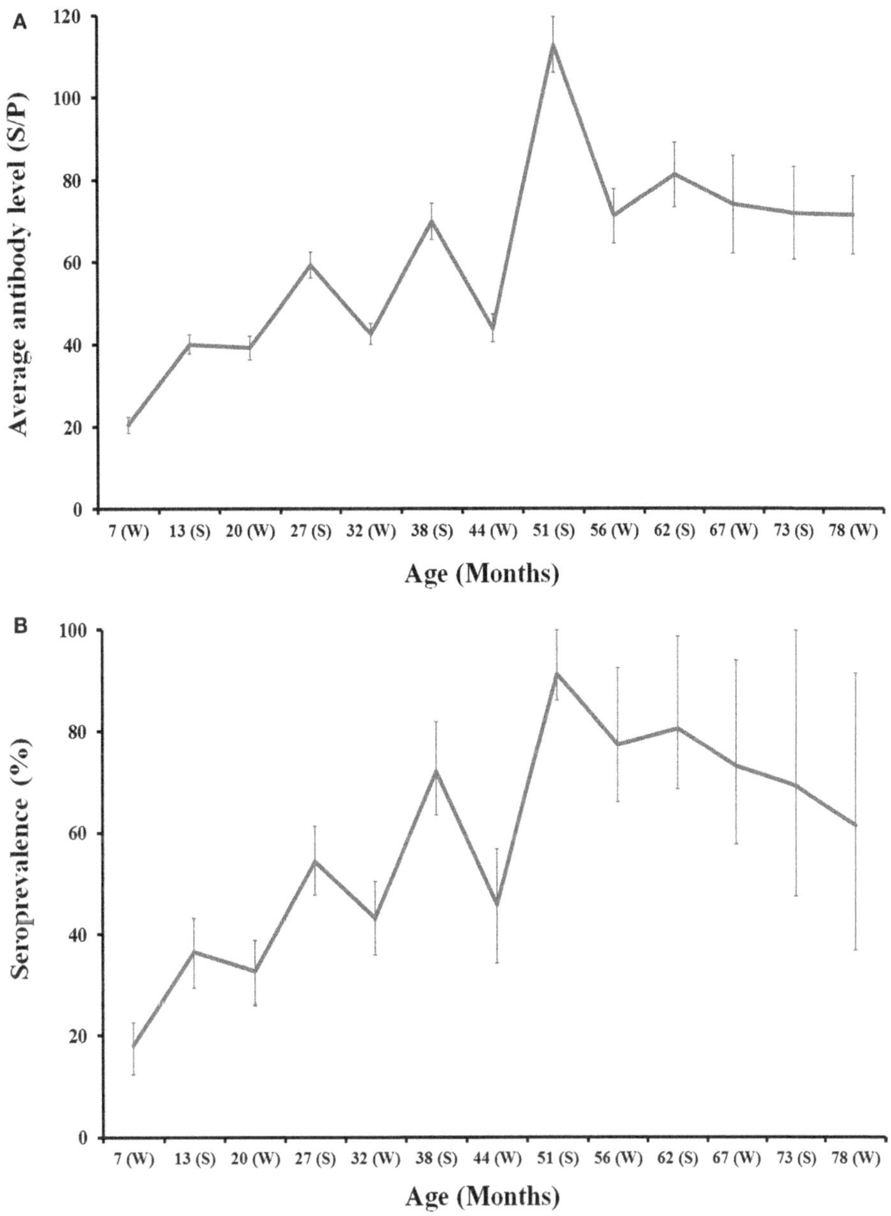

FIGURE 2 | Age-related evolution of *C. burnetii* level of antibodies (A) and seroprevalence (B) for 2008, 2009, and 2010 deer cohorts together. Season is depicted in the *x*-axis of each chart (W: Winter; S: Summer). Exact 95% confidence intervals for seroprevalence and SE for average antibody levels are displayed in the charts.

ruminants (supplementary feeding, fencing, translocations) but lacking appropriate sanitary control (34). Changes in livestock production schemes in the Netherlands – increasing number of goat herds without *C. burnetii* control – led to the 2007–2010 epidemics of human Q fever (35), demonstrating how important demographic changes of a single host may be to increase the risk of infection by *C. burnetii*. Interestingly, farmed and free-roaming Iberian red deer populations display similar population and individual seroprevalence values to livestock (15, 24). Furthermore, increasing geographic distribution and population density of red deer in Europe may increase the implication of this wild species in future Q fever epidemics. Prevention would only be possible if accurate scientific knowledge is available. Our study provides insights into poorly studied epidemiological aspects of the dynamics of *C. burnetii* in red deer populations.

Long-Term Dynamics of *C. burnetii* in Farmed Red Deer

There is a main question to answer in relation to the dynamics of *C. burnetii*: Does the status of *C. burnetii* change with time in an endemic ruminant herd? Our results for 12 consecutive

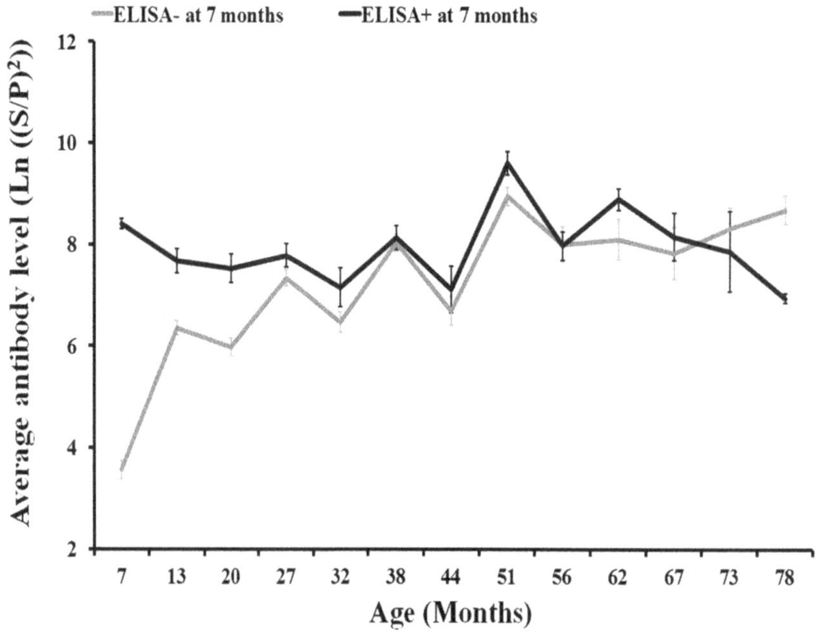

FIGURE 3 | Evolution of antibody levels (and associated SE) with individuals' age according to the presence/absence of anti-*C. burnetii* antibodies by ELISA (SP > 40) at 7 months of age for 2008, 2009, and 2010 deer cohorts together.

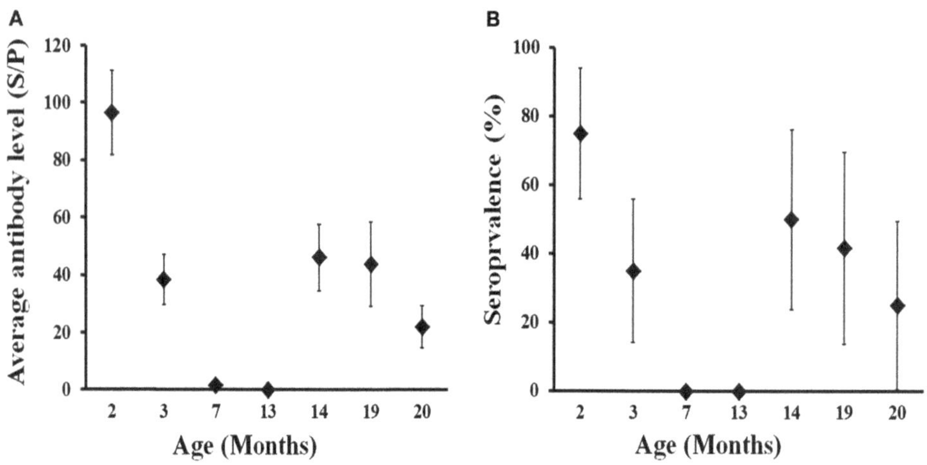

FIGURE 4 | Age-related evolution of *C. burnetii* level of specific antibodies (A) and seroprevalence (B) in farmed red deer (2013 cohort). Exact 95% confidence intervals for seroprevalence and SE for average antibody levels are displayed in the charts.

years show fluctuation in the status of *C. burnetii* prevalence in a ruminant herd in which the pathogen circulates endemically. Piñero et al. (20) also provided evidence of inter-annual variation in endemic dairy cattle herds but within a shorter time period.

Inter-annual variation of the status of an endemic pathogen in a herd could be the consequence of the trade-off between pathogen burden and host immunity if we assume that there are no changes in the composition of the herd – e.g. size, culling and import rates, age, and sex structures – and the influence of external pathogen sources remains constant (14, 20). Those features remained constant along the study period in the deer farm. Even the potential influence of other sources of *C. burnetii* such as European rabbits – *O. cuniculus* – remained similar along the study period, with *C. burnetii* seroprevalence from 2005 to 2013 above 50% (13). Therefore, herd immunity effects seem to be the most probable cause of changes in the epidemiological status of *C. burnetii* in the herd. However, in spite of the observed negative trend in the relationship between incidence in yearling females - probably associated with infection pressure - and seroprevalence in adult females, relationships were not statistically significant. Increasing incidence in yearling females from 2009 to 2012 coincided with a period of lower seroprevalence values in adult females in comparison to 2005–2007. By contrast, there was a steep decrease in incidence in yearlings from 2012 to 2014 when seroprevalence in adult (non-vaccinated) females was again high. This observation could potentially be linked to herd vaccination against *C. burnetii* (the authors, unpublished data) or alternatively be the consequence of a natural period of high humoral immunity in the herd; but in any case, it indicates variation in infection pressure. Interestingly, an outstanding rate of reproductive failure in the herd in 2011 - that was presumably caused by Q fever (7) - coincided with the increasing incidence observed in yearlings in 2009–2012.

It was unfortunately impossible to monitor the presence and burden of *C. burnetii* in the environment in the farm (aerosols, soil, water, food, pastures) along the study period in order to accurately estimate the evolution of infection pressure with time. However, this has been carried out in dairy cattle and changes in the epidemiological status of *C. burnetii* in dairy cattle herds are linked to the detection of *C. burnetii* in manure, air, and dust samples (20). According to Piñero et al. (20) high herd humoral immunity levels would reduce shedding of large burdens of *C. burnetii* to the environment, therefore, reducing infection pressure. This would result in a reduced incidence in naïve (yearling) individuals in the herd. Another observation that may support variation in infection pressure with time is that 30.9% (30/97) and 9.9% (9/91) of deer calves born in 2008 and 2009, respectively, were seropositive to *C. burnetii* at 7 months of age (naturally infected in their first year of life) in contrast to 0% (0/21) in 2013. This pattern paralleled observations in incidence in yearling females. These changes could be linked to the implementation of vaccination in the herd from 2012 onward since vaccinated and unvaccinated deer coexist in existing enclosures in the farm.

Short-Term Herd Effects on the Dynamics of *C. burnetii* in Red Deer

Intra-annual variation in exposure to *C. burnetii* has been previously suggested in wildlife studies (36). Ruminant females shed *C. burnetii* mainly around parturition and, therefore, in species with a defined breeding season shedding should be concentrated. In contrast to dairy cattle, which breed along the year, the breeding season of the red deer is concentrated at the end of spring (37). This fact implies that, within a year, there is a predominant shedding season during which the risk of exposure of individuals is higher. The short half-life of *C. burnetii* antibodies allowed differentiating that the risk of exposure in winter is much lower than by the end of spring-early summer, which is consistent with a predominant shedding season in deer than coincides with the breeding season. This particularity of the epidemiology of *C. burnetii* in farmed red deer may favor the implementation of control strategies since adequate management measures in liaison with medical treatments can significantly reduce the exposure of individuals around the breeding season.

Host Individual Traits Influencing *C. burnetii* Dynamics in Red Deer

Host individual traits may modulate the relationship that a host establishes with *C. burnetii* and age-related effects have been described frequently (25). In this study, we found a significant increase in seroprevalence and antibody level with the individuals' age. This may be caused by cumulative effects of continuous exposure to *C. burnetii* with time or may be linked to increasing immune competence with the individual's age. Two observations point to an effect of host immune competence as the causal factor for this age-related increase in seroprevalence and antibody levels: (i) the increasing trend in both parameters up to the fourth year of life (similar to findings in cattle, 27) and the decreasing pattern thereafter; and (ii) the low average half-life of anti-*C. burnetii* antibodies observed (discussed below).

Acquired immunity after natural infection by *C. burnetii* at early ages may have a protective effect over the outcome of future infections since reproductive failure caused by Q fever is more evident in primiparous females and decreases with age (22, 32). However, we observed that in calves exposed to *C. burnetii* at 7 months of age the average humoral immune response induced by infections in adulthood did not differ from that observed in non-exposed calves at that age. Whether the effect derived from natural infection is similar to what we would expect from vaccination is difficult to predict, but this finding suggests that acquired immunity at early ages does not prevent re-infection by *C. burnetii* in the future. This could be linked to the short average half-life of *C. burnetii* antibodies observed in deer. Vaccination of deer at early ages with an appropriate re-vaccination calendar would perhaps induce long-lasting protection against infection by *C. burnetii*.

The pattern of antibody levels in the 2013 cohort suggest that deer calves get antibodies from their mothers early in their lives that then disappear before their seventh month of life. Maternal-acquired antibodies have also been reported from cattle calves (23). Dairy cows infected with *C. burnetii* maintain detectable levels of antibodies along the gestation period and even after partum (38) that are transmitted to new-born calves with the colostrum. Whether maternal antibodies protect against infection by *C. burnetii* is unknown. Results from the 2013 cohort suggest that maternal antibodies protect calves in their first year of life - perhaps in association with the concentrated shedding season in late spring, but the presence of antibodies in 7-month-old animals of the 2008/2009 cohorts contradicts that observation. If we assume - on the basis of incidence rates - that infection pressure was higher in 2008/2009 than in 2013 and that a high percentage of calves born every year acquire maternal antibodies, we may hypothesize that under high infection pressure in the herd a percentage of the calves are not protected during their first year of life. Only proper experimental approaches with a controlled challenge would offer information to understand the effect of humoral immunity on protection (39). Nonetheless, our findings suggest that deer calves should be vaccinated for the first time when they are around 5–6 months of life. The exact timing for vaccination should be determined through future experiments with a higher sampling frequency.

An interesting finding that should be born in mind when planning vaccination protocols in deer farms is that any protection linked to humoral immunity would last only around 6 months. Maternal antibodies in the 2013 cohort were high at 2 months of age and completely disappeared 5 months later. This observation and the sharp decrease of antibodies from natural infection from months 14–19 to month 20 suggest an average half-life of anti-*C. burnetii* antibodies of 5–6 months without natural re-infections. Therefore, re-vaccination every 6 months would be recommendable to maintain humoral immunity in deer. The average half-life of antibodies in other species may be higher since antibodies can be detected even a year after infection in humans (40).

CONCLUSION

Red deer are able to maintain *C. burnetii* and transmit it to other wildlife, livestock, pets, and humans. Current knowledge on the status of *C. burnetii* in red deer in Iberia together with results obtained in this study points to this species as a source of Q fever that needs to be considered by animal and public health authorities.

In endemic herds, *C. burnetii* inter-annual dynamics may be modulated by host herd and individual factors that should be considered for planning efficient control approaches. Particular host life-history traits (e.g., concentrated breeding) also have an important effect on the intra-annual variation in the dynamics of *C. burnetii*. Naturally acquired humoral immunity seems to have no effect on future re-infection of deer by *C. burnetii*, perhaps linked to the observed short average half-life of antibodies in red deer.

AUTHOR CONTRIBUTIONS

DG-B and FR-F designed the study and wrote the manuscript; DG-B, IF-M, JO, JQ, and FR-F collected samples; DG-B performed serological analyses; DG-B and FR-F analyzed data; DG-B, IF-M, JO, JQ, and FR-F critically reviewed the manuscript.

ACKNOWLEDGMENTS

We are grateful to people who contributed to sample collection, including farm keepers and members of the SaBio group at IREC (Tania Carta, Joaquín Vicente, Mauricio Durán and Óscar Rodríguez). We thank Dr. Ursula Höfle for reviewing the English grammar and expression of the manuscript.

FUNDING

The research was funded by "Centro para el Desarrollo Tecnológico Industrial" (CDTI) of the Spanish Ministry for the Economy and Competitiveness (MINECO) and by EU-FP7 "Antigone" project. FR-F acknowledges funding by the 'Ramón y Cajal' programme of MINECO. IF-M is funded by the University of Castilla – La Mancha.

REFERENCES

1. Oporto B, Barandika JF, Hurtado A, Aduriz G, Moreno B, Garcia-Perez AL. Incidence of ovine abortion by *Coxiella burnetii* in northern Spain. *Ann N Y Acad Sci* (2006) **1078**:498–501. doi:10.1196/annals.1374.095
2. D'amato F, Million M, Edouard S, Delerce J, Robert C, Marrie T, et al. Draft genome sequence of *Coxiella burnetii* Dog Utad, a strain isolated from a dog-related outbreak of Q fever. *New Microbes New Infect* (2014) **2**:136–7. doi:10.1002/nmi2.55
3. Kosatsky T. Household outbreak of Q-fever pneumonia related to a parturient cat. *Lancet* (1984) **2**:1447–9. doi:10.1016/S0140-6736(84)91633-7
4. Lloyd C, Mark F, Stidworthy MA, Wernery U. *Coxiella burnetii* abortion in captive dama gazelle (*Gazella dama*) in the United Arab Emirates. *J Zoo Wildl Med* (2010) **41**:83–9. doi:10.1638/2009-0005.1
5. Kersh GJ, Lambourn DM, Self JS, Akmajian AM, Stanton JB, Timothy V, et al. *Coxiella burnetii* infection of a steller sea lion (*Eumetopias jubatus*) found in Washington State. *J Clin Microbiol* (2010) **48**:3428–31. doi:10.1128/JCM.00758-10
6. Kreizinger Z, Szeredi L, Bacsadi A, Nemes C, Sugár L, Varga T, et al. Occurrence of *Coxiella burnetii* and Chlamydiales species in abortions of domestic ruminants and in wild ruminants in Hungary, Central Europe. *J Vet Diagn Invest* (2015) **27**:206–10. doi:10.1177/1040638714563566
7. González-Barrio D, Almería S, Caro MR, Salinas J, Ortiz JA, Gortázar C, et al. *Coxiella burnetii* shedding by farmed red deer (*Cervus elaphus*). *Transbound Emerg Dis* (2015) **62**:572–4. doi:10.1111/tbed.12179
8. Agerholm JS. *Coxiella burnetii* associated reproductive disorders in domestic animals-a critical review. *Acta Vet Scand* (2013) **55**:13. doi:10.1186/1751-0147-55-13
9. Kirchgessner MS, Dubovi EJ, Whipps CM. Disease risk surface for *Coxiella burnetii* seroprevalence in white-tailed deer. *Zoonoses Public Health* (2013) **60**:457–60. doi:10.1111/zph.12023
10. Meredith AL, Cleaveland SC, Denwood MJ, Brown JK, Shaw DJ. *Coxiella burnetii* (Q-Fever) seroprevalence in prey and predators in the United Kingdom: evaluation of infection in wild rodents, foxes and domestic cats using a modified ELISA. *Transbound Emerg Dis* (2014) **62**(6):639–49. doi:10.1111/tbed.12211
11. Reusken C, van der Plaats R, Opsteegh M, de Bruin A, Swart A. *Coxiella burnetii* (Q fever) in *Rattus norvegicus* and *Rattus rattus* at livestock farms and urban locations in the Netherlands; could *Rattus* spp. represent reservoirs for (re)introduction? *Prev Vet Med* (2011) **101**:124–30. doi:10.1016/j.prevetmed.2011.05.003
12. Astobiza I, Barral M, Ruiz-Fons F, Barandika JF, Gerrikagoitia X, Hurtado A, et al. Molecular investigation of the occurrence of *Coxiella burnetii* in wildlife and ticks in an endemic area. *Vet Microbiol* (2011) **147**:190–4. doi:10.1016/j.vetmic.2010.05.046
13. González-Barrio D, Maio E, Vieira-Pinto M, Ruiz-Fons F. European rabbits as reservoir for *Coxiella burnetii*. *Emerg Infect Dis* (2015) **21**:1055–8. doi:10.3201/eid2106.141537
14. González-Barrio D, Martín-Hernando MP, Ruiz-Fons F. Shedding patterns of endemic Eurasian wild boar (*Sus scrofa*) pathogens. *Res Vet Sci* (2015) **102**:206–11. doi:10.1016/j.rvsc.2015.08.014
15. González-Barrio D, Velasco Ávila AL, Boadella M, Beltrán-Beck B, Barasona JA, Santos JPV. Host and environmental factors modulate the exposure of free-ranging and farmed red deer (*Cervus elaphus*) to *Coxiella burnetii*. *Appl Environ Microbiol* (2015) **81**:6223–31. doi:10.1128/AEM.01433-15
16. Gortazar C, Reperant LA, Kuiken T, de la Fuente J, Boadella M, Martínez-Lopez B, et al. Crossing the interspecies barrier: opening the door to zoonotic pathogens. *PLoS Pathog* (2014) **10**:e1004129. doi:10.1371/journal.ppat.1004129
17. Chaber AL, Lloyd C, O'Donovan D, McKeown S, Wernery U, Bailey T. A serologic survey for *Coxiella burnetii* in semi-wild ungulates in the Emirate of Dubai, United Arab Emirates. *J Wildl Dis* (2012) **48**:220–2. doi:10.7589/0090-3558-48.1.220
18. Hussein MF, Al-Khalifa IM, Aljumaah RS, Elnabi AG, Mohammed OB, Omer SA, et al. Serological prevalence of *Coxiella burnetii* in captive wild ruminants in Saudi Arabia. *Comp Clin Pathol* (2012) **21**:33–8. doi:10.1007/s00580-010-1061-y
19. Hoffman LC, Wiklund E. Game and venison – meat for de modern consumer. *Meat Sci* (2008) **74**:197–208. doi:10.1016/j.meatsci.2006.04.005

20. Piñero A, Ruiz-Fons F, Hurtado A, Barandika JF, Atxaerandio R, García-Pérez AL. Changes in the dynamics of *Coxiella burnetii* infection in dairy cattle: an approach to match field data with the epidemiological cycle of *C. burnetii* in endemic herds. *J Dairy Sci* (2014) **97**:2718–30. doi:10.3168/jds.2013-7229
21. Maurin M, Raoult D. Q fever. *Clin Microbiol Rev* (1999) **12**:518–53.
22. Astobiza I, Barandika JF, Ruiz-Fons F, Hurtado A, Povedano I, Juste RA, et al. *Coxiella burnetii* shedding and environmental contamination at lambing in two highly naturally-infected dairy sheep flocks after vaccination. *Res Vet Sci* (2011) **91**:e58–63. doi:10.1016/j.rvsc.2010.11.014
23. Tutusaus J, López-Gatius F, Almería S, Serrano B, Monleón E, Badiola J, et al. No detectable precolostral antibody response in calves born from cows with cotyledons positive for *Coxiella burnetii* by quantitative PCR. *Acta Vet Hung* (2013) **61**:4432–41. doi:10.1556/AVet.2013.026
24. Woldehiwet Z. Q fever (coxiellosis): epidemiology and pathogenesis. *Res Vet Sci* (2004) **77**:93–100. doi:10.1016/j.rvsc.2003.09.001
25. Ruiz-Fons F, Astobiza I, Barandika J, Hurtado A, Atxaerandio R, Juste R, et al. Seroepidemiological study of Q fever in domestic ruminants in semi-extensive grazing systems. *BMC Vet Res* (2010) **6**:3. doi:10.1186/1746-6148-6-3
26. Capuano F, Perugini AG, Parisi A, Montagna CO, Nilvelli M. Improved detection of *Coxiella burnetii* in cows milk by immunomagnetic separation and PCR. *Vet Res Commun* (2004) **28**:279–82. doi:10.1023/B:VERC.0000045426.44521.24
27. Guatteo R, Beaudeau F, Joly A, Seegers H. *Coxiella burnetii* shedding by dairy cows. *Vet Res* (2007) **38**:849–60. doi:10.1051/vetres:2007038
28. Ruiz-Fons F, Rodríguez O, Torina A, Naranjo V, Gortázar C, de La Fuente J. Prevalence of *Coxiella burnetti* infection in wild and farmed ungulates. *Vet Microbiol* (2008) **126**:282–6. doi:10.1016/j.vetmic.2007.06.020
29. De Cremoux R, Rousset E, Touratier A, Audusseau G, Nicollet P, Ribaud D. *Coxiella burnetii* vaginal shedding and antibody responses in dairy goat herds in a context of clinical Q fever outbreaks. *FEMS Immunol Med Microbiol* (2012) **64**:120–2. doi:10.1111/j.1574-695X.2011.00893.x
30. Van den Brom R, van Engelen E, Roest HIJ, van der Hoek W, Vellema P. *Coxiella burnetii* infections in sheep or goats: an opinionated review. *Vet Microbiol* (2015) **181**(1–2):119–29. doi:10.1016/j.vetmic.2015.07.011
31. Guatteo R, Seegers H, Joly A, Beaudeau F. Prevention *of Coxiella burnetii* shedding in infected dairy herds using a phase I *C. burnetii* inactivated vaccine. *Vaccine* (2008) **26**:4320–8. doi:10.1016/j.vaccine.2008.06.023
32. Astobiza I, Barandika JF, Ruiz-Fons F, Hurtado A, Povedano I, Juste RA, et al. Four-year evaluation of the effect of vaccination against *Coxiella burnetii* on reduction of animal infection and environmental contamination in a naturally infected dairy sheep flock. *Appl Environ Microbiol* (2011) **77**:7405–7. doi:10.1128/AEM.05530-11
33. Apollonio M, Andersen R, Putman R. *European Ungulates and Their Management in the 21st Century*. Cambrigde: Cambrigde University Press (2010).
34. Gortázar C, Acevedo A, Ruiz-Fons F, Vicente J. Disease risk and overabundance of game species. *Eur J Wildl Res* (2006) **52**:81–7. doi:10.1007/s10344-005-0022-2
35. Roest HIJ, Tilburg JJHC, van der Hoek W, Vellema P, van Zijderveld FG, Klassen CHW, et al. The Q fever epidemic in the Netherlands: history, onset, response and reflection. *Epidemiol Infect* (2011) **139**:1–12. doi:10.1017/S0950268810002268
36. Pioz M, Loison A, Gauthier D, Gibert P, Jullien JM, Artois M. Diseases and reproductive success in a wild mammal: example in the alpine chamois. *Oecologia* (2008) **155**:691–704. doi:10.1007/s00442-007-0942-5
37. Clutton-Brock TH, Guinness FE, Albon SP. *Red Deer: Behaviour and Ecology of Two Sexes*. Chicago, IL: University of Chicago Press (1982).
38. Garcia-Ispierto I, Almería S, López-Gatius F. *Coxiella burnetii* seropositivity is highly stable throughout gestation in lactating high-producing dairy cows. *Reprod Domest Anim* (2011) **46**:1067–72. doi:10.1111/j.1439-0531.2011.01788.x
39. Roest HIJ, Post J, van Gelderen B, van Zijderveld FG, Rebel JMJ. Q fever in pregnant goats: humoral and cellular immune responses. *Vet Res* (2013) **44**:67. doi:10.1186/1297-9716-44-67
40. Angelakis E, Raoult D. Q fever. *Vet Microbiol* (2010) **140**:297–309. doi:10.1016/j.vetmic.2009.07.016

Conflict of Interest Statement: The authors declare that the research was conducted in the absence of any commercial or financial relationships that could be considered as a potential conflict of interest.

15

West Nile Virus Challenge Alters the Transcription Profiles of Innate Immune Genes in Rabbit Peripheral Blood Mononuclear Cells

Muhammad J. Uddin[1], Willy W. Suen[1], Natalie A. Prow[2], Roy A. Hall[3,4] and Helle Bielefeldt-Ohmann[1,3,4]*

[1] School of Veterinary Science, University of Queensland, Gatton, QLD, Australia, [2] QIMR Berghofer Medical Research Institute, Brisbane, QLD, Australia, [3] Australian Infectious Diseases Research Centre, University of Queensland, St Lucia, QLD, Australia, [4] School of Chemistry and Molecular Biosciences, University of Queensland, St Lucia, QLD, Australia

Edited by:
Guillermo Tellez, University of Arkansas, USA

Reviewed by:
Kieran G. Meade, Teagasc, Ireland
Amanda Jane Gibson, Royal Veterinary College, UK

***Correspondence:**
Muhammad J. Uddin
m.uddin2@uq.edu.au

The peripheral innate immune response to West Nile virus (WNV) is crucial for control of virus spread to the central nervous system. Therefore, transcriptomes encoding the innate immune response proteins against WNV were investigated in peripheral blood mononuclear cells (PBMCs) of New Zealand White rabbits, a recently established novel rabbit model for WNV pathogenesis studies. PBMCs were challenged with an Australian WNV strain, $WNV_{NSW2011}$, *in vitro*, and mRNA expression of selected immune response genes were quantified at 2-, 6-, 12-, and 24-h post-infection (pi) using qRT-PCR. Compared to mock-inoculated PBMCs, WNV-stimulated PBMCs expressed high levels of interferon (IFN) alpha (IFNA), gamma (IFNG), IL6, IL12, IL22, CXCL10, and pentraxin 3 (PTX3) mRNA. Likewise, TLR1, 2, 3, 4, 6, and 10 mRNA became up-regulated with the highest expression seen for TLR3, 4, and 6. TLRs-signaling downstream genes (MyD88, STAT1, TRAF3, IRF7, and IRF9) subsequently became up-regulated. The high expression of IFNs, TLR3, TLR4, TRAF3, STAT1, IRF7, and IRF9 are in accordance with antiviral activities, while expression of TNFA, HO1, iNOS, caspase 3, and caspase 9 transcripts suggests the involvement of oxidative stress and apoptosis in WNV-stimulated rabbit PBMCs, respectively. The level of $WNV_{NSW2011}$ RNA increased at 24-h pi in PBMCs challenged with virus *in vitro* compared to input virus. The expression dynamics of selected genes were validated in PBMCs from rabbits experimentally infected with WNV *in vivo*. Higher expression of IFNA, IFN beta (IFNB), IFNG, TNFA, IL6, IL22, PTX3, TLR3 and TLR4, IRF7, IRF9, STST1, TRAF3, caspase 3, and caspase 9 were seen in PBMCs from WNV-infected rabbits on day 3 post-intradermal virus inoculation compared to PBMCs from uninfected control rabbits. This study highlights the array of cytokines and TLRs involved in the host innate immune response to WNV in the rabbit leukocytes and suggests that these cells may be a useful *in vitro* model for WNV infection study.

Keywords: West Nile virus, rabbit, PBMCs, innate immune response, cytokines, TLRs

INTRODUCTION

Since the first isolation of the Australian strain of West Nile virus, the Kunjin strain (WNV_{KUN}), in 1960 in North Queensland (1), it has been found to be endemic in Australia (2). WNV_{KUN} belongs to lineage 1 of WNV, which also includes the highly pathogenic neuro-invasive New York 99 strain (WNV_{NY99}) (3). WNV_{KUN} causes mainly asymptomatic infection and only a small number of mild human cases have been documented with no reported fatalities in Australia (2). In contrast, since its introduction into New York in 1999, WNV_{NY99} has spread rapidly throughout the USA with close to 40,000 human cases of WNV disease and more than 1,600 deaths reported in the USA between 1999 and 2014 (4). WNV has also spread to other parts of the Americas, and also to Europe, Asia, and the Middle East (5). In addition to human infections, the WNV_{NY99} virus has caused significant morbidity and mortality in horses and birds, with more than 20,000 equine cases and hundreds of thousands of avian deaths (6). Relative to the WNV_{NY99} strain, WNV_{KUN} exhibits much reduced virulence in humans, animals, and birds (2). Equine disease associated with WNV_{KUN} infection was rare, however, in early 2011 following extensive flooding in the Murray–Darling river basin and other inland river systems, an unprecedented outbreak of equine encephalitis occurred in south-eastern Australia involving more than 1,000 horses (7). Genomic sequencing of viruses isolated from a horse succumbing to encephalitis in the 2011 outbreak revealed the etiological agent to be a variant strain of WNV, most closely related to WNV_{KUN} and subsequently named $WNV_{NSW2011}$ (7). As the virus strain may still be circulating and the human and equine populations in Eastern Australia remain susceptible to WNV_{KUN} (8, 9), it is important to get a better understanding of the host response to this virus.

Peripheral blood mononuclear cells (PBMCs) are among the first immune components to encounter WNV following a mosquito bite. It has been postulated that the PBMC may serve as target cells for initial replication of WNV and play a role in subsequent viral dissemination (10). Additionally, primary PBMC cell culture has been proposed to be a potentially useful model of a natural WNV host (10). To survive virus infection, the host must recognize invasion and develop an effective antiviral immune response. This response is initiated in infected cells after detection of non-self pathogen-associated molecular patterns (PAMPs). PAMPs motifs are detected by specific, conserved host molecular patterns - pathogen recognition receptors (PRRs), such as Toll-like receptors (TLRs), which trigger signaling cascades that induce the activation of interferon (IFN) regulatory factors (IRFs) and nuclear factor kappa B (NFκB), leading to expression of antiviral molecules, including type I IFNs (IFNA and IFNB), and hundreds of different IFN-stimulated effector genes (ISGs). ISG products include additional antiviral effector molecules and immunomodulatory cytokines that serve to restrict virus replication and modulate the immune response (11).

The signaling pathways thought to detect entry and infection by WNV and initiate a protective IFN response have mostly been studied in mice (12–18) with only limited studies in the horse (19). Based on those studies, a partial signaling pathway has been proposed by which WNV and other flaviviruses are detected, and the effector mechanisms that contribute to protective cell-intrinsic immunity executed (11, 20). Nevertheless, there appears to be some discrepancies between the protective immune mechanisms between humans and mice (21, 22) and even more so between mice and horses (23, 24). In order to overcome the latter problem, we have recently established a New Zealand White (NZW) rabbit model for WNV-infection (25). Physiologically, rabbits resemble horses by being hindgut fermenters and 10–20% of feral rabbits may be exposed to WNV in any season throughout Australia (8). Previously, gene expression has been performed in selected tissues (thalamus and cerebrum) of horse (19), mouse (26), NZW rabbits (25), and in human cells and tissues infected with WNV (27). However, there is a gap in knowledge of the expression patterns of immune-related genes during the early time points following infection. Therefore, this study aimed to characterize the innate immune response in rabbit PBMCs, exposed *in vitro* to $WNV_{NSW2011}$ using transcriptomic analysis of immunologically important genes. Selected transcripts were subsequently confirmed in the *in vivo* WNV-infection model, supporting the contention that *in vitro* studies of PBMCs responses are a useful surrogate model for acute WNV infection in natural hosts and relevant animal model.

MATERIALS AND METHODS

Preparation of WNV

The $WNV_{NSW2011}$ strain used in this study was isolated from a 10% weight/volume brain homogenate of an encephalitic horse during the 2011 Australian arboviral outbreak. The virus isolate was passaged initially in C6/36 cells (*Aedes albopictus* mosquito cells), followed by 1× in Vero (African green monkey kidney) cells and 3× final passages in C6/36 cells cultured with 10% fetal bovine serum (FBS) at 28°C before use. Detailed characterization of the mouse virulence of $WNV_{NSW2011}$ has been described in Frost et al. (7). The mock inoculum consisted of tissue culture medium only. The virus stock was stored at −80°C. The titer of the stock was quantified using standard plaque assay on Vero cells, as described previously (25, 28). The $WNV_{NSW2011}$ was diluted to 1×10^6 PFU/50 μL for use in PBMCs infection *in vitro* experiments.

PBMCs Isolation, Culture, and Challenged with Viruses

EDTA-stabilized blood samples were collected from WNV-seronegative NZW rabbits ($n = 3$) (25). All animal procedures had received prior approval from the University of Queensland

---

Abbreviations: ACTB, actin, beta; CXCL10, C–X–C motif chemokine 10 [also known as Interferon gamma-induced protein 10 (IP-10)]; GAPDH, glyceraldehyde 3-phosphate dehydrogenase; HO1, heme oxygenase 1; IFNα, interferon alpha; IFNβ, interferon beta; IFNγ, interferon gamma; IL12, interleukin IL22; IL6, interleukin 6; iNOS, inducible nitric oxide synthase; IRF, interferon regulatory factor; Kunjin, australian strain of west nile virus; MyD88, myeloid differentiation 88; PPIA, peptidylprolyl isomerase A (also known as cyclophilin A); PTX3, pentraxin 3; STAT1, signal transducer and activator of transcription 1; TLR, toll-like receptor; TNFα, tumor necrosis factor alpha; TRAF3, TNF receptor-associated factor 3.

Animal Ethics Committee (SVS/369/12/ARC), and all procedures were performed under xylazine sedation and anesthesia (25). Blood was collected by cardiac bleed of anesthetized rabbits into EDTA-coated collection tubes (Vacuette®, Greiner Bio One, Australia) immediately prior to their euthanasia. The PBMCs were isolated from the blood using Ficoll-Histopaque (Sigma) as described previously (29). The viability of the purified PBMCs was assessed using the trypan blue exclusion method and was always >90%. The cells were counted using a hemocytometer and the concentration was adjusted to 1×10^6 cells/0.5 ml in RPMI-1460 supplemented with L-glutamine (2 nM), streptomycin (50 μg/mL), penicillin (50 U/mL), and 10% FBS (29). The cells were cultured in 24-well cell culture plates (Costar Corning, the Netherlands) seeded with 500 μL of cell suspension per well and incubated at 37°C with 5% CO_2. Remaining PBMCs (fresh-isolated PBMCs) were pelleted and kept at −80°C for RNA isolation. After 1 h of incubation, the PBMCs were challenged by adding 50 μL of $WNV_{NSW2011}$ to each well to give a final multiplicity of infection (MOI) of one. The dose of virus was chosen based on the typical dose inoculated by mosquitoes (30). Additional 450 μL medium was added to each well to make up the final volume of 1 ml. One well of PBMCs per animal was harvested at 2, 6, 12, and 24 h after virus infection, respectively. The harvested cells (WNV-stimulated PBMCs) were pelleted and kept at −80°C until subjected to RNA isolation. For complete harvesting of adherent PBMCs, detachment with lidocaine HCl (12 mM) was performed (31). To ensure the complete harvesting of cells, wells were checked using an inverted microscope. Duplicate wells of uninfected cells (mock-inoculated PBMCs) were cultured in 500 μL of RPMI culture media supplemented with 10% FBS. They were harvested and treated in a similar manner at each time point.

PBMCs Isolation from Infected Rabbits

In order to compare the transcriptional profile of in vitro challenged PBMCs against those from in vivo challenged rabbits blood samples were obtained from $WNV_{NSW2011}$-infected New Zealand White (NZW) rabbits ($n = 3$) on day 3 pi, and mock-infected NZW rabbits ($n = 3$) on day 6 post-mock (medium only) inoculation (25). Collected blood was immediately processed for PBMCs isolation, as described above.

RNA Isolation and Transcriptome Quantification

Total RNA was isolated from PBMCs using miRNeasy RNA isolation kit (Qiagen Pty Ltd., Australia) and on-column DNA digestion (Qiagen) was performed following the manufacturer's instructions. The quantity and quality of RNA was measured using NanoDrop 1000 spectrophotometer (Thermo Scientific, Australia). The isolated RNA was subjected to PCR with GAPDH primers without a reverse transcription step and run in gel to check for DNA-contamination. None was found to be contaminated (data not shown). The isolated RNA was kept at −80°C for further transcriptome analysis using quantitative real time PCR (qRT-PCR). Primers for cytokines, TLRs and downstream genes, apoptosis and oxidative stress-related genes, and two normalizer genes (*GAPDH* and *PPIA*) were designed from FASTA products of the GenBank mRNA sequences for *Oryctolagus cuniculus* using the Primer3 program (32). No suitable normalizer genes has been reported in rabbits PBMCs yet, but *GAPDH* and *PPIA* are reported to be appropriate stably expressed normalizer genes in PBMCs in pigs (33). The $WNV_{NSW2011}$ (WNV_{KUN})-specific primers (34) and primers of some cytokines (35) were described earlier. Details of the primers are given in **Table 1**.

To quantify the mRNA expression for target and reference genes, qRT-PCR was performed using the Rotor Gene Corbett 6000 quantitative real-time PCR system (Qiagen). A one step qRT-PCR was performed using Rotor-Gene SYBR Green RT-PCR Kit (Qiagen). Each run contained each RNA sample and a no-template control. qRT-PCR was set up using 1 μL of RNA template, 5.25 μL of deionized RNase free H_2O, 0.5 μM of upstream and downstream primers, 0.25 μL Rotor-Gene RT mix (RT mix), and 12.5 μL of 2× Rotor-Gene SYBR Green RT-PCR master mix (MM) (Qiagen) in a total reaction volume of 20 μL. The cycling conditions included reverse transcription step (10 min at 55°C), PCR initial activation step (5 min at 95°C), and a two-step cycling protocol with a denaturation step and a combined annealing/extension step. The two-step thermal cycling conditions were 5 s at 95°C followed by 10 s at 60°C (40 cycles). An amplification-based auto-threshold (Rotor-Gene Q Series Software, Qiagen) and adaptive baseline were selected as algorithms. Melting curve analysis was performed to detect the specificity of the PCR reaction. Each sample was run twice, and the average value was used as expression value. The qRT-PCR products of selected genes (e.g., GAPDH) on agarose gel. The gel documentation showed amplification only at the anticipated product length (i.e., 126 bp for GAPDH) (data not shown). Gene-specific expression was measured as relative to the geometric mean of the expression of two normalizer genes (*GAPDH* and *PPIA*) (**Table 1**). The delta Ct (ΔCt) ($\Delta Ct = Ct_{target} - Ct_{normaliser\ genes}$) values were calculated as the difference between target gene and reference genes, and expression was calculated as $2^{(-\Delta\Delta Ct)}$ (36). To compare the magnitude of gene expression, the fold change was calculated. For this purpose, the delta delta Ct ($\Delta\Delta$Ct) values were calculated as follows: $\Delta\Delta Ct = \Delta Ct_{WNV} - \Delta Ct_{mock}$. The bar graphs (**Figures 1–5A; Figure 7**) show the expression of genes in WNV-stimulated PBMCs over mock-inoculated PBMCs (fold change: the normalized expression value of a gene in WNV-stimulated cells/the normalized expression value of a gene in mock-inoculated cells). In addition, accounting for the effects of culture conditions on gene transcription in WNV- and mock-inoculated rabbit PBMCs, the normalized expression of genes from PBMCs harvested at each time point was compared to their respective expression levels before either WNV inoculation or mock inoculation. The $\Delta\Delta$Ct values were calculated by subtracting ΔCt of genes in fresh-isolated PBMCs from the ΔCt of genes in WNV- or mock-inoculated PBMCs at each time-point. The average expression values of the mRNA levels were considered for further analysis.

Statistical Analysis

The technical replications were averaged. The impact of virus-challenge (treatment) and duration of incubation (time points) were evaluated using the SAS software package v. 9.2 (SAS Institute, Cary, NC, USA). For this purpose, the GLM (general

TABLE 1 | List of primer sequences used in this study.

Gene	Primer set[a]	Amplicon size (bp)	GenBank accession number
Kunjin	F: AACCCCAGTGGAGAAGTGGA[b] R: TCAGGCTGCCACACCAAA	70	D00246
IFNA	F: TGCTTGCAGGACAGACATGA R: ATCTCGTGGAGCACAGAGAT	95	XM_002708065.1
IFNB	F:TCCAACTATGGCACGGAAGTCT[b] R:TTCTGGAGCTGTTGTGGTTCCT	89	XM_002707968
IFNG	F:TGCCAGGACACACTAACCAGAG[c] R:TGTCACTCTCCTCTTTCCAATTCC	127	NM_001081991
TNFA	F:CTGCACTTCAGGGTGATCG[c] R:CTACGTGGGCTAGAGGCTTG	94	NM_001082263
IL6	F: CTACCGCTTTCCCCACTTCAG[c] R: TCCTCAGCTCCTTGATGGTCTC	135	NM_001082064.2
IL12/IL23P40	PS211: CTCCGAAGAAGATGGCATTACC[c] PS212: TCTCCTTTGTGGCAGGTGTATTG	126	XM_002710347
IL22	PS567: ACCTCACCTTCATGCTGGCTAA PS568: CATGGAACAGCTCATTCCCAAT	84	XM_002711248
CXCL10	F: ATAGAAGCATCCTGAGCCCA R: GAACTGCAAACTGAGGCCAA	86	XM_002717106.1
PTX3	F: TTCCCCATGCGTTCCAAGAA R: GTGGCTTTGACCCAAATGCA	95	XM_002716328.1
HO1	F: ACTGCCGAGGGTTTTAAGCT R: GGTTCTCCTTGTTGTGCTCA	88	XM_002711415.1
iNOS	F: GACGTCCAGCGCTACAATATCC[c] R: GATCTCTGTGACGGCCTGATCT	102	XM_002718780
Caspase 3	F: AAGCCGACTTCCTGTATGCA R: CGTACTCTTTCAGCATGGCA	111	NM_001082117.1
Caspase 9	F: AAACGTGGATTTGGCGTACG R: TGCTGCTGAAGTTCACGTTG	80	XM_002722329.1
TLR1	F: TGTGTCCCACAATGAGCTGT R: GGCAGAGCATCAAACGCATT	93	XM_002709270.1
TLR2	F: GCTGCGCAAGATCATGAACA R: TTTATGGCGGCCCTCAAGTT	96	NM_001082781.1
TLR3	F: ATGACCTGCCCACCAACATA R: TTCTGGCTCCAGCTTTGAGA	140	NM_001082219.1
TLR4	F: AGGCTGTTGGTGGAAGTTGA R: TGCTTATCTGACAGGTGGCA	91	NM_001082732.2
TLR6	F: CATTGAGCACAACGCAGTGT R: AGCTCGCATGTACAGTGGAA	108	XM_002709388.1
TLR10	F: ACACCGGTAATGCACTTGGA R: TAAGCAAGGTGTCTGGCCAT	85	XM_002709387.1
MyD88	F: GCCAGTGAGCTCATCGAGAA R: TCACACTCCTTGCTCTGCAG	80	XM_002723869.1
IRF1	F: AGCACTGTCACCACATAGCA R: TCATCTGTCGCAGCTTCAGA	120	NM_001171347.1
IRF7	F: AAGTGCAAGGTGTACTGGGA R: AGCTCTTGGAAGAAGGTGCT	119	XM_002724304.1
IRF9	F: TAACTGAGGCTGCTGTGCAA R: ACACGCCCGTTGTAGATGAA	103	XM_002718097.1
TRAF3	F: TGGCTATAAGATGTGCGCCA R: ACTCTCCACGCATGATGACA	95	XM_002721716.1

(Continued)

TABLE 1 | Continued

Gene	Primer set[a]	Amplicon size (bp)	GenBank accession number
STAT1	F: TTCAACATCCTGGGCACACA R: TGCCAGCGTTCTTCTGTTCT	112	XM_002712346.1
GAPDH	F: TGACGACATCAAGAAGGTGGTG** R: GAAGGTGGAGGAGTGGGTGTC	126	NM_001082253
PPIA	F: AGGGCATGAGCATTGTGGAA R: TCCACAGTTGGCAATGGTGA	86	NM_001082057.1

[a]*Annealing temperature was 60°C for all the primer sets.*
[b]*Primer set is adopted from Ref. (34).*
[c]*Primer set are adopted from Ref. (35).*

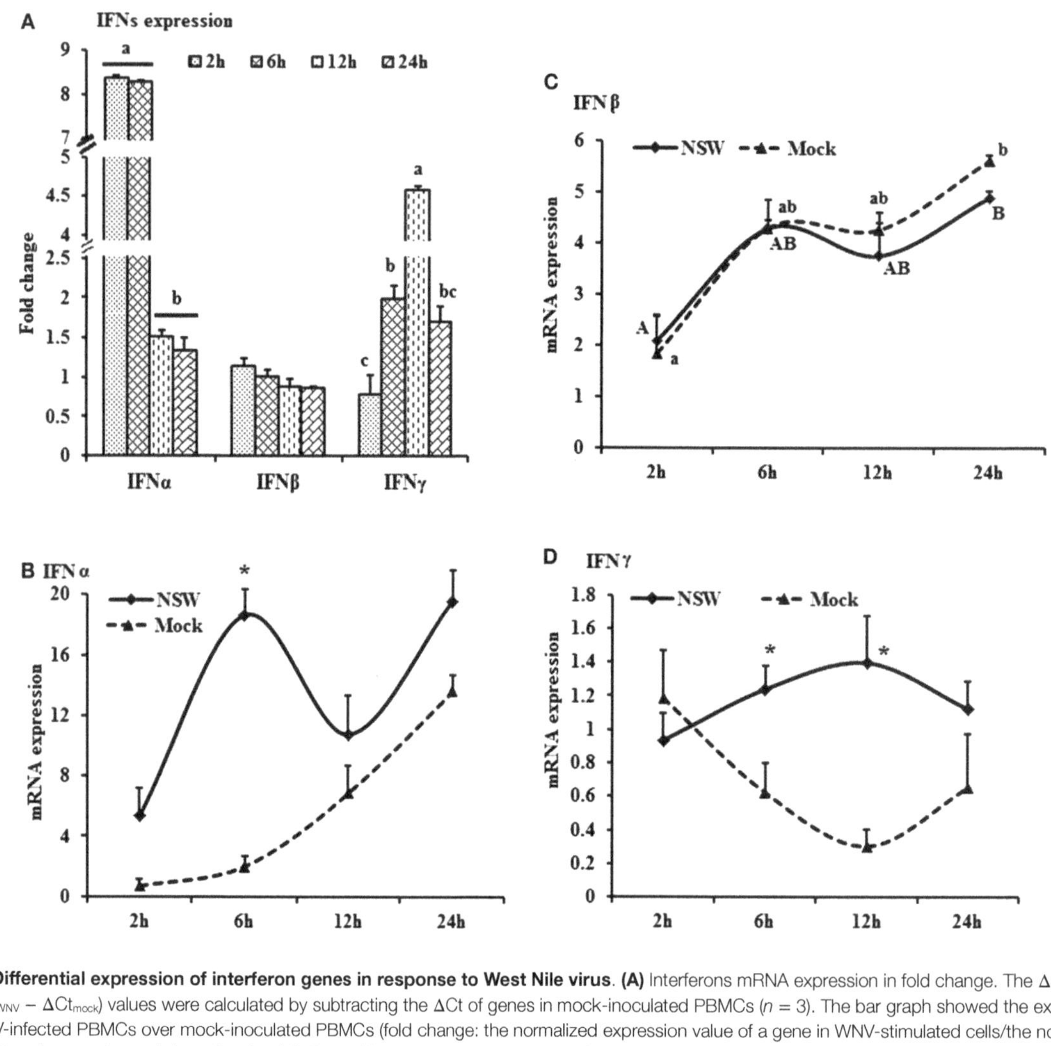

FIGURE 1 | Differential expression of interferon genes in response to West Nile virus. (A) Interferons mRNA expression in fold change. The $\Delta\Delta Ct$ ($\Delta\Delta Ct = \Delta Ct_{WNV} - \Delta Ct_{mock}$) values were calculated by subtracting the ΔCt of genes in mock-inoculated PBMCs ($n = 3$). The bar graph showed the expression of genes in WNV-infected PBMCs over mock-inoculated PBMCs (fold change: the normalized expression value of a gene in WNV-stimulated cells/the normalized expression value of a gene in mock-inoculated cells). Bars without common superscripts (a,b; a,c; b,c) denote statistical difference among time points ($p < 0.05$). **(B–D)** Relative expression of interferons mRNA, accounting for the effects of culture conditions on gene transcription in WNV- and mock-inoculated rabbit PBMCs ($n = 3$). To compare the normalized expression of IFNs genes from PBMCs harvested at each time point to their respective expression levels before either WNV inoculation or mock inoculation, the $\Delta\Delta Ct$ values were calculated by subtracting ΔCt of genes in fresh-isolated PBMCs from the ΔCt of genes in WNV- or mock-inoculated PBMCs at each time-point (for WNV-stimulated PBMCs, $\Delta\Delta Ct_{WNV} = \Delta Ct_{WNV} - \Delta Ct_{fresh}$; and for mock-inoculated PBMCs, $\Delta\Delta Ct_{mock} = \Delta Ct_{mock} - \Delta Ct_{fresh}$). A time-dependent relative expression patterns of **(B)** *IFNA*, **(C)** *IFNB*, and **(D)** *IFNG* mRNA in WNV-stimulated rabbit PBMCs at different time points. Line graphs without common superscript differ significantly ($p < 0.05$). Upper case letter denotes difference of a gene expression among the time points in WNV-challenged cells; lower case letter denotes difference of a gene expression among the time points in mock-inoculated cells. *indicates the difference of a gene expression between WNV- and mock-challenged cells in the same time point ($p < 0.05$).

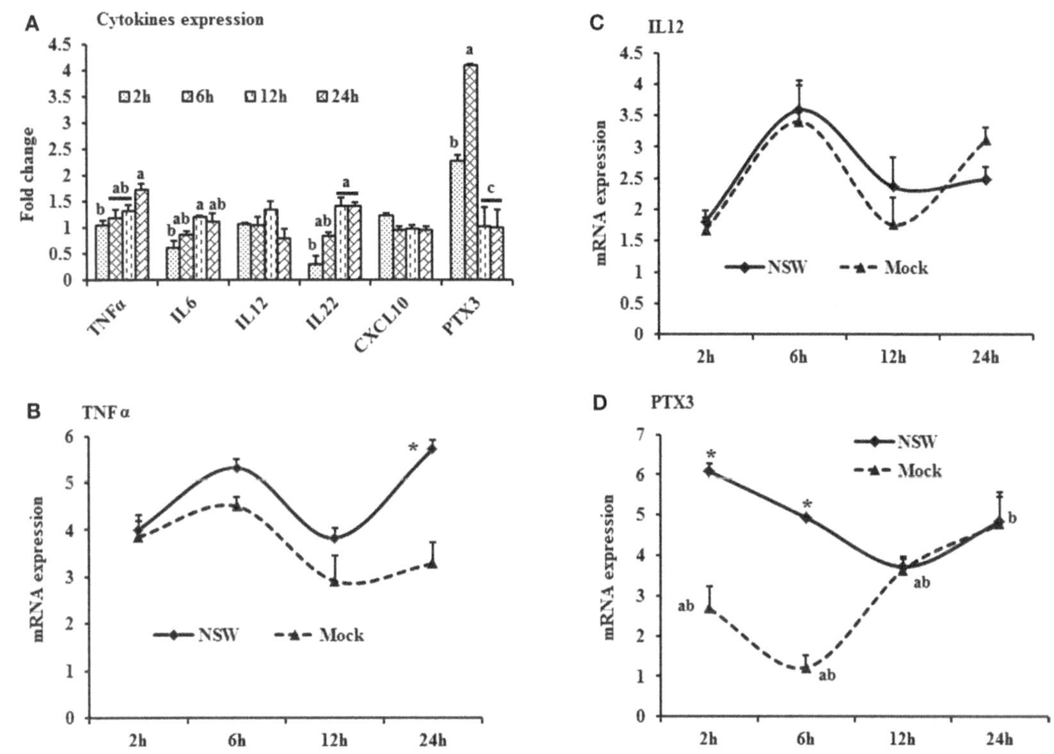

FIGURE 2 | Differential expression of inflammatory cytokine genes in response to West Nile virus. (A) Cytokines mRNA expression in fold change. The ΔΔCt ($\Delta\Delta Ct = \Delta Ct_{WNV} - \Delta Ct_{mock}$) values were calculated by subtracting the ΔCt of genes in mock-inoculated PBMCs ($n = 3$). The bar graph showed the expression of genes in WNV-infected PBMCs over mock-inoculated PBMCs (fold change: the normalized expression value of a gene in WNV-stimulated cells/the normalized expression value of a gene in mock-inoculated cells). Bars without common superscripts (a,b; a,c; b,c) denote statistical difference among time points ($p < 0.05$). **(B–D)** Relative expression of cytokines mRNA, accounting for the effects of culture conditions on gene transcription in WNV- and mock-inoculated rabbit PBMCs ($n = 3$). To compare the normalized expression of cytokine genes from PBMCs harvested at each time point to their respective expression levels before either WNV inoculation or mock inoculation, the ΔΔCt values were calculated by subtracting ΔCt of genes in fresh-isolated PBMCs from the ΔCt of genes in WNV- or mock-inoculated PBMCs at each time-point (for WNV-stimulated PBMCs, $\Delta\Delta Ct_{WNV} = \Delta Ct_{WNV} - \Delta Ct_{fresh}$; and for mock-inoculated PBMCs, $\Delta\Delta Ct_{mock} = \Delta Ct_{mock} - \Delta Ct_{fresh}$). A time-dependent relative expression patterns of **(B)** *TNFA*, **(C)** *IL12*, and **(D)** *PTX3* mRNA in WNV-challenged rabbit PBMCs at different time points. Line graphs without common superscript differ significantly ($p < 0.05$). Upper case letter denotes difference of a gene expression among the time points in WNV-challenged cells; lower case letter denotes difference of a gene expression among the time points in mock-inoculated cells. *indicates the difference of a gene expression between WNV- and mock-challenged cells in the same time point ($p < 0.05$).

linear model; Proc GLM) procedure and the implemented analysis of variance (ANOVA) statistic were used. Pairwise comparisons were performed between the time points and treatment groups using Tukey's multiple comparisons in SAS, where *P* value was simultaneously adjusted. Besides, student's *t*-test was applied when treatment groups were compared. The data were expressed as means ±SD and values of $p < 0.05$ were considered to indicate statistically significant differences.

RESULTS

Expression Dynamics of Cytokines

The mRNA levels of cytokine *IFNA*, *IFNB*, *IFNG*, *IL6*, *IL12*, *CXCL10*, *IL22*, and *TNFA* showed a time-dependent expression pattern in rabbit PBMCs in response to WNV infection (**Figures 1A** and **2A**). When gene expressions in WNV-infected PBMCs were expressed in fold change with regards to the expression of genes in control (mock-inoculated) PBMCs (**Figures 1A** and **2A**), *IFNA* expression was up-regulated (8.4-folds) between 2- and 6-h pi and then declined (**Figure 1A**). The highest expression of *IFNB* gene was detected at the beginning of PBMCs–virus interaction and then declined gradually over time (**Figure 1A**). *IFNG* mRNA expression was increased over time and peaked (4.6 times) at 12-h pi (**Figure 1A**). While *IL6* and *IL22* mRNA expression increased over time, pentraxin 3 (*PTX3*) expression was significantly increased at the earlier hours of virus stimulation (**Figure 2A**).

When cytokine mRNA expressions in WNV-infected and mock-inoculated PBMCs were calculated with regards to the expression in freshly isolated PBMCs (fresh-PBMCs), *IFNA* mRNA expression was significantly higher at 6 h, then declined to the expression level in control at 12-h pi (**Figure 1B**). *IFNB* mRNA showed similar expression pattern in both infected and control cell lines (**Figure 1C**). With the exception at initial cell–pathogen interaction, *IFNG* (**Figure 1D**) and *TNFA* (**Figure 2B**) mRNA expression in virus-infected PBMCs was greater than in the mock-inoculated PBMCs. *IL12* expression in both the infected- and mock-inoculated PBMCs exhibited a similar pattern

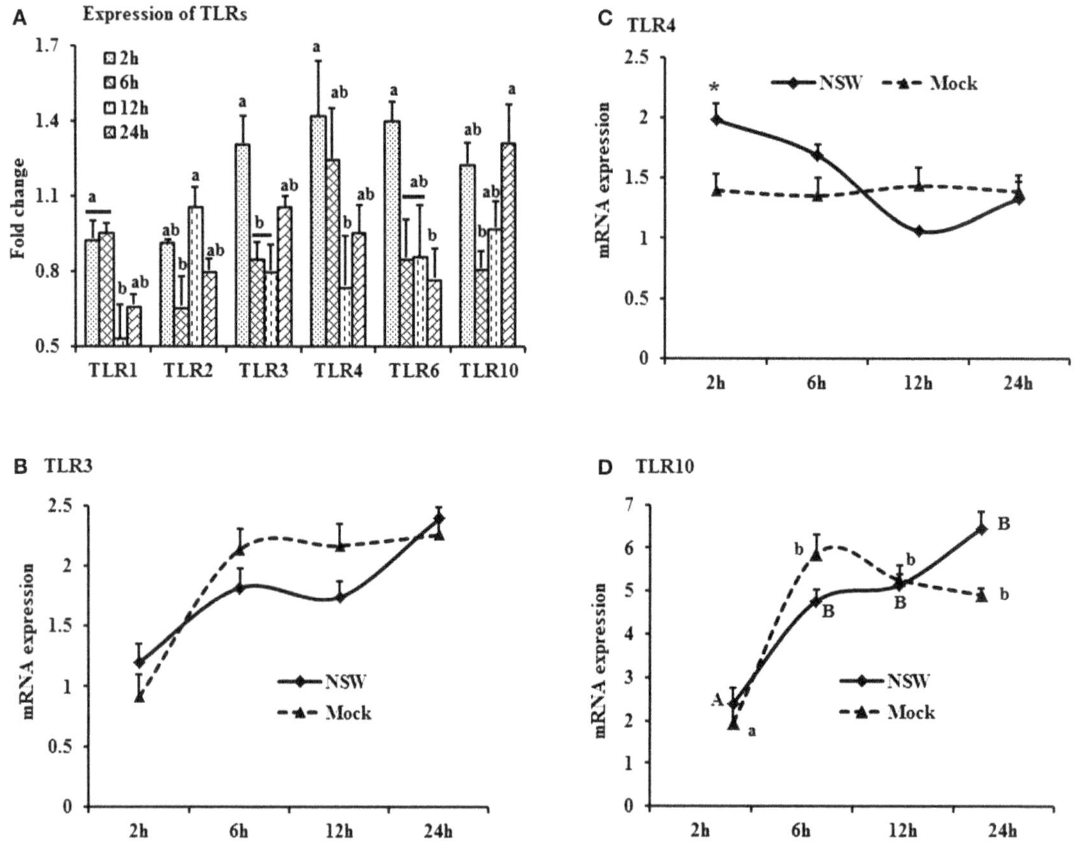

FIGURE 3 | Differential expression of Toll-like receptor genes in response to West Nile virus. (A) TLrs mRNA expression in fold change. The $\Delta\Delta Ct$ ($\Delta\Delta Ct = \Delta Ct_{WNV} - \Delta Ct_{mock}$) values were calculated by subtracting the ΔCt of genes in mock-inoculated PBMCs ($n = 3$). The bar graph showed the expression of genes in WNV-infected PBMCs over mock-inoculated PBMCs (fold change: the normalized expression value of a gene in WNV-stimulated cells/the normalized expression value of a gene in mock-inoculated cells). Bars without common superscripts (a,b; a,c; b,c) denote statistical difference among time points ($p < 0.05$). **(B–D)** Relative expression of TLRs mRNA, accounting for the effects of culture conditions on gene transcription in WNV- and mock-inoculated rabbit PBMCs ($n = 3$). To compare the normalized expression of TLRs genes from PBMCs harvested at each time point to their respective expression levels before either WNV inoculation or mock inoculation, the $\Delta\Delta Ct$ values were calculated by subtracting ΔCt of genes in fresh-isolated PBMCs from the ΔCt of genes in WNV- or mock-inoculated PBMCs at each time-point (for WNV-stimulated PBMCs, $\Delta\Delta Ct_{WNV} = \Delta Ct_{WNV} - \Delta Ct_{fresh}$; and for mock-inoculated PBMCs, $\Delta\Delta Ct_{mock} = \Delta Ct_{mock} - \Delta Ct_{fresh}$). A time-dependent relative expression patterns of **(B)** *TLR3*, **(C)** *TLR4*, and **(D)** *TLR10* mRNA in WNV-challenged rabbit PBMCs at different time points. Line graphs without common superscript differ significantly ($p < 0.05$). Upper case letter denotes difference of a gene expression among the time points in WNV-challenged cells; lower case letter denotes difference of a gene expression among the time points in mock-inoculated cells. *indicates the difference of a gene expression between WNV- and mock-challenged cells in the same time point ($p < 0.05$).

of expression, peaking at 6-h pi then declined (**Figure 2C**). *PTX3* gene expression was significantly up-regulated in the early hours of WNV infection, then declined to the expression level in mock-inoculated PBMCs (**Figure 2D**).

Expression Patterns of TLRs and Associated Genes

The TLR-family genes showed similar patterns of expression characteristics with higher genes involvement at the beginning as well as at 24 h of post-virus stimulation, except *TLR2* and *TLR6* (**Figure 3A**). *TLR3*, *4*, and *6* mRNA expressions was higher in virus-stimulated PBMCs, compared to the mock-inoculated PBMCs (**Figure 3A**). When mRNA expressions in WNV-stimulated and mock-inoculated PBMCs were calculated with regards to the expression in fresh PBMCs, *TLR3* and *TLR4* expression was up-regulated at the initial hour pi in virus-stimulated PBL compared to mock-inoculated PBMCs, then declined (**Figures 3B,C**). *TLR10* mRNA expression was up-regulated in both WNV-stimulated and mock-inoculated PBMCs (**Figure 3D**).

When mRNA expressions in WNV-stimulated PBMCs were expressed in fold change with regards to the expression of mRNA in mock-inoculated PBMCs, *MyD88* expression was initially up-regulated then declined, whereas *IRF7* mRNA expression increased over time (**Figure 4A**). *STAT1* mRNA expression peaked at 24-h pi in WNV-stimulated PBMCs compared to mock-inoculated PBMCs (**Figure 4A**). *TRAF3* mRNA expression increased over time, peaking at 24-h pi (**Figure 4B**), and *STAT1* mRNA expression was significantly up-regulated at 24-h pi (**Figure 4C**) in virus-stimulated PBMCs. *IRF7* mRNA expression

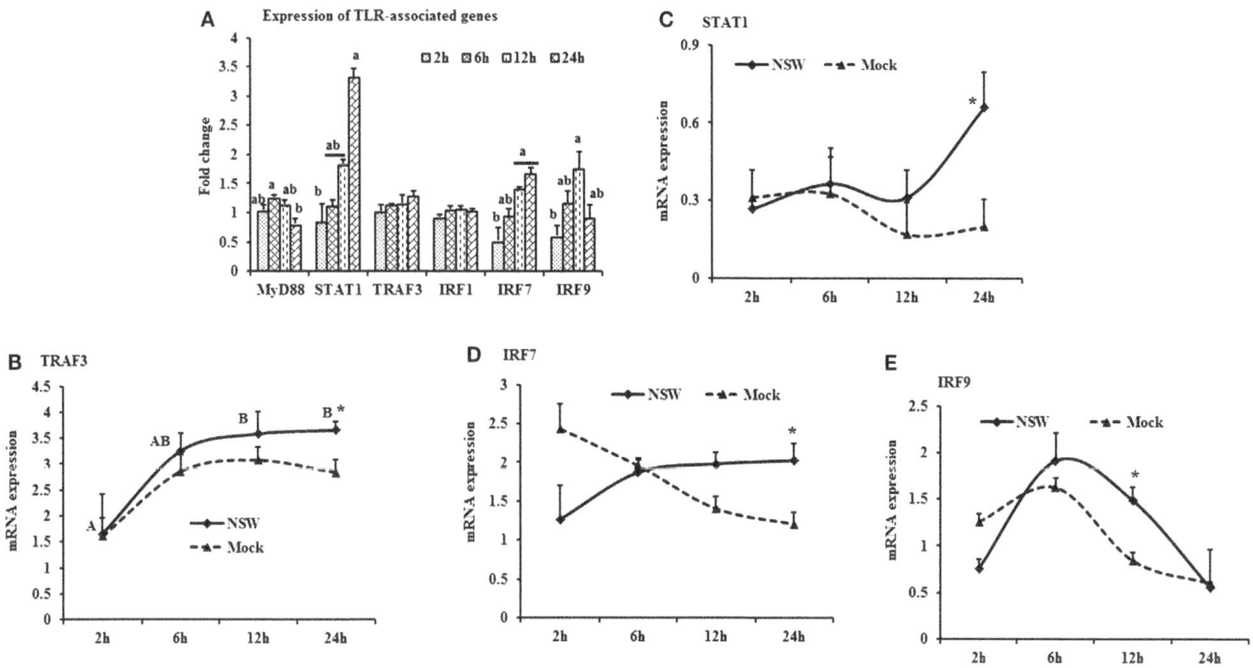

FIGURE 4 | Differential expression of the TLR downstream genes in response to West Nile virus. **(A)** TLR-associated genes mRNA expression in fold change. The $\Delta\Delta Ct$ ($\Delta\Delta Ct = \Delta Ct_{WNV} - \Delta Ct_{mock}$) values were calculated by subtracting the ΔCt of genes in mock-inoculated PBMCs ($n = 3$). The bar graph showed the expression of genes in WNV-infected PBMCs over mock-inoculated PBMCs (fold change: the normalized expression value of a gene in WNV-stimulated cells/the normalized expression value of a gene in mock-inoculated cells). Bars without common superscripts (a,b) denote statistical difference among time points ($p < 0.05$). **(B–E)** Relative expression of TLRs-associated genes mRNA, accounting for the effects of culture conditions on gene transcription in WNV- and mock-inoculated rabbit PBMCs ($n = 3$). To compare the normalized expression of TLR-associated genes from PBMCs harvested at each time point to their respective expression levels before either WNV inoculation or mock inoculation, the $\Delta\Delta Ct$ values were calculated by subtracting ΔCt of genes in fresh-isolated PBMCs from the ΔCt of genes in WNV- or mock-inoculated PBMCs at each time-point (for WNV-stimulated PBMCs, $\Delta\Delta Ct_{WNV} = \Delta Ct_{WNV} - \Delta Ct_{fresh}$; and for mock-inoculated PBMCs, $\Delta\Delta Ct_{mock} = \Delta Ct_{mock} - \Delta Ct_{fresh}$). A time-dependent relative expression patterns of **(B)** *TRAF3*, **(C)** *STAT1*, **(D)** *IRF7*, and **(E)***IRF9* mRNA in WNV-challenged rabbit PBMCs at different time points. Line graphs without common superscript differ significantly ($p < 0.05$). Upper case letter denotes difference of a gene expression among the time points in WNV-challenged cells; lower case letter denotes difference of a gene expression among the time points in mock-inoculated cells. *indicates the difference of a gene expression between WNV- and mock-challenged cells in the same time point ($p < 0.05$).

between the earlier and later hours of stimulation showed opposite pattern in response to WNV stimulation in rabbit PBMCs (**Figure 4D**). *IRF9* showed a similar pattern of expression both in WNV-stimulated and mock-inoculated PBMCs with a significant upregulation at 12-h pi (**Figure 4E**).

Oxidative Stress and Apoptosis-Related Genes Expressions

Oxidative stress-related *HO1* gene expression became up-regulated over time, whereas iNOS mRNA expression decreased over time after a slight peak at 6-h pi in virus-stimulated PBMCs (**Figure 5A**). The expression of the apoptosis-associated gene *caspase 3* increased over time, whereas *caspase 9* mRNA expression was up-regulated at initial hours pi, then declined (**Figure 5A**).

When mRNA expressions in WNV-stimulated and mock-inoculated PBMCs were calculated with regards to the expression in fresh-PBMCs, *HO1* mRNA expression increased over time in both WNV-stimulated and mock-inoculated PBMCs (**Figure 5B**), whereas *iNOS* expression was higher in virus-stimulated PBMCs at 6-h pi (**Figure 5C**). Both *caspase 3* and *9* mRNA expressions were higher in virus-stimulated PBMCs at 12-h pi, then declined (**Figures 5D,E**).

Kinetics of Virus-Specific Gene Expression in Rabbit PBMCs

When viral RNA expression was compared among the virus-stimulated PBMCs samples, the WNV-specific transcript expression was increased at 24-h pi compared to the expression at 2- and 6-h pi (**Figure 6**). Notably, viral RNA could not be detected in *in vitro* mock-inoculated PBMCs or in fresh PBMCs samples or in PBMCs collected from *in vivo* virus infected or control rabbits.

Validation of Transcripts Expressions in PBMCs from Virus-Infected Rabbits

Despite the lack of detectable viral RNA in PBMCs collected on day 3 pi from $WNV_{NSW2011}$-infected rabbits, the cells had upregulation of *IFNA*, *IFNB*, *TNFA*, *IL22* and *PTX3* (**Figure 7A**), *TLR3* and *IRF7* (**Figure 7B**), and *caspase 9* (**Figure 7C**) mRNA expression when compared to PBMCs from mock-infected control rabbits. *IFNA*, *IFNB*, *TNFA*, and *PTX3* mRNA expression was 8-,

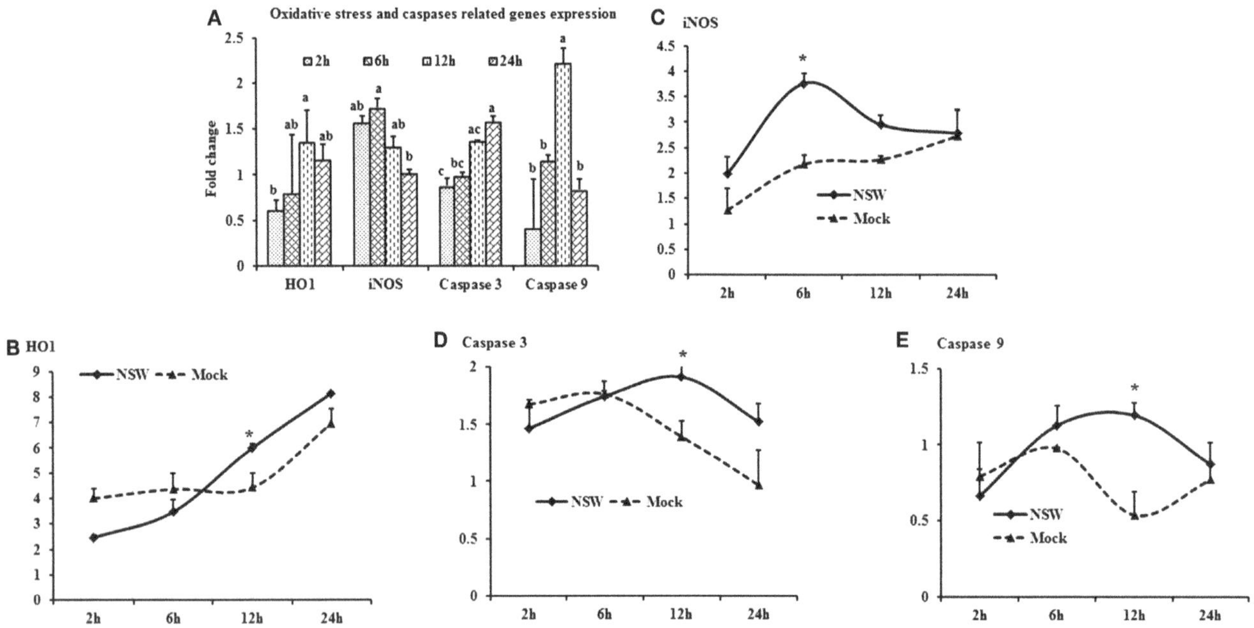

FIGURE 5 | Differential expression of oxidative stress and apoptosis-related genes in response to West Nile virus. (A) Oxidative stress and apoptosis-related genes mRNA expression in fold change. The ΔΔCt ($\Delta\Delta Ct = \Delta Ct_{WNV} - \Delta Ct_{mock}$) values were calculated by subtracting the ΔCt of genes in mock-inoculated PBMCs ($n = 3$). The bar graph showed the expression of genes in WNV-infected PBMCs over mock-inoculated PBMCs (fold change: the normalized expression value of a gene in WNV-stimulated cells/the normalized expression value of a gene in mock-inoculated cells). Bars without common superscripts (a,b; a,b,c) denote statistical difference of a gene expression among time points ($p < 0.05$). **(B–E)** Relative expression of oxidative stress and apoptosis-related genes mRNA, accounting for the effects of culture conditions on gene transcription in WNV- and mock-inoculated rabbit PBMCs ($n = 3$). To compare the normalized expression of oxidative stress- and apoptosis-related genes from PBMCs harvested at each time point to their respective expression levels before either WNV inoculation or mock inoculation, the ΔΔCt values were calculated by subtracting ΔCt of genes in fresh-isolated PBMCs from the ΔCt of genes in WNV- or mock-inoculated PBMCs at each time-point (for WNV-stimulated PBMCs, $\Delta\Delta Ct_{WNV} = \Delta Ct_{WNV} - \Delta Ct_{fresh}$; and for mock-inoculated PBMCs, $\Delta\Delta Ct_{mock} = \Delta Ct_{mock} - \Delta Ct_{fresh}$). A time-dependent relative expression patterns of **(B)** *HO1*, **(C)** *iNOS*, **(D)** *Caspase 3* and **(E)** *Caspase 9* mRNA in WNV-challenged rabbit PBMCs at different time points. Line graphs without common superscript differ significantly ($p < 0.05$). Upper case letter denotes difference of a gene expression among the time points in WNV-challenged cells; lower case letter denotes difference of a gene expression among the time points in mock-inoculated cells. *indicates the difference of a gene expression between WNV- and mock-challenged cells in the same time point ($p < 0.05$).

2.8-, 3.2-, and 3.5-folds, respectively, higher in PBMCs from the virus-infected rabbits compared to the PBMCs from the control animals (**Figure 7A**). Remarkably, *TLR3* and *IRF7* transcripts were up-regulated by 13 and 44 times, respectively, in PBMCs from $WNV_{NSW2011}$-infected rabbits compared to PBMCs from mock-infected rabbits (**Figure 7B**).

DISCUSSION

The economic burden of non-lethal WNV disease in horses and humans is substantial (37–39). Due to the cost and logistic limitations of using horses for pathogenesis studies, we have recently established an alternative small animal model in laboratory NZW rabbits to study the host-pathogen interactions (25). Tracking changes in the gene expression following viral infection is paramount to understand the host-pathogen interactions including the host-immune responses and pathogenesis. In this study, the expression patterns of selected genes involved in the innate immune response are documented in rabbit blood mononuclear cells following *in vitro* and *in vivo* challenge with an equine-virulent, Australian strain of WNV. The innate immune component includes Toll-like receptors, acute phase proteins, and cytokines expressed by different cell types including blood leukocytes. Among the ten members of the TLR family (TLR1-10), TLR3, 7, 8, and 9 are reported to recognize viral genomic components (40). TLR3 has been associated with the direct recognition of double-stranded viral RNA, while TLR7 and TLR8 target single-stranded viral RNA (40). The involvement of TLR3 (12) and TLR7 (18) have been extensively studied for WNV infection and recognition in mice (15), however, TLR7 and TLR8 are reported to be absent and pseudogenized, respectively, in rabbit (*O. cuniculus*) (41). Furthermore, TLR9 recognizes unmethylated viral-CpG DNA leaving TLR3 the only available TLR for the recognition of viral RNA in the rabbit. In case of WNV infection, peripheral inflammatory responses are initiated through the TLR3 (11, 15). In this study, upregulation of *TLR3* mRNA in *in vitro* virus challenged rabbit PBMCs was detected, suggestive of the involvement of this molecule in the WNV-induced innate immune response.

Although there was only a marginal and transient upregulation of the expression of *MyD88* mRNA under the present culture conditions, a study documented that MyD88 is involved in the restriction and spread of WNV in mice (16). *MyD88*-deficient mice showed elevated viral burden, and increased WNV replication was observed in *MyD88* deficient macrophages and subsets

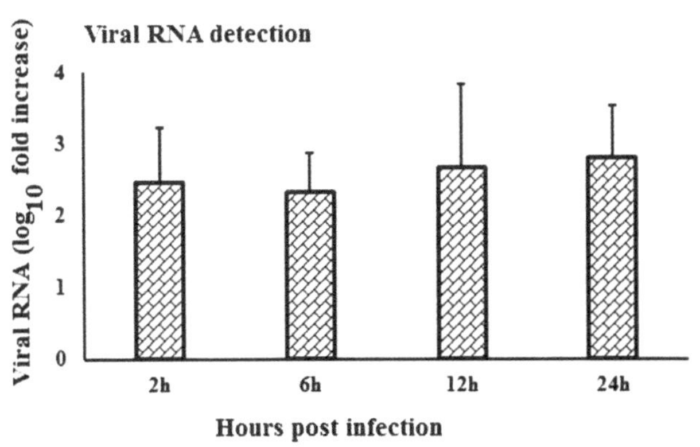

FIGURE 6 | Kinetics of viral RNA expression in *in vitro* WNV-infected PBMCs. $WNV_{NSW2011}$ RNA expression in *in vitro* virus-infected PBMCs at different time points was been quantified using qRT-PCR. The ΔΔCt ($\Delta\Delta Ct = \Delta Ct_{WNV} - \Delta Ct_{mock}$) values were calculated by subtracting the ΔCt of genes in mock-inoculated PBMCs ($n = 3$). Ct for the mock-inoculated PBMCs (undetected) was set to 40. The bar graph showed the expression of genes in WNV-infected PBMCs over mock-inoculated PBMCs (fold change: the normalized expression value of a gene in WNV-stimulated cells/the normalized expression value of a gene in mock-inoculated cells).

of neurons in cell culture [reviewed by Ref. (11)]. This implies that WNV, after being recognized by TLRs, initiates the downstream signaling cascades of the MyD88 and TRAF dependent pathways. Even in the face of some disparity in the utilization of adaptor proteins by different TLRs, their downstream signaling cascades converge on the transcription factor NFκB. TLR engagement initiates rapid signaling events that lead to activation of the transcription factors NFκB and IRF3, and production of cytokines including type I IFNs (11). The upregulation of *IFNA* was only transient in the *in vitro* WNV-stimulated PBMCs compared to mock-inoculated PBMCs. Induction of IFNα genes occurs mainly via the transcriptional activity of IRF7 (11). Recently, over expression of *TLR2*, *TLR3*, *TLR5*, *MyD88*, *STAT1*, *CXCL10*, *IL6*, *IL12*, and *TNFA* has been quantified in various tissues collected from *in vivo* WNV-infected mice (26). Higher mRNA expression of adaptor molecule MyD88, STAT1, TRAF3, IRF7, and 9 is suggestive of the involvement of these molecules in the rabbit PBMCs innate immune response to WNV. STAT1 is the key molecule controlling the course of IFN stimulation and kinetics of ISG expression. The type I IFN response depends on the phosphorylation patterns of STAT1 and is important for the WNV-induced immune response (42). Our results corroborate this, as *STAT1* mRNA increased over time in the *in vitro* WNV-infected rabbit PBMCs. WNV has been reported to block the phosphorylation of STAT1 as a means of immune evasion (11), leading to the blocking of IRF9 expression. However, IRF9 mRNA expression was up-regulated in *in vitro* WNV-stimulated rabbit PBMCs, suggesting that the reported immune evasion mechanisms either do not occur in rabbit PBMCs or at least not under the present culture conditions.

Productive replication of WNV has previously been demonstrated in *in vitro*-infected horse PBMCs by viral growth curve and qRT-PCR for WNV RNA (10). These authors reported that

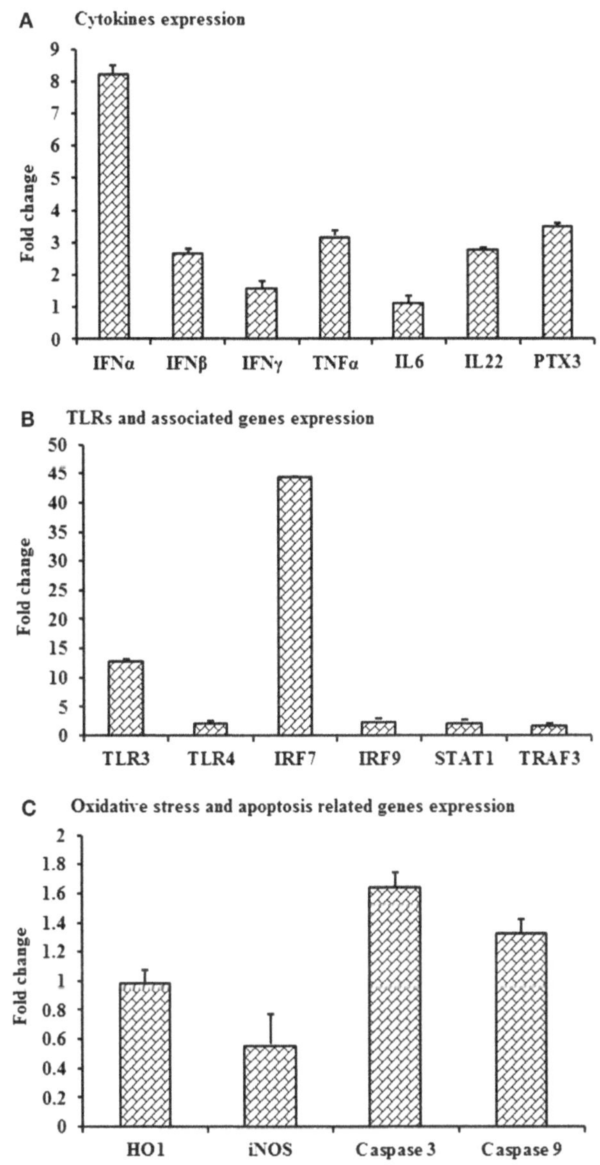

FIGURE 7 | Differential expression of mRNA level of selected immune molecules in *in vivo* WNV-infected rabbits. Expression of **(A)** *IFNA*, *IFNB*, *IFNG*, *TNFA*, *IL6*, *IL22* and *PTX3*, **(B)** *TLR3*, *TLR4*, *IRF7*, *IRF9*, *STAT1*, and *TRAF3*, and **(C)** *HO1*, *iNOS*, *Caspase 3*, and *Caspase 9* mRNA in $WNV_{NSW2011}$-infected rabbit PBMCs at day 3 post-inoculation in fold change. The ΔΔCt ($\Delta\Delta Ct = \Delta Ct_{WNV} - \Delta Ct_{mock}$) values were calculated by subtracting the ΔCt of genes in uninfected control rabbit PBMCs ($n = 3$). The bar graph showed the expression of genes in WNV-infected PBMCs over uninfected control rabbit PBMCs (fold change: the normalized expression value of a gene in *in vivo* WNV-infected rabbit cells/the normalized expression value of a gene in uninfected control rabbit cells). Data are presented as mean ± SD.

peak virus titer was reached at 6-day pi and high titers were maintained through 10- to 15-day pi (10). Rawle et al. (43) compared the growth kinetics of $WNV_{NSW2011}$ and WNV_{NY99} using plaque assay and found that $WNV_{NSW2011}$ did not replicate in human blood monocyte-derived dendritic cells as they extended the experiment from 24- to 72-h pi, whereas WNV_{NY99} successfully replicated in these cells during the entire duration of the experiment. Since other studies (10, 43) did not quantify viral RNA during the first 24-h pi, a comparison to our findings of viral RNA detection is precluded. These differences in growth kinetics in leukocytes between $WNV_{NSW2011}$ and WNV_{NY99} may be ascribed to virus characteristics *sensu stricto* or may be explained by their respective ability to induce protective innate immune responses. In case of *in vivo* NZW rabbit infection, the draining lymph node was found to be the main site for peripheral replication of $WNV_{NSW2011}$ following foodpad inoculation, with peak levels reached on day 3 pi (25). In addition, virus antigen was detected in pleomorphic leukocytes, macrophages, and/or dendritic cells in the paracortical zone of draining popliteal lymph nodes and in the leukocytes in multiple sites of the deep dermis of the injected footpad (25). It is important to note that the present study was limited to 24 h post-*in vitro* stimulation of rabbit PBMCs, as the study aimed to decipher the patterns of early responses of selected genes involved in innate immune response to WNV. Further studies will be required to characterize the virus growth kinetics in rabbit PBMCs over extended time periods but that was beyond the scope of the present study.

Higher expression of IRF7 mRNA *in vitro* stimulation of PBMCs and in PBMCs from rabbits 3 days post-*in vivo* infection is suggestive of its involvement in WNV-induced innate immune responses in the rabbit. TLR3 activation leads to the induction of IRF7 which triggers IRF3 and NFκB to produce IFNs (11). A deficiency of *IRF7* completely abrogated the *IFNα* response while no effect on *IFNB* gene induction was observed in IRF7−/− macrophages in mouse (13). *IFNB* mRNA expression was unaffected in *in vitro* virus-induced PBMCs, which may be explained by the previous findings that *IRF3* and *IRF7* only partially regulate the *IFNB* gene and ISG expression in macrophages (13). The upregulation of *IRF7* and IFNA mRNA expression was significantly higher in *in vitro* WNV-stimulated rabbit PBMCs compared to mock-inoculated PBMCs, suggesting the involvement of these downstream molecules in WNV infection.

Unexpectedly, mRNA expression of *TLR4* and *TLR6*, which recognizes bacterial pathogens, was found to be significantly up-regulated in this study. Antiviral activity of TLR3 and TLR4 has been detected in human microglial cells (44). Single-stranded RNA viruses such as respiratory syncytial virus (RSV) are documented to activate the innate immune response through TLR2 and TLR6 in murine macrophages (45). However, an irregular pattern of *TLR2* expression was found in WNV-stimulated rabbit PBMCs. Nevertheless, this is in agreement with previous studies that demonstrated varying TLR expression in different cell types (46). TLR2 is reported to recognize Epstein–Barr virus (EBV) in human monocyte (47). It is important to note that RSV and EBV are negative sense ssRNA and DNA virus, respectively, whereas WNV is a positive sense ssRNA virus. Recently, upregulation of TLR2 and TLR3 within 1-day pi has been reported in WNV-infected mouse tissues (26), which coincided with our findings in PBMCs.

Recognition of WNV through TLR signaling pathways via MyD88 and TRIF adaptor molecules induced the IRF family and NF-κB genes. NF-κB binds to transcription sites and induces an array of genes that are responsible for production of acute phase proteins, iNOS, coagulation factors, and pro-inflammatory cytokines. Some of the major immune pathways identified to be up-regulated by microarray in the equine brain following experimental WNV infection included the *IL15*, *IL22*, *IL9*, and *IFN* signaling pathways (19), while in mice *IFNB*, *TNFA*, and *IL6* may be key factors (17). In this study, *TNFA* mRNA was up-regulated in *in vitro* WNV-stimulated rabbit PBMCs, suggesting that *TNFA* may be an important component of the WNV-induced innate immune response. Although rabbit PBMCs have not been studied before, the role of macrophages in WNV infection has been reviewed earlier (11). Activation of macrophages in response to WNV infection also promotes the release of type I IFN, TNFA, IL1B, IL8, and other cytokines, thus reducing viral replication in cell culture [reviewed by Ref. (11)]. TNFα is strongly induced by TLR activation and consequently, cellular activation by TNFα could potentially induce TLR gene expression and provide a means for enhancing cellular responsiveness to microbial ligands recognized by those TLRs (40). TNFα mRNA expression was found to be up-regulated over time and peaked at 24-h pi, which is similar to findings by Kwon et al. (48), who found that *TNFA* was significantly up-regulated in horse monocytes 12 and 20 h after challenge with synthetic poly I:C.

IFNG mRNA expression was up-regulated from 6 to 24 h after *in vitro* WNV stimulation of rabbit PBMCs. A dominant protective antiviral role of IFNG against WNV has been documented to occur in peripheral lymphoid tissues (49). A notable difference in the levels of type I and II interferon was reported in the brain in $WNV_{NSW2011}$-infected rabbits, but their expressions were invariable in draining lymph nodes (25). A lack of IFNG production or signaling was reported to increase vulnerability to lethal WNV infection in mice, with a rise in mortality, a decrease in survival time, higher viremia and greater viral replication in lymphoid tissues (49). γδT cells require IFNG to limit the dissemination of WNV and treatment of primary dendritic cells with IFNG-reduced WNV replication (49). However, it remains to be determined which cell subset in the rabbit PBMCs were responsible for the IFNG mRNA expression. *IL22* mRNA was up-regulated over time in rabbit PBMCs in response to *in vitro* WNV stimulation. IL22 is expressed by a wide range of immune cells, including T and NK cells, and engagement of the IL22 receptor leads to STAT3 and STAT1 signaling (50). Notably, relatively high expression of *IL22* mRNA by rabbit PBMCs following *in vivo* infection of the animals may help explain that no viral RNA was detected in their PBMCs at 3-day pi. The expression of *IL22* was consistent with a previous study detecting upregulation of *IL22* mRNA in WNV infected horse lymphoid tissues (19).

PTX3 was one of the most (4.2-folds) up-regulated genes in rabbit PBMCs infected with WNV *in vitro*. Microarray expression analysis showed that *PTX3* was the gene displaying the most pronounced expression in thalamus and cerebrum of horses experimentally infected with WNV (19). PTX3 is a soluble, acute phase protein (soluble pattern recognition receptor; PRMs) and recognizes PAMPs (51). PTX3 is produced by a variety of cells and tissues, most notably dendritic cells and macrophages, in response to TLR engagement and inflammatory cytokines. This molecule has many functions, including an integral role in the pathway of PRRs in recognition of viruses and bacteria (52). The *PTX3* gene is induced by *IL1B* and *TNFA*, and functions in phagocytosis and opsonization of antigens, as well as in the inflammatory response (52). Human and murine PTX3 bound to influenza virus and mediated a range of antiviral activities, including inhibition of hemagglutination, neutralization of virus infectivity, and inhibition of viral neuraminidase (53). The exact role of *PTX3* in WNV-infection remains to be elucidated, but our results suggest a potential antiviral role in some species, notably rabbit (**Figure 2**).

Apoptosis is a highly conserved mode of programed cell death, mediated by the activation of caspases. WNV is reported to induce apoptosis in human brain derived glia cells in culture by the activation of caspase 3, 8, and 9 (54). WNV proteins such as envelope (E) and non-structural protein 3 (NS3) have been shown to induce caspase-dependent apoptosis when transfected into cells (55). Apoptosis is induced through the mitochondrial pathway resulting in caspase 9 and caspase 3 activation in mouse brain cells *in vitro* (55). WNV NS3 induced host cell apoptotic pathways involving caspase 8 and 3 in different cell types (56), but so far there has been no study of caspase expressions either in rabbit or equine PBMCs following WNV infection. Higher expression of *caspase 3* and *9* mRNA both in *in vitro*-infected rabbit PBMCs and in PBMCs from the *in vivo* rabbit model are in accordance with other studies establishing that caspase 3, 8, and 9-dependent apoptosis is involved in WNV infection. It remains to be shown that the rabbit cells proceed to undergo apoptosis following WNV exposure *in vitro*.

HO1 mRNA expression was increased at 12- to 24-h post-WNV infection of PBMCs *in vitro*, whereas iNOS mRNA expression was up-regulated at 6-h pi. In contrast, neither *iNOS* nor *HO1* appeared to be affected in the PBMCs from WNV-infected rabbits. The discrepancy might be due to the time difference between the *in vitro* and the *in vivo* study. Monocytes infiltrating into the brain of mice in WNV-induced encephalitis produced nitric oxide (NO) (57). Macrophages have been reported to control JEV infection directly through the production of NO and other reactive oxygen intermediates (58). Activation of HO1 by a natural substrate, hemin, effectively enhanced the ability of human macrophages to resist infections by several pathogens, including dengue virus, WNV and poxvirus (59). Similarly high expression of *TNFA* and *HO1* might suggest that oxidative stress protects rabbit PBMCs from WNV infection both *in vitro* and *in vivo*.

CONCLUSION

Expression patterns of selected genes involved in the innate immune response to WNV have been documented in this study using rabbit PBMCs as an *in vitro* model. Expression of selected genes was validated in the WNV-infected rabbit *in vivo*. A rabbit model has several advantages over the mouse model, the more commonly used model for WNV, by mimicking the course of infection in the horse better, including viremia, virus distribution, and morbidity. Therefore, the presented data on the genes pivotal in WNV infection in a novel rabbit cell model will help to focus on candidate markers for further study. Specifically, a pan-genomic approach using Next-Generation Sequencing would have yielded much deeper insights into the differential expression in response to WNV.

AUTHOR CONTRIBUTIONS

MU conceived and designed the experiments, performed the experiments, analyzed the data, drafted, and edited the manuscript. WS conceived and designed the experiments, performed the experiments, analyze the data, and edited the manuscript. NP and RH conceived and designed the experiments and edited the manuscript. HB-O conceived and designed the experiments, analyzed the data, drafted, and edited the manuscript.

FUNDING

This study was supported by a grant from the Australian Research Council (ARC-LP120100686; RH, HB-O et al.). MU is supported by a UQ Postdoctoral Fellowship. WS is supported by an Australian Postgraduate Award.

REFERENCES

1. Doherty RL, Carley JG, Mackerras MJ, Marks EN. Studies of arthropod-borne virus infections in Queensland. III. Isolation and characterization of virus strains from wild-caught mosquitoes in North Queensland. *Aust J Exp Biol Med Sci* (1963) **41**:17–39. doi:10.1038/icb.1963.2
2. Hall RA, Broom AK, Smith DW, Mackenzie JS. The ecology and epidemiology of Kunjin virus. *Curr Top Microbiol Immunol* (2002) **267**:253–69. doi:10.1007/978-3-642-59403-8_13
3. Lanciotti RS, Ebel GD, Deubel V, Kerst AJ, Murri S, Meyer R, et al. Complete genome sequences and phylogenetic analysis of West Nile virus strains isolated from the United States, Europe, and the Middle East. *Virology* (2002) **298**(1):96–105. doi:10.1006/viro.2002.1449
4. CDC. West Nile virus disease cases and deaths reported to CDC by year and clinical presentation, 1999–2012. (2012). Available from: http://www.cdc.gov/westnile/resources/pdfs/cummulative/99_2013_CasesAndDeathsClinicalPresentationHumanCases.pdf
5. Bakonyi T, Ferenczi E, Erdelyi K, Kutasi O, Csorgo T, Seidel B, et al. Explosive spread of a neuroinvasive lineage 2 West Nile virus in Central Europe, 2008/2009. *Vet Microbiol* (2013) **165**(1–2):61–70. doi:10.1016/j.vetmic.2013.03.005
6. Petersen LR, Brault AC, Nasci RS. West Nile virus: review of the literature. *JAMA* (2013) **310**(3):308–15. doi:10.1001/jama.2013.8042
7. Frost MJ, Zhang J, Edmonds JH, Prow NA, Gu X, Davis R, et al. Characterization of virulent West Nile virus Kunjin strain, Australia, 2011. *Emerg Infect Dis* (2012) **18**(5):792–800. doi:10.3201/eid1805.111720
8. Prow NA, Hewlett EK, Faddy HM, Coiacetto F, Wang W, Cox T, et al. The Australian public is still vulnerable to emerging virulent strains of West Nile Virus. *Front Public Health* (2014) **2**:146. doi:10.3389/fpubh.2014.00146
9. Prow NA, Tan CS, Wang W, Hobson-Peters J, Kidd L, Barton A, et al. Natural exposure of horses to mosquito-borne flaviviruses in south-east Queensland,

Australia. *Int J Environ Res Public Health* (2013) **10**(9):4432–43. doi:10.3390/ijerph10094432

10. Garcia-Tapia D, Loiacono CM, Kleiboeker SB. Replication of West Nile virus in equine peripheral blood mononuclear cells. *Vet Immunol Immunopathol* (2006) **110**(3–4):229–44. doi:10.1016/j.vetimm.2005.10.003
11. Diamond MS, Gale M Jr. Cell-intrinsic innate immune control of West Nile virus infection. *Trends Immunol* (2012) **33**(10):522–30. doi:10.1016/j.it.2012.05.008
12. Daffis S, Samuel MA, Suthar MS, Gale M Jr, Diamond MS. Toll-like receptor 3 has a protective role against West Nile virus infection. *J Virol* (2008) **82**(21):10349–58. doi:10.1128/JVI.00935-08
13. Daffis S, Samuel MA, Suthar MS, Keller BC, Gale M Jr, Diamond MS. Interferon regulatory factor IRF-7 induces the antiviral alpha interferon response and protects against lethal West Nile virus infection. *J Virol* (2008) **82**(17):8465–75. doi:10.1128/JVI.00918-08
14. Lazear HM, Pinto AK, Vogt MR, Gale M Jr, Diamond MS. Beta interferon controls West Nile virus infection and pathogenesis in mice. *J Virol* (2011) **85**(14):7186–94. doi:10.1128/JVI.00396-11
15. Suthar MS, Diamond MS, Gale M Jr. West Nile virus infection and immunity. *Nat Rev Microbiol* (2013) **11**(2):115–28. doi:10.1038/nrmicro2950
16. Szretter KJ, Daffis S, Patel J, Suthar MS, Klein RS, Gale M Jr, et al. The innate immune adaptor molecule MyD88 restricts West Nile virus replication and spread in neurons of the central nervous system. *J Virol* (2010) **84**(23):12125–38. doi:10.1128/JVI.01026-10
17. Wang T, Town T, Alexopoulou L, Anderson JF, Fikrig E, Flavell RA. Toll-like receptor 3 mediates West Nile virus entry into the brain causing lethal encephalitis. *Nat Med* (2004) **10**(12):1366–73. doi:10.1038/nm1140
18. Welte T, Reagan K, Fang H, Machain-Williams C, Zheng X, Mendell N, et al. Toll-like receptor 7-induced immune response to cutaneous West Nile virus infection. *J Gen Virol* (2009) **90**(Pt 11):2660–8. doi:10.1099/vir.0.011783-0
19. Bourgeois MA, Denslow ND, Seino KS, Barber DS, Long MT. Gene expression analysis in the thalamus and cerebrum of horses experimentally infected with West Nile virus. *PLoS One* (2011) **6**(10):e24371. doi:10.1371/journal.pone.0024371
20. Arjona A, Wang P, Montgomery RR, Fikrig E. Innate immune control of West Nile virus infection. *Cell Microbiol* (2011) **13**(11):1648–58. doi:10.1111/j.1462-5822.2011.01649.x
21. Mestas J, Hughes CC. Of mice and not men: differences between mouse and human immunology. *J Immunol* (2004) **172**(5):2731–8. doi:10.4049/jimmunol.172.5.2731
22. Graham JB, Thomas S, Swarts J, McMillan AA, Ferris MT, Suthar MS, et al. Genetic diversity in the collaborative cross model recapitulates human West Nile virus disease outcomes. *MBio* (2015) **6**(3):e493–415. doi:10.1128/mBio.00493-15
23. Karagianni AE, Kapetanovic R, McGorum BC, Hume DA, Pirie SR. The equine alveolar macrophage: functional and phenotypic comparisons with peritoneal macrophages. *Vet Immunol Immunopathol* (2013) **155**(4):219–28. doi:10.1016/j.vetimm.2013.07.003
24. Bielefeldt-Ohmann H, Prow NA, Wang W, Tan CS, Coyle M, Douma A, et al. Safety and immunogenicity of a delta inulin-adjuvanted inactivated Japanese encephalitis virus vaccine in pregnant mares and foals. *Vet Res* (2014) **45**:130. doi:10.1186/s13567-014-0130-7
25. Suen WW, Uddin MJ, Wang W, Brown V, Adney D, Broad N, et al. Experimental West Nile virus infection in rabbits: an alternative model for studying mechanism of non-lethal meningoencephalitis and virus control. *Pathogens* (2015) **4**(3):529–58. doi:10.3390/pathogens4030529
26. Pena J, Plante JA, Carillo AC, Roberts KK, Smith JK, Juelich TL, et al. Multiplexed digital mRNA profiling of the inflammatory response in the West Nile Swiss Webster mouse model. *PLoS Negl Trop Dis* (2014) **8**(10):e3216. doi:10.1371/journal.pntd.0003216
27. Munoz-Erazo L, Natoli R, Provis JM, Madigan MC, King NJ. Microarray analysis of gene expression in West Nile virus-infected human retinal pigment epithelium. *Mol Vis* (2012) **18**:730–43.
28. Prow NA, Setoh YX, Biron RM, Sester DP, Kim KS, Hobson-Peters J, et al. The West Nile virus-like flavivirus Koutango is highly virulent in mice due to delayed viral clearance and the induction of a poor neutralizing antibody response. *J Virol* (2014) **88**(17):9947–62. doi:10.1128/JVI.01304-14
29. Uddin MJ, Nuro-Gyina PK, Islam MA, Tesfaye D, Tholen E, Looft C, et al. Expression dynamics of Toll-like receptors mRNA and cytokines in porcine peripheral blood mononuclear cells stimulated by bacterial lipopolysaccharide. *Vet Immunol Immunopathol* (2012) **147**(3–4):211–22. doi:10.1016/j.vetimm.2012.04.020
30. Styer LM, Kent KA, Albright RG, Bennett CJ, Kramer LD, Bernard KA. Mosquitoes inoculate high doses of West Nile virus as they probe and feed on live hosts. *PLoS Pathog* (2007) **3**(9):1262–70. doi:10.1371/journal.ppat.0030132
31. Ohmann HB, Gilchrist JE, Babiuk LA. Effect of recombinant DNA-produced bovine interferon alpha (BoIFN-alpha 1) on the interaction between bovine alveolar macrophages and bovine herpesvirus type 1. *J Gen Virol* (1984) **65**(Pt 9):1487–95. doi:10.1099/0022-1317-65-9-1487
32. Rozen S, Skaletsky H. Primer3 on the WWW for general users and for biologist programmers. *Methods Mol Biol* (2000) **132**:365–86.
33. Cinar MU, Islam MA, Proll M, Kocamis H, Tholen E, Tesfaye D, et al. Evaluation of suitable reference genes for gene expression studies in porcine PBMCs in response to LPS and LTA. *BMC Res Notes* (2013) **6**:56. doi:10.1186/1756-0500-6-56
34. Pyke AT, Smith IL, van den Hurk AF, Northill JA, Chuan TF, Westacott AJ, et al. Detection of Australasian Flavivirus encephalitic viruses using rapid fluorogenic TaqMan RT-PCR assays. *J Virol Methods* (2004) **117**(2):161–7. doi:10.1016/j.jviromet.2004.01.007
35. Schnupf P, Sansonetti PJ. Quantitative RT-PCR profiling of the rabbit immune response: assessment of acute *Shigella flexneri* infection. *PLoS One* (2012) **7**(6):e36446. doi:10.1371/journal.pone.0036446
36. Pfaffl MW. A new mathematical model for relative quantification in real-time RT-PCR. *Nucleic Acids Res* (2001) **29**(9):e45. doi:10.1093/nar/29.9.e45
37. Lindsey NP, Staples JE, Lehman JA, Fischer M. Surveillance for human West Nile virus disease – United States, 1999–2008. *MMWR Surveill Summ* (2010) **59**(2):1–17.
38. Nielsen CF, Reisen WK, Armijos MV, Maclachlan NJ, Scott TW. High subclinical West Nile virus incidence among nonvaccinated horses in northern California associated with low vector abundance and infection. *Am J Trop Med Hyg* (2008) **78**(1):45–52.
39. Nolan MS, Schuermann J, Murray KO. West Nile virus infection among humans, Texas, USA, 2002-2011. *Emerg Infect Dis* (2013) **19**(1):137–9. doi:10.3201/eid1901.121135
40. Kawai T, Akira S. Toll-like receptors and their crosstalk with other innate receptors in infection and immunity. *Immunity* (2011) **34**(5):637–50. doi:10.1016/j.immuni.2011.05.006
41. Abrantes J, Areal H, Esteves PJ. Insights into the European rabbit (*Oryctolagus cuniculus*) innate immune system: genetic diversity of the toll-like receptor 3 (TLR3) in wild populations and domestic breeds. *BMC Genet* (2013) **14**:73. doi:10.1186/1471-2156-14-73
42. Perwitasari O, Cho H, Diamond MS, Gale M Jr. Inhibitor of kappaB kinase epsilon (IKK(epsilon)), STAT1, and IFIT2 proteins define novel innate immune effector pathway against West Nile virus infection. *J Biol Chem* (2011) **286**(52):44412–23. doi:10.1074/jbc.M111.285205
43. Rawle DJ, Setoh YX, Edmonds JH, Khromykh AA. Comparison of attenuated and virulent West Nile virus strains in human monocyte-derived dendritic cells as a model of initial human infection. *Virol J* (2015) **12**:46. doi:10.1186/s12985-015-0279-3
44. Suh HS, Zhao ML, Choi N, Belbin TJ, Brosnan CF, Lee SC. TLR3 and TLR4 are innate antiviral immune receptors in human microglia: role of IRF3 in modulating antiviral and inflammatory response in the CNS. *Virology* (2009) **392**(2):246–59. doi:10.1016/j.virol.2009.07.001
45. Murawski MR, Bowen GN, Cerny AM, Anderson LJ, Haynes LM, Tripp RA, et al. Respiratory syncytial virus activates innate immunity through Toll-like receptor 2. *J Virol* (2009) **83**(3):1492–500. doi:10.1128/JVI.00671-08
46. Uddin MJ, Kaewmala K, Tesfaye D, Tholen E, Looft C, Hoelker M, et al. Expression patterns of porcine Toll-like receptors family set of genes (TLR1-10) in gut-associated lymphoid tissues alter with age. *Res Vet Sci* (2013) **95**(1):92–102. doi:10.1016/j.rvsc.2013.01.027
47. Gaudreault E, Fiola S, Olivier M, Gosselin J. Epstein-Barr virus induces MCP-1 secretion by human monocytes via TLR2. *J Virol* (2007) **81**(15):8016–24. doi:10.1128/JVI.00403-07

48. Kwon S, Vandenplas ML, Figueiredo MD, Salter CE, Andrietti AL, Robertson TP, et al. Differential induction of Toll-like receptor gene expression in equine monocytes activated by Toll-like receptor ligands or TNF-alpha. *Vet Immunol Immunopathol* (2010) **138**(3):213–7. doi:10.1016/j.vetimm.2010.07.015
49. Shrestha B, Wang T, Samuel MA, Whitby K, Craft J, Fikrig E, et al. Gamma interferon plays a crucial early antiviral role in protection against West Nile virus infection. *J Virol* (2006) **80**(11):5338–48. doi:10.1128/JVI.00274-06
50. Lejeune D, Dumoutier L, Constantinescu S, Kruijer W, Schuringa JJ, Renauld JC. Interleukin-22 (IL-22) activates the JAK/STAT, ERK, JNK, and p38 MAP kinase pathways in a rat hepatoma cell line. Pathways that are shared with and distinct from IL-10. *J Biol Chem* (2002) **277**(37):33676–82. doi:10.1074/jbc.M204204200
51. Moalli F, Jaillon S, Inforzato A, Sironi M, Bottazzi B, Mantovani A, et al. Pathogen recognition by the long pentraxin PTX3. *J Biomed Biotechnol* (2011) **2011**:830421. doi:10.1155/2011/830421
52. Bottazzi B, Garlanda C, Salvatori G, Jeannin P, Manfredi A, Mantovani A. Pentraxins as a key component of innate immunity. *Curr Opin Immunol* (2006) **18**(1):10–5. doi:10.1016/j.coi.2005.11.009
53. Reading PC, Bozza S, Gilbertson B, Tate M, Moretti S, Job ER, et al. Antiviral activity of the long chain pentraxin PTX3 against influenza viruses. *J Immunol* (2008) **180**(5):3391–8. doi:10.4049/jimmunol.180.5.3391
54. Kleinschmidt MC, Michaelis M, Ogbomo H, Doerr HW, Cinatl J Jr. Inhibition of apoptosis prevents West Nile virus induced cell death. *BMC Microbiol* (2007) **7**:49. doi:10.1186/1471-2180-7-49
55. Yang JS, Ramanathan MP, Muthumani K, Choo AY, Jin SH, Yu QC, et al. Induction of inflammation by West Nile virus capsid through the caspase-9 apoptotic pathway. *Emerg Infect Dis* (2002) **8**(12):1379–84. doi:10.3201/eid0812.020224
56. Ramanathan MP, Chambers JA, Pankhong P, Chattergoon M, Attatippaholkun W, Dang K, et al. Host cell killing by the West Nile Virus NS2B-NS3 proteolytic complex: NS3 alone is sufficient to recruit caspase-8-based apoptotic pathway. *Virology* (2006) **345**(1):56–72. doi:10.1016/j.virol.2005.08.043
57. Getts DR, Terry RL, Getts MT, Muller M, Rana S, Deffrasnes C, et al. Targeted blockade in lethal West Nile virus encephalitis indicates a crucial role for very late antigen (VLA)-4-dependent recruitment of nitric oxide-producing macrophages. *J Neuroinflammation* (2012) **9**:246. doi:10.1186/1742-2094-9-246
58. Saxena SK, Singh A, Mathur A. Antiviral effect of nitric oxide during Japanese Encephalitis virus infection. *Int J Exp Pathol* (2000) **81**(2):165–72. doi:10.1046/j.1365-2613.2000.00148.x
59. Dhawan S. Heme oxygenase-1 induction stimulates host defense mechanism against infections. *J Immunol* (2011) **186**:110.113.

Conflict of Interest Statement: All authors read and approved the final manuscript. The authors declare that they have no competing interests.

16

Iron and ferritin levels in the serum and milk of bovine leukemia virus-infected dairy cows

Star A. Schnell[1], Hiromichi Ohtsuka[2], Seiichi Kakinuma[3], Yasunaga Yoshikawa[1], Kiyotaka Watanabe[1] and Koichi Orino[1]*

[1] Laboratory of Veterinary Biochemistry, School of Veterinary Medicine, Kitasato University, Towada, Japan, [2] Large Animal Clinical Sciences, School of Veterinary Medicine, Rakuno Gakuen University, Ebetsu, Japan, [3] Kakinuma Veterinary Hospital, Honjou, Japan

Iron metabolism was examined in 15 bovine leukemia virus (BLV)-infected dairy cows (2.6–7.8 years old). BLV infection was detected by measuring serum antibody titer against BLV virus antigen (gp51). The anti-BLV antibody titers of the BLV-infected cows were significantly higher in serum than in milk; a single serum-positive animal lacked detectable anti-BLV antibodies in its milk. Iron and ferritin concentrations also were significantly higher in serum than in milk. Although most of the BLV-infected dairy cows had past or present anamneses (such as inflammatory diseases, including intramammary infection), the milk ferritin concentrations of the infected cows were significantly lower than those of normal cows; serum ferritin concentrations did not differ significantly between these two groups. The anti-BLV antibody titers in milk samples showed significant correlation with serum iron concentrations. These results suggest that BLV infection affects iron homeostasis through iron metabolism in the dairy cow mammary gland.

Keywords: bovine leukemia virus, dairy cow, iron, milk, serum

Edited by:
Nobuko Mori, Nippon Veterinary and Life Science University, Japan

Reviewed by:
Gebin Li, China Agricultural University, China
Takeshi Ohkubo, Ibaraki University, Japan

****Correspondence:***
Koichi Orino, Laboratory of Veterinary Biochemistry, School of Veterinary Medicine, Kitasato University, 23-35-1 Higashi, Towada, Aomori 034-8628, Japan
orino@vmas.kitasato-u.ac.jp

Introduction

Bovine leukosis is classified into two types: sporadic bovine leukosis (SBL, characterized by T-cell leukosis) and enzootic bovine leukosis (EBL, characterized by B-cell leukosis) (1–5). EBL, which occurs at a much higher frequency than SBL, and is an infectious disease caused by bovine leukemia virus (BLV) (4). This virus belongs to the genus *Deltaretrovirus* in the family *Retreviridae* (1, 3). BLV infection affects cellular functions in transcription, translation, RNA processing, signal transduction, cell growth, apoptosis, stress response, and immune response (3, 6–12). BLV is a unique retrovirus related to human T-cell leukemia virus type 1 (HTLV-1), which is a causative agent of adult T-cell leukemia (1, 13). In the BLV and HTLV-1 systems, cell transformation may be the result of the expression of the Tax protein (5, 6, 13). Molecular understanding of the leukemogenesis induced by BLV infection may provide insights for the development of novel and effective antiretroviral therapeutics applicable for HTLV (1).

Bovine leukemia virus infection is frequently asymptomatic; in many cases, infected animals remain virus carriers for life without exhibiting signs of infection (1, 13). Approximately 30% of infected cattle develop persistent lymphocytosis (PL), which is characterized by permanent and relatively stable increases in the number of B lymphocytes in the peripheral blood while resulting in fatal leukemia or lymphoma in fewer than 5% of the infected cows (5, 6). BLV is transmitted horizontally through transfer of biological fluids contaminated with BLV-infected B-lymphocytes, such as inappropriate re-use of needles and gloves for rectal examination; through milk; and possibly via insect bites (1, 5). BLV-infected cows with subclinical mastitis may be sources of infectious transmission, since these animals produce milk that contains BLV-infected lymphocytes (14, 15).

Serum ferritin is the best indicator for estimating body iron stores, whereas serum ferritin provides a marker for malignant and inflammatory conditions (16). Significantly higher serum ferritin levels were observed in leukemic cows compared to normal animals (17). Although BLV-infected dairy cow may appear healthy, BLV infection may cause economic loss in cattle production and export (1, 3, 5, 18). Although the association between BLV infection and mastitis in dairy cows remains controversial (14, 15, 19), BLV infection is believed to induce mastitis due to the virus' immunosuppressive effects (14). Additionally, serum iron levels are decreased in animals suffering from inflammatory diseases, an effect that results from IL-6 mediated hypoferremia (20). By contrast, serum ferritin can be an inflammatory marker of acute-phase infection, although elevated serum ferritin levels can lead to misdiagnosis of anemia (21). Furthermore, milk ferritin levels are increased in response to intramammary infection (22).

Despite this previous work in bovids, iron metabolism of BLV-infected dairy cows has not been studied. There is still controversial in the relation between BLV-infection and mastitis (14, 15, 19). Serum ferritin may be indicator of BLV infection stage as in tumor marker (23). The purpose of this study was to elucidate the effect of BLV infection on iron metabolism in dairy cows.

Materials and Methods

Chemicals

Bovine leukemia antibody test kit was purchased from Japan New Chisso Corp., Tokyo, Japan. Ferrozine was purchased from Sigma (St. Louis, MO, USA). Immuno Plate Maxisorp F96, Alkaline phosphatase (ALP)-conjugated NeutrAvidin, and EZ-link™ sulfo-NHS-biotin were purchased from Thermo Fisher Scientific (Waltham, MA, USA). Other reagents used were of analytical grade. Pure water (Elix water) was produced from tap water using an Elix Advantage Water Purification System (Millipore, Billerica, MA, USA).

Blood and Milk from BLV-Infected Dairy Cows

Peripheral blood samples were collected from the jugular veins of dairy cows on dairy farms maintained in the Saitama prefecture of Japan. All cows including normal dairy cows more than 2 years old were reared to the Japanese feeding standard for dairy cattle but at different sampling date. Following recovery from centrifuged coagulated blood, serum was stored at −20°C in the presence of 0.1% sodium azide until analysis. Serum samples were assessed for the presence anti-BLV antibody by ELISA kit. ELISA titers (S/P values) were calculated as follows: Absorbances (at 405 nm; A_{405}) were determined per the kit instructions and corrected by subtracting background (A_{405} for reaction wells not coated with antigen). Corrected A_{405} values for experimental samples were normalized against corrected A_{405} values for the positive control (hence S/P). BLV-infected cows were identified based on ELISA titers (S/P values) over 0.3. Milk samples also were collected from the respective cows, and were defatted by centrifugation prior to ELISA testing.

All experiments were conducted following the established guidelines for animal welfare and were approved by the Committee on the Ethics of Animal Experiments of Kitasato University (Permit Number: 14-027).

Iron Measurement

Serum and milk samples were diluted twofold with Elix water, and (for each sample) a 150-μL aliquot was mixed with an equal volume of a solution of a reducing and iron-dissolving reagent (2 M thioglycolate, 2 M HCl, and 10% (w/w) trichloroacetic acid). The mixture was kept at room temperature for 15 min followed by a centrifugation at 16,000 × *g* for 15 min. Each resulting supernatant (150 μL) was neutralized by addition of 150 μL of neutralizing reagent [30% (w/w) sodium acetate], followed by addition of 15 μL of 10 mM ferrozine solution as a chromogen reagent. After incubation for 30 min, the absorbance of the mixture in each well was measured using a spectrophotometer at a wavelength of 562 nm. Iron concentration was determined using the molar extinction coefficient (εmM = 27.9) of the ferrous ferrozine complex at 562 nm (24).

Ferritin Preparation and Antibodies to Ferritin

Bovine spleen was collected at slaughterhouse and frozen for the preparation of ferritin until use. Bovine spleen ferritin was purified from the frozen spleen according to the previously described method (25). Rabbit antiserum to bovine spleen ferritin was prepared and partially purified by affinity chromatography as described previously (25). A portion of the affinity-purified antibody to the bovine spleen ferritin was biotinylated with EZ-link™ sulfo-NHS-biotin according to manufacturer's instructions.

Ferritin Measurement

Ferritin in serum and defatted milk samples was measured by sandwich ELISA according to a previously described method (22, 25). Briefly, anti-bovine spleen ferritin antibody (100 μL at 200 ng/mL) in phosphate buffered-saline (PBS: 150 mM NaCl, 20 mM sodium phosphate, pH 7.2) was added to each well of a microtiter plate. After wells were washed with PBS containing 0.5% Tween 20 (PBST), a 300-μL aliquot of ELISA buffer (PBS containing 0.1% Tween 20 and 0.1% gelatin, pH 7.2) was added to each well, and the plate was held at room temperature for 1 h to block non-specific adsorption of ferritin protein with gelatin. Following another wash with PBST, 100-μL aliquots of bovine spleen ferritin standards (0.156–10 ng/mL) in ELISA buffer containing 0.5 M $(NH_4)_2SO_4$ were added, and the plate was incubated at 37°C for 2 h. Serum and milk samples were diluted 6- or 10-fold with the same buffer used to prepare the standard solution. The diluted milk sample was heat-treated at 60°C for 20 min followed by centrifugation at 14,000 × *g* for 15 min, and the resulting supernatant was used to determine the ferritin concentration as previously described (22). Aliquots (100 μL) of serum samples and heat-treated milk samples were pipetted to wells of the plate along with the ferritin standard series. After washing with PBST, 100 μL of biotinylated rabbit anti-bovine spleen ferritin antibody (125 ng/mL) diluted in ELISA buffer was added to each well, and

TABLE 1 | Age, anamnesis, and ferritin and iron concentrations, and S/P value in serum and milk of BLV-i nfected dairy cows.

Sample no.	Age (year)	Anamnesis	Serum			Milk		
			S/P	Fe (ppm)	Ferritin (ng/mL)	S/P	Fe (ppm)	Ferritin (ng/mL)
1	2.6		1.5	1.4	16	0.3	0.14	1.7
2	2.8		1.7	1.3	54	0.1	0.07	4.9
3	3.5	Injury of parturient canal	2.2	1.6	37	0.8	0.39	1.6
4	3.7	Mastitis	2.7	2.6	23	1.8	0.07	0.8
5	3.8	Mastitis	2.3	1.4	42	1.4	0.35	5.7
6	4.0	Mastitis	2.0	1.9	53	1.2	0.12	13.8
7	4.0	Ketosis, pneumonia	2.8	1.2	42	0.7	0.10	1.3
8	4.2	Mastitis	2.4	1.2	28	1.1	0.24	2.9
9	4.8	Mastitis	2.3	1.2	32	1.1	0.14	1.8
10	4.9	Mastitis, dystocia	2.3	1.8	20	1.4	0.20	1.4
11	5.4	Abomasal displacement, pneumothorax	2.3	2.0	57	0.9	0.20	1.6
12	5.5	Mastitis, ketosis	2.3	1.4	39	NT	NT	1.2
13	5.7	Bronchitis	2.8	1.5	62	0.8	0.14	1.0
14	7.4	Dystocia, abomasal displacement	2.2	0.2	53	0.4	0.06	2.3
15	7.8	Mastitis	2.3	1.0	39	1.1	0.41	3.0
Mean ± SD	4.7 ± 1.5		2.3 ± 0.1	1.5 ± 0.5	40 ± 14	0.9 ± 0.5**	0.2 ± 0.1*	3.1 ± 3.4**

** and **: P < 0.01 and P < 0.001; significantly different from serum samples, respectively.*
NT: not tested.

the plate was incubated at 37°C for 1.5 h. After washing, 100 μL of ALP-conjugated NeutrAvidin (1 μg/mL) diluted in ELISA buffer was added to each well, and the plate was incubated at 37°C for 1.5 h. After washing, the ALP enzyme reaction was carried out using disodium *p*-nitrophenyl phosphate as previously described (25). The concentration of *p*-nitrophenol produced by the ALP reaction was determined by measuring the absorbance at 405 nm.

Statistical Analysis

All data obtained are presented as mean ± SD. The statistical significance of the differences in means between two groups was determined by Student's *t*-test according to the distribution of data. A *P*-value <0.05 was considered significant for all tests.

Results

Effect of BLV Infection on Iron Metabolism in Dairy Cows

In this study, 15 BLV-infected dairy cows were selected according to the criteria of antibody titer against gp51 protein by ELISA kit. The antibody to gp51 antigen also was detected in the 13 milk samples, all but one of the cows that were BLV-positive by serum criteria. The antibody titers in the milk specimens were significantly lower ($P < 0.001$) than those in the sera of the BLV-positive cows (**Table 1**). The iron and ferritin concentrations in the milk of these cows also were significantly lower than the respective values in the sera ($P < 0.01$ and $P < 0.001$ in the iron and ferritin concentrations, respectively). The only significant correlation observed was that between serum iron concentration and milk S/P value (**Figure 1**). No significant difference was observed in serum ferritin concentrations between BLV-infected dairy cows (40 ± 14 ng/mL; $n = 15$) and normal dairy cows older than 2 years of age (37 ± 5 ng/mL; $n = 20$). By contrast, milk ferritin concentrations of BLV-infected cows (3.1 ± 3.4 ng/mL; $n = 14$) were significantly lower than those of normal dairy cows (7.2 ± 5.0 ng/mL; $n = 17$) (**Table 1; Figure 2**).

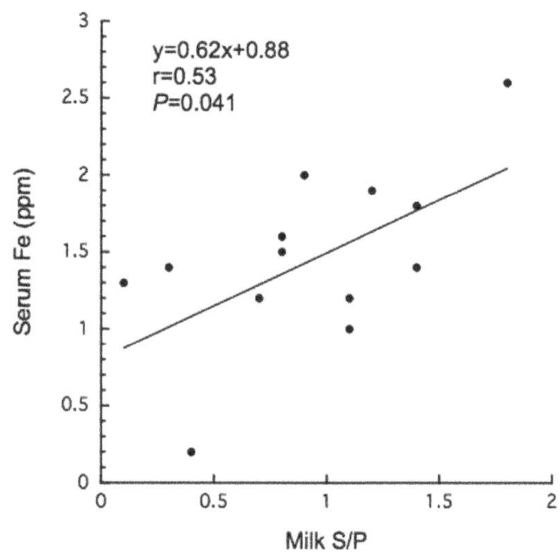

FIGURE 1 | Significant correlation between serum iron concentration and milk S/P value in BLV-infected dairy cows.

Discussion

Bovine leukemia virus -infected cows often remain asymptomatic or aleukemic, presumably following establishment of proviral infection (1, 5, 6). Only one-third of infected cattle develop PL, a polyclonal expansion of B lymphocytes coexpressing CD5, high levels of surface immunoglobulin M (sIgM), and myeloid markers (1, 5–7). In the present study, antibodies to BLV antigen (gp51) were detected in all but one of the milk samples obtained from animals that were BLV-positive by serum titers. Notably, however, antibody titers in the milk of these cows were significantly lower

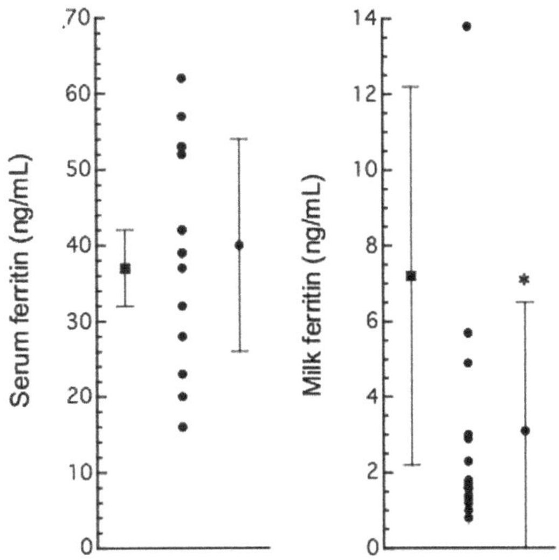

FIGURE 2 | Serum and milk ferritin concentrations in normal (solid boxes) and BLV-infected (solid circles) dairy cows. Serum ($n = 20$) and milk ($n = 15$) ferritin concentrations are presented as mean ± SD from non-pregnant cows over 2 years old. Serum and milk ferritin concentrations are plotted as data from individual animals; vertical bars indicate mean ± SD (from **Table 1**). *: $P < 0.05$, compared to normal cows.

than those in the respective sera. BLV particles may be found in the mammary glands of cows with subclinical mastitis (3, 15). Moreover, the presence of BLV proteins in the bovine milk exosome has been reported to correlate with the presence of anti-BLV antibodies in the milk (26). BLV-infected cows may release BLV particles or BLV proteins via the milk, providing a potential mechanism of BLV transmission. However, further studies will be needed to determine whether anti-BLV antibodies in the milk are sufficient to neutralize BLV particles and so prevent transmission via this biological fluid.

Bovine leukemia virus infection also has been shown to alter the expression of cytokines such as IL-2, IL-6, IL-10, and IL-12 (1). IL-6 may play a contributory role in viral latency due to the elevation of its level in blood circulation (1). IL-6 mediates hypoferremia of inflammation by the reduction of hepcidin, which in turn causes a decrease in intestinal iron absorption and the release of iron from macrophages (20). Most BLV-infected dairy cows exhibit past and present anamnesis, including inflammatory disease such as intrammamary disease. Although BLV infection may affect immune response to pathological agents due to immunosuppressive effects (1), it remains unclear how BLV provirus infection is associated with other pathological conditions. However, reports of an association between BLV infection and mastitis remain controversial (14, 15, 19). Previous reports indicated that zinc and iron levels in milk were significantly higher in California Mastitis Test-positive cows than in normal ones (27). BLV infection may activate cytokine receptor as well as B-cell growth cytokine (IL-4, IL-6, and IL-10) (11). On the other hand, in the comparison with previous report (28, 29), we failed to detect a significant difference in serum or milk iron concentrations when comparing between BLV-infected and normal dairy cows. Taken together, mammary gland is likely to affect systemic iron homeostasis for unknown reason. High ferritin levels were found in the sera of cows with leukemia (17). In humans, ferritin can be tumor marker and factors to monitor the effectiveness of treatment (23). However, it is unlikely to lead to the increase of serum ferritin when transformation does not occur. Interestingly, in the present study, milk ferritin levels were decreased in BLV-infected cows, even though the infected cows displayed inflammatory conditions (e.g., intramammary infection). This work also suggested the existence of a positive correlation between serum iron concentration and milk S/P value (**Figure 1**). Although the secretory mechanism of milk ferritin and iron in mammary gland remains to be resolved for individual viral stages, mammary gland infection by BLV appears to affect systemic iron homeostasis, seemingly independent of inflammatory condition, as described above.

Bovine leukemia virus infection can cause immune suppression in affected animals through multiple mechanisms (18). The results of this study suggest that BLV provirus infection also may disrupt iron metabolism. Further study will be needed to elucidate the relationship of iron metabolism between the whole body and the mammary gland.

References

1. Gillet N, Florins A, Boxus M, Burteau C, Nigro A, Vandermeers F, et al. Mechanisms of leukemogenesis induced by bovine leukemia virus: prospects for novel anti-retroviral therapies in human. *Retrovirology* (2007) **4**:18. doi:10.1186/1742-4690-4-18
2. Ishiguro N, Matsui T, Shinagawa M. Differentiation analysis of bovine T-lymphosarcoma. *Vet Immunol Immunopathol* (1994) **41**:1–17. doi:10.1016/0165-2427(94)90053-1
3. Kettmann R, Burny A, Callebaut I, Droogmans L, Mammerikx M, Willems L, et al. Bovine leukemia virus. In: Levy JA, editor. *The Retroviridae*. (Vol. 3), New York, NY: Plenum Press (1994). p. 39–81.
4. Onuma M, Honma T, Mikami T. Studies on the sporadic and enzootic forms of bovine leucosis. *J Comp Pathol* (1979) **89**:159–67. doi:10.1016/0021-9975(79)90055-0
5. Schwartz I, Levy D. Pathobiology of bovine leukemia virus. *Vet Res* (1994) **25**:521–36.
6. Aida Y, Murakami H, Takahashi M, Takeshima S-H. Mechanisms of pathogenesis induced by bovine leukemia virus as a model for human T-cell leukemia virus. *Front Microbiol* (2013) **4**:1–11. doi:10.3389/fmicb.2013.00328
7. Cantor GH, Pritchard SM, Dequiedt F, Willems L, Kettmann R, Davis WC. CD5 is dissociated from the B-cell receptor-mediated apoptosis. *J Virol* (2001) **75**:1689–96. doi:10.1128/JVI.75.4.1689-1696.2001
8. Connor TJ, Leonard BE. Depression, stress and immunological activation: the role of cytokines in depressive disorders. *Life Sci* (1998) **65**:583–606. doi:10.1016/S0024-3205(97)00990-9
9. Dequiedt F, Cantor GH, Hamilton VT, Pritchard SM, Davis WC, Kerkhofs P, et al. Bovine leukemia virus-induced persistent lymphocytosis in cattle does not correlate with increased *ex vivo* survival of B lymphocytes. *J Virol* (1999) **73**:1127–37.
10. Derse D. trans-acting regulation of bovine leukemia virus mRNA processing. *J Virol* (1988) **62**:1115–9.
11. Keefe RG, Choi Y, Ferrick DA, Stott JL. Bovine cytokine expression during different phases of bovine leukemia virus infection. *Vet Immunol Immunopathol* (1997) **56**:39–51. doi:10.1016/S0165-2427(96)05727-3
12. Yacobson B, Brenner J, Ungar-Waron H, Trainin Z. Short-termed expression of interleukin-12 during experimental BLV infection may direct disease

progression to persistent lymphocytosis. *Vet Immunol Immunopathol* (1998) **64**:207–18. doi:10.1016/S0165-2427(98)00136-6

13. Burny A, Cleuter T, Kettmann R, Mammerickx G, Marbaix G, Portetelle D, et al. Bovine leukemia: facts and hypotheses derived from the study of an infectious cancer. *Vet Microbiol* (1988) **17**:197–218. doi:10.1016/0378-1135(88)90066-1
14. Wellenberg GJ, van der Poel WHM, Oirschot V. Viral infections and bovine mastitis: a review. *Vet Microbiol* (2002) **88**:27–45. doi:10.1016/S0378-1135(02)00098-6
15. Yoshikawa H, Xie B, Oyamada T, Hiraga A, Yoshikawa T. Infection of bovine leukemia virus (BLV) in mammary tissues of BLV-antibody positive cows affected by subclinical mastitis. *J Vet Med Sci* (1997) **59**:301–301. doi:10.1292/jvms.59.301
16. Orino K, Watanabe K. Molecular, physiological and clinical aspects of the iron storage protein ferritin. *Vet J* (2008) **178**:191–201. doi:10.1016/j.tvjl.2007.07.006
17. Orino K. Biochemical studies on bovine ferritin. *Jpn J Vet Res* (1998) **46**:96–7.
18. Frie MC, Coussens PM. Bovine leukemia virus: a major silent threat to proper immune responses in cattle. *Vet Immunol Immunopathol* (2015) **153**:103–14. doi:10.1016/j.vetimm.2014.11.014
19. Fetrow J, Ferrer JF. Bovine leukemia virus infection and mastitis. *J Dairy Sci* (1981) **65**:881–2. doi:10.3168/jds.S0022-0302(82)82282-0
20. Nemeth E, Rivera S, Gabayan V, Keller C, Taudorf S, Pedersen BK, et al. IL-6 mediates hypoferremia of inflammation by inducing the synthesis of the iron regulatory hormone hepcidin. *J Clin Invest* (2014) **113**:1271–8. doi:10.1172/JCI200420945
21. Lorrier MA, Herron JL, Carrell RW. Detecting iron deficiency by serum tests. *Clin Chem* (1985) **31**:337–8.
22. Orino K, Watanabe S, Ohtsuka H, Kohiruimaki M, Watanabe K. Measurement of ferritin in bovine milk and its clinical significance. *J Dairy Sci* (2006) **89**:3842–5. doi:10.3168/jds.S0022-0302(06)72426-2
23. Akanni EO, Mabayoje VO, Oseni BSA, Ajani OO. C-reactive protein and tumor marker (ferritin) levels in chronic myeloid leukaemia patients. *Am Eurasian J Sci Res* (2010) **5**:31–8.
24. Stookey LL. Ferrozine-a new spectrophotometric reagent for iron. *Anal Chem* (1970) **42**:779–81. doi:10.1021/ac60289a016
25. Orino K, Ishiji T, Yamamoto S, Watanabe K. Characterization of bovine serum ferritin-binding proteins. *Comp Biochem Physiol* (2004) **137A**:375–81. doi:10.1016/j.cbpb.2003.10.018
26. Yamada T, Shigemura H, Ishiguro N, Inoshima Y. Cell infectivity in relation to bovine leukemia virus gp51 and p24 in bovine milk exosomes. *PLoS One* (2013) **8**:e7359. doi:10.1371/journal.pone.0077359
27. Yirdiz H, Kaygusuzoglu E. Investigation of Ca, Zn, Mg, Fe, and Cu concentrations in blood and milk of cows with negative and positive CMT results. *Bull Vet Inst Pulawy* (2005) **49**:209–13.
28. Oliveira MAA, Osorio MM. Cow's milk consumption and iron deficiency anemia in children. *J Pediatr (Rio J)* (2005) **81**:361–7. doi:10.1590/S0021-75572005000600004
29. Senturk S, Metcitoglu Z, Ulgen M, Borum E, Temiziel E, Kasap S. Evaluation of serum iron and iron binding capacity in cows with paratuberculosis. *Tierarztl Prax Ausg G Grosstiere Nutztiere* (2009) **37**:375–8.

Conflict of Interest Statement: The authors declare that the research was conducted in the absence of any commercial or financial relationships that could be construed as a potential conflict of interest.

17

Selection of *Bacillus* spp. for cellulase and xylanase production as direct-fed microbials to reduce digesta viscosity and *Clostridium perfringens* proliferation using an *in vitro* digestive model in different poultry diets

Edited by:
Ryan Arsenault,
University of Delaware, USA

Reviewed by:
Jason Kindrachuk,
Frederick Integrated Research Facility, USA
Ramesh Selvaraj,
Ohio Agricultural Research and Development Center, USA

***Correspondence:**
Guillermo Tellez,
Department of Poultry Science,
Center of Excellence for Poultry Science, University of Arkansas,
1260 West Maple, POSC 0-114,
Fayetteville, AR 72701, USA
gtellez@uark.edu

Juan D. Latorre[1], Xochitl Hernandez-Velasco[2], Vivek A. Kuttappan[1], Ross E. Wolfenden[3], Jose L. Vicente[3], Amanda D. Wolfenden[1], Lisa R. Bielke[1], Omar F. Prado-Rebolledo[4], Eduardo Morales[5], Billy M. Hargis[1] and Guillermo Tellez[1]*

[1] Department of Poultry Science, University of Arkansas, Fayetteville, AR, USA, [2] Departamento de Medicina y Zootecnia de Aves, Facultad de Medicina Veterinaria y Zootecnia, Universidad Nacional Autonoma de Mexico, Mexico City, Mexico, [3] Pacific Vet Group-USA, Inc., Fayetteville, AR, USA, [4] Facultad de Medicina Veterinaria y Zootecnia, Universidad de Colima, Colima, Mexico, [5] Departamento de Produccion Agricola y Animal, Universidad Autonoma Metropolitana, Mexico City, Mexico

Previously, our laboratory has screened and identified *Bacillus* spp. isolates as direct-fed microbials (DFM). The purpose of the present study was to evaluate the cellulase and xylanase production of these isolates and select the most appropriate *Bacillus* spp. candidates for DFM. Furthermore, an *in vitro* digestive model, simulating different compartments of the gastrointestinal tract, was used to determine the effect of these selected candidates on digesta viscosity and *Clostridium perfringens* proliferation in different poultry diets. Production of cellulase and xylanase were based on their relative enzyme activity. Analysis of 16S rRNA sequence classified two strains as *Bacillus amyloliquefaciens* and one of the strains as *Bacillus subtilis*. The DFM was included at a concentration of 10^8 spores/g of feed in five different sterile soybean-based diets containing corn, wheat, rye, barley, or oat. After digestion time, supernatants from different diets were collected to measure viscosity, and *C. perfringens* proliferation. Additionally, from each *in vitro* simulated compartment, samples were taken to enumerate viable *Bacillus* spores using a plate count method after heat-treatment. Significant ($P < 0.05$) DFM-associated reductions in supernatant viscosity and *C. perfringens* proliferation were observed for all non-corn diets. These results suggest that antinutritional factors, such as non-starch polysaccharides from different cereals, can enhance viscosity and *C. perfringens* growth. Remarkably, dietary inclusion of the DFM that produce cellulase and xylanase reduced both viscosity and *C. perfringens* proliferation compared with control diets. Regardless of diet composition, 90% of the DFM spores germinated during the first 30 min in the crop compartment of the digestion model, followed by a noteworthy increased in the intestine compartment by ~$2\log_{10}$, suggesting a full-life cycle development. Further studies to evaluate *in vivo* necrotic enteritis effects are in progress.

Keywords: *Clostridium perfringens*, *Bacillus*-DFM, spore, enzymes, viscosity

Introduction

Necrotic enteritis (NE) in broilers is a multi-factorial disease with severe economic implications (1). It is caused by type A strains of *Clostridium perfringens* that are specific to poultry with toxin types alpha and NetB (2, 3). Coccidia infections are the most common pre-requisite for NE to occur (4), however, dysbacteriosis associated with diet ingredients, changes in feed ration, immunosuppression, *Salmonella* infections, and/or removal of the use of quimioterapeutics are known to predispose birds to NE (1–5). Antibiotic growth promoters (AGPs) are commonly used to mitigate the incidence of enteric diseases, such as NE. Nevertheless, concerns regarding the development of antibiotic-resistant microorganisms and social pressures have led to a tendency to ban AGPs in poultry production (6). In this scenario, there is an imperative necessity to find feasible alternatives for AGPs to maintain poultry health (7). In fact, the use of selected strains of various beneficial microorganisms from the genus *Bacillus* and *Lactobacillus* have shown to be a suitable option for the poultry industry (8). *Bacillus* spp. are Gram-positive, aerobe, motile, and usually found in soil and water sources, as well as in the gastrointestinal tract of animals and humans (9). Different *Bacillus* spp. have already been studied and extensively used as a source of industrial enzymes as well as antibiotics by biotechnology companies (10). However, the production of most of these enzymes depends on the intense metabolic changes associated with environmental conditions (11–13). During extreme environmental conditions, vegetative cells of *Bacillus* spp. form endospores, which are considered, the toughest way of life on Earth (14).

The use of spores from selected *Bacillus* strains, as direct-fed microbials (DFM), are shown to have the capacity to germinate and sporulate in the gastrointestinal tract of different animal species including poultry. Thus, they become metabolically active *in vivo*, imparting numerous nutritional benefits including the production of extracellular enzymes, such as protease, lipase, cellulase, xylanase, phytase, and keratinase (15, 16), and other chemical compounds beneficial for the host (17).

In most of the USA and other countries, including Brazil, broiler feed is based primarily on corn and soybean meal. However, sometimes it is difficult to formulate least-cost diets using corn. Consequently, other cereals or ethanol by-products with variable concentrations of antinutritional factors are used as alternatives. When chickens are fed alternative grains with high levels of non-starch polysaccharides (NSP), an increase in digesta viscosity, poor nutrient digestibility, reduced bone mineralization, and occurrence of enteric diseases, such as NE, have been reported (18, 19). Hence, utilization of these feedstuffs in poultry diets usually result in decreased growth performance, intestinal dysbacteriosis, and detrimental litter conditions caused by sticky droppings (20, 21). For that reason, the inclusion of enzymes, such as carbohydrases, is a routine practice in poultry diets that contain grains with elevated NSP concentration values in comparison to corn (22, 23). However, there are inconveniences related to dietary inclusion of some enzymes, due to denaturation and lost of activity under high-pelletization temperatures commonly used in poultry rations. Therefore, the objective of the present study was to perform a selection of *Bacillus* spp. for cellulase and xylanase production as DFM, and evaluate them on digesta viscosity and *C. perfringens* proliferation in different poultry diets using an *in vitro* digestive model. The practical implication of the results will be to utilize cost-effective alternative grains in poultry feed formulation, and at the same time improve digestibility as well as production performance in birds using a more thermostable DFM product.

Materials and Methods

Diets

Five mash soybean-based broiler grower diets containing different cereals, such as corn, wheat, rye, barley, or oat, were used as substrate for bacterial growth during the *in vitro* digestive model. Experimental diets were formulated to approximate the nutritional requirements of broiler chickens as recommended by the NRC (24), and adjusted to breeder's recommendations (25). No antibiotics, coccidiostats, or enzymes were added to the feed (**Table 1**). All diets were autoclaved and confirmed negative for *Bacillus* spp. spores. Later, these diets were inoculated with the respective spores (10^8 spores/g of feed) of the *Bacillus*-DFM candidate according to various treatments.

In Vitro Assessment of Cellulase and Xylanase Production

Previous research conducted in our laboratory focused on isolation of several *Bacillus* spp. from environmental and poultry sources (26, 27). Isolates were then screened for production of cellulase and xylanase. For evaluation of cellulase activity, the cellulose-Congo red agar was used and consisted of 0.50 g of K_2HPO_4 (Fisher Scientific, San Francisco, CA, USA), 0.25 g of $MgSO_4$ (Sigma Chemical Co, St. Louis, MO, USA), 1.88 g of ashed, acid-washed cellulose powder (J. T. Baker Chemical Inc, Phillipsburg, NJ, USA), 0.20 g of Congo red (J. T. Baker Chemical Inc, Phillipsburg, NJ, USA), 20 g of noble agar (Difco Laboratories, Detroit, MI, USA), and 1000 mL of distilled water (15). For evaluation of xylanase activity, the medium used to screen *Bacillus* isolates contained 3 g of $NaNO_3$, 0.5 g of K_2HPO_4, 0.2 g of $MgSO_4{\cdot}7H_2O$, 0.02 g of $MnSO_4{\cdot}H_2O$, 0.02 g of $FeSO_4{\cdot}H_2O$, 0.02 g of $CaCl_2{\cdot}2H_2O$ with 20 g of noble agar (Difco Laboratories, Detroit, MI, USA), and 1000 mL of distilled water. Besides, 1 g yeast extract and 5 g beechwood xylan (Sigma Chemical Co, St. Louis, MO, USA) were used as carbon sources (28). During the screening process, 10 μL of each *Bacillus* isolate were placed on the center of each plate containing cellulose or xylan media. After 24 h of incubation at 37°C, all plates were evaluated and the diameters of the zones of clearance were measured removing the diameter of the bacterial colony. The relative enzyme activity (REA) was calculated by using the formula: REA = diameter of zone of clearance divided by the diameter of the bacterial colony in millimeters. Based on REA test in each group, organisms were categorized in to excellent (REA > 5.0), good (REA > 2.0 to 5.0), or poor (REA < 2.0) REA (29). Each *Bacillus* strain was evaluated by triplicate, and the average measurements are presented in **Table 2**.

DFM Culture Identification

Based on the REA results, three *Bacillus*-DFM candidates with excellent to good REA were selected. These candidates were then

TABLE 1 | Ingredient composition and nutrient content of different broiler chicken diets used for *in vitro* digestion with or without inclusion of *Bacillus*-DFM candidate spore on as-is basis[a].

Item	Corn-based diet	Wheat-based diet	Barley-based diet	Rye-based diet	Oat-based diet
INGREDIENTS (g/kg)					
Corn (80 g/kg CP)	619.6	–	–	–	–
Wheat (135 g/kg CP)	–	711.0	–	–	–
Barley (113 g/kg CP)	–	–	654.3	–	–
Rye (126 g/kg CP)	–	–	–	622.6	–
Oats (98 g/kg CP)	–	–	–	–	638.0
Soybean meal (475 g/kg CP)	298.2	203.9	241.9	264.6	260.0
Poultry oil	39.1	42.8	65.0	70.0	70.0
Dicalcium phosphate	16.9	17.1	17.0	16.6	16.4
Calcium carbonate	10.6	8.5	8.2	10.4	10.0
Salt	3.8	3.0	3.0	5.7	2.0
DL-Methionine	3.3	2.5	3.0	3.0	3.2
L-Lysine HCL	2.8	4.6	2.0	2.0	1.6
Threonine	1.2	2.1	1.1	0.6	0.6
Choline chloride 60%	2.0	2.0	2.0	2.0	2.0
Vitamin premix[b]	1.0	1.0	1.0	1.0	1.0
Mineral premix[c]	1.0	1.0	1.0	1.0	1.0
Antioxidant[d]	0.5	0.5	0.5	0.5	0.5
CALCULATED ANALYSIS					
Metabolizable energy (MJ/kg)	13.0	13.0	12.3	12.2	11.9
Crude protein (g/kg)	195.0	200.0	190.0	205.0	186.4

[a]*Inclusion of 10^8 spore/g of feed mixed with calcium carbonate.*
[b]*Vitamin premix supplied per kilogram of diet: retinol, 6 mg; cholecalciferol, 150 μg; DL-α-tocopherol, 67.5 mg; menadione, 9 mg; thiamine, 3 mg; riboflavin, 12 mg; pantothenic acid, 18 mg; niacin, 60 mg; pyridoxine, 5 mg; folic acid, 2 mg; biotin, 0.3 mg; cyanocobalamin, 0.4 mg.*
[c]*Mineral premix supplied per kg of diet: Mn, 120 mg; Zn, 100 mg; Fe, 120 mg; copper, 10–15 mg; iodine, 0.7 mg; selenium, 0.2 mg; and cobalt, 0.2 mg.*
[d]*Ethoxyquin.*

TABLE 2 | Relative enzyme activity values (REA) and *Clostridium perfringens* zone of inhibition produced by different *Bacillus* spp. strains present in the *Bacillus*-DFM candidate treatment.

Measurements	AM1002	AM0938	JD17
CELLULASE ACTIVITY AT 24 h			
Colony size (mm)	5.7 ± 0.33[a]	6.0 ± 0.58[a]	6.3 ± 0.33[a]
Zone of clearance (mm)	35.2 ± 1.76[a]	30.7 ± 0.67[a,b]	29.3 ± 2.19[b]
REA[c]	6.2 ± 0.12[a]	5.1 ± 0.49[a,b]	4.7 ± 0.29[b]
XYLANASE ACTIVITY AT 24 h			
Colony size (mm)	5.0 ± 0.58[b]	6.7 ± 0.33[a,b]	7.3 ± 0.67[a]
Zone of clearance (mm)	31.7 ± 0.88[a]	32.0 ± 1.15[a]	29.0 ± 1.53[a]
REA[c]	6.3 ± 0.87[a]	4.9 ± 0.43[a,b]	4.0 ± 0.15[b]
***C. perfringens* AT 24 h**			
Zone of inhibition (mm)[d]	12.3 ± 1.45[a]	14.0 ± 1.00[a]	8.0 ± 1.15[b]

[a,b]*Superscripts within a row with no common superscript differ significantly $P < 0.05$.*
[c]*Relative enzyme activity values (REA) reflect the capacity to produce cellulase and xylanase enzymes by Bacillus spp. REA was calculated dividing the diameter of area of clearance by the diameter of the Bacillus colony. Based on REA test, organism can be categorized into three groups showing excellent (REA > 5.0), good (REA > 2.0–5.0), or poor (REA < 2.0) relative enzyme activity. All Bacillus spp. isolates were tested by triplicate. Data expressed as mean ± SE.*
[d]*Represents the diameter of the zone of inhibition observed at 24 h of incubation without the diameter of the bacterial colony. All Bacillus spp. isolates were tested by triplicate. Data expressed as mean ± SE.*

identified and characterized using a bioMerieux API 50 CHB test kit (bioMerieux, Marcy l'Etoile, FRA). Individual strain was also subjected to 16S rRNA sequence analysis to a specialized laboratory (Midi labs, Newark, DE, USA). Generally recognized as safe (GRAS) status of these three isolates was affirmed, as described by Wolfenden et al. (30). One of the three *Bacillus* strains (AM1002) was identified as *Bacillus subtilis*, and the other two isolates (AM0938 and JD17) were identified as *B. amyloliquefaciens* (**Table 3**). Following the identification, all three *Bacillus* candidate strains were sporulated and mixed in equal amounts during the *Bacillus*-DFM preparation process as described below and incorporated to the experimental diets.

Preparation of Spore-Based DFM

In an effort to grow high numbers of viable spores, modified version of a solid state fermentation media (SS) developed by Zhao et al. (31) was used. Briefly, to prepare the SS fermentation media, ammonia broth was added to a mixture of 70% rice straw and 30% wheat bran at the rate of 40% by weight. Then, the SS fermentation media was added to 250 mL Erlenmeyer flasks and sterilized by autoclaving for 30 min at 121°C. Each of the three *Bacillus* strains candidates was grown, individually, overnight at 37°C in test tubes containing 10 mL of tryptic soy broth (TSB, Becton Dickinson, Sparks, MD, USA). After incubation, 2 mL of each candidate culture were added separately to the previously prepared SS fermentation media flasks. The inoculated flasks were incubated for 24 h at 37°C to promote growth of the *Bacillus* spp. candidates, and incubated for another 72 h at 30°C to trigger the initiation of the sporulation process. Following this, the inoculated SS fermentation media was removed from the Erlenmeyer flasks, placed onto Petri dishes, and dried at 60°C for 18 h. Then, the SS fermentation media was aseptically ground into a fine powder that contained stable *Bacillus* spores (~10^{11} spores/g). One gram of spores from each isolate (1:1:1) was combined to produce the *Bacillus*-DFM candidate final product containing ~3×10^{11} spores/g. *Bacillus*-DFM candidate was included into each experimental diet to reach a final concentration of 10^8 spores/g using a rotary mixer for 15 min.

TABLE 3 | Identification of *Bacillus* spp. isolates by bioMerieux API 50 CHB[a] and 16S rRNA sequence analyses[b] present in the *Bacillus*-DFM candidate treatment.

Isolate	API50 CHB		16S rRNA sequence analysis	
	Taxon	% ID	Closest match	% ID
AM1002	*Bacillus subtilis/amyloliquefaciens*	99.2	*Bacillus subtilis*	100.0
AM0938	*Bacillus subtilis/amyloliquefaciens*	99.0	*Bacillus amyloliquefaciens*	99.7
JD17	*Bacillus subtilis/amyloliquefaciens*	99.4	*Bacillus amyloliquefaciens*	99.6

[a] *BioMerieux API 50 CHB test kit.*
[b] *16S rRNA sequence analysis.*

Samples of feed containing the DFM candidate were subjected to 100°C for 10 min to eliminate vegetative cells and validate the amount of spores per gram of feed after inclusion and mixing steps. Following heat-treatment, 10-fold dilutions of the same feed samples from the glass tubes were plated on tryptic soy agar plates (TSA, Becton Dickinson, Sparks, MD, USA); letting spores in the feed sample germinate to vegetative cells after incubation at 37°C for 24 h, hence representing the number of spores present per gram of feed.

Clostridium perfringens Strain

A strain of *C. perfringens* previously described in a NE challenge model was kindly donated by Dr. Jack. L. McReynolds, USDA-ARS, College Station, TX, USA (32). A frozen aliquot was shipped on ice to our laboratory and was amplified in TSB with sodium thioglycolate (Sigma-Aldrich, St Louis, MO, USA). The broth culture was plated on phenylethyl alcohol agar plates (PEA, Becton Dickinson, Sparks, MD, USA) with 5% sheep blood (Remel, Lenexa, KS, USA) to confirm purity, aliquots were made with 25% sterile glycerol and stored at −80°C until further use. A single aliquot was individually amplified in TSB with sodium thioglycolate overnight for the *in vitro* proliferation studies and the final dose was confirmed by plating 10-fold dilutions on TSA plates with sodium thioglycolate.

In Vitro Assessment of Antimicrobial Activity Against *Clostridium perfringens*

The three *Bacillus* isolates present in the *Bacillus*-DFM candidate treatment were individually cultured aerobically overnight on TSA and screened for *in vitro* antimicrobial activity against *C. perfringens* as reported previously (33). Briefly, 10 µL of each *Bacillus* isolate were placed on the center of TSA plates, and incubated for 24 h at 37°C. Then, the plates with visible *Bacillus* colonies were overlaid with TSA with sodium thioglycolate containing 10^6 cfu/mL of *C. perfringens*, and all plates were incubated anaerobically at 37°C. After 24 h of incubation, all plates were evaluated and the diameters of the zones of inhibition were measured removing the diameter of the bacterial colony. Each *Bacillus* strain was evaluated by triplicate, and the average measurements of antimicrobial activity against *C. perfringens* are presented in **Table 2.**

In Vitro Digestion Assay

The *in vitro* digestion model used in the present study was based on previous publications, with minor modifications (34, 35), and the assay was performed with five different experimental diets, with or without *Bacillus*-DFM candidate, in quintuplicates. Briefly, for all the gastrointestinal compartments simulated during the *in vitro* digestion model, a biochemical oxygen demand incubator (VWR, Houston, TX, USA) set at 40°C (to simulate poultry body temperature), customized with an standard orbital shaker (19 rpm; VWR, Houston, TX, USA) was used for mixing the feed content. Additionally, all tube samples were held at an angle of 30° inclination to facilitate proper blending of feed particles and the enzyme solutions in the tube. The first gastrointestinal compartment simulated was the crop, where 5 g of feed and 10 ml of 0.03M hydrochloric acid (HCL, EMD Millipore Corporation, Billerica, MA, USA) were placed in 50 mL polypropylene centrifuge tubes and mixed vigorously reaching a pH value around 5.2. Tubes were then incubated for 30 min. Following this time, all tubes were removed from the incubator. To simulate the proventriculus as the next gastrointestinal compartment, 3000 U of pepsin per gram of feed (Sigma-Aldrich, St Louis, MO, USA) and 2.5 mL of 1.5M HCl were added to each tube to reach a pH of 1.4–2.0. All tubes were incubated for additional 45 min. The third and the final steps were intended to simulate the intestinal section of the gastrointestinal tract. For that, 6.84 mg of 8× pancreatin (Sigma-Aldrich, St Louis, MO, USA) in 6.5 mL of 1.0M sodium bicarbonate (Sigma-Aldrich, St Louis, MO, USA) were added, and the pH was adjusted to range between 6.4 and 6.8 with 1.0M sodium bicarbonate. All tube samples were further incubated for 2 h. Hence, the complete *in vitro* digestion process took 3 h and 15 min. After the digestion, supernatants from all the diets were obtained by centrifugation for 30 min at 2000 × *g*. All supernatants were then tested for viscosity and *C. perfringens* proliferation, as described below.

Viscosity

Viscosity was measured using a Brookfield digital cone-plate viscometer fitted with a CP-40 spindle (Brookfield Engineering Laboratories Inc., Stoughton, MA, USA). From each supernatant, 0.5 mL was taken to measure viscosity at a shear rate of 42.5/s at 40°C to mimic body temperature of poultry. Viscosity was evaluated by quintuplicate per diet with or without inclusion of the *Bacillus*-DFM candidate and reported in centipoise (cP = 1/100 dyne s/cm^2).

Clostridium perfringens Proliferation

Proliferation of *C. perfringens* was performed according to previously published methods (35), with minor modifications. A suspension of 10^5 cfu/mL of *C. perfringens* was added to five replicates of each of the following groups: (1) 6 mL TSB with sodium thioglycolate as a positive control group; (2) 3 mL TSB with sodium thioglycolate plus 3 mL supernatant from each digested control non-DFM diet; (3) 3 mL TSB with sodium thioglycolate plus 3 mL supernatant from digested diets supplemented with *Bacillus*-DFM. Samples were incubated anaerobically at 40°C, with tubes set at 30° angle with constant shaking (200 rpm) for 4 h. After incubation, 10-fold serial dilutions were made from all treatment groups in 0.85% sterile saline. Then, 10 µL was plated on TSA with sodium thioglycolate and incubated for 24 h at 40°C, anaerobically. Results were expressed as $\log_{10}$ cfu of *C. perfringens*/mL.

In Vitro Determination of Spore Persistence

Persistence of the *Bacillus*-DFM spores in the *in vitro* digestive model was also evaluated (five replicates per diet treatment). At each time point during the digestive simulation process (crop, proventriculus, and intestine), 0.2 mL was immediately loaded into 0.5 mL sterile centrifuge tubes and heat-treated (pasteurized) at 75°C for 10 min to eliminate the presence of vegetative cells (36). After pasteurization, samples were loaded into sterile 96-well flat bottom plate and 10-fold dilutions were made and plated on TSA. Plates were incubated for 24 h at 37°C on aerobic conditions to enumerate spores per gram of sample.

Statistical Analysis

Data from all measurements were subjected to One-way analysis of variance as a completely randomized design using the General Linear Models procedure of SAS (SAS version 9.1) (37). Means were separated with Duncan's multiple-range test at $P < 0.05$ considered as significant. Data were reported as mean ± SE.

Results

Isolates AM1002, AM0938, and JD17 were selected from a pooled of *Bacillus* isolates in our laboratory, based on the REA values for cellulose and xylanase, and the zone of inhibition for *C. perfringens* (**Table 2**). Isolate AM1002 showed a REA value of 6.2 and AM0938 showed a REA value of 5.1, both considered excellent REA values (>5.0) for cellulase activity (29); additionally, isolate JD17 showed a REA value of 4.7, which is considered good (>2.0–5.0) for cellulase production. A similar trend was observed for xylanase activity where isolate AM1002 showed a REA value of 6.3 (excellent); AM0938 showed a REA value of 4.8 (good), and isolate JD17 showed a REA value of 4.0 (good) for xylanase production. In the case of antimicrobial activity against *C. perfringens*, isolate AM0938 generated the largest diameter of the zone of inhibition with 14 mm, followed by isolates AM1002 and JD17 with 12 and 8 mm, respectively. Although enzyme production and antimicrobial activity were observed for all the isolates, individual differences were evident even in bacteria of the same species (**Table 2**). The API 50 CHB system characterized all three isolates as *B. subtilis/amyloliquefaciens* (**Table 3**). Analysis of 16S rRNA sequence classified two strains (AM0938, JD17) as *B. amyloliquefaciens* and one of the strains (AM1002) as *B. subtilis*, which was consistent with the results observed by the carbohydrate fermentation profile of the biochemical test.

The results of the evaluation of digesta viscosity of different diets with or without inclusion of a *Bacillus*-DFM candidate after *in vitro* digestion are summarized in **Table 4**. An evident increase in viscosity was observed in soybean-based diets containing wheat, barley, rye, and oats when compared to corn, being rye, and oat diets with the highest viscosity values. However, it was noteworthy to observe that dietary inclusion of the *Bacillus*-DFM candidate significantly ($P < 0.05$) reduced viscosity in all diets containing cereals different to corn in comparison to control diets without DFM inclusion (**Table 4**).

Table 5 summarizes the results of the proliferation of *C. perfringens* in the supernatant from different digested diets with or without inclusion of a *Bacillus*-DFM candidate. A significant increase in *C. perfringens* proliferation was observed in supernatants collected from control diets that contained wheat, barley, rye, and oat compared to the TSB positive control group. Startlingly, dietary inclusion of a *Bacillus*-DFM candidate in non-corn diets significantly reduced *C. perfringens* proliferation when compared to the control non-DFM supplemented diets. The corn-based diet showed similar cfu values of *C. perfringens* with or without inclusion of the *Bacillus*-DFM candidate.

Persistence of the *Bacillus*-DFM candidate spores in the different gastrointestinal compartments simulated in the *in vitro* digestive model is presented in **Table 6**. Regardless of diet composition, on average, a reduction of more than half of a $\log_{10}$ was observed in the crop compartment during the first 30 min of incubation, and it was followed by a further significant ~2$\log_{10}$ reduction of spore counts in the proventriculus. Remarkably, in all diets, a significant increment in spore numbers, ~2$\log_{10}$ was observed during the final digestion step simulating intestinal conditions (**Table 6**).

TABLE 4 | Evaluation of *in vitro* viscosity of different diets with or without inclusion of a *Bacillus*-DFM candidate.

Diet	Viscosity (cP)[c]	
	Control	*Bacillus*-DFM
Corn-based	0.96 ± 0.01[a]	0.97 ± 0.01[a]
Wheat-based	1.55 ± 0.02[a]	1.28 ± 0.01[b]
Barley-based	1.75 ± 0.02[a]	1.34 ± 0.03[b]
Rye-based	8.40 ± 0.37[a]	2.39 ± 0.04[b]
Oat-based	36.9 ± 2.15[a]	1.34 ± 0.01[b]

[a,b]*Superscripts within a row with no common superscript differ significantly P < 0.05.*
[c]*Viscosity was measured after 3 h and 15 min of in vitro digestion at 40°C. Data expressed as mean ± SE.*

TABLE 5 | Proliferation of *Clostridium perfringens*[d] in different digested diets with or without inclusion of *Bacillus*-DFM candidate spore[e].

Diet[c]	TSB + Thio	Control diet	*Bacillus*-DFM
Corn-based	6.38 ± 0.13[a]	6.44 ± 0.19[a]	6.68 ± 0.08[a]
Wheat-based	6.12 ± 0.24[b]	7.12 ± 0.07[a]	5.20 ± 0.18[b]
Barley-based	6.36 ± 0.06[c]	7.50 ± 0.13[a]	6.86 ± 0.11[b]
Rye-based	6.05 ± 0.21[c]	7.15 ± 0.09[a]	6.68 ± 0.12[b]
Oat-based	6.12 ± 0.07[b]	6.96 ± 0.13[a]	5.76 ± 0.07[c]

[a,b]*Superscripts within a row with no common superscript differ significantly P < 0.05.*
[c]*Supernatant from each diet was used as part of the broth for C. perfringens growth. Data expressed as mean ± SE.*
[d]*Inoculum used 10^5 cfu of C. perfringens and 10^8 spores/g of Bacillus-DFM candidate.*
[e]*Data expressed in $\log_{10}$ cfu/mL.*

TABLE 6 | Persistence of *Bacillus*-DFM candidate[c] spore during *in vitro* digestion[f] in different diets under variable biochemical conditions simulating different sections of the gastrointestinal tract of poultry[e].

Diet[d]	Crop (30 min)	Proventriculus (45 min)	Intestine (120 min)
Corn-based	7.32 ± 0.10^a	5.43 ± 0.17^b	7.20 ± 0.09^a
Wheat-based	7.54 ± 0.06^a	5.58 ± 0.10^b	7.33 ± 0.19^a
Barley-based	7.45 ± 0.16^a	4.95 ± 0.21^b	7.27 ± 0.08^a
Rye-based	7.28 ± 0.10^a	5.60 ± 0.22^b	7.09 ± 0.17^a
Oat-based	7.66 ± 0.07^a	5.06 ± 0.15^b	7.30 ± 0.15^a

[a,b]*Superscripts within a row with no common superscript differ significantly $P < 0.05$.*
[c]*Inclusion of 10^8 spore/g of feed*
[d]*Heat shock was induced by placing a sample of each simulated compartment in a water bath at 75°C for 10 min. Data expressed as mean ± SE.*
[e]*Data expressed in log_{10} cfu/mL.*
[f]*pH and time of incubation varied according to the simulated organ.*

Discussion

High-energy diets have been utilized to maximize growth during starter, grower, and finisher phases of production. Consequently, the primary dietary energy sources in commercial broiler diets have been traditional cereal grains such as corn and sorghum. However, with the recent price volatility of common feed ingredients, the animal industry seeks alternative grains or industry by-products to include in diet formulations (38, 39). Wheat, barley, rye, and oat contain lower bioavailable energy, and elevated NSP levels in comparison to corn (40) are alternative options. However, these cereals have limited use in monogastric diets, because often high-inclusion results in relatively poor performance, detrimental litter conditions, and increase predisposition for NE (41–43). Hence, supplemental carbohydrases, such as NSP-degrading enzymes, have allowed to increase the utilization of these alternative ingredients by reducing their antinutritional effects (40, 44, 45). The carbohydrase market is accounted by two dominant enzymes: xylanases and cellulases. Other commercially available carbohydrases include α-amylase, α-galactosidase, β-glucanase, β-mannanase, and pectinase (46).

In the present study, the *Bacillus spp.* strains that conform the DFM candidate treatment were identified as either *B. subtilis* or *B. amyloliquefaciens* (**Table 3**), therefore being feasible for *in vivo* evaluation studies as they are GRAS candidates (12, 26–28). Furthermore, the three selected *Bacillus spp.* isolates showed a variable ability to produce cellulase and xylanase (**Table 2**), hence, in addition to the benefits that spores or vegetative cells can provide as probiotics (9, 12), they may improve the digestibility of cereals with high-soluble NSP (47).

The *Bacillus*-DFM candidate treatment also demonstrated effective antimicrobial properties against *C. perfringens*, which could be due to production of antimicrobial-like compounds and/or competition for nutrients (**Tables 2** and **5**). Little is known about the mechanisms underlying the higher incidence of NE in broilers fed diets containing cereals with elevated levels of NSP, but it could be related to a prolonged feed rate of passage and a reduction in the digestion of nutrients that later in the hind gut will be available for bacteria to growth (48). For *in vitro* evaluation of *C. perfringens* proliferation, TSB with sodium thioglycolate (positive control) groups were included. In the TSB group (positive control), the *C. perfringens* inoculum was increased ~0.5$\log_{10}$, after 4 h of incubation. However, it was interesting to observe a significant increase in *C. perfringens* proliferation in the supernatants collected from control non-DFM diets that contained wheat, barley, rye, and oat, compared with the enrichment TSB medium with sodium thioglycolate group (**Table 5**).

These results suggest that partial digestion of NSP grains and increased digesta viscosity provides a favorable nutritional environment that supports the growth of *C. perfringens*. Interestingly, dietary inclusion of a *Bacillus*-DFM candidate in non-corn diets significantly reduced both viscosity (**Table 4**) and *C. perfringens* proliferation (**Table 5**), when compared to control diets without DFM inclusion. This result shows the capacity of certain *Bacillus* isolates to inhibit the growth of pathogenic bacteria like *C. perfringens*, probably due to competition for nutrients, production of antimicrobial-like compounds, or changes in environmental conditions. Proliferation of *C. perfringens* in the corn-based diet remained constant with or without the inclusion of the *Bacillus*-DFM candidate and in the TSB positive control group (**Table 5**). This outcome could be related to the lower concentration of NSP usually found in corn grains in comparison to other cereals, which was also supported by low digesta viscosity values (**Table 4**). These results are in accordance with previous reports (35), however, it is important to mention that diet ingredients are just one of the multiple predisposing factors that could affect the incidence of NE in commercial conditions (49, 50).

Beneficial bacterial spores are popular as DFM, though little is known about their mode of action. Previous studies conducted in our laboratory, have demonstrated that ~90% of *Bacillus* spores of a selected strain germinate within 30 min under *in vitro* and *in vivo* model conditions, with relatively constant numbers of spores in each gastrointestinal compartment evaluated, hence, suggesting that full-life cycle may occurs (51). In the present study, regardless of the diet, similar *in vitro* persistence of the *Bacillus*-DFM candidate spores was observed in the different simulated compartments (**Table 6**). On average, a half $\log_{10}$ reduction in spore numbers were detected in the crop compartment suggesting spore germination. In the proventriculus compartment, a further ~2$\log_{10}$ reduction was shown, supporting our previous findings (27, 51), which suggest that further germination of spores occurs even at low pH environments. However, it was particularly interesting to observe a ~2$\log_{10}$ increment in spore counts in the intestinal simulated compartment (**Table 6**). The increment in the numbers of spores could be a response to bacterial metabolites, competition for oxygen and nutrients available, resulting in resporulation (17). The above observations also support previous reports suggesting that spore transiting through the gastrointestinal tract could potentially undergo a full-life cycle of germination and resporulation (36, 52). Moreover, it has been demonstrated that germination of spores into metabolically and functionally active vegetative cells, within a similar time frame, produced beneficial metabolic and immunological effects in different animal species (53–57).

In summary, our results confirm that poultry diets containing cereal grains with a higher content of NSP in comparison to corn can enhance viscosity and *C. perfringens* growth (18–21). Remarkably, the dietary inclusion of a selected *Bacillus*-DFM candidate in non-corn-based diets significantly reduced both viscosity and *C. perfringens* proliferation when compared with the control non-supplemented-diets. Additionally, *Bacillus*-DFM candidate spore persisted and change their amount according to the variable biochemical conditions of the *in vitro* digestive model; therefore, supporting the hypothesis of the possible full-life cycle development in the gastrointestinal tract. The results from the present *in vitro* study encourage us to further evaluate the utilization of this *Bacillus*-DFM candidate in an *in vivo* NE model that we have developed in our laboratory (5), as well as to purify, characterize, and measure the international units of cellulase and xylanase that these *Bacillus* isolates produce. This knowledge will provide a valuable tool to use a stable DFM that produce exogenous enzymes in poultry diets.

References

1. Hofacre CL. Necrotic enteritis, currently a billion dollar disease: is there anything new on the horizon? In: Lyons TP, Jacques KA, editors. *Science and Technology in the Feed Industry: Proceedings of Alltech's 17th Annual Symposium*. Nottingham: Nottingham University Press (2001). p. 79–86.
2. Keyburn AL, Sheedy SA, Ford ME, Williamson MM, Awad MM, Rood JI, et al. Alpha-toxin of *Clostridium perfringens* is not an essential virulence factor in necrotic enteritis in chickens. *Infect Immun* (2006) **74**:6496–500. doi:10.1128/IAI.00806-06
3. Keyburn AL, Boyce JD, Vaz P, Bannam TL, Ford ME, Parker D, et al. NetB, a new toxin that is associated with avian necrotic enteritis caused by *Clostridium perfringens*. *PLoS Pathog* (2008) **4**:e26. doi:10.1371/journal.ppat.0040026
4. Schoepe H, Pache C, Neubauer A, Potschka H, Schlapp T, Wieler LH, et al. Naturally occurring *Clostridium perfringens* nontoxic alpha-toxin variant as a potential vaccine candidate against alpha-toxin-associated diseases. *Infect Immun* (2001) **69**:7194–6. doi:10.1128/IAI.69.11.7194-7196.2001
5. Shivaramaiah S, Wolfenden RE, Barta JR, Morgan MJ, Wolfenden AD, Hargis BM, et al. The role of an early *Salmonella typhimurium* infection as a predisposing factor for necrotic enteritis in a laboratory challenge model. *Avian Dis* (2011) **55**:319–23. doi:10.1637/9604-112910-ResNote.1
6. Castanon JI. History of the use of antibiotic as growth promoters in European poultry feeds. *Poult Sci* (2007) **86**:2466–71. doi:10.3382/ps.2007-00249
7. Alvarez-Olmos MI, Oberhelman RA. Probiotic agents and infectious diseases: a modern perspective on a traditional therapy. *Clin Infect Dis* (2001) **32**:1567–76. doi:10.1086/320518
8. Tellez G, Pixley C, Wolfenden R, Layton S, Hargis B. Probiotics/direct fed microbials for *Salmonella* control in poultry. *Food Res Int* (2012) **45**:628–33. doi:10.1016/j.foodres.2011.03.047
9. Hong HA, Khaneja R, Tam NM, Cazzato A, Tan S, Urdaci M, et al. *Bacillus subtilis* isolated from the human gastrointestinal tract. *Res Microbiol* (2009) **160**:134–43. doi:10.1016/j.resmic.2008.11.002
10. Kunst F, Ogasawara N, Moszer I, Albertini AM, Alloni G, Azevedo V, et al. The complete genome sequence of the Gram-positive bacterium *Bacillus subtilis*. *Nature* (1997) **390**:249–56. doi:10.1038/36786
11. González-Pastor JE, Hobbs EC, Losick R. Cannibalism by sporulating bacteria. *Science* (2003) **301**:510–3. doi:10.1126/science.1086462
12. Hong HA, Duc LH, Cutting SM. The use of bacterial spore formers as probiotics. *FEMS Microbiol Rev* (2005) **29**:813–35. doi:10.1016/j.femsre.2004.12.001
13. López D, Vlamakis H, Losick R, Kolter R. Cannibalism enhances biofilm development in *Bacillus subtilis*. *Mol Microbiol* (2009) **74**:609–18. doi:10.1111/j.1365-2958.2009.06882.x
14. Vreeland RH, Rosenzweig WD, Powers DW. Isolation of a 250 million-year-old halotolerant bacterium from a primary salt crystal. *Nature* (2000) **407**:897–900. doi:10.1038/35038060
15. Hendricks CW, Doyle JD, Hugley B. A new solid medium for enumerating cellulose-utilizing bacteria in soil. *Appl Environ Microbiol* (1995) **61**:2016–9.
16. Sen S, Ingale SL, Kim YW, Kim JS, Kim KH, Lohakare JD, et al. Effect of supplementation of *Bacillus subtilis* LS 1-2 to broiler diets on growth performance, nutrient retention, caecal microbiology and small intestinal morphology. *Res Vet Sci* (2012) **93**:264–8. doi:10.1016/j.rvsc.2011.05.021
17. Jadamus A, Vahjen W, Simon O. Growth behaviour of a spore forming probiotic strain in the gastrointestinal tract of broiler chicken and piglets. *Arch Tierernahr* (2001) **54**:1–17. doi:10.1080/17450390109381962
18. MacAuliffe T, Pietraszek A, McGinnis J. Variable rachitogenic effects of grain and alleviation by extraction or supplementation with Vitamin D, fat and antibiotics. *Poult Sci* (1976) **55**:2142–7. doi:10.3382/ps.0552142
19. Choct M, Hughes RJ, Wang J, Bedford MR, Morgan AJ, Annison G. Increased small intestinal fermentation is partly responsible for the anti-nutritive activity of non-starch polysaccharides in chickens. *Br Poult Sci* (1996) **37**:609–21. doi:10.1080/00071669608417891
20. Fengler AI, Marquardt RR. Water-soluble pentosans from rye: II. Effects on rate of dialysis and on the retention of nutrients by the chick. *Cereal Chem* (1988) **65**:298–302.
21. Bedford MR, Classen HL. An *in vitro* assay for prediction of broiler intestinal viscosity and growth when fed rye-based diets in the presence of exogenous enzymes. *Poult Sci* (1993) **72**:137–43. doi:10.3382/ps.0720137
22. Adeola O, Cowieson AJ. Board-invited review: opportunities and challenges in using exogenous enzymes to improve nonruminant animal production. *J Anim Sci* (2011) **89**:3189–218. doi:10.2527/jas.2010-3715
23. Slominski BA. Recent advances in research on enzymes for poultry diets. *Poult Sci* (2011) **90**:2013–23. doi:10.3382/ps.2011-01372
24. NRC. *Nutrient Requirements of Poultry*. 9th rev. ed. Washington, DC: National Academy Press (1994).
25. Cobb-Vantress, Inc. *Cobb 500 Broiler Performance and Nutrition Supplement* (2013). Available from: http://www.cobb-vantress.com/docs/default-source/cobb-500-guides/cobb500-broiler-performance-nutrition-supplement-(english).pdf
26. Shivaramaiah S, Pumford NR, Morgan MJ, Wolfenden RE, Wolfenden AD, Torres-Rodríguez A, et al. Evaluation of *Bacillus* species as potential candidates for direct-fed microbials in commercial poultry. *Poult Sci* (2011) **90**:1574–80. doi:10.3382/ps.2010-00745
27. Menconi A, Morgan MJ, Pumford NR, Hargis BM, Tellez G. Physiological properties and *Salmonella* growth inhibition of probiotic *Bacillus* strains isolated from environmental and poultry sources. *Int J Bacteriol* (2013) **2013**:1–8. doi:10.1155/2013/958408
28. Monisha R, Uma MV, Murthy VK. Partial purification and characterization of *Bacillus pumilus* xylanase from soil source. *KUSET* (2009) **5**:137–48.
29. Jani SA, Chudasama CJ, Patel DB, Bhatt PS, Patel HN. Optimization of extracellular protease production from alkali thermos tolerant *Actinomycetes: Sacharomonospora viridis* SJ-21. *Bull Environ Pharmacol Life Sci* (2012) **1**:84–92.
30. Wolfenden RE, Pumford NR, Morgan MJ, Shivaramaiah S, Wolfenden AD, Pixley CM, et al. Evaluation of selected direct-fed microbial candidates on live performance and *Salmonella* reduction in commercial turkey brooding houses. *Poult Sci* (2011) **90**:2627–31. doi:10.3382/ps.2011-01360
31. Zhao S, Deng L, Hu N, Zhao B, Liang Y. Cost-effective production of *Bacillus licheniformis* using simple netting bag solid bioreactor. *World J Microbiol Biotechnol* (2008) **24**:2859–63. doi:10.1007/s11274-008-9820-5
32. McReynolds JL, Byrd JA, Anderson RC, Moore RW, Edrington TS, Genovese KJ, et al. Evaluation of immunosuppressants and dietary mechanisms in an experimental disease model for necrotic enteritis. *Poult Sci* (2004) **83**:1948–52. doi:10.1093/ps/83.12.1948
33. Layton SL, Hernandez-Velasco X, Shivaramaiah C, Xavier J, Menconi A, Latorre JD, et al. The effect of a *Lactobacillus*-based probiotic for the control of necrotic enteritis in broilers. *Food Nutr Sci* (2013) **4**:1–7. doi:10.4236/fns.2013.411A001
34. Zyla K, Ledoux DR, Garcia A, Veum TL. An *in vitro* procedure for studying enzymic dephosphorylation of phytate in maize-soybean feeds for turkey poults. *Br J Nutr* (1995) **74**:3–17. doi:10.1079/BJN19950102
35. Annett CB, Viste JR, Chirino-Trejo M, Classen HL, Middleton DM, Simko E. Necrotic enteritis: effect of barley, wheat and corn diets on proliferation of *Clostridium perfringens* type A. *Avian Pathol* (2002) **31**:598–601. doi:10.1080/0307945021000024544
36. Barbosa TM, Serra CR, La Ragione RM, Woodward MJ, Henriques AO. Screening for *Bacillus* isolates in the broiler gastrointestinal tract. *Appl Environ Microbiol* (2005) **71**:968–78. doi:10.1128/AEM.71.2.968-978.2005
37. SAS Institute. *SAS User Guide. Version 9.1*. Cary, NC: SAS Institute Inc (2002).
38. Friesen OD, Guenter W, Marquardt RR, Rotter BA. The effect of enzyme supplementation on the apparent metabolizable energy and nutrient digestibilities

of wheat, barley, oats, and rye for the young broiler chick. *Poult Sci* (1992) **71**:1710–21. doi:10.3382/ps.0711710
39. Kiarie E, Romero LF, Nyachoti CM. The role of added feed enzymes in promoting gut health in swine and poultry. *Nutr Res Rev* (2013) **26**:71–88. doi:10.1017/S0954422413000048
40. Bach Kundsen KE. Carbohydrate and lignin contents of plant materials used in animal feeding. *Anim Feed Sci Technol* (1997) **67**:319–38. doi:10.1016/S0377-8401(97)00009-6
41. Bedford MR, Classen HL, Campbell GL. The effect of pelleting, salt, and pentosanase on the viscosity of intestinal contents and the performance of broilers fed rye. *Poult Sci* (1991) **70**:1571–7. doi:10.3382/ps.0701571
42. Choct M, Hughes RJ, Trimble RP, Angkanaporn K, Annison G. Non-starch polysaccharide-degrading enzymes increase the performance of broiler chickens fed wheat of low apparent metabolizable energy. *J Nutr* (1995) **125**:485–92.
43. Mahmood K, Rahman SU, Hussain I, Abbas RZ, Khaliq T, Arif J, et al. Non-antibiotic strategies for the control of necrotic enteritis in poultry. *Worlds Poult Sci J* (2014) **70**:865–79. doi:10.1017/S0043933914000919
44. Shirzadi H, Moravej H, Shivazad M. Influence of non starch polysaccharide-degrading enzymes on the meat yield and viscosity of jejunal digesta in broilers fed wheat/barley-based diet. *Afr J Biotechnol* (2010) **9**:1517–22. doi:10.5897/AJB09.1483
45. Zou J, Zheng P, Zhang K, Ding X, Bai S. Effects of exogenous enzymes and dietary energy on performance and digestive physiology of broilers. *J Anim Sci Biotechnol* (2013) **4**:14. doi:10.1186/2049-1891-4-14
46. Bedford MR, Schulze H. Exogenous enzymes for pigs and poultry. *Nutr Res Rev* (1998) **11**:91–114. doi:10.1079/NRR19980007
47. Wang ZR, Qiao SY, Lu WQ, Li DF. Effects of enzyme supplementation on performance, nutrient digestibility, gastrointestinal morphology, and volatile fatty acid profiles in the hindgut of broilers fed wheat-based diets. *Poult Sci* (2005) **84**:875–81. doi:10.1093/ps/84.6.875
48. Palliyeguru MWCD, Rose SP. Sub-clinical necrotic enteritis: its aetiology and predisposing factors in commercial broiler production. *Worlds Poult Sci J* (2014) **70**:803–16. doi:10.1017/S0043933914000865
49. Murphy TC, McCracken JK, McCann ME, George J, Bedford MR. Broiler performance and *in vivo* viscosity as influenced by a range of xylanases, varying in ability to effect wheat *in vitro* viscosity. *Br Poult Sci* (2009) **50**:716–24. doi:10.1080/00071660903389950
50. Lee KW, Lillehoj HS, Jeong W, Jeoung HY, An DJ. Avian necrotic enteritis: experimental models, host immunity, pathogenesis, risk factors, and vaccine development. *Poult Sci* (2011) **90**:1381–90. doi:10.3382/ps.2010-01319
51. Latorre JD, Hernandez-Velasco X, Kallapura G, Menconi A, Pumford NR, Morgan MJ, et al. Evaluation of germination, distribution, and persistence of *Bacillus subtilis* spore through the gastrointestinal tract of chickens. *Poult Sci* (2014) **93**:1793–800. doi:10.3382/ps.2013-03809
52. Cartman ST, La Ragione RM, Woodward MJ. *Bacillus subtilis* spore germinate in the chicken gastrointestinal tract. *Appl Environ Microbiol* (2008) **74**:5254–8. doi:10.1128/AEM.00580-08
53. Hoa TT, Duc LH, Isticato R, Baccigalupi L, Ricca E, Van PH, et al. Fate and dissemination of *Bacillus subtilis* spore in a murine model. *Appl Environ Microbiol* (2001) **67**:3819–23. doi:10.1128/AEM.67.9.3819-3823.2001
54. La Ragione RM, Woodward MJ. Competitive exclusion by *Bacillus subtilis* spore of *Salmonella enterica* serotype enteritidis and *Clostridium perfringens* in young chickens. *Vet Microbiol* (2003) **94**:245–56. doi:10.1016/S0378-1135(03)00077-4
55. Leser TD, Knarreborg A, Worm J. Germination and outgrowth of *Bacillus subtilis* and *Bacillus licheniformis* spore in the gastrointestinal tract of pigs. *J Appl Microbiol* (2008) **104**:1025–33. doi:10.1111/j.1365-2672.2007.03633.x
56. Huang JM, Hong HA, Van Tong H, Hoang TH, Brisson A, Cutting SM. Mucosal delivery of antigens using adsorption to bacterial spore. *Vaccine* (2010) **28**:1021–30. doi:10.1016/j.vaccine.2009.10.127
57. Xu X, Huang Q, Mao Y, Cui Z, Li Y, Huang Y, et al. Immunomodulatory effects of *Bacillus subtilis* (*natto*) B4 spore on murine macrophages. *Microbiol Immunol* (2012) **56**:817–24. doi:10.1111/j.1348-0421.2012.00508.x

Conflict of Interest Statement: The authors declare that the research was conducted in the absence of any commercial or financial relationships that could be construed as a potential conflict of interest.

18

An introduction to the avian gut microbiota and the effects of yeast-based prebiotic-type compounds as potential feed additives

*Stephanie M. Roto, Peter M. Rubinelli and Steven C. Ricke**

Department of Food Science, Center for Food Safety, University of Arkansas, Fayetteville, AR, USA

Edited by:
Michael Kogut, United States Department of Agriculture, Agricultural Research Service, USA

Reviewed by:
Kenneth James Genovese, United States Department of Agriculture, Agricultural Research Service, USA
Sherry Layton, Vetanco, Argentina

***Correspondence:**
Steven C. Ricke, Department of Food Science, Center for Food Safety, University of Arkansas, Fayetteville, AR 72704, USA
sricke@uark.edu

The poultry industry has been searching for a replacement for antibiotic growth promoters in poultry feed as public concerns over the use of antibiotics and the appearance of antibiotic resistance has become more intense. An ideal replacement would be feed amendments that could eliminate pathogens and disease while retaining economic value via improvements on body weight and feed conversion ratios. Establishing a healthy gut microbiota can have a positive impact on growth and development of both body weight and the immune system of poultry while reducing pathogen invasion and disease. The addition of prebiotics to poultry feed represents one such recognized way to establish a healthy gut microbiota. Prebiotics are feed additives, mainly in the form of specific types of carbohydrates that are indigestible to the host while serving as substrates to select beneficial bacteria and altering the gut microbiota. Beneficial bacteria in the ceca easily ferment commonly studied prebiotics, producing short chain fatty acids, while pathogenic bacteria and the host are unable to digest their molecular bonds. Prebiotic-like substances are less commonly studied, but show promise in their effects on the prevention of pathogen colonization, improvements on the immune system, and host growth. Inclusion of yeast and yeast derivatives as probiotic and prebiotic-like substances, respectively, in animal feed has demonstrated positive associations with growth performance and modification of gut morphology. This review will aim to link together how such prebiotics and prebiotic-like substances function to influence the native and beneficial microorganisms that result in a diverse and well-developed gut microbiota.

Keywords: poultry, microbiota, lactobacillus, *Bifidobacterium*, yeast

Introduction

Poultry production in the past century has transitioned from predominantly breeding layers to breeding a mixture of both layers and broilers, based on the evolution of consumer demand (1–3). Success in the optimization of different broiler lines is due to genetics as well as optimizing diets with more precise nutritional formulations (4, 5). Comparison of individual genetic lines has revealed differing intestinal development, feed intake, and digestibility traits among other characteristics, which may impact performance (6–9). Improved diets have allowed broilers to reach their optimum body weight and feed conversion rate while minimizing mortality. Comparing poultry diets from the 1950s to those of the 1990s and 2000s illustrates the progress made (10, 11). For example, broiler chickens raised on a typical diet in 1957 had an average weight of 1,430 g at 84 days of age, whereas broilers fed a diet from 2001 yielded an average weight of 5,520 g at the same age. The feed conversion ratio in 2001 (2.68) was also considerably better compared to 1957 (3.26) (11). The current poultry diet contains the appropriate balance of amino acids, fatty acids, major and trace minerals, energy, and protein necessary for optimum growth (12).

Supplementation of various biologics have been attempted to enhance poultry feed for maximum growth development and health. Antibiotics enhance growth and reduce pathogens and although the exact mechanisms remain unclear, numerous working hypotheses have been offered (13–17). Antibiotic incorporation into poultry feed has since been tightly restricted and/or omitted due to microbial antibiotic resistance, presumably originating from both poultry (among other livestock) and humans (18–20). Since the exclusion of antibiotics in diets, a number of alternative supplements have been tried (**Table 1**), including prebiotics (21).

A prebiotic, as defined by Gibson and Roberfroid (35), is "a non-digestible food ingredient that beneficially affects the host by selectively stimulating the growth and/or activity of one or a limited number of bacteria in the colon and thus improves health." This definition has been subsequently refined to include the requirements for resistance to the acidic gastric environment, gastric enzymes, gastrointestinal absorption, and fermentation by the gastrointestinal microbiota while stimulating growth of beneficial intestinal bacteria (22). Being indigestible by the upper gastrointestinal tract (GIT) enables it to enter the lower GIT as a substrate for health-promoting bacteria, such as bifidobacteria and lactobacilli, thereby modulating the microbiota (35). Many feed additives currently used do not fit wholly into the strict prebiotic classification; they may lack one or more of the criteria set by Roberfroid (22). Although these substances have differing modes of action compared to prebiotics, they have a similar end result of a healthy and mature GIT microbiome. They may inhibit pathogenic invasion, reduce pathogens in the environment, modulate the host immune response, or enhance the host GIT morphology to enable the host to better limit pathogens in the GIT lumen. These substances will be referred to as prebiotic-like substances for the remainder of this review.

The objective of this review is to provide an overview of the effects of prebiotic-like substances, particularly those that are yeast-derived, while assessing the influence on microbial diversity of the poultry gut microbiota when using single or complex mixtures. In order to achieve this, both the gut microbiota as well as prebiotics is reviewed. Additionally, the characteristics of complex mixtures of prebiotic-like substances are assessed, including their effects on the gut development and physiology, the interactions that occur between host and microorganisms, and the potential use of prebiotic-like substances in creating a more healthy gut microbiota. This review includes findings from not only poultry but also human and animal models, which may provide insight into potential effects in poultry.

Gut Microbiome: Terminology and Definitions

The microbiota is defined as the diverse population of microorganisms in a given environment, while the microbiome can be defined by either its genetic or ecological capacities (36). Genetic diversity is the entire collection of genes of the microorganisms in an environment, while the ecological diversity is all the microorganisms that make up an ecosystem (36). The term "microflora," once commonly used, is now often replaced by "microbiota" to avoid the plant connotation from the suffix "flora." (36). Regardless of the term used, it is essential to use a modifying adjective when referring to a specific anatomical region. For example, "gut microbiome" is indicating only the microorganisms in the GIT. There are numerous microbiome sites in addition to the gut microbiome, as they can be any shared anatomical sites between a community of microorganisms (commensal, pathogenic, or symbiotic) (37–39). An oral microbiome, for example, is the community of microorganisms that interact with and live within the oral cavity. It has several distinct microbial habitats within the oral cavity (gingival, tongue, and teeth) and extensions of the oral cavity (esophagus, middle ear, and nasal passages). Each different habitat within the oral cavity has its own distinct bacterial

TABLE 1 | Commonly researched feed additives for host health, including growth promotion and pathogen prevention, used in animal feed, their modes of action, and reviews for references.

Compound	What they do	How they work	Reviews for reference
Prebiotic	Food ingredient to act as substrate for beneficial bacteria in the host GIT microbiota	Host consumes prebiotic and it endures through the GIT relatively intact to the lower intestines where it selectively acts as substrate for beneficial bacteria	(22–24)
Probiotic	Live microbial feed supplements that beneficially impact intestinal microbial balance	Competes with pathogenic bacteria to colonize the intestines; ferments substrates to produce short-chain fatty acids; stimulates the immune response of the host	(23, 25, 26)
Mannan-oligosaccharide	Specific oligosaccharide that inhibits pathogenic bacteria from binding the mucosal epithelial lining	Pathogens have receptors specific for mannan residues, the pathogenic bacteria binds the mannan and does not bind to the host epithelial cells	(27–29)
Organic acid	Reduce the number of pathogens	Undissociated form traverses the bacterial cell membrane; once inside the bacterial cell, the organic acid dissociates to produce H^+ ions, which lowers the pH. The bacterial cell then has to expend its energy to restore it natural balance rather than promote its own growth	(30–34)

population in the form of complex biofilms (40). Research has shown that even the distinctive sites of the tongue - the dorsal and the lateral regions - possess differing bacterial profiles (41). Other frequently studied sites of microbiomes are the skin and the respiratory tract (42–44). The various regions and diversity among bacterial communities of the microbiota are indicative of the inherent complexity of microbiome research.

The gut microbiome is a widely studied topic because of its impact on health as well as its characteristic intricacy. The gut microbiome is home to one of the densest bacterial populations on earth, with numbers ranging from 10^8 to 10^{14}/g of digesta (45, 46). The microbiome encompasses biochemical and metabolic pathways not found in the host genome; this attests to the extent to which the microbiome has evolved (47). Microorganisms that comprise the gut microbiota have been found to directly impact the health of the host, providing protection against epithelial damage, aiding in digestion, and promoting development of a healthy immune system (48, 49). Commensal bacteria, in the GIT of animals, aid in absorption of nutrients as well as enhance nutrient utilization (50). Additionally, research conducted thus far has shown that earlier development of a mature and diversified microbiota leads to better growth and fewer health issues, such as obesity, allergies, and asthma (51, 52). This is in part due to healthy competition among microorganisms.

Avian Gut Anatomy, Structure, and Functionality

For a thorough understanding of the microbial communities that inhabit the GIT of poultry and the effects they may have, a brief description of the poultry GI system is warranted. The GIT of poultry, chickens specifically, begins at the esophagus and continues down past the crop, proventriculus, and gizzard, through the intestines (duodenum, jejunum, ileum, and ceca), and ends at the colon and cloaca (53, 54). The gut microbiota generally refers to the intestinal regions and the studies included in this review focus on the duodenum, jejunum, ileum, ceca, and fecal contents as well as the structural characteristics to illustrate the gut microbiome of poultry. The ceca and their contents are most often studied based on their slow passage rate [comparatively, gut transit time from mouth to the lower ileum is approximately 3 h, while contents may be retained in the ceca as long as 35 h (55–57)] as it exhibits the most diversification in the bacterial communities it harbors, in turn, indicating its impact on host health (54).

The intestines are multi-layered tubes, containing epithelial, muscular, and mucosal layers (58). Each section of the intestine, from the most proximal duodenum passing through the jejunum and out to the most distal ileum, contains numerous folds and is lined with villi and crypts. The villi are finger-like projections on the surface of the mucosal lining responsible for increasing surface area to maximize nutrient absorption and containing a meshwork of capillaries to allow nutrients entry into the bloodstream (59). When moving in the distal direction from the duodenum down toward the ileum, the mucosal lining reduces in thickness. The villi length and crypt depth also decrease in a continual gradation, which supports the notion of the majority of nutrient absorption occurring in the small intestine (58). Reduced intestinal weight is associated with improved nutrient absorption (60). Microscopic analysis has revealed that the reduction of intestinal weight is due to thinning of the epithelial lining rather than to the reduction in intestinal length, which is suggested to allow for improved nutrient absorption (61, 62).

The pancreas functions in hydrolysis of macromolecules, releasing digestive enzymes into the duodenum responsible for the hydrolysis of proteins, carbohydrates, and lipids supplied by the diet. In addition to enzyme production, the pancreas also produces hormones and bicarbonate that aid in metabolism regulation and buffer the intestinal pH, respectively (59, 63). The addition of enzymes to the duodenum allows for the small intestine to be the primary site of nutrient digestion and absorption. Having a general understanding of the digestive system of poultry allows for a more thorough insight into how microorganisms may impact GIT physiology. Turk (58) provides a more encompassing review of the entire avian GIT.

Avian Gut Microbiome Characterization

Characterization of microbial communities native to the poultry GIT began in 1901 and has since revealed these communities to be both diverse and dynamic (64). As biased culture-based methods advanced to molecular and sequencing techniques, a broader, more comprehensive representation of the microbiome has been recognized (64, 65). Researchers have attempted to determine a bacteriological profile of the poultry GIT via 16S rRNA gene-based studies; the findings have demonstrated that the majority of the 16S rRNA sequences in the cecal contents are not-yet-identified bacterial species (64, 66, 67). These discoveries uncovered the shortcomings of previously employed culture-based methods. For example, comparison of results obtained from Zhu et al. (64) and Rada et al. (68) found differing levels of *Bifidobacteria*-species present in untreated chicken cecal contents. Zhu et al. (64) used temporal temperature gradient gel electrophoresis followed by sequencing of the 16S rRNA fragments, while Rada et al. (68) used selective media; the experimental designs of both were comparable. The works of Zhu et al. (64) and Rada et al. (68) are two such examples for the characterization of the GIT microbiome; various techniques have been attempted to ascertain the microbial populations present in the different regions of the intestinal tract (**Table 2**).

Each area of the intestinal tract harbors distinct microbial communities. For example, the cecal contents exhibit greater levels of *Clostridiaceae*-related sequences as opposed to the ileum where more abundance of *Lactobacillus*-related sequences occurs (75). Apajalhti et al. (70) used G + C content to demonstrate similar results: the measurement of bacterial communities present in the ceca and ileum exhibited considerable variation when comparing the two G + C profiles. Variation in microbial communities is not only limited to differing organs, there is also a temporal factor in the nature of the microbiome (76). The cecal contents of younger birds appeared to possess more transient communities that matured into communities with much greater complexity, while the ileum indicated an overall constant microbiome except at days 3 and 49 (the youngest and oldest sampling points) (75). The response to newly introduced microorganisms also appears

TABLE 2 | Research conducted on commensal bacteria in poultry GIT based on location.

Host	Site(s)	Age(s)	Commensal or pathogenic	Method of investigation	Reference
Chicken	Ileum, cecum	7, 13 days	Commensal	PCR-based DGGE; 16S rRNA gene library analysis; qPCR	(69)
Chicken	Ileum	4, 8, 14, 21, 35 days	Commensal	DGGE; RFLP	(6)
Chicken	Ileum, cecum	4 weeks	Commensal	Percent G + C profiling	(70)
Chicken	Cecum, intestines	4, 14, 25 days	Pathogenic	Primers (species-specific) of 16S rDNA	(71)
Chicken	Cecum	1 day, 1, 2, 4, 6 weeks	Commensal	TTGE; 16S rRNA gene sequencing	(64)
Chicken	Crop, ileum, cecum, rectum	40, 41 days[a]	Commensal	16S rDNA sequencing	(72)
Chicken	Ileum, cecum	28 days	Commensal	FISH with 16S rRNA oligonucleotides	(73)
Chicken	Crop, duodenum, colon	2 months	Commensal	FCM-FISH	(74)

[a]*Indicates differing rearing methods: conventionally raised and organically raised, respectively.*

to be dependent on sex of the host when analyzed in a mouse model; male and female GIT microbiota influence the metabolic activities and immune system differently (77). The concept of host factors affecting microbial diversity offers the opportunity to use established and healthy microbiomes to generate a working GIT microbial profile. However, this may prove to be quite challenging as it has been found that chickens interacting together in the same conditions, receiving the same feed, and of the same age and sex still display uniquely dominant bacterial communities (78). Although the exact quantities and qualities of a healthy microbiota have yet to be determined, a relationship appears to exist between the establishment of a mature intestinal microbiome and positive impacts on the host, resulting in improved growth and health (79).

Avian Gut Microbiome-Metabolic Activities

The poultry GIT is essentially coated in a dense layer of commensal bacteria in a diverse array of niches. Generally, the most complex microbial communities are found in the crop and the ceca. There is less colonization in the intestines based on the unfavorable environment. For example, the duodenum contains numerous enzymes, high concentrations of antimicrobial compounds, such as bile salts, and also has a rapidly changing environment due to reflux from the jejunum up to the gizzard (80). Traveling further down the GIT, the ileum and ceca become more favorable environments with fewer enzymes and antimicrobial compounds; this is reflected in the increased concentrations of commensal bacteria, around 10^9 and 10^{11} bacteria/g, respectively (46). The unique anatomical structure of the cecum allows for the occupancy of fermentable substrates not widely available in different areas of the GIT; this enables differing microorganisms to reside and produce large amounts of energy metabolites to aid in achieving the bird's energy requirements (81).

Research profiling whole body energy consumption patterns has attributed 22.8% to being utilized by the GIT and liver (82), but not all of that energy is actually being used by and for the host. It was reported that the presence of GIT microbiota significantly increased the dietary metabolizable energy in the broiler chicken host, indicating that the microbiota are responsible for utilizing the additional dietary energy (83). The commensal bacterial communities utilize nutrients from the host's diet as energy sources, making those nutrients unavailable to the host. However, they are able to produce short-chain fatty acids (SCFAs) from the fermentation of those nutrients (84). Research suggests the GIT microbiota aid in digestion and energy release from starch and fibrous contents, especially in the ceca. It is proposed that the amounts and types of SCFAs that are generated in the ceca are in proportion to differing starches that enter the ceca (85). Although SCFAs serve as additional energy sources for the host, it is suggested that only a proportion (up to 25%) of the overall SCFA energy is recovered by the bird (85, 86). In high-fiber and low-energy diets, bacterial digestion of the fiber also releases energy in the form of SCFA (84, 87). Along with generating accessible energy, the gut microbiome is associated with conservation of energy when nutrient sources (proteins, fats, and sugars) are low (88, 89). The production and absorption of SCFAs in the intestine are occurring continuously, with more or less being produced due to alterations in the diet or cecal microbiome (85).

Conversely, the resident microbiome has also been associated with unfavorable effects to the host's utilization of dietary energy. Although the presence of the GIT microbiota has indicated a significant increase in levels of metabolizable energy in conventionally raised broiler chickens when compared to germfree (89), the metabolizable energy is attributed to the products generated by the GIT microbiota. The variation can be associated with the digestibility of those energy sources (dietary fiber and starches) being broken down into monosaccharides and SCFA. The SCFA are portrayed as possessing a high metabolic energy value, yet they are inefficiently utilized by the host. Therefore the levels of SCFA present are not reflective of the net deposition of energy to the host (86, 89). Another potential explanation may be that the presence of the gut microbiota increases the cost of energy by altering the rate of energy-consuming reactions (89, 90). For example, pathogens attach to the epithelial lining, alter its integrity and function, and in turn stimulate the renewal of epithelial lining, which increases the amount of dietary energy spent on gut maintenance (27, 91). It has also been observed that conventionally raised birds have higher energy requirements for maintenance when compared to germfree birds (92). This may be due to the addition of the host's microbiota usage of metabolizable energy, or the host's microbiota making dietary energy unavailable to the host (92).

Avian Microbiome and Foodborne Pathogens

The complex lining of the lower intestines with bacteria serves as a barrier against colonization of pathogenic bacteria, which if allowed to occur, could lead to infection. The bacteria that settle first in the lining of the intestines necessitate that any other microorganisms in search of new residence must compete for space and nutrients in order to survive and colonize (80, 93, 94). Establishing the early foundation of a mature GIT microbiota has been associated with prevention of infection with pathogens, namely *Salmonella*, by beneficial bacteria outcompeting the pathogenic bacteria for space and nutrients (95–98). In nature, chicks are hatched in the presence of maternal fecal contents, allowing rapid colonization of members from the maternal gut microbiome (25). In an attempt to colonize newly hatched chicks with a mature and healthy microbiome that will discourage pathogenic bacteria from colonizing, chicks have been experimentally inoculated with competitive exclusion culture mixtures (97, 99–102). Introduction of the competitive exclusion cultures has proven to be effective in protecting young chicks from enteric pathogens and several reviews have been written on various aspects of this research (103–106).

As previously mentioned, commensal bacteria produce SCFA, which are recognized as having growth-inhibiting effects on enterobacteriaceae (107–109). The presence of the SCFA causes a drop in cytoplasmic pH, which is recognized as a contributing factor to the inhibition of pathogen growth (110). Although the mechanisms of SCFAs are not well understood, they are known to exhibit bactericidal and bacteriostatic properties (30–32, 111). Russell (30) suggested that it is not only the result of a drop in pH caused by the SCFA but also the uncoupling reactions produced by the translocation of protons by SCFA that contribute to the growth inhibition effects seen. In accordance with this notion, Davidson et al. (112) suggested that because the fatty acids produced are weak acids, they are effective as antimicrobials in their undissociated forms as they are able to easily diffuse through the cytoplasmic membrane of the microorganism. The fatty acids dissociate into anions and protons once in the cytoplasm of the microorganism (maintained relatively neutral or slightly alkaline), in turn decreasing the pH and causing conformational changes of cytoplasmic proteins, enzymes, and nucleic acids. In an attempt to reestablish a neutral/slightly alkaline pH, microorganisms utilize ATP-dependent pump systems to transport the anions and protons outside of the cell. This is in accordance with findings of Cherrington et al. (113), where incubation of *Escherichia coli* with propionic and formic acids resulted in reduced rates of macromolecular synthesis initially, yet it partially regained synthesis rates after continued incubation.

Anion accumulation is suspected to be another factor in uncoupling reactions that attributes to growth inhibition of bacteria in the presence of SCFA. It is suggested that the accumulation of acid anions causes an uncoupling effect of the electron transport chain from oxidative respiration (via the passage of molecules in their dissociated and undissociated forms, transferring protons into the cell to dissipate the proton motive force) as well as a chaotropic effect (disrupting hydrogen bonding in water causing macromolecules in solution to lose stability) that are accountable for the increased hydrogen ion leakage into the cell. The cell is unable to excrete hydrogen ions rapidly enough, making it difficult for the cell to regain its neutral/slightly alkaline intracellular pH (30, 110, 114, 115). The intracellular increase in hydrogen is unable to counteract the accumulation of acid anions (116). Another inhibitor of bacterial growth by SCFA is the disruption of the membrane of a microorganism by means of permeabilization or intercalation, allowing for the release of macromolecules and the destabilization of the membrane (117, 118). However, there are instances of pathogenic bacteria acquiring resistance to SCFAs (32). For example, pre-incubation of *Salmonella* with high concentrations of SCFA at neutral pH resulted in an acid tolerance response and has also been demonstrated to be responsible for modulation of virulence gene expression and attachment/invasion of *in vitro* tissue culture cells (119–122).

While the production of fatty acids is inhibitory to invading bacteria, studies suggested that the fatty acids are inactive against the species that produced them (123). Smulders et al. (124) found that acid-producing bacteria are tolerant to acids and in turn, the acidic environments that they generate. Therefore, the influences of the SCFAs produced by autochthonous bacteria may provide protection against pathogenic bacteria – *Salmonella*, coliforms, and *Campylobacter* – intent on colonizing in the intestine while leaving commensal bacteria unscathed (125). However, little else has been reported on the effects of the fatty acids on the producing species.

Key Players in the Gut Microbiota

In the past, the microorganisms colonizing the GIT were thought to be commensal, neither beneficial nor harmful to the host, as opposed to being mutualistic (37). However, numerous germfree experiments in various animal models have indicated the value of these indigenous microorganisms (126–128). There has been overwhelming data collected revealing the beneficial impacts on both host physiology as well as immunology (75, 129). Several studies have indicated that introducing a balance of beneficial microorganisms to the poultry microbiota improves body weight gain and feed conversion ratio as well as warding off common diseases in poultry, such as Newcastle disease and infectious bursal disease (130–132). However, in order to better promote strategies for increasing the presence of beneficial bacteria, those bacteria and their interacting counterparts must be identified.

Although being incredibly diverse, the most abundant microorganisms in the gut microbiota of poultry are primarily anaerobic (54). This is somewhat expected since there is little to no oxygen available as an electron acceptor in the lumen, although the concentration of oxygen is greater toward the epithelium, thus forcing bacteria to use fermentation to produce pockets of organic acids within the lumen (133). Moreover, Sun and O'Riordan (133) suggest that as a result of this environment, it is necessary to investigate SCFAs more in depth because bulk analysis does not reveal the true nature and spatial arrangement of these acids (which would further indicate the location and family of anaerobic bacteria). There is no consistent data available indicating the overall Gram status of poultry GIT microbiota. Investigation into the commensal bacteria present in an untreated chicken ceca has resulted in an array of bacterial communities (Gram-positive Y-branched, Gram-positive non-sporulating, Gram-negative) and may be attributed to the rearing conditions, chicken breed, diet, or even the cultivation and enumeration methods applied for bacterial characterization (125). Nevertheless, there are trends observed in available data investigating the microbial populations in broiler chickens grown in a conventional poultry flock and those raised under laboratory conditions (76, 134).

Lactobacilli and bifidobacteria are two of the more well-known beneficial bacteria, however, there are numerous others: *Bacillus*, *Enterococcus*, *E. coli*, *Lactococcus*, *Streptococcus* as well as undefined mixed cultures (**Table 3**) (23). These bacteria are indigenous to the GIT, occupy space, and consume nutrients along the intestinal tract, limiting the colonization of pathogenic bacteria. In addition to competing for space and nutrients, these bacteria have been recognized for exporting bacteriocins, which can target and kill invading pathogens (133). All of these microorganisms fit under the umbrella term probiotics. Like prebiotics, probiotics also have specified criteria and characteristics: (1) non-pathogenic and of host origin, (2) resistant to gastric pH and processing/storage, allowing them to persist in the intestinal tract, (3) able to adhere to epithelial and mucosal membranes, (4) modulate immune responses, and (5) produce inhibitory compounds (23). It is the complexity and broad diversity of the beneficial microorganisms that make up the microbiome and allow for a mature and healthy host (51, 52).

Bacteria may be beneficial to the host by aiding in degradation of polysaccharides otherwise indigestible to the host. The monosaccharides produced can be subsequently broken down further into SCFAs and lactic acid (37). As previously mentioned, both lactobacilli and bifidobacteria are beneficial and indigenous to the human and chicken GIT (145). Lactobacilli are members of a group collectively referred to as lactic acid bacteria, which metabolize carbohydrates to produce lactic acid as the primary end product (146). Oligosaccharides are their main nutritional source, which is reflected in their residence in ecological niches rich in carbohydrate-containing substrates, most commonly plant material, spoiled or fermented foodstuffs, and mucosal membranes of humans and animals (147). Along with their broad range of habitats, lactobacilli are able to adapt to various conditions by altering their strictly fermentative metabolism accordingly; they may be obligately homofermentative, facultatively homofermentative, or obligately heterofermentative (148). Their fermentative status is based on the levels and proportions of end products they generate from fermentation of differing substrates (although other factors, such as chemical and physical environment, play a role in determining fermentative status). Obligately homofermentative indicates that their primary fermentation product is lactic acid (>85%) generated by fermenting hexoses (149). Facultatively homofermentative indicates that they are capable of fermenting hexoses and pentoses using different pathways to generate lactic acid (although under low substrate concentration and strictly anaerobic conditions, they are capable of producing acetic acid, ethanol, and formic acid). Obligately heterofermentative lactobacilli ferment hexoses generating equimolar amounts of lactic acid, CO_2, and acetic acid (148–150). Although the end products produced are a fair indication of fermentative status, they are not the sole factor. These microorganisms are aerotolerant and acidophilic, allowing for the GIT to be an optimal residence (146, 151).

Bifidobacteria are another well-documented example of beneficial bacteria. They are often associated with lactic acid bacteria for their production of lactic acid, however, they are phylogenetically distinct. Bifidobacteria are Gram-positive, heterofermentative, and non-motile (152). Like lactobacilli, bifidobacteria digest oligosaccharides to use as carbon and energy sources, to produce lactic acid, acetic acid, ethanol, and formic acid (153). They are not exclusive to the utilization of dietary compounds, they can also digest carbohydrates produced by other members of the GIT (154). Additionally, they are capable of internalizing simple sugars remaining in the environment, thus preventing pathogenic bacteria from utilizing them as a nutrient source (155).

Both lactobacilli and bifidobacteria are known to be members of the intestinal microbiota in animals and humans; their presence is important for the maintenance of the GIT microbiota (156–158). Being that lactobacilli and bifidobacteria are autochthonous and dominant in the GIT, they can be utilized as a control method of pathogenic bacteria by competition, for example *Clostridium perfringens* (156). Lactobacilli and bifidobacteria possess characteristics that allow them to out-compete pathogenic bacteria. Various strains of lactobacilli adhere to intestinal epithelial-like cells and exhibit antimicrobial activity against bacteria typically found in the (human) GIT (157). A link between the lactobacillus strain's pH tolerance and antimicrobial properties has been reported, both *in vitro* and *in vivo* (157).

TABLE 3 | Suggested microorganisms for potential probiotic use based on various characteristics.

Microorganism	Host	Site isolated	Rationale	Reference
Enterococcus faecium	Chicken	Intestines	Bacteriocin-producing ability	(135)
Pediococcus pentosaceus	Chicken	Intestines	Bacteriocin-producing ability	(135)
Mixed culture[a]	Chicken	Cecum	Inhibition ability of *Salmonella*	(99, 136–139)
Lactobacillus reuteri	Chicken	GIT	β-glucanase gene enhances growth and nutrient digestion	(140)
Lactobacillus fermentum	Chicken	GIT	Intestinal adherence, pathogen inhibition, tolerance to gastric enzymes	(141)
Bifidobacterium longum	Chicken	GIT	Anti-Campylobacter activity	(142)
Streptococcus faecium	Chicken	GIT	Impacts of body weight, feed conversion, carcass yield, *Salmonella* colonization	(143)
Streptococcus bovis	Cattle	Rumen	Inhibition ability of *Salmonella*	(144)

[a]*Mixed culture composed of 29 cecal bacterial strains that have shown to inhibit Salmonella colonization.*

Different species of lactobacilli and bifidobacteria produce various antimicrobial agents, which allow them to be inhibitory toward pathogenic bacteria. Many species of lactobacilli and bifidobacteria produce SCFA; the production of these acids causes a drop in intestinal pH. The lowered pH level extends the lag phase for sensitive microorganisms (124). The undissociated forms of these acids are able to penetrate the microbial cell and hinder metabolic functions (further information on the mechanisms of these acids was discussed in a previous section of the current review). Another end product generated from lactobacilli and bifidobacteria is CO_2, which has demonstrated inhibition of microbial growth (149). The inhibitory mechanism of CO_2 is unclear, although Eklund (159) was able to rule out the proposed mechanism of CO_2 accumulation in the membrane of the microorganisms, physically interrupting the bacterial membrane. Growth of *E. coli*, *Bacillus subtilis*, *Pseudomonas aeruginosa*, and *Bacillus cereus* has been shown to be inhibited in the presence of CO_2 at various concentrations (159). Succinic acid is produced by both lactobacilli and bifidobacteria, although at minimal levels (160, 161), and is associated with antibacterial activities in a multitude of environments (162, 163). Diacetyl is an end product of lactobacilli that exhibits antimicrobial effects. It is suggested that diacetyl is more effective in a lower pH (≤ 7) causing it to be lethal to Gram-negative bacteria and inhibitory of yeasts (164). Bacteriocins, produced by lactobacilli, may have a narrow or broad range of activity. Lindegren and Dobrogosz (149) have reviewed the various antimicrobial agents produced by lactic acid bacteria in more detail.

Overgrowth of any single type of bacteria can have unfavorable effects on the host. Lactobacilli are considered beneficial bacteria, however, antibiotic growth promoters that stimulate improved growth of broilers were also associated with heightened sensitivity of lactobacilli to those antibiotics (165). Although the host may benefit from the commensal bacteria competing with pathogenic bacteria, an overgrowth of commensal bacteria can be detrimental to the host by excessive uptake of nutrients making them unavailable to the host (166). Additionally, overgrowth of lactobacilli can impair host fat absorption by not allowing proper biotransformation – deconjugation and dehydroxylation – of bile acids (14). Overgrowth of bacteria can also lead to overproduction of fermentation end products to the detriment of the host. For example, overgrowth of *Streptococcus bovis*, a commensal lactic acid-producing bacteria can generate considerable acid production and a concomitant lowering of the surrounding environment pH. This sequence can be advantageous for competing against pathogens. Consequently, under *in vitro* incubation conditions in co-culture with *Salmonella typhirmurium* growth of *S. bovis* can behave as a probiotic and directly limit *Salmonella* growth as a function of carbon source and time of inoculation (144). However, when easily fermented carbohydrates are fed to ruminants, excessive *S. bovis* growth can occur in the rumen resulting in rapid lactic acid overproduction, subsequent lowering of the ruminal pH, and the eventual development of a harmful ruminal lactic acidosis condition in the animal (167). Therefore, even though *S. bovis* might be considered a gut commensal organism, and in some cases a probiotic candidate, it can also be associated with host clinical disease states, such as bacterial endocarditis and colon cancer in humans (144).

Introduction and History of Prebiotics

The most widely accepted definition of prebiotics are non-digestible feed ingredients that are selectively fermented by beneficial bacteria in the lower GIT (capable of withstanding harsh conditions in the upper GIT) so as to provide energy to promote bacterial growth and metabolism in the colon which contributes to specific changes that lead to improved host health (22, 35, 168). Colonic food is a non-digestible ingredient that makes it past the upper GIT and into the colon, serving as a substrate for non-specific bacterial inhabitants, both beneficial and harmful (169, 170). Not all colonic foods are necessarily prebiotics; the rationale for designating a compound as a prebiotic or not depends upon whether beneficial bacteria alone are able to digest it. Some miscellaneous compounds that serve as colonic food, but do not fall into the category of prebiotics because of the non-specific targeting of microbiome bacteria include resistant starch, non-starch polysaccharides, non digestible oligosaccharides, and yeast fermentation products (171). There have been numerous studies conducted and reviews written covering common prebiotics and their beneficial impacts; therefore they will not be discussed in detail here (**Table 4**) (35, 172–174).

Some lesser-studied prebiotic-like compounds are *Saccharomyces cerevisiae* fermentation products (SCFPs) or yeast culture (YC) components; these compounds do not fall

TABLE 4 | Published reviews on the considerations of common prebiotics in various hosts.

Prebiotic	Considerations	Host	Reference
Inulin-type	Structure overview	Not applicable	(172)
Short-chain carbohydrates	Gut function and health	Human	(175)
Inulin-type	Bifidogenic, resistant to digestion	Non-specific	(176)
Resistant starch	Production of SCFA, microbiome modulation, gut-associated immunomodulation	Human	(177)
Mannan-oligosaccharides	Modulation of gut microbiome	Poultry	(27)
Fructo-oligosaccharide, galacto-oligosaccharide, lactulose	Criteria for prebiotic classification	Human	(168)
Inulin-type, oligofructose	Quantification of inulin and oligofructose in Western diet	Human	(173)
Fructo-oligosaccharide	Bifidogenic, lack carcinogenic and toxic effects	Poultry, swine	(174)
Fructo-oligosaccharide, inulin-type	Selective to beneficial bacteria, prevent pathogen colonization	Poultry	(178)

into the precise definition of prebiotics as set by Roberfroid (22), among other classical definitions. However, they have prebiotic-like effects in that they have been shown to enhance nutrient utilization and digestibility, as well as improving the immune system and inhibiting pathogen-intestinal cell interaction by modifying the GIT microbiome (179–181). The fermentation of *S. cerevisiae* – undefined strains – produces SCFP. They include the fermentation products and metabolites, the media used in the fermentation to preserve fermentation activity, and both the yeast cell wall fragments and residual live yeast cells; thus, they share characteristics in both probiotic and prebiotic realms (179). There are commercial YC products available that are being more thoroughly investigated to identify their exact effects and maximize the directed influence(s) they may have.

Because yeasts are most often associated with the wine making, brewing, baking, and other fermenting industries, it is critical to consider why these unique organisms were initially promoted for use in improvements of animal and human health. In order to do this, a brief review of the history of yeast that led to its usage as a feed additive is discussed in the following section.

Introduction to Yeast: History and Background

To understand the current use of yeast and yeast products in food and agricultural settings, it is important to at least briefly describe the history of yeast in scientific applications and the evidence for the close relationship among yeast strains originally uncovered and those used in today's laboratory-based research. Humans began using yeast over 7,000 years ago, with its earliest usage dating back to the Neolithic times for wine making (182, 183). In the past century, yeasts have been investigated on a genetic level after the Carlsberg Laboratory introduced scientific concepts to the brewing industry, as discussed by Greig and Leu (184). In the 1930s, the genetic analysis of yeast became accepted based on its potential as an experimental organism; it was pioneered by Øjvind Winge and Carl Lindegren (185). Winge used a strain isolated from the Carlsberg Laboratory, while Lindegren used a strain, EM93, isolated from rotting Californian figs (182). Yeast continued gaining popularity in the scientific field for its ease in gene manipulation (182). In the 1950s, Robert Mortimer constructed the strain S288C, which has been purported to share more than 85% of its genome with EM93, Lindegren's original strain (most laboratories involved in the analysis of yeast use a derivative of EM93 – a strain of *S. cerevisiae*). This strain was subsequently sequenced in 1996, making it the first fully sequenced yeast genome (186, 187). For further purposes of the current review, *S. cerevisiae* is the main species of yeast discussed unless otherwise indicated.

Yeast in the Laboratory

A renowned model organism, yeast is a single-celled fungal eukaryote that most often divides by budding. Yeasts are used in various industries because of their ability to ferment sugars in the absence of oxygen to produce CO_2 and alcohol. In a laboratory setting, yeasts are most often used for analysis as a model template to study higher eukaryotic organisms. Yeasts are ideal for studying processes known to occur in more complex eukaryotic organisms because even though yeasts are unicellular, they encode similar proteins and are thus representative of more complex organisms at the cellular level (188). When comparing all yeast protein sequences to mammalian sequences, of the potential protein encoding regions in yeast, "statistically robust" homology among the two was observed (189). Because of the lack of mammalian protein families and proteins sequenced, there may be much greater similarities between the two.

Part of the attraction of yeast as an experimental model is the ability to easily manipulate and mutate genes, either on plasmids or in the yeast chromosome itself, to view the resulting phenotypic effects (182). An insight into its fairly simple manipulation is evident in research performed by both Caspeta et al. (190) and Liu et al. (191). Caspeta et al. (190) manipulated *S. cerevisiae* into expressing thermotolerance to temperatures $\geq$34°C (typical response to these temperatures is serious impairment of function) by exposing the isolate for short stretches of time to increased heat followed by serial batch transfers. This resulted in non-inheritable heat tolerant strains that exhibited increased growth rates as well as increased glucose consumption rates at higher temperatures when compared to thermolabile strains (190). Thermotolerance has also been bestowed upon *S. cerevisiae* by the introduction of genes from organisms that are naturally thermotolerant. This transfer of genes allows for inheritable alteration in future generations of *S. cerevisiae*. Duina et al. (182) illustrated the extent to which yeast has proven its efficacy as a model organism, discussing research advancements and accolades (Nobel Prize and Lasker Award) in an array of fields achieved by utilizing yeast.

Although great progress has resulted from the study of yeast, it has also stimulated further inquiry. Yeast researchers began with the goal of determining functions of single genes and proteins, but now seek a "systems level" approach. The benefit of understanding how proteins interact to maintain cellular functions (metabolism, reproduction, growth, regulation, signaling, and homeostasis) is now at the forefront for yeast biology (192). Yeast's position as a model organism for various scientific fields is reviewed more thoroughly in several articles and therefore will not be further discussed here (192–194). A review by Siddiqui et al. (195) encompasses the potential of engineering yeasts to contain secondary metabolite pathways for pharmacological purposes. Additionally, Sherman (196) has generated a comprehensive review (both extended and truncated versions available) on the biological basics of yeast, which includes a section on a variety of outside literature references for yeast.

Yeast Metabolism

Yeasts are capable of cellular respiration in the presence and absence of oxygen; for this review, we will discuss respiration only in the absence of oxygen, as it is most applicable to the topic of the current review. Anaerobic respiration, or fermentation, is the process of breaking down sugars to generate energy for carrying out cellular processes. In anaerobic cellular respiration, sugars are broken down into pyruvate and subsequently decarboxylated and reduced to form CO_2 and ethanol. For fermentation to begin, any complex sugars must be broken down into simple sugars (e.g., sucrose to glucose and fructose) via enzymes from yeasts, adding an additional step to the fermentation process (197). In the process of understanding this, it is recognized that complex carbohydrates (starches and fiber) are more challenging for yeasts to ferment than simple sugars. Investigation into the types of sugars and environments yeasts are capable of fermenting is necessary to optimize the production and utilization of yeast fermentation products. By understanding the conditions in which yeast fermentation is optimized, they can be engineered to generate additional metabolites that may prove to be beneficial for use in animal feed.

Yeast as an Animal Feed Additive

The usage of live yeast and yeast products in animal feed is not a new concept, although pinpointing the exact point of its conception has proven to be challenging. It is suggested that the introduction of YC in animal feed was not until the 1980s (198). It appears that the majority of research has been dedicated toward ruminants, while equine, porcine, poultry, and companion animals received attention to a lesser extent. Initially, yeast was used in an array of modes because of the large quantities of yeast biomass waste generated by distilleries (and other yeast utilizing industries) (199). It was used as a feed additive because it was a rich source of protein, fiber, and minerals. It has been hypothesized that both viable and non-viable yeast cells provide essential B vitamins and organic acids (200). In the past, both viable and non-viable yeast cells have been added to animal feed - including poultry feed - and resulted in increased host growth and improved health (199).

It is essential to have a precise definition for YC, so it is not confused with using live yeast (probiotic/direct fed microbial form) or yeast extract (only soluble portion of yeast autolysis) products (201). As described in a previous section of the current review, YC contains the cellular constituents as well as residual viable cells. It is effective when used because it contains lysed yeast cells; this allows for the nutrients within the yeast cells to be available for digestion and absorption (202). These yeast cells are lysed by autolysis; they are subjected to temperature or osmotic shock, thereby killing the yeast cell while leaving the endogenous enzymes undamaged. The yeast cell's own enzymes begin to degrade the yeast cell, releasing its contents and further degrading its proteins into amino acids (203). Some yeast cells that are capable of tolerating the temperature or osmotic shock, do not autolyze, and remain metabolically active.

The mode of action of YC is seen to enhance digestive and fermentative functions of the GIT, while modifying activities of the GIT microbiota, although the mechanisms are less clear (198). Based on *in vitro* and *in vivo* studies, supplemented YCs appear to have several impacts on the rumen microbiota including increased numbers of beneficial bacteria and fiber digesting bacteria as well as shifting away from hydrogen consuming methanogens and toward bacteria capable of converting hydrogen and CO_2 to acetic acid, all of which could, in turn, potentially benefit the ruminant host animal either directly or indirectly (204, 205). Enhanced growth performance resulting from the supplementation of YC with probiotics (*Lactobacillus acidophilus* and *Streptococcus faecium*) has indicated its potential effect of increasing digestion and absorption of the GIT microbiota occurring in broiler chickens (206). de Oliva Neto et al. (207) conducted studies on the antibacterial properties of YC supernatant, which indicated a reduction of pathogenic bacterial growth when tested against a common distillery bacterial species. Interestingly, the supernatants were tested as both fresh and post freeze/thaw, and reported similar results indicating the antimicrobial activity could withstand freezing. Conversely, when heat (90°C for 20 min) was applied, the antibacterial activity was destroyed. Accordingly, YC and yeast extract have yielded varying results, which suggests the necessity for metabolically active yeast cells. When supplementing heat-treated inactive yeast cells to steer diets, there was no effect on the concentrations of cellulolytic bacteria, while supplementing live, metabolically active yeast cells increased the concentration of cellulolytic bacteria (208).

In addition to their ability to interfere with bacteria due to their relative large size, supplementation with live yeast products has led to a few suggested modes of action (209). One mechanism suggested by Jouany et al. (204) involves metabolic competition with bacteria that may be adhering to and digesting fiber or starch molecules. In this scenario, the yeasts ferment the carbohydrates produced, prohibiting their usage by other bacteria. Another mechanism of action of live yeast cells is their ability to produce protective products with antitoxin effects (210). Yeast intake has resulted in a stimulation of activity of host intestinal brush border enzymes, which has counteractive effects to those of pathogens, along with supplying the host with additional enzymes (211). Elimination of oxygen has been deemed the most influential mode of action in ruminants (212). Although there is little oxygen present in the GIT, live yeast cells scavenge for excess oxygen introduced by food and water intake; this allows for a more optimal environment for anaerobic bacteria (204, 212). Most all implications regarding the mechanism of oxygen elimination have been derived from studies conducted on ruminants.

As noted previously, the majority of the studies on the effects and mechanisms of YC have been performed on ruminants. Although such studies may be a good indicator of the potential use of YC in other animals, it can also be expected that there will be differences seen among ruminants and non-ruminants. For example, considerable research has been conducted on the effects of milk production in cattle, while this is beneficial for other lactating animals, the information gleaned from these studies holds little merit for poultry researchers. Instead, conducting *in vitro* and *in vivo* studies on specific animal subjects of interest would be more useful in identifying the mechanisms of YC in those animals rather than projecting ruminant/rumen microbiota results onto non-ruminant species.

Impact of YC on Host–Microorganism Interactions

The effects of YC on the intestinal morphology in swine have indicated increased jejunal villi width, which allows for greater digestive and absorptive intestinal capacity leading to better body weight gain when compared to controls (180). In contrast, poultry data obtained has thus far indicated significant differences in intestinal morphology (213–215). Supplementation of YC has resulted in more shallow crypt depths, indicating less necessity for cell renewal and turn-over, allowing for decreased host energy utilization for intestinal epithelial maintenance (216). Feed efficiency and body weight gain have both resulted in significant increases when YC, yeast derivatives, and live yeast cells are added to the poultry diet (215, 217, 218).

Inclusion of YC in animal feed has led to suggestions that they may aid in the clearing of pathogens from infected animals. A study involving the inoculation of pigs with *Salmonella* suggested that the inclusion of YC in the diet allowed for rapid shedding of the pathogen from the GIT (180). Supplementation of broiler feed with YC has also been seen to enhance adaptive immune system T lymphocytes, allowing for better clearing of the pathogens (181). El-Husseiny et al. (219) observed that commercial YC were able to significantly increase antibody production against SRBC, much in agreement with the findings of Al-Homidan and Fahmy (220), who reported significantly higher antibody titer concentrations in response to Newcastle disease in broilers fed YC.

Further examination into the components of yeasts' cell walls indicates the beneficial structural polysaccharides present and released into culture when yeast cells autolyze. Mannan-oligosaccharide (MOS) is included in the YC as it is derived from the outer cell wall of *S. cerevisiae*. MOSs bind to pathogenic bacteria in the GIT, preventing their attachment to the mannan residues on intestinal epithelia (221). This not only protects the host from pathogens but also allows for host energy reserves to be utilized for their own growth rather than to the repair and regeneration of the epithelial lining (222). β-glucans are also released when the yeast cell wall is degraded; presence of these molecules can lead to pathogen inhibition along with immunomodulating effects. Similar to MOS, β-glucans act by preventing pathogens from binding to the villi of the gut mucosa (214, 216). Additionally, β-glucans are known to activate phagocytes, natural killer cells and B and T lymphocytes as well as increase cytokine production and phagocytic activity of macrophages (223).

Mannan-oligosaccharide supplementation has been reported to increase broiler growth performance when supplemented in their diet (224, 225). *In vitro* experimentation has indicated that addition of MOS inhibits the attachment of enteropathogenic *E. coli* to the gut mucosa as well as removing attached *E. coli* from the mucosa (226). Inclusion of yeast fermentation products, like MOS, appears to reduce pathogenic bacterial populations. The mechanism is unclear, although the agglutination of the pathogens with sugars from the yeast cell wall occurs rather than attachment to the host intestinal lining is one hypothesized mechanism (227). Yang et al. (228) indicated MOS altered the gut microbiota of broilers and reduced the number of mucosal-associated coliforms.

Although some studies suggest a positive association between yeast and growth promotion (229, 230), other studies have indicated no positive effects on inclusion of YC in broiler diets (231). Paryad and Mahmoudi (229) indicated that inclusion of 2% yeast (*Saccharomyces cerevisae*) in broiler chicken diets resulted in significant differences in body weight gain, feed intake, and feed conversion rate when compared to controls. Similarly, investigation into YC on growth promotion in lambs suggested its efficacy, resulting in increased feed intake and growth by 8 and 26%, respectively. Conversely, similar research conducted on lambs evaluating the efficacy of three yeast strains and a mixed culture resulted in little consistency and lacked an overall effect when compared among yeast strains (232). Adebiyi et al. (231) also showed no significant differences in body weight gain in broiler chickens when fed varying percentages of YC.

Yeast Metabolites and Metabolism as Prebiotic-Like Substances

In addition to the structural polysaccharides derived from the yeast cell wall, yeasts generate a number of metabolites that may offer benefits to the host animal when supplemented to animal feed. Metabolites include carotenoids, vitamins, enzymes, amino acids, and some miscellaneous products (200). Several yeast species are naturally capable of producing carotenoids (including β-carotenes), which are subsequently metabolized into vitamin A (200). Vitamin A aids in cellular differentiation and proliferation, making it critical for intestinal maintenance and health (233). The enzyme responsible for the synthesis of vitamin A from β-carotene is β,β-carotene 15,15′-monooxygenase, which has been isolated and characterized from the intestines of poultry, among other animals (234, 235). Although *S. cerevisiae* is not capable of naturally producing carotenoids, it is capable of and has been engineered to express a biosynthetic pathway for the production of β-carotene (236).

Other vitamins (vitamin precursors) produced by yeasts include ergosterol, L-ascorbic acid, and D-erythroascorbic acid. Ergosterol is particularly abundant in *S. cerevisiae*, accounting for up to 90% of the total sterols (237). It is located in the membrane of yeasts and is responsible for its fluidity, structure, permeability, and activity of membrane-bound enzymes (238). Ergosterol is a precursor to both vitamin D_2 and cortisone (239). Vitamin D_2 is responsible for the proper absorption and transport of calcium, among other minerals (240). D-Erythroascorbic acid is also synthesized by *S. cerevisiae* and depending on the substrates available, that pathway can be manipulated into producing L-ascorbic acid (vitamin C) (241). The ingestion of vitamin C has been suggested to alleviate some of the repercussions of heat stress: poor immune function and growth performance (242). However, instances of supplementation of L-ascorbic acid in poultry diets have had varying results; some resulted in increased levels of superoxide dismutase in 45-week-old broilers, while others revealed no effect on the activities of antioxidative enzymes, superoxide dismutase included in 7-week-old broilers (243, 244).

Yeasts are recognized for their production of enzymes expressing various activities (245). Jones (246) wrote a comprehensive review documenting the activities of the proteolytic systems in *S. cerevisiae*, along with mentioning other enzymes elucidated in *S. cerevisiae* (carboxypeptidases, aminopeptidases, and dipeptidyl aminopeptidases). An enzyme in *Saccharomyces boulardii*, a subtype of *S. cerevisiae*, was found to degrade the ileal receptors in rats for toxin A generated from *Clostridium difficile* (a food-associated pathogen causing gastroenteritis; one study isolated *C. difficile* from 2.3% of broiler chickens tested) (247, 248). The degradation of the receptors prohibits the toxin from binding and prevents infection from occurring (249, 250). There have been multiple other proposed mechanisms of action for yeast on the immunoprotective effect in the GIT, specifically the prevention of *C. difficile* infection: (1) *S. boulardii* releases proteases that hydrolyze toxins and prevent its binding to the intestinal receptor (250),

(2) *S. boulardii* is capable of stimulating the activity of disaccharidases in the intestinal brush border with no additional alterations of the intestinal mucosa (211), and (3) *S. boulardii* increased the production and secretion of glycoproteins, namely the secretory component of immunoglobulin A (251). Potentially, by narrowing the focus on the exact mechanism of action, *S. cerevisiae* could be engineered to confer said mechanism and supplemented into animal (poultry) feed to prevent colonization of *C. difficile*.

Invertase is another enzyme produced by *S. cerevisiae*; it hydrolyzes sucrose into glucose and fructose (252). Invertase efficiency and sucrose availability allows for glucose to be a carbon source for *S. cerevisiae* (252). Ideally, provided the diet contained appropriate levels of sucrose, one could engineer *S. cerevisiae* to overproduce invertase and subsequently add it to poultry feed. This would allow increased production of glucose, available not only for its own needs but also for other microorganisms in the surrounding environment. This mode of action would not be selective toward beneficial bacteria in the microbiome.

Yeasts have multiple amino acid transport systems; amino acids are incorporated into proteins or they are broken down and utilized as nitrogen and carbon sources to promote growth (253). Yeasts and yeast derivatives are capable of producing amino acids; therefore supplementation to animal feed would provide both the host and the microbiome with amino acids. Almquist (254) reviewed the essential amino acid requirements in young chicks, laying hens, and turkeys; Almquist included a table outlining the percentages of each amino acid to reach a specific protein level. Amino acids are necessary for poultry to have proper growth and promote efficient weight gain and feed conversion ratios (255). Lysine appears to be one such amino acid that plays a significant role in the body composition of poultry (256). Mutants of *S. cerevisiae* have been revealed to produce up to 17 times as much lysine as wildtype; thus this rich source of lysine may prove to be valuable to the growth and development of poultry (257).

Miscellaneous metabolites are also produced in *S. cerevisiae*, including toxins responsible for the "killer phenomenon." Originally, this phenomenon was considered to be lethal only toward members of the same species; however, further investigation has led to the recognition of these toxic species to have destructive consequences reaching both prokaryotic and eukaryotic organisms (258–261). Polonelli and Morace (261) acknowledge that the inhibition of outside species may not be a direct impact on the toxins secreted, but more of a concerted effort from multiple metabolites. Nevertheless, these toxic species of *S. cerevisiae* are displaying lethality toward unrelated species. This can be utilized to the advantage of commercial poultry production, provided further research is conducted on characterizing whether this toxicity also occurs toward beneficial bacteria.

Conclusions: Impact on Poultry Industry and Future Directions

In the search for a replacement to antibiotic growth promoters, the poultry broiler industry has two main objectives, a substance that (1) increases the growth of broiler chickens (body weight gain and feed conversion ratio) and (2) prevents the colonization of invading pathogens. Ideally, a single feed additive would prevent pathogen colonization while developing beneficial microbiota to aid in bird growth and feed conversion (262). Multiple feed additives have been attempted: antimicrobial agents, probiotics, prebiotics, and prebiotic-like substances. Probiotics need to be clearly identified and carefully analyzed to understand the influence they may have on the poultry GIT microbiota. As discussed previously, lactobacilli and bifidobacteria are two known groups that provide the host health and well-being based on their end products. These bacteria both ward off pathogens by creating an unfavorable environment against pathogen retention in the gut and also generally aid host GIT health, in turn resulting in enhanced bird growth (133).

To increase the efficacy of supplying probiotics to the host, the concept of synbiotics has been suggested. Synbiotics entail equipping the beneficial bacteria with substrates specific to their metabolic needs (23). Potentially, this allows for the greatest impact as it reduces the substrates taken by the probiotics from the host. Prebiotic-like substances are often times non-selective, therefore, combining a probiotic and a prebiotic-like substance does not fit into the synbiotic definition (263). Understanding the effects and specificity of probiotics, prebiotics, and prebiotic-like substances will allow for the best match of known commensal bacterial communities and substrates for a given host.

Yeast cells and YC products developed thus far have been extensively examined for their effects as supplements in animal feed. Numerous studies report the positive association with growth performance, immunostimulation, and microbiome modulation in animals and humans (209). In addition to being explored for their positive impacts as supplements in animal feed, yeasts and their derivatives have been investigated for their low risk and assurances of safety in their usage. Yeasts are cost efficient in both production and formulation (200). They do not have the ability to transfer genes they may acquire to pathogenic or commensal bacteria, or to the host. Yeasts are able to resist acquisition of antimicrobial resistance as well as not allowing for the transfer of such resistance (209). This also allows yeast to be safely used in parallel with antibacterial agents. Yeasts also have multiple mechanisms of action, allowing them to be productive in a range of environments (200).

A more thorough understanding of the microbiome can elucidate the mechanisms of prebiotics and prebiotic-like substances. The GIT microbiome is distinct and unique in its functionality relying on the presence of a definable, and potentially identifiable, microbial consortia. Understanding the influences of the members of the microbiome and also the microbiome as a single entity will allow for a more directed approach in the search of therapeutics and growth promoters. The GIT microbiome may be more appropriately considered as an additional organ; it has impact on host growth and development, and host health.

The limitations in previous research conducted have made future research necessary to resolve unanswered questions. It is imperative to define universal and standardized detection methodology to identify the bacterial communities present in the healthy, mature poultry microbiome. This would alleviate the issue of having varying results based on detection methods utilized. In addition, evaluating the currently suggested probiotic candidate organisms (**Table 3**) indicates the potential advantages of involving multiple potential probiotic bacterial and yeast strains to exhibit a concerted effort in maintaining GIT health. This would allow for the identification of potentially more uniform mixed probiotic cultures consisting of functionally well-defined individual bacterial members that when used to inoculate newly hatched chicks ensures more rapid development of a mature beneficial microbiome.

Further work with yeast, YC, and yeast extracts needs to be conducted on poultry. Much of the discussion in the current review was based on the results from yeast products applied to animals and humans but not poultry. To gain an accurate sense of the effects in poultry, such experimentation needs to be conducted in poultry (*in vitro* and *in vivo*). Additionally, many of the metabolites mentioned previously were investigated independent of yeast, YC, or yeast extract. It would be beneficial to assess the impact of metabolites and components from yeast individually as well as when combined. This would allow for the identification of beneficial metabolites and their respective individual and combined functional impacts on the corresponding host.

Funding

Funding is provided internally by Dr. Steven Ricke's lab.

Acknowledgments

We thank the University of Arkansas, Fayetteville, Department of Food Science program for supporting SR with a graduate student assistantship. We would also like to acknowledge Dr. Jeffrey Lewis, Department of Biological Sciences, University of Arkansas, Fayetteville, AR, USA for his input on yeast biology.

References

1. US EPA. *Background of Poultry Production. Poultry Production Ag 101* (2013) [cited 2015 Aug 24]. Available from: http://www.epa.gov/oecaagct/ag101/poultry.html
2. Daniel CR, Cross AJ, Koebnick C, Sinha R. Trends in meat consumption in the USA. *Public Health Nutr* (2010) **14**:575–83. doi:10.1017/S1368980010002077
3. USDA Office of Communications. Ch 2: profiling food consumption in America. *Agriculture Fact Book 2001–2002*. Washington, DC (2003) [cited 2015 Aug 24]. Available from: http://www.usda.gov/factbook/chapter2.pdf
4. Emmerson DA. Commercial approaches to genetic selection for growth and feed conversion in domestic poultry. *Poult Sci* (1997) **76**:1121–5. doi:10.1093/ps/76.8.1121
5. Cherry JA, Siegel PB, Beane WL. Genetic-nutritional relationships in growth and carcass characteristics of broiler chickens. *Poult Sci* (1978) **57**:1482–7. doi:10.3382/ps.0571482
6. Lumpkins BS, Batal AB, Lee MD. Evaluation of the bacterial community and intestinal development of different genetic lines of chickens. *Poult Sci* (2010) **89**:1614–21. doi:10.3382/ps.2010-00747
7. de Verdal H, Narcy A, Bastianelli D, Chapuis H, Meme N, Urvoix S, et al. Improving the efficiency of feed utilization in poultry by selection. 2. Genetic parameters of excretion traits and correlations with anatomy of the gastro-intestinal tract and digestive efficiency. *BMC Genet* (2011) **12**:71. doi:10.1186/1471-2156-12-71
8. Norris D, Ngambi JW. Genetic parameters estimates for body weight in local Venda chickens. *Trop Anim Health Prod* (2006) **38**:605–9. doi:10.1007/s11250-006-4420-6
9. Leeson S, Caston L, Summer JD. Layer performances of four strains of *Leghorn pullets* subjected to various rearing programs. *Poult Sci* (1997) **76**:1–5. doi:10.1093/ps/76.1.1
10. Havenstein GB, Ferket PR, Scheideler SE, Rives DV. Carcass composition and yield of 1991 vs 1957 broilers when fed "typical" 1957 and 1991 broiler diets. *Poult Sci* (1994) **73**:1795–804. doi:10.3382/ps.0731795
11. Havenstein GB, Ferket PR, Qureshi MA. Growth, livability, and feed conversion of 1957 versus 2001 broilers when fed representative 1957 and 2001 broiler diets. *Poult Sci* (2003) **82**:1500–8. doi:10.1093/ps/82.10.1500
12. Ravindran A. FAO Poultry Development Review. Poultry Feed Availability and Nutrition in Developing Countries: Main Ingradients Used in Poultry Feed Formulations. (2013) [cited 2015 Aug 24]. Available from: http://www.fao.org/docrep/019/i353ie.pdf
13. Bunyan J, Jeffries L, Sayers JR, Gulliver AL, Coleman K. Antimicrobial substances and chick growth promotion: the growth-promoting activities of antimicrobial substances, including fifty-two used either in therapy or as dietary additives. *Br Poult Sci* (1977) **18**:283–94. doi:10.1080/00071667708416364
14. Feighner SD, Dashkevicz MP. Subtherapeutic levels of antibiotics in poultry feeds and their effects on weight gain, feed efficiency, and bacterial cholyltaurine hydrolase activity. *Appl Environ Microbiol* (1987) **53**:331–6.
15. Gaskins HR, Collier CT, Anderson DB. Antibiotics as growth promotants: mode of action. *Anim Biotechnol* (2002) **13**:29–42. doi:10.1081/ABIO-120005768
16. Dibner JJ, Richards JD. Antibiotic growth promoters in agriculture: history and mode of action. *Poult Sci* (2005) **84**:634–43. doi:10.1093/ps/84.4.634
17. Jones FT, Ricke SC. Observations on the history of the development of antimicrobials and their use in poultry feeds. *Poult Sci* (2003) **82**:613–7. doi:10.1093/ps/82.4.613
18. HHS. *National Action Plan for Combating Antibiotic-Resistant Bacteria*. Washington, DC: Presidential Advisory Council on Combating Antibiotic-Resistant Bacteria (2015).
19. Castanon JIR. History of the use of antibiotic as growth promoters in European poultry feeds. *Poult Sci* (2007) **86**:2466–71. doi:10.3382/ps.2007-00249
20. CDC. *Antibiotic Resistance Threats in the United States, 2013*. Altanta, GA: Center for Disease Control and Prevention (2013) [cited 2015 Aug 24] Available from: http://www.cdc.gov/drugresistance/pdf/ar-threats-2013-508.pdf
21. Huyghebaert G, Ducatelle R, Van Immerseel F. An update on alternatives to antimicrobial growth promoters for broilers. *Vet J* (2011) **187**:182–8. doi:10.1016/j.tvjl.2010.03.003
22. Roberfroid MB. Prebiotics: the concept revisisted. *J Nutr* (2007) **137**:830S–7S.
23. Patterson JA, Burkholder KM. Application of prebiotics and probiotics in poultry production. *Poult Sci* (2003) **82**:627–31. doi:10.1093/ps/82.4.627
24. Flickinger EA, Van Loo J, Fahey GC Jr. Nutritional responses to the presence of inulin and oligofructose in the diets of domesticated animals: a review. *Crit Rev Food Sci Nutr* (2003) **43**:19–60. doi:10.1080/10408690390826446
25. Lutful Kabir SM. The role of probiotics in the poultry industry. *Int J Mol Sci* (2009) **10**:3531–46. doi:10.3390/ijims10083531
26. Fuller R. Probiotics in man and animals. *J Appl Bacteriol* (1989) **66**:365–78. doi:10.1111/j.1365-2672.1989.tb05105.x
27. Yang Y, Iji PA, Choct M. Dietary modulation of gut microflora in broiler chickens: a review of the role of six kinds of alternatives to in-feed antibiotics. *Worlds Poult Sci J* (2009) **65**:97–114. doi:10.1017/S0043933909000087
28. Ferket PR, Parks CW, Grimes JL. *Benefits of Dietary Antibiotic and Mannanoligosaccharide Supplementation for Poultry* (2002). Available from: http://www.feedinfo.com/files/multi2002-ferket.pdf
29. Flickinger EA, Fahey GC Jr. Pet food and feed applications of inulin, oligofructose and other oligosaccharides. *Br J Nutr* (2002) **87**:S297–300. doi:10.1079/BJN/2002552
30. Russell JB. Another explanation for the toxicity of fermentation acids at low pH: anion accumulation versus uncoupling. *J Appl Bacteriol* (1992) **73**:363–70. doi:10.1111/j.1365-2672.1992.tb04990.x
31. Ricke SC. Perspectives on the use of organic acids and short chain fatty acids as antimicrobials. *Poult Sci* (2003) **82**:632–9. doi:10.1093/ps/82.4.632
32. Van Immerseel F, Russell JB, Flythe MD, Gantois I, Timbermont L, Pasmans F, et al. The use of organic acids to combat *Salmonella* in poultry: a mechanistic explanation of the efficacy. *Avian Pathol* (2006) **35**:182–8. doi:10.1080/03079450600711045

33. Thompson JL, Hinton M. Antibacterial activity of formic and propionic acids in diet of hens on salmonellas in the crop. *Br Poult Sci* (1997) **38**:59–65. doi:10.1080/00071669708417941
34. Ganguly S. Supplementation of prebiotics, probiotics and acids on immunity in poultry feed: a brief review. *Worlds Poult Sci J* (2013) **69**:639–48. doi:10.1017/S0043933913000640
35. Gibson GR, Roberfroid MB. Dietary modulation of the human colonic microbiota: introducing the concept of prebiotics. *J Nutr* (1995) **125**:1401–12.
36. AAM. *Human Microbiome FAQ*. Washington, DC: American Academy of Microbiology of American Society for Microbiology (2013).
37. Bäckhed F, Ley RE, Sonnenburg JL, Peterson DA, Gordon JL. Host-bacterial mutualism in the human intestine. *Science* (2005) **307**:1915–20. doi:10.1126/science.1104816
38. Xu J, Gordon JI. Honor thy symbionts. *Proc Natl Acad Sci U S A* (2003) **100**:10452–9. doi:10.1073/pnas.1734063100
39. Farthing MJ. Bugs and the gut: an unstable marriage. *Best Pract Res Clin Gastroenterol* (2004) **18**:233–9. doi:10.1016/j.bpg.2003.11.001
40. Hall-Stoodley L, Costerton JW, Stoodley P. Bacterial biofilms: from the natural environment to infectious diseases. *Nat Rev Microbiol* (2004) **2**:95–108. doi:10.1038/nrmicro821
41. Aas JA, Paster BJ, Stokes LN, Olsen I, Dewhirst FE. Defining the normal bacterial flora of the oral cavity. *J Clin Microbiol* (2005) **43**:5721–32. doi:10.1128/JCM.43.11.5721-5732.2005
42. Costello E, Lauber CL, Hamady M, Fierer N, Gordon JI, Knight R. Bacterial community variation in human body habitats across space and time. *Science* (2009) **326**:1694–7. doi:10.1126/science.1177486
43. Han MK, Huang YJ, Lipuma JJ, Boushey HA, Boucher RC, Cookson WO, et al. Significance of the microbiome in obstructive lung disease. *Thorax* (2012) **67**:456–63. doi:10.1136/thoraxjnl-2011-201183
44. Huang YJ, Lunch SV. The emerging relationship between the airway microbiota and chronic respiratory disease: clinical implications. *Expert Rev Respir Med* (2011) **5**:809–21. doi:10.1586/ers.11.76
45. Gill SR, Pop M, DeBoy RT, Eckburg PB, Turnbaugh PJ, Samuel BS, et al. Metagenomic analysis of the human distal gut microbiome. *Science* (2006) **312**:1355–9. doi:10.1126/science.1124234
46. Apajalahti JHA, Kettunen A, Graham H. Characteristics of the gastrointestinal microbial communities, with special reference to chicken. *Worlds Poult Sci J* (2004) **60**:223–32. doi:10.1079/WPS200415
47. Egert M, De Graaf AA, Smidt H, De Vos WM, Venema K. Beyond diversity: functional microbiomics of the human colon. *Trends Microbiol* (2006) **14**:86–91. doi:10.1016/j.tim.2005.12.007
48. Hoffmann C, Hill DA, Minkah N, Kirn T, Troy A, Artis D, et al. Community-wide response of the gut microbiota to enteropathogenic *Citrobacter rodentium* infection revealed by deep sequencing. *Infect Immun* (2009) **77**:4668–78. doi:10.1128/IAI.00493-09
49. Brisbin JT, Gong J, Sharif S. Interactions between commensal bacteria and the gut-associated immune system of the chicken. *Anim Health Res Rev* (2008) **9**:101–10. doi:10.1017/S146625230800145X
50. Delzenne NM, Cani PD. Interaction between obesity and the gut microbiota: relevance in nutrition. *Annu Rev Nutr* (2011) **31**:15–31. doi:10.1146/annurev-nutr-072610-145146
51. Munyaka PM, Khafipour E, Ghia J. External influence of early childhood establishment of gut microbiota and subsequent health implications. *Front Pediatr* (2014) **2**:109. doi:10.3389/fped.2014.00109
52. Arrieta M, Stiemsma LT, Amenyogbe N, Brown EM, Finlay B. The intestinal microbiome in early life: health and disease. *Front Immunol* (2014) **5**:427. doi:10.3389/fimmu.2014.00427
53. Mabelebele M, Alabi OJ, Ng'ambi JW, Norris D, Ginindza MM. Comparison of gastrointestinal tracts and pH values of digestive organs of Ross 308 broiler and indigenous Venda chickens fed the same diet. *Asian J Anim Vet Adv* (2014) **9**:71–6. doi:10.3923/ajava.2014.71.76
54. Pan D, Yu Z. Intestinal microbiome of poultry and its interaction with host and diet. *Gut Microbes* (2014) **5**:108–19. doi:10.4161/gmic.26945
55. Scanes CG, Brant G, Ensminger ME. Poultry biology. 4th ed. *Poultry Science*. Upper Saddle River, NJ: Prentice Hall (2004). p. 22–45.
56. Duke GE, Petrides GA, Ringer RK. Chromium-51 in food metabolizability and passage rate studies with the ring-necked Pheasant. *Poult Sci* (1968) **47**:1356–64. doi:10.3382/ps.0471356
57. Clarke PL. Coccidial infection with *Eimeria tenella* and caecal defaecation in chicks. *Br Poult Sci* (1979) **20**:317–22. doi:10.1080/00071667908416586
58. Turk DE. The anatomy of the avian digestive tract as related to feed utilization. *Poult Sci* (1982) **61**:1225–44. doi:10.3382/ps.0611225
59. Gelis S. Evaluating and treating the gastrointestinal system. *Clin Avian Med* (2013) **1**:411–40.
60. Izat AL, Colberg M, Reiber MA, Adams MH, Skinner JT, Cabel MC, et al. Effects of different antibiotics on performance, processing characteristics and parts yield of broiler chickens. *Poult Sci* (1990) **69**:1787–91. doi:10.3382/ps.0691787
61. Jukes HG, Hill DC, Branion HD. Effect of feeding antibiotics on the intestinal tract of the chick. *Poult Sci* (1956) **35**:716–23. doi:10.3382/ps.0350716
62. Henry PR, Ammerman CB, Campbell DR, Miles RD. Effect of antibiotics on tissue trace mineral concentration and intestinal tract weight of broiler chicks. *Poult Sci* (1987) **66**:1014–8. doi:10.3382/ps.0661014
63. Jacob J. *Avian Digestive System [Internet]. Extension America's Research-Based Learning Network* (2015) [cited 2015 Apr 14]. Available from: http://www.extension.org:80/pages/65376/avian-digestive-system
64. Zhu XT, Zhong T, Pandya Y, Joerger RD. 16S rRNA-based analysis of microbiota from the cecum of broiler chickens. *Appl Environ Microbiol* (2002) **68**:124–37. doi:10.1128/AEM.68.1.124-137.2002
65. Lan PTN, Hayashie H, Sakamoto M, Benno Y. Phylogenetic analysis of cecal microbiota in chicken by the use of 16S rDNA clone libraries. *Microbiol Immunol* (2002) **46**:371–82. doi:10.1111/j.1348-0421.2002.tb02709.x
66. Apajalahti JHA, Kettunen A, Bedford MR, Holben WE. Percent G+C profiling accurately reveals diet-related difference in the gastrointestinal microbial community of broiler chickens. *Appl Environ Microbiol* (2001) **67**:5656–67. doi:10.1128/AEM.67.12.5656-5667.2001
67. Gong J, Forster RJ, Yu H, Chambers JR, Wheatcroft R, Sabour PM, et al. Molecular analysis of bacterial populations in the ileum of broiler chickens and comparison with bacteria in the cecum. *FEMS Microbiol Ecol* (2002) **41**:171–9. doi:10.1111/j.1574-6941.2002.tb00978.x
68. Rada V, Sirotek K, Petr J. Evaluation of selective media for bifidobacteria in poultry and rabbit caecal samples. *Zentralbl Veterinarmed B* (1999) **46**:369–73. doi:10.1046/j.1439-0450.1999.00241.x
69. Malmuthuge N, Li M, Chen Y, Fried P, Griebel PJ, Bushansingh B, et al. Distinct commensal bacteria associated with ingest and mucosal epithelium in the gastrointestinal tract of calves and chickens. *FEMS Microbiol Ecol* (2012) **79**:337–47. doi:10.1111/j.1574-6941.2011.01220.x
70. Apajalahti JHA, Sarkilahti LK, Maki BRE, Heikkinen JP, Nurminen PH, Holben WE. Effective recovery of bacterial DNA and percent-guanine-plus-cytosine-based analysis of community structure in the gastrointestinal tract of broiler chickens. *Appl Environ Microbiol* (1998) **64**:4084–8.
71. Amit-Romach E, Sklan D, Uni Z. Microflora ecology of the chicken intestine using 16S ribosomal DNA primers. *Poult Sci* (2004) **83**:1093–8. doi:10.1093/ps/83.7.1093
72. Bjerrum L, Enberg RM, Leser TD, Jensen BB, Finster K, Pedersen K. Microbial community composition of the ileum and cecum of broiler chickens as revealed by molecular and culture-based techniques. *Poult Sci* (2006) **85**:1151–64. doi:10.1093/ps/85.7.1151
73. Olsen KN, Henriksen M, Bisgaard M, Nielsen OL, Christensen H. Investigation of chicken intestinal bacterial communities by 16S rRNA targeted fluorescence in situ hybridization. *Antonie Van Leeuwenhoek* (2008) **94**:423–37. doi:10.1007/s10482-008-9260-0
74. Collado MC, Sanz Y. Characterization of the gastrointestinal mucosa-associated microbiota of pigs and chickens using culture-based and molecular methodologies. *J Food Prot* (2007) **70**:2799–804.
75. Lu J, Idris U, Harmon B, Hofacre C, Mauer JJ, Lee MD. Diversity and succession of the intestinal bacterial community of the maturing broiler chicken. *Appl Environ Microbiol* (2003) **69**:6816–24. doi:10.1128/AEM.69.11.6818-6824.2003
76. Mead GC, Adams BW. Some observations on the caecal microflora of the chick during the first two weeks of life. *Br Poult Sci* (1975) **16**:169–76. doi:10.1080/00071667508416174
77. Karunasena E, McMahon KW, Chang D, Brashears MM. Responses to the pathogen *Mycobacterium avium* subsp. *paratuberculosis* and beneficial microbes exhibit host sex specificity. *Appl Environ Microbiol* (2014) **80**:4481–90. doi:10.1128/AEM.01229-14

78. Van der Wielen PW, Keuzenkamp DA, Lipman LJA, van Knapen F, Biesterveld S. Spatial and temporal variation of the intestinal bacterial community in commercially raised broiler chickens during growth. *Microb Ecol* (2002) **44**:286–93. doi:10.1007/s00248-002-2015-y
79. Patterson JA. The commensal microbiota. In: Callaway TR, Ricke SC, editors. *Direct-Fed Microbials and Prebiotics for Animals*. New York, NY: Springer Science+Business Media, LLC (2011). p. 3–11.
80. Gabriel I, Lessire M, Mallet SG, Guillot JF. Microflora of the digestive tract: critical factors and consequences for poultry. *Worlds Poult Sci J* (2006) **62**:499–512. doi:10.1017/S0043933906001115
81. Lei F, Yin Y, Wang Y, Deng B, Yu HD, Li L, et al. Higher-level production of volatile fatty acids *in vitro* by chicken gut microbiotas than by human gut microbiotas as determined by functional analyses. *Appl Environ Microbiol* (2012) **78**:5763–72. doi:10.1128/AEM.00327-12
82. McBride BW, Kelly JM. Energy cost of absorption and metabolism in the ruminant gastrointestinal tract and liver: a review. *J Anim Sci* (1990) **68**:2997–3010.
83. Hedge SN, Roll BA, Coates ME. The effects of gut microflora and dietary fibre on energy utilization by the chick. *Br J Nutr* (1982) **48**:73–80. doi:10.1079/BJN19820089
84. Lan Y, Verstegen M, Tammings S, Williams B. The role of the commensal gut microbial community in broiler chickens. *Worlds Poult Sci J* (2005) **61**:95–104. doi:10.1079/WPS200445
85. Annison EF, Hill KJ, Kenworthy R. Volatile fatty acids in the digestive tract of the fowl. *Br J Nutr* (1968) **22**:207–16. doi:10.1079/BJN19680026
86. Bolton W, Dewar WA. The digestibility of acetic, propionic and butyric acids by the fowl. *Br Poult Sci* (1965) **6**:103–5. doi:10.1080/00071666508415562
87. Muramatsu T, Kodama H, Morishita T, Furuse M, Okumura J. Effect of intestinal microflora on digestible energy and fiber digestibility in chickens fed a high fiber diet. *Am J Vet Res* (1991) **52**:1178–81.
88. Muramatsu T, Nakajima S, Furuse M, Tasaki I, Okumura J. Influence of the gut microflora on fasting heat production in chicks. *Br Poult Sci* (1988) **29**:301–9. doi:10.1080/00071668808417055
89. Muramatsu T, Nakajima S, Okumura J. Modification of energy metabolism by the presence of the gut microflora in the chicken. *Br J Nutr* (1994) **71**:709–17. doi:10.1079/BJN19940178
90. Choct M. Soluble non-starch polysaccharides affect net utilization of energy by chickens. *Rec Adv Anim Nutr Aust* (1999) **12**:31–5.
91. Gaskins HR. Immunological development and mucosal defense in the pig intestine in progress. In: Wiseman J, Varley MA, Chadwick JP, editors. *Progress in Pig Science*. Nottingham: Nottingham University Press (1998). p. 81–101.
92. Furuse M, Yokota H. Protein and energy utilization in germ-free and conventional chicks given diets containing different levels of dietary protein. *Br J Nutr* (1984) **51**:255–64. doi:10.1079/BJN19840030
93. Hardin G. The competitive exclusion principle. *Science* (1960) **131**:1292–7. doi:10.1126/science.131.3409.1292
94. Lawley TD, Walker AW. Intestinal colonization resistance. *Immunology* (2012) **138**:1–11. doi:10.1111/j.1365-2567.2012.03616.x
95. Crhanova M, Hradecka H, Faldynova M, Matulova M, Havlickova H, Sisak F, et al. Immune response of chicken gut to natural colonization by gut microflora and to *Salmonella enterica* serovar enteritidis infection. *Infect Immun* (2011) **79**:2755–63. doi:10.1128/IAI.01375-10
96. Al-Zenki SF, Al-Nasser AY, Al-Saffar AE, Abdullah FK, Al-Bahouh ME, Al-Haddad AS, et al. Effects of using a chicken-origin competitive exclusion culture and probiotic cultures on reducing *Salmonella* in broilers. *J Appl Poult Res* (2009) **18**:23–9. doi:10.3382/japr.2008-00036
97. Nurmi E, Rantala M. New aspects of *Salmonella* infection in broiler production. *Nature* (1973) **241**:210–1. doi:10.1038/241210a0
98. Gleeson TM, Stravic S, Blanchfield B. Protection of chicks against *Salmonella* infection with a mixture of pure culture of intestinal bacteria. *Avian Dis* (1989) **33**:636–42. doi:10.2307/1591137
99. Nisbet D. Defined competitive exclusion cultures in the prevention of enteropathogen colonization in poultry and swine. *Antonie Van Leeuwenhoek* (2002) **81**:481–6. doi:10.1023/A:1020541603877
100. Lloyd AB, Cummings RB, Kent RD. Prevention of *Salmonella typhimurium* infection in poultry by pre-treatment of chickens and poults with intestinal extracts. *Aust Vet J* (1997) **53**:82–7. doi:10.1111/j.1751-0813.1977.tb14891.x
101. Barnes EM, Impey CS, Cooper DM. Manipulation of the crop and intestinal flora of the crop and intestinal flora of the newly-hatched chick. *Am J Clin Nutr* (1980) **33**:2426–33.
102. Corrier DE, Hinton A, Ziprin RL, Beier RC, DeLoach JR. Effect of dietary lactose on cecal pH, bacteriostatic volatile fatty acids, and *Salmonella typhimurium* colonization of broiler chicks. *Avian Dis* (1990) **34**:617–25. doi:10.2307/1591254
103. Stavric S. Defined cultures and prospects. *Int J Food Microbiol* (1992) **15**:245–63. doi:10.1016/0168-1605(92)90056-9
104. Schleifer JH. A review of the efficacy and mechanism of competitive exclusion for the control of *Salmonella* in poultry. *Worlds Poult Sci J* (1985) **41**:72–83. doi:10.1079/WPS19850007
105. Mead GC. Prospects for 'competitive exclusion' treatment to control salmonellas and other foodborne pathogens in poultry. *Vet J* (2000) **159**:111–23. doi:10.1053/tvjl.1999.0423
106. Stavric S, D'Aoust JY. Undefined and defined bacterial preparations for the competitive exclusion of *Salmonella* in poultry – a review. *J Food Prot* (1993) **56**:173–80.
107. Paul B, Hirshfield I. The effect of acid treatment on survival and protein expression of a laboratory K-12 strain *Escherichia coli*. *Res Microbiol* (2003) **154**:115–21. doi:10.1016/S0923-2508(02)00011-6
108. Levison ME. Effect of colon flora and short-chain fatty acids on growth in vitro of *Pseudomonas aeruginosa* and *Enterobacteriaceae*. *Infect Immun* (1973) **8**:30–5.
109. Lee A, Gemmell E. Changes in the mouse intestinal mictoflora during weaning: role of volatile fatty acids. *Infect Immun* (1972) **5**:1–7.
110. Mani-López E, García HS, López-Malo A. Organic acids as antimicrobials to control *Salmonella* in meat and poultry products. *Food Res Int* (2012) **45**:713–21. doi:10.1016/j.foodres.2011.04.043
111. Cherrington CA, Hinton M, Mead GC, Chopra I. Organic acids: chemistry, antibacterial activity and practical applications. *Adv Microb Phys* (1991) **32**:88–108. doi:10.1016/S0065-2911(08)60006-5
112. Davidson PM, Taylor TM, Schmidt SE. Chemical preservatives and natural antimicrobial compounds. In: Doyle MP, editor. *Food Microbiology: Fundamentals and Frontiers*. Washington, DC: ASM Press (2007). p. 765–801.
113. Cherrington CA, Hinton M, Chopra I. Effect of short-chain organic acids on macromolecular synthesis in *Escherichia coli*. *J Appl Bacteriol* (1990) **68**:69–74. doi:10.1111/j.1365-2672.1990.tb02550.x
114. Axe DD, Bailey JE. Transport of lactate and acetate through the energized cytoplasmic membrane of *Escherichia coli*. *Biotechnol Bioeng* (1995) **47**:8–19. doi:10.1002/bit.260470103
115. Kashket ER. Bioenergetics of lactic acid bacteria: cytoplasmic pH and osmotolerance. *FEMS Microbiol Lett* (1987) **46**:233–44. doi:10.1111/j.1574-6968.1987.tb02463
116. Diez-Gonzalez F, Russell JB. Effects of carbonylcyanide-*m*-chlorophenylhydrazone (CCCP) and acetate on *Escherichia coli* O157:H7 and K-12: uncoupling versus anion accumulation. *FEMS Microbiol Lett* (1997) **151**:71–6. doi:10.1111/j.1574-6968.1997.tb10396.x
117. Alakomi H-L, Skyttä E, Saarela M, Mattila-Sandholm T, Latva-Kala K, Helander IM. Lactic acid permeabilizes Gram-negative bacteria by disrupting the outer membrane. *Appl Environ Microbiol* (2000) **66**:2001–5. doi:10.1128/AEM.66.5.2001-2005.2000
118. Alakomi H-L, Puupponen-Pimiä R, Aura A-M, Helander IM, Nohynek L, Oksman-Caldentey K-M, et al. Weakening of *Salmonella* with selected microbial metabolites of berry-derived phenolic compounds and organic acids. *J Agric Food Chem* (2007) **55**:3905–12. doi:10.1021/jf070190y
119. Kwon YM, Ricke SC. Induction of acid resistance of *Salmonella typhimurium* by exposure to short-chain fatty acids. *Appl Environ Microbiol* (1998) **64**:3458–63.
120. Foster JW. Low pH adaptation and the acid tolerance response of *Salmonella typhimurium*. *Crit Rev Microbiol* (1995) **21**:215–37. doi:10.3109/10408419509113541
121. Durant JA, Lowry VK, Nisbet DJ, Stanker LH, Corrier DE, Ricke SC. Short chain fatty acids alter HEp-2 cell association and invasion by stationary growth phase *Salmonella typhimurium*. *J Food Sci* (2000) **65**:1206–9. doi:10.1111/j.1365-2621.2000.tb10266.x
122. Durant JA, Corrier DE, Ricke SC. Short-chain volatile fatty acids modulate the expression of the *hilA* and *invF* genes of *Salmonella typhimurium*. *J Food Prot* (2000) **63**:573–8.

123. Huang CB, Alimova Y, Myers TM, Ebersole JL. Short- and medium-chain fatty acids exhibit antimicrobial activity for oral microorganisms. *Arch Oral Biol* (2011) **56**:650–4. doi:10.1016/j.archoralbio.2011.01.011
124. Smulders FJM, Barendsen P, van Logtestijn JG, Mossel DAA, van der Marel GM. Review: lactic acid: considerations in favour of its acceptance as a meat decontaminant. *Int J Food Sci Technol* (1986) **21**:419–36. doi:10.111/j.1365-2621.1986.tb00420.x
125. van Der Wielen PW, Biesterveld S, Notermans S, Hofstra H, Urlings BA, van Knapen F. Role of volatile fatty acids in development of the cecal microflora in broiler chickens during growth. *Appl Environ Microbiol* (2000) **66**:2536–40. doi:10.1128/AEM.66.6.2536-2540.2000
126. Cook RH, Bird FH. Duodenal villus area and epithelial cellular migration in conventional and germ-free chicks. *Poult Sci* (1973) **52**:2276–80. doi:10.3382/ps.0522276
127. Gordon HA, Bruckner-Kardoss E. Effect of normal microbial flora on intestinal surface area. *Am J Physiol* (1961) **201**:175–8.
128. Naqi SA, Lewis DH, Hall CF. The intestinal microflora of turkeys. *Avian Dis* (1970) **14**:620–5.
129. Round JL, Mazmanian SK. The gut microbiota shapes intestinal immune responses during health and disease. *Nat Rev Immunol* (2009) **9**:313–23. doi:10.1038/nri2515
130. Talebi A, Amirzadeh B, Mokhtari B, Gahri H. Effects of a multi-strain probiotic (PrimaLac) on performance and antibody responses to Newcastle disease virus and infectious bursal disease virus vaccination in broiler chickens. *Avian Pathol* (2008) **37**:509–12. doi:10.1080/03079450802356995
131. Salianeh N, Shirzad MR, Seifi S. Performance and antibody response of broiler chickens fed diets containing probiotic and prebiotic. *J Appl Anim Res* (2011) **39**:65–7. doi:10.1080/09712119.2011.565222
132. Mohan B, Kadirvel R, Natarjan A, Bhaskaran M. Effect of probiotic supplementation on growth, nitrogen utilization and serum cholesterol in broilers. *Br Poult Sci* (1996) **37**:395–401. doi:10.1080/00071669608417870
133. Sun Y, O'Riordan MX. Regulation of bacterial pathogenesis by intestinal short-chain fatty acids. *Adv Appl Microbiol* (2013) **85**:93–118. doi:10.1016/B978-0-12-407672-3.00003-4
134. Barnes EM, Mead GC, Barnum DA, Harry EG. The intestinal flora of the chicken in the period 2 to 6 weeks of age, with particular reference to the anaerobic bacteria. *Br Poult Sci* (1972) **13**:311–26. doi:10.1080/00071667208415953
135. Shin MS, Han SK, Ji AR, Kim KS, Lee WK. Isolation and characterization of bacteriocin-producing bacteria from the gastrointestinal tract of broiler chickens for probiotic use. *J Appl Microbiol* (2008) **105**:2203–12. doi:10.1111/j.1365-2672.2008.03935.x
136. Corrier DE, Nisbet DJ, Scanlan CM, Hollister AG, DeLoach JA. Control of *Salmonella typhimurium* colonization in broiler chicks with a continuous-flow characterized mixed culture of cecal bacteria. *Poult Sci* (1995) **74**:916–24. doi:10.3382/ps.0741093
137. Nisbet DJ, Corrier DE, Ricke SC, Hume ME, Byrd JA II, DeLoach JR. Cecal propionic acid as a biological indicator of the early establishment of a microbial ecosystem inhibitory to *Salmonella* in chicks. *Anaerobe* (1996) **2**:345–50. doi:10.1006/anae.1996.0044
138. Nisbet DJ, Corrier DE, Ricke SC, Hume ME, Byrd JA II, DeLoach JR. Maintenance of the biological efficacy in chicks of a cecal competitive-exclusion culture against *Salmonella* by continuous-flow fermentation. *J Food Prot* (1996) **59**:1279–83.
139. Durant JA, Young CR, Nisbet DJ, Stanker LH, Ricke SC. Detection and quantification of poultry probiotic bacteria in mixed culture using monoclonal antibodies in an enzyme-linked immunosorbent assay. *Int J Food Microbiol* (1997) **38**:181–9. doi:10.1016/S0168-1605(97)00102-5
140. Yu B, Liu JR, Hsiao FS, Chiou PWS. Evaluation of *Lactobacillus reuteri* Pg4 strain expressing heterologous β-glucanase as a probiotic in poultry diets based on barley. *Anim Feed Sci Technol* (2008) **141**:82–91. doi:10.1016/j.anifeedsci.2007.04.010
141. Lin W-H, Yu B, Jang S-H, Tsen H-Y. Different probiotic properties for *Lactobacillus fermentum* strains isolated from swine and poultry. *Anaerobe* (2007) **13**:107–13. doi:10.1016/j.anaerobe.2007.04.006
142. Santini C, Baffoni L, Gaggia F, Granata M, Gasbarri R, Di Gioia D, et al. Characterization of probiotic strains: an application as feed additives in poultry against *Campylobacter jejuni*. *Int J Food Microbiol* (2010) **141**:S98–108. doi:10.1016/j.ijfoodmicro.2010.03.039
143. Owings WJ, Reynolds DL, Hasiak RJ, Ferket PR. Influence of dietary supplementation with *Streptococcus faecium* M-74 on broiler body weight, feed conversion, carcass characteristics, and intestinal microbial colonization. *Poult Sci* (1990) **69**:1257–64. doi:10.3382/ps.0691257
144. Herrera P, O'Bryan CA, Crandall PG, Ricke SC. Growth response of *Salmonella enterica* typhimurium in co-culture with ruminal bacterium *Streptococcus bovis* is influenced by time of inoculation and carbohydrate substrate. *Food Res Int* (2012) **45**:1054–7. doi:10.1016/j.foodres.2011.07.001
145. Walter J. Ecological role of lactobacilli in the gastrointestinal tract: implications for fundamental and biomedical research. *Appl Environ Microbiol* (2008) **74**:4985–96. doi:10.1128/AEM.00753-08
146. Tannock GW. A special fondness for lactobacilli. *Appl Environ Microbiol* (2004) **70**:3189–94. doi:10.1128/AEM.70.6.3189-3194.2004
147. Barnardeau M, Vernoux JP, Henri-Dubernet S, Guéguen M. Safety assessment of dairy microorganisms: the *Lactobacillus* genus. *Int J Food Microbiol* (2007) **126**:278–85. doi:10.1016/j.ijfoodmicro.2007.08.015
148. Pot B, Tsakalidou E. Taxonomy and metabolism of *Lactobacillus*. In: Ljungh A, Wadström T, editors. *Lactobacillus Molecular Biology: From Genomics to Probiotics*. Norfolk: Caister Academic Press (2009). p. 3–58.
149. Lindegren SE, Dobrogosz WJ. Antagonistic activities of lactic acid bacteria in food and feed fermentations. *FEMS Microbiol Rev* (1990) **87**:149–64. doi:10.1111/j.1574-6968.1990.tb04885.x
150. Hammes WP, Vogel RF. The genus *Lactobacillus*. In Wood BJB and Holzapfel WH, editors. *The Genera of Lactic Acid Bacteria*, (Vol. **2**) New York, NY: Chapman and Hall (1995). p. 19–54.
151. Bobillo M, Marshall VM. Effect of acidic pH and salt on acid end-products by *Lactobacillus plantarum* in aerated, glucose-limited continuous culture. *J Appl Microbiol* (2008) **73**:67–70. doi:10.1111/j.1365-2672.1992.tb04971.x
152. Pokusaeva K, Fitzgerald GF, van Sinderen D. Carbohydrate metabolism in *Bifidobacteria*. *Genes Nutr* (2011) **6**:285–306. doi:10.1007/s12263-010-0206-6
153. Van der Meulen R, Avonts L, De Vuyst L. Short fractions of oligofructose are preferentially metabolized by *Bifidobacterium animalis* DN-173 010. *Appl Environ Microbiol* (2004) **70**:1923–30. doi:10.1128/AEM.70.4.1923-1930.2004
154. Korakli M, Ganzle MG, Vogel RF. Metabolism by bifidobacteria and lactic acid bacteria of polysaccharides from wheat and rye, and exopolysaccharides produced by *Lactobacillus sanfranciscensis*. *J Appl Microbiol* (2002) **92**:958–65. doi:10.1046/j.1365-2672.2002.01607.x
155. Lorenzoni G. Prebiotics. In: Lorenzoni G, editor. *Poultry Diseases Influenced by Gastrointestinal Health: Traditional Treatments and Innovative Solutions*. Nottingham: Nottingham University Press (2010). p. 36–8.
156. Stephenson DP, Moore RJ, Allison GE. *Lactobacillus* strain ecology and persistence within broiler chickens fed different diets: identification of persistent strains. *Appl Environ Microbiol* (2010) **76**:6494–503. doi:10.1128/AEM.01137-10
157. Jacobsen CN, Rosenfeldt-Nielsen V, Hayford AE, Møller PL, Micharlsen KF, Pærregaard A, et al. Screening of probiotics activities of forty-seven strains of *Lactobacillus* spp. by *in vitro* techniques and evaluation of the colonization ability of five selected strains in humans. *Appl Environ Microbiol* (1999) **65**:4949–56.
158. Sandine WE. Role of *Lactobacillus* in the intestinal tract. *J Food Prot* (1979) **42**:259–62.
159. Eklund T. The effect of carbon dioxide on bacterial growth and on uptake processes in bacterial membrane vesicles. *Int J Food Microbiol* (1984) **1**:179–85. doi:10.1016/0168-1605(84)90014-X
160. Kaneuchi C, Seki M, Komagata K. Production of succinic acid from citric acid and related acids by *Lactobacillus* strains. *Appl Environ Microbiol* (1988) **54**:3053–6.
161. Van der Meulen R, Adriany T, Verbrugghe K, De Vuyst L. Kinetic analysis of bifidobacterial metabolism reveals a minor role for succinic acid in the regeneration of NAD^+ through its growth-associated production. *Appl Environ Microbiol* (2006) **72**:5204–10. doi:10.1128/AEM.00146-06
162. Gao Z, Shao J, Sun H, Zhong W, Zhuang W, Zhang Z. Evaluation of different kinds of organic acids and their antibacterial activity in Japanese apricot fruits. *Afr J Agric Res* (2012) **7**:4911–8. doi:10.5897/AJAR12.1347
163. Yang LH, Lau SCK, Lee OO, Tsoi MMY, Qian PY. Potential roles of succinic acid against colonization by a tubeworm. *J Exp Mar Bio Ecol* (2007) **349**:1–11. doi:10.1016/j.jembe.2007.03.016

164. Jay JM. Antimicrobial properties of diacetyl. *Appl Environ Microbiol* (1982) **44**:525–32.
165. Eyssen H, De Prins V, De Somer P. The growth-promoting action of virginiamycin and it influence on the crop flora in chickens. *Poult Sci* (1962) **41**:227–33. doi:10.3382/ps.0410227
166. Zaidel O, Lin HC. Uninvited guests: the impact of small intestinal bacterial overgrowth on nutritional status. *Pract Gastroenterol* (2003) **7**:27–34.
167. Herrera P, Kwon YM, Ricke SC. Ecology and pathogenicity of gastrointestinal *Streptococcus bovis*. *Anaerobe* (2009) **15**:44–54. doi:10.1016/j.anaerobe.2008.11.003
168. Gibson GR, Probert HM, Van Loo J, Rastall RA, Roberfroid MB. Dietary modulation of the human colonic microbiota: updating the concept of prebiotics. *Nutr Res Rev* (2004) **17**:259–75. doi:10.1079/NRR200479
169. Roberfroid MB. Prebiotics and probiotics: are they functional foods? *Am J Clin Nutr* (2000) **71**:1682–7.
170. Wang X, Gibson GR. Effects of the in vitro fermentation of oligofructose and inulin by bacteria growing in the human large intestine. *J Appl Bacteriol* (1993) **75**:373–80. doi:10.1111/j.1365-2672.1993.tb02790.x
171. Delzenne NM, Roberfroid MB. Physiological effects of non-digestible oligosaccharides. *LWT Food Sci Technol* (1994) **27**:1–6. doi:10.1006/fstl.1994.1001
172. Marchessault RH, Blahe T, Deslandes Y, Revol J-F. Conformation and crystalline structure of (2◊1)-β-D-fructofuranan (inulin). *Can J Chem* (1980) **58**:2415–22. doi:10.1139/v80-390
173. Van Loo J, Coussement P, Leenheer LD, Hoebregs H, Smits G. On the presence of inulin and oligofructose as natural ingredients in the western diet. *Crit Rev Food Sci Nutr* (1995) **35**:525–52. doi:10.1080/10408399509527714
174. Fishbein L, Kaplan M, Gough M. Fructooligosaccharides: a review. *Vet Hum Toxicol* (1988) **30**:104–7.
175. Macfarlane S, Macfarlane GT, Cummings JH. Review article: prebiotics in the gastrointestinal tract. *Aliment Pharmacol Ther* (2006) **24**:701–14. doi:10.1111/j.1365-2036.2006.03042.x
176. Kelly G. Inulin-type prebiotics – a review: part 1. *Altern Med Rev* (2008) **13**:315–29.
177. Fuentes-Zaragoza E, Sánchez-Zapata E, Sendra E, Sayas E, Navarro C, Fernández-López J, et al. Resistant starch as prebiotic: a review. *Starch* (2011) **63**:402–15. doi:10.1002/star.20100009
178. Ricke SC. Potential of fructooligosaccharide prebiotics in alternative and nonconventional poultry production systems. *Poult Sci* (2015) **94**:1411–8. doi:10.3382/ps/pev049
179. Shen YB, Carroll JA, Yoon I, Mateo RD, Kim SW. Effects of supplementing *Saccharomyces cerevisiae* fermentation product in sow diets on performance of sows and nursing piglets. *J Anim Sci* (2011) **89**:2462–71. doi:10.2527/jas.2010-3642
180. Price KL, Totty HB, Lee HB, Utt MD, Fitzner GE, Yoon I, et al. Use of *Saccharomyces cerevisiae* fermentation product on growth performance and microbiota of weaned pigs during *Salmonella* infection. *J Anim Sci* (2010) **88**:3896–908. doi:10.2527/jas.2009-2728
181. Gao J, Zhang HJ, Wu SG, Yu SH, Yoon I, Moore D, et al. Effect of *Saccharomyces cerevisiae* fermentation product on immune functions of broilers challenged with *Eimeria tenella*. *Poult Sci* (2009) **88**:2141–51. doi:10.3382/ps.2009-00151
182. Duina A, Miller ME, Keeney JB. Budding yeast for budding geneticists: a primer on the *Saccharomyces cerevisiae* model system. *Genetics* (2014) **197**:33–48. doi:10.1534/genetics.114.163188
183. Mortimer R. Evolution and variation of the yeast (*Saccharomyces*) genome. *Genome Res* (2000) **10**:403–9. doi:10.1101/gr.10.4.403
184. Greig D, Leu JY. Natural history of budding yeast. *Curr Biol* (2009) **19**:R886–90. doi:10.1016/j.cub.2009.07.037
185. Mortimer RK, Johnston JR. Genealogy of principal strains of the yeast genetic stock center. *Genetics* (1986) **113**:35–43.
186. Winston F, Dollard C, Ricupero-Hovasse SL. Construction of a set of convenient *Saccharomyces cerevisiae* strains that are isogenic to S288C. *Yeast* (1995) **11**:53–5. doi:10.1002/yea.320110107
187. Goffeau A, Barrell BG, Bussey H, Davis RW, Dujun B, Feldmann H, et al. Life with 6000 genes. *Science* (1996) **274**: 563–6. doi:10.1126/science.274.5287.546
188. Botstein D, Fink GR. Yeast: an experimental organism for modern biology. *Science* (1988) **240**:1439–43. doi:10.1126/science.3287619
189. Botstein D, Chervitz SA, Cherry JM. Yeast as a model organism. *Science* (1997) **277**:1259–60. doi:10.1126/science.277.5330.1259
190. Caspeta L, Chen Y, Ghiaci P, Feizi A, Buskov S, Hallström BM. Altered sterol composition renders yeast thermotolerant. *Science* (2014) **346**:75–8. doi:10.1126/science.1258137
191. Liu Y, Zhang G, Sun H, Sun X, Jiang N, Rasool A, et al. Enhanced pathway efficiency of *Saccharomyces cerevisiae* by introducing thermo-tolerant devices. *Bioresour Technol* (2014) **170**:38–44. doi:10.1016/j.biortech.2014.07.063
192. Botstein D, Fink GR. Yeast: an experimental organism for 21st century biology. *Genetics* (2011) **189**:695–704. doi:10.1534/genetics.111.130765
193. Gershon H, Gershon D. The budding yeast, *Saccharomyces cerevisiae*, as a model for aging research: a critical review. *Mech Ageing Dev* (2000) **120**:1–22. doi:10.1016/S0047-6374(00)00182-2
194. Mager WH, Winderickx J. Yeast as a model for medical and medicinal research. *Trends Pharmacol Sci* (2005) **26**:265–73. doi:10.1016/j.tips.2005.03.004
195. Siddiqui MS, Thodey K, Trenchard I, Smolke CD. Advancing secondary metabolite biosynthesis in yeast with synthetic biology tools. *FEMS Yeast Res* (2012) **12**:144–70. doi:10.1111/j.1567-1364.2011.00774.x
196. Sherman F. Getting started with yeast. *Methods Enzymol* (2002) **250**:3–41. doi:10.1016/S0076-6879(02)50954-X
197. Bisson LF. Yeast-metabolism of sugars. In: Fleet GH, editor. *Wine Microbiology and Biotechnology*. Chur: Harwood Academic Publishers (1993). p. 55–75.
198. Denev SA, Peeva T, Radulova P, Stancheva P, Staykova G, Beev G, et al. Yeast cultures in ruminant nutrition. *Bulg J Agric Sci* (2007) **13**:357–74.
199. Lyons TP, Jacques KA, Dawson KA. Miscellaneous products from yeasts. 2nd ed. In: Rose AH, Harrison JS, editors. *The Yeasts, Volume 5. Yeast Technology*. London: Academis (2012). p. 293–325.
200. Buzzini P, Vaughn-Martini A. Yeast biodiversity and biotechnology. In: Rosa CA, Péter G, editors. *Biodiversity and Ecophysiology of Yeasts*. Berlin: Springer (2006). p. 533–60.
201. Grant CL, Pramer D. Minor element composition of yeast extract. *J Bacteriol* (1962) **84**:869–70.
202. Charpentier C, Feuillat M. Yeast autolysis. In: Fleet GH, editor. *Wine Microbiology and Biotechnology*. Chur: Harwood Academic Publishers (1993). p. 225–42.
203. Moon S-K, Lee J, Song H, Cho J-H, Choi G-W, Seung D. Characterization of ethanol fermentation waste and its application to lactic acid production by *Lactobacillus paracasei*. *Bioprocess Biosyst Eng* (2013) **36**:547–54. doi:10.1007/s00449-012-0810-5
204. Jouany JP. A new look at yeast cultures as probiotics for ruminants. *Feed Mix* (2001) **9**:17–9.
205. Fonty G, Chaucheyras-Durand F. Effects and modes of action of live yeasts in the rumen. *Biologia* (2006) **61**:741–50. doi:10.2478/s11756-006-0151-4
206. Singh SK, Niranjan PS, Singh UB, Koley S, Verma DN. Effects of dietary supplementation of probiotics on broiler chicken. *Anim Nutr Feed Technol* (2009) **9**:85–90.
207. de Oliva Neto P, Amorim Ferreira M, Yokoya F. Screening for yeast with antibacterial properties from an ethanol distillery. *Bioresour Technol* (2004) **92**:1–6. doi:10.1016/j.biortech.2003.08.005
208. Dawson KA, Newman KE, Boling JA. Effects of microbial supplements containing yeast and lactobacilli on roughage-fed ruminal microbial activities. *J Anim Sci* (1990) **68**:3392–8.
209. Czerucka D, Piche T, Rampal P. Review article: yeast as probiotics – *Saccharomyces boulardii*. *Aliment Pharmacol Ther* (2007) **26**:767–78. doi:10.1111/j.1365-2036.2007.03442.x
210. Elmer GW, Corthier G. Modulation of *Clostridium difficile* induced mortality as a function of the dose and the viability of the *Saccharomyces boulardii* used as a preventative agent in gnotobiotic mice. *Can J Microbiol* (1991) **37**:315–7. doi:10.1139/m91-049
211. Buts J-P, Bernasconi P, Van Craynest M-P, Maldague P, De Meyer R. Response of human and rat small intestinal mucosa to oral administration of *Saccharomyces boulardii*. *Pediatr Res* (1986) **20**:192–6. doi:10.1203/00006450-198602000-00020

212. Newbold CJ, Wallace RJ, McIntosh FM. Mode of action of the yeast *Saccharomyces cerevisiae* as a feed additive for ruminants. *Br J Nutr* (1996) **76**:249–61. doi:10.1079/BJN19960029
213. Santin E, Maiorka A, Macari M, Grecco M, Sanchez JC, Okada TM. Performance and intestinal mucosa development of broiler chickens fed diets containing *Saccharomyces cerevisiae* cell wall. *J Appl Poult Res* (2001) **10**:236–44. doi:10.1093/japr/10.3.236
214. Zhang AW, Lee BD, Lee SK, Lee KW, An GH, Song KB, et al. Effects of yeast (*Saccharomyces cerevisiae*) cell components on growth performance, meat quality, and ileal mucose development of broiler chicks. *Poult Sci* (2005) **84**:1015–21. doi:10.1093/ps/84.7.1015
215. Firman JD, Moore D, Broomhead J, McIntyre D. Effects of dietary inclusion of a *Saccharomyces cerevisiae* fermentation product on performance and gut characteristics of male turkeys to market weight. *Int J Poult Sci* (2013) **12**:141–3. doi:10.3923/ijps.2013.141.143
216. Gao J, Zhang HJ, Yu SH, Wu SG, Yoon I, Quigley J, et al. Effects of yeast culture in broiler diets on performance and immunomodulatory functions. *Poult Sci* (2008) **87**:1377–84. doi:10.3382/ps.2007-00418
217. Shareef AM, Al-Dabbagh ASA. Effect of probiotic (*Saccharomyces cerevisiae*) on performance of broiler chicks. *Iraqi J Vet Sci* (2009) **23**:23–9. doi:10.3382/ps.2012-02846
218. Bradley GL, Savage TF, Timm KI. The effects of supplementing diets with *Saccharomyces cerevisiae* var. *boulardii* on male poult performance and ileal morphology. *Poult Sci* (1994) **73**:1766–70. doi:10.3382/ps.0731766
219. El-Husseiny OM, Abdallah AG, Abdel-Latiff KO. The influence of biological feed additives on broiler performance. *Int J Poult Sci* (2008) **7**:862–71. doi:10.3923/ijps.2008.862.871
220. Al-Homidan A, Fahmy MO. The effect of dried yeast (*Saccharomyces cerevisiae*) supplementation on growth, performance, carcass chemical analysis, immunity, ileum villi heights and bacterial counts of broiler chickens. *Egypt Poult Sci J* (2007) **27**:613–23.
221. Spring P, Wenk C, Dawson KA, Newman KE. The effects of dietary mannanoligosaccharides on cecal parameters and the concentrations of enteric bacteria in the ceca of *Salmonella*-challenged broiler chicks. *Poult Sci* (2000) **79**:205–11. doi:10.1093/ps/79.2.205
222. Loddi MM, Nakaghi LSO, Edens F, Tucci FM, Hannas MI, Moraes VMB, et al. Mannanoligosaccharides and organic acids on intestinal morphology integrity of broilers evaluated by scanning electron microscopy. In: *Proceedings of the 11th European Poultry Science Conference*, Bremen (2002). p. 121.
223. Hoffman OA, Olson EJ, Limper AH. Fungal beta-glucans modulate macrophage release of tumor necrosis factor-alpha in response to bacterial lipopolysaccharide. *Immunol Lett* (1993) **37**:19–25. doi:10.1016/0165-2478(93)90127-N
224. Hooge D. Meta-analysis of broiler chicken pen trials evaluating dietary mannan oligosaccharide, 1993-2003. *Int J Poult Sci* (2004) **3**:163–71. doi:10.3923/ijps.2004.163.174
225. Rosen GD. Holo-analysis of the efficacy of Bio-Mos® in broiler nutrition. *Br Poult Sci* (2007) **48**:21–6. doi:10.1080/00071660601050755
226. Peuranen S, Kogher A, Dawson KA. Yeast cell wall preparations prevent the attachment of enteropathogenic *Escherichia coli* on broiler gut mucus. *Reprod Nutr Dev* (2006) **46**:S111.
227. Line JE, Bailey JS, Cox NA, Stern NJ, Tompkins T. Effect of yeast-supplemented feed on *Salmonella* and *Campylobacter* populations in broilers. *Poult Sci* (1998) **77**:405–10. doi:10.1093/ps/77.3.405
228. Yang Y, Iji PA, Kocher A, Thomson E, Mikkelsen LL, Choct M. Effects of mannanoligosaccharide in broiler chicken diets on growth performance, energy utilization, nutrient digestibility and intestinal microflora. *Br Poult Sci* (2008) **49**:186–94. doi:10.1080/00071660801998613
229. Paryad A, Mahmoudi M. Effect of different levels of supplemental yeast (*Saccharomyces cerevisiae*) on performance, blood constituents and carcass characteristics of broilers chicks. *Afr J Agric Res* (2008) **3**:835–42.
230. Tripathi MK, Karim SA. Effect of individual and mixed live yeast culture feeding on growth performance, nutrient utilization and microbial crude protein synthesis in lambs. *Anim Feed Sci Technol* (2010) **155**:163–71. doi:10.1016/j.anifeedsci.2009.11.007
231. Adebiyi OA, Makanjuola BA, Bankole TO, Adeyori AS. Yeast culture (*Saccharomyces cerevisiae*) supplementation: effect on the performance and gut morphology of broiler birds. *Global J Sci Front Res Biol Sci* (2012) **12**:25–9.
232. Tripathi MK, Karim SA, Chaturvedi OH, Verma DL. Effect of different liquid cultures of live yeast strains on performance, ruminal fermentation and microbial protein synthesis in lambs. *J Anim Physiol Anim Nutr* (2007) **92**:631–9. doi:10.1111/j.1439-0396.2007.00759.x
233. Sporn MB, Dunlop NM, Newton DL, Smith JM. Prevention of chemical carcinogenesis by vitamin A and its synthetic analogs (retinoids). *Fed Proc* (1976) **35**:1332–8.
234. Wyss A, Wirtz G, Woggon W-D, Brugger R, Wyss M. Cloning and expression of β,β-carotene 15,15′-dioxygenase. *Biochem Biophys Res Commun* (2000) **271**:334–6. doi:10.1006/bbrc.2000.2619
235. Wyss A. Carotene oxygenases: a new family of double bond cleavage enzymes. *J Nutr* (2004) **134**:246S–50S.
236. Yamano S, Ishii T, Nakagawa M, Ikenaga H, Misawa N. Metabolic engineering for production of β-carotene and lycopene in *Saccharomyces cerevisiae*. *Biosci Biotechnol Biochem* (1993) **58**:1112–4. doi:10.1271/bbb.58.1112
237. Arnezeder C, Hampel WA. Influence of growth rate on the accumulation of ergosterol in yeast-cells. *Biotechnol Lett* (1990) **12**:277–82. doi:10.1007/BF01093521
238. Parks LW, Casey WM. Physiological implications of sterol biosynthesis in yeast. *Annu Rev Microbiol* (1995) **49**:95–116. doi:10.1146/annurev.mi.49.100195.000523
239. Shang F, Wen S, Wang X, Tan T. Effect of nitrogen limitation on the ergosterol production by fed-batch culture of *Saccharomyces cerevisiae*. *J Biotechnol* (2006) **122**:285–92. doi:10.1016/j.jbiotec.2005.11.020
240. Scanes CG, Harvey S, Marsh JA, King DB. Hormones and growth in poultry. *Poult Sci* (1984) **63**:2062–74. doi:10.3382/ps.0632062
241. Hancock RD, Galpin JR, Viola R. Biosynthesis of L-ascorbic acid (vitamin C) by *Saccharomyces cerevisiae*. *FEMS Microbiol Lett* (2000) **186**:245–50. doi:10.1111/j.1574-6968.2000.tb09112.x
242. Ferket PR, Qureshi MA. Performance and immunity of heat-stressed broilers fed vitamin- and electrolyte-supplemented drinking water. *Poult Sci* (1992) **71**:88–97. doi:10.3382/ps.0710088
243. Öztürk-Ürek R, Bozkaya LA, Tarhan L. The effects of some antioxidant vitamin- and trace element-supplemented diets on activities of SOD, CAT, GSH-Px and LPO levels in chicken tissues. *Cell Biochem Funct* (2001) **19**:125–32. doi:10.1002/cbf.905
244. Young JF, Stagsted J, Jensen SK, Karlsson AH, Henckel P. Ascorbic acid, α-tocopherol, and oregano supplements reduce stress-induced deterioration of chicken meat quality. *Poult Sci* (2003) **82**:1343–51. doi:10.1093/ps/82.8.1343
245. Jakobsen M, Narvhus J. Yeasts and their possible beneficial and negative effects on the quality of dairy products. *Int Dairy J* (1996) **6**:755–68. doi:10.1016/0958-6946(95)00071-2
246. Jones EW. Three proteolytic systems in the yeast *Saccharomyces cerevisiae*. *J Biol Chem* (1991) **266**:7963–6.
247. Harvey RB, Norman KN, Andrews K, Hume ME, Scanlan CM, Callaway TR, et al. *Clostridium difficile* in poultry and poultry meat. *Foodborne Pathog Dis* (2011) **8**:1321–3. doi:10.1089/fpd.2011.0936
248. McCullough MJ, Clemons KV, McHusker JH, Stevens DA. Species identification and virulence attributes of *Saccharomyces boulardii* (nom. inval.). *J Clin Microbiol* (1998) **36**:2613–7.
249. Pothoulakis C, Kelly CP, Joshi MA, Gao N, O'Keane CJ, Castagliuolo I, et al. *Saccharomyces boulardii* inhibits *Clostridium difficile* toxin A binding and enterotoxicity in rat ileum. *Gastroenterology* (1993) **104**:1108–15.
250. Castagliuolo I, LaMont JT, Nikulasson ST, Pothoulakis C. *Saccharomyces boulardii* protease inhibits *Clostridium difficile* toxin A effects in the rat ileum. *Infect Immun* (1996) **64**:5225–32.
251. Buts J-P, Bernasconi P, Vaerman J-P, Dive C. Stimulation of secretory IgA and secretory component of immunoglobulins in small intestine of rats treated with *Saccharomyces boulardii*. *Dig Dis Sci* (1990) **35**:251–6. doi:10.1007/BF01536771
252. Shankar T, Thangamathi P, Rama R, Sivakumar T. Optimization of invertase production using *Saccharomyces cerevisiae* MK under varying cultural conditions. *Int J Biochem Biophys* (2013) **1**:47–53. doi:10.13189/ijbb.2013.0101301
253. Walker GM. *Yeast Physiology and Biotechnology*. Chichester: Wiley (1998). 78 p.

254. Almquist HJ. Amino acid requirements of chickens and turkeys – a review. *Poult Sci* (1952) **31**:966–81. doi:10.3382/ps.0310966
255. Aletor VA, Hamid II, Nieß E, Pfeffer E. Low-protein amino acid-supplemented diets in broiler chickens: effects on performance, carcass characteristics, whole body composition and efficiencies of nutrient utilisation. *J Sci Food Agric* (2000) **80**:547–54. doi:10.1002/(SICI)1097-0010(200004)80:5<547::AID-JSFA531>3.0.CO;2-C
256. Sibbald IR, Wolynetz MS. Effects of dietary lysine and feed intake on energy utilization and tissue synthesis by broiler chicks. *Poult Sci* (1986) **65**:98–105. doi:10.3382/ps.0650098
257. Gasent-Ramírez JM, Benítez T. Lysine-overproducing mutants of *Saccharomyces cerevisiae* baker's yeast isolated in continuous culture. *Appl Environ Microbiol* (1997) **63**:4800–6.
258. Bevan EA, Makower M. The physiological basis of the killer character in yeast. *Proc 11th Int Conf Genet* (1963). **1**:202–3.
259. Walker GM, McLeod AH, Hodgson VJ. Interactions between killer yeasts and pathogenic fungi. *FEMS Microbiol Lett* (1995) **127**:213–22. doi:10.1111/j.1574-6968.1995.tb07476.x
260. Marquina D, Santos A, Peinado JM. Biology of killer yeasts. *Int Microbiol* (2002) **5**:65–71. doi:10.1007/s10123-002-0066-z
261. Polonelli L, Morace G. Reevaluation of the yeast killer phenomenon. *J Clin Microbiol* (1986) **24**:866–9.
262. Stanley D, Hughes RJ, Moore RJ. Microbiota of the chicken gastrointestinal tract: influence on health, productivity and disease. *Appl Microbiol Biotechnol* (2014) **98**:4301–10. doi:10.1007/s00253-014-5646-2
263. Schrezemmeir J, de Vrese M. Probiotics, prebiotics, and synbiotics – approaching a definition. *Am J Clin Nutr* (2001) **73**:361S–4S.

Conflict of Interest Statement: The authors declare that the research was conducted in the absence of any commercial or financial relationships that could be construed as a potential conflict of interest.

19

Potential of plant essential oils and their components in animal agriculture – *in vitro* studies on antibacterial mode of action

*Corliss A. O'Bryan, Sean J. Pendleton†, Philip G. Crandall and Steven C. Ricke**

Department of Food Science, Center for Food Safety, University of Arkansas, Fayetteville, AR, USA

Edited by:
Michael D. Flythe, USDA-Agricultural Research Service, USA

Reviewed by:
Takeshi Ohkubo, Ibaraki University, Japan
Sung Woo Kim, North Carolina State University, USA

***Correspondence:**
Steven C. Ricke, Department of Food Science, Center for Food Safety, University of Arkansas, 2650 Young Avenue, Fayetteville, AR 72704, USA
sricke@uark.edu

†Present address:
Sean J. Pendleton, Department of Food Science and Technology, University of Tennessee, Knoxville, TN, USA

The antimicrobial activity of essential oils and their components has been recognized for several years. Essential oils are produced as secondary metabolites by many plants and can be distilled from all different portions of plants. The recent emergence of bacteria resistant to multiple antibiotics has spurred research into the use of essential oils as alternatives. Recent research has demonstrated that many of these essential oils have beneficial effects for livestock, including reduction of foodborne pathogens in these animals. Numerous studies have been made into the mode of action of essential oils, and the resulting elucidation of bacterial cell targets has contributed to new perspectives on countering antimicrobial resistance and pathogenicity of these bacteria. In this review, an overview of the current knowledge about the antibacterial mode of action of essential oils and their constituents is provided.

Keywords: essential oils, foodborne pathogens, mode of action, quorum sensing, antibacterial

Introduction

Plant materials including flowers, roots, bark, leaves, seeds, peel, fruits, and wood can be used to extract aromatic and volatile liquids known as essential oils (EOs) (1–3). These EOs have a long history of use for medical purposes, in perfumes and cosmetics, and as herbs and spices for foods. EOs are considered to be secondary metabolites in plants; secondary metabolites are organic compounds that are not directly involved in the normal growth, development, or reproduction of the plant (4). These secondary metabolites are often involved in plant defense and thus may possess antimicrobial properties (4, 5). The first experiment to determine the bactericidal properties of EOs is said to have been carried out by de la Croix in 1881 (6). In more recent years, many EOs, or their components, have been shown to possess broad-range antibacterial properties (7).

Increased resistance to infectious diseases, including parasitic infections such as coccidiosis, has been noted when plant phytonutrients were fed to animals. For instance, Lee et al. (8) found that feeding plum powder to laying hens increased their immune response as well as conferring immunity to coccidiosis. Lillehoj et al. (9) determined the effects of feeding capsicum oleoresin or cinnamaldehyde on the global gene expression profiles of broilers. Capsicum oleoresin induced gene changes in genes associated with metabolism and immunity, whereas cinnamaldehyde affected genes related to antigen presentation, humoral immune response, and inflammatory disease. Feeding of these compounds also protected the birds against infection with live coccidiosis parasites. Mathlouthi et al. (10) found that oregano or rosemary EOs had different antimicrobial effects *in vitro* against pathogenic and non-pathogenic bacteria but had the same growth promoting effects as avilamycin when added to broiler diets. Authors speculated that the *in vivo* growth promotion effects were due to ecological changes in the bacterial gut flora rather than antibacterial effects against a single bacterial genus and species. Betancourt et al. (11) confirmed a shift in gut flora in the foregut but not ceca and colon in broilers fed oregano EOs during a 42-day grow out period.

Alali et al. (12) tested a mixture of carvacrol, thymol, eucalyptol, and lemon for the ability to prevent colonization and shedding in broilers intentionally fed *Salmonella* Heidelberg. They determined that feeding 0.05% (v/v) of the EO mixture significantly reduced the colonization of the crops of challenged birds as well as lowering feed conversion and improving weight gain in the birds. However, cecal colonization and shedding were not significantly decreased. Cerisuelo et al. (13) fed an EO mixture composed of cinnamaldehyde and thymol to broilers, either with or without butyric acid. They determined that the EO blend reduced cecal numbers of *Salmonella*, especially when combined with butyric acid, as compared to control feed. Ricke et al. (14) provide an overview of the anti-*Salmonella* effects of EOs in agriculture.

Benchaar et al. (15) investigated the effects of EOs *in vitro* rumen microbial fermentation. They determined that only the phenolic compounds, carvacrol, thymol, and eugenol affected ruminal fermentation, relative to the control, increasing pH and butyrate and decreasing propionate, indicating antibacterial activity which was not nutritionally beneficial. Callaway et al. (16) studied the *in vitro* effects of orange peel and orange pulp, both sources of EOs, against *Escherichia coli* O157:H7 and *Salmonella typhimurium* in rumen fluid. Growth of both pathogens was reduced by addition of 0.002 g/ml of orange pulp or orange peel. Callaway et al. (17) were able to demonstrate that the orange peel products when fed to experimentally inoculated sheep reduced *S. typhimurium* populations in the gut, with a significant reduction reached in the ceca.

The antimicrobial properties of EOs are a recent focus for agricultural applications because of a desire on the part of many consumers to reduce the use of "hazardous or unnatural chemicals" in their food (18–20). Although there are many studies on the antimicrobial activities of EOs, few take the next step and determine the mode of action of these compounds. However, application of EOs as antibacterial substances for food animals or as food preservatives requires detailed knowledge about their properties, including the mode of action. The purpose of this review is to provide an overview of current knowledge about the antimicrobial mode of action of EOs and their constituents.

Effects on Cell Wall and Membrane

Antimicrobial activity of EOs is strongly linked to their hydrophobicity (21–28). The cell walls of Gram-positive bacteria are made up predominantly of peptidoglycan linked with other molecules such as proteins or teichoic acid (29). On the other hand, Gram-negative bacteria possess an outer membrane of containing hydrophilic lipopolysaccharides (LPS), which creates a barrier toward hydrophobic compounds such as those found in EOs (30, 31). Gram-negative bacteria are thus considered to be less susceptible to the effects of EOs than Gram-positive bacteria (32). However, the hydrophobic constituents of EOs are able to gain access to the periplasm of Gram-negative bacteria through the porin proteins of their outer membrane (24), through which they can slowly travel (33) See **Table 1** for an overview of the bacterial targets of select EOs and their constituents.

TABLE 1 | Target of antibacterial action of some essential oils.

Target	Essential oil or component	Reference
Cell wall or membrane	Carvacrol	Helander et al. (24), Ultee et al. (28, 34), Fitzgerald et al. (37), Xu et al. (48)
	Cinnamon	Bouhdid et al. (40)
	Cinnamaldehyde	Gill and Holley (57)
	Cymene	Ultee et al. (28)
	Eugenol	Walsh et al. (36)
	Farnesol	Inoue et al. (38)
	Nerolidol	Inoue et al. (38)
	Oregano	Bouhdid et al. (43), De Souza et al. (53)
	Plaunotol	Inoue et al. (38)
	Rosemary	De Souza et al. (53)
	Tea tree oil	Cox et al. (26)
	Thymol	Helander et al. (24), Walsh et al. (36), Xu et al. (48)
	Vanillin	Fitzgerald et al. (37)
Respiration	Cinnamon	Bouhdid et al. (40)
	Tea tree oil	Cox et al. (26)
	Vanillin	Fitzgerald et al. (37)
Quorum sensing	Clove	Khan et al. (64)
	Geranium	Szabo et al. (65)
	Lavender	Szabo et al. (65)
	Oregano	Alvarez et al. (66)
	Rose	Szabo et al. (65)
	Rosemary	Szabo et al. (65)

Potassium Leakage from Cells

The leakage of potassium into the extracellular space is considered an indicator for an increase in membrane permeability and ultimate loss of viability for the cell. This particular result was observed in multiple studies (22, 26, 34–40). Carvacrol is a fraction of many EOs and is the major component of oregano EO, which consists of 60–74% carvacrol and thyme EO which consists of 45% carvacrol (41, 42). Ultee et al. (34) examined carvacrol for its antimicrobial properties against *Bacillus cereus* and determined that, at a concentration of 0.15 ml/l, carvacrol caused an immediate decrease in intracellular potassium and an increase in the extracellular potassium. Fitzgerald et al. (37) studied the effects of carvacrol and vanillin on *E. coli*, *Lactobacillus plantarum*, and *Listeria innocua*. At concentrations of 7.6 and 0.496 ml/l of vanillin and carvacrol, respectively, they saw that intracellular potassium levels decreased and the extracellular potassium levels increased in all organisms. Both thymol and eugenol were able to increase extracellular potassium at concentrations of 0.50 ml/l in *E. coli* and *Staphylococcus aureus* (36). Tea tree oil at 2.50 ml/l caused the release of 100% of the total cellular potassium in *E. coli* within 30 min, but only approximately 20% was released by *S. aureus* in the same time (26), which is in contrast to the reported greater susceptibility of Gram-positives (32) and illustrates the great diversity in efficacy of EOs. Bouhdid et al. (43) demonstrated that oregano EO caused potassium leakage in both *Pseudomonas aeruginosa* and *S. aureus*. Oil-treated cells were examined by transmission electron microscopy (TEM), which revealed mesosome-like structures, coagulated cytoplasmic material, and intracellular material outside the cell; these effects were more noticeable in *P. aeruginosa* compared with *S. aureus* (43). Bouhdid et al. (40) determined the effects of EO of *Cinnamomum verum* on *P. aeruginosa* and *S. aureus* and discovered that a concentration of 1.25 ml/l was able to increase extracellular potassium levels in both bacteria. Inoue et al. (38) tested the terpene alcohols farnesol, nerolidol, and plaunotol for their antimicrobial effects on *S. aureus*. All three compounds increased the extracellular potassium levels when applied to *S. aureus* at a concentration of 0.020 ml/l. Togashi et al. (39) found that when geraniol was added to farnesol in a ratio of 0.010:0.005 ml/l, the ability of farnesol to cause potassium leakage was enhanced, while geranylgeraniol inhibited the potassium leakage activity of farnesol. Bajpai et al. (44) used scanning electron micrographs of *B. cereus* and *E. coli* to demonstrate that cells treated with *Ginkgo biloba* EO (250 and 500 μg/ml, respectively) had disruption of cell membranes and swelling of the cells which led to leakage of potassium from the cells. The studies discussed in this section indicate that these EOs and components act in a similar fashion on the membrane to cause the bacterial cell to lose the ability to regulate potassium transfer across the membrane, leading to an outpouring of potassium from the cell and a subsequent loss of viability.

Leakage of Other Cell Components

The release of other cellular components has also been an object of study for those seeking to determine microbial action of EOs. Carboxyfluorescein diacetate is commonly used as a probe for viable cells (45, 46). Carboxyfluorescein diacetate was used to stain live cells of *L. innocua* which were then exposed to the EOs of *Cymbopogon citratus*, *Ocimum gratissimum*, or *Thymus vulgaris* (47). Loss of fluorescence was taken to be indicative of leakage of carboxyfluorescein from within the cell and thus a measure of the disruption of the cell membrane. EOs of *C. citratus* (7.80 ml/l), *O. gratissimum* (5.0 ml/l), and *T. vulgaris* (4.30 ml/l) were adjusted to a concentration of 1.04×10^4 arbitrary units (AUs) for treatment; AUs were determined by the formula AU ml^{-1} = mean diameter (mm) of the minimal inhibition zone × dilution factor × 50. All EOs were shown to cause a decrease in fluorescence as compared to an unexposed control (47). Xu et al. (48) also examined the leakage of carboxyfluorescein by *E. coli* after exposure to components of thyme EO, carvacrol and thymol, at different concentrations (0.10 and 0.20 ml/l). They found that both carvacrol and thymol caused an increase in carboxyfluorescein released by *E. coli* cells. Trombetta et al. (32) assessed the release of carboxyfluorescein from large unilamellar vesicles (LUVs) that were exposed to (+) menthol, thymol, and linalyl acetate at several concentrations (0.10, 0.25, and 0.50 ml/l). They concluded that (+) menthol and thymol were both effective in causing the release of carboxyfluorescein from the LUVs, but linalyl acetate was only slightly effective. Helander et al. (24) researched the release of fatty acids from *E. coli* cells treated with thymol, carvacrol, (+)-carvone, or *trans*-cinnamaldehyde. Thymol and carvacrol were shown to release a significant amount of fatty acids into the supernatant, while (+)-carvone and *trans*-cinnamaldehyde were ineffective at releasing fatty acids. The results produced by Helander et al. (24) demonstrated that thymol and carvacrol actually break down the cell membrane. Proteins absorb light at 280 nm; therefore, release of 280 nm materials was considered indicative of macromolecular leakage by the cell; *E. coli* and *S. aureus* exposed to tea tree oil were found to leak 280 nm absorbing material, but at levels lower than potassium leakage (35). Nucleic acids, on the other hand, absorb light at 260 nm, and the release of 260 nm material from bacterial cells would be indicative of macromolecular leakage by the cell. Ifesan et al. (49); Carson et al. (50), and Oussalah et al. (51) all examined the release of 260 nm absorbing material. Strains of *S. aureus* exposed to a crude extract of a perennial herb, *Eleutherine americana*, had a peak release of 260 nm absorbing materials after 8 h of exposure to 2.50–10.0 ml/l of the extract (49). After 22 h of exposure, the absorbance decreased from the levels seen after 8 h, most likely due to denaturation of the materials, which caused them to become unreactive to the light at 260 nm (49). A significant amount of 260 nm material was released by *S. aureus* cells after an hour of exposure to tea tree oil or its components (50). Oussalah et al. (52) examined Spanish oregano, Chinese cinnamon, and savory EOs against *E. coli* O157:H7 and *Listeria monocytogenes*. They found that at 0.25 ml/l each EO was able to cause an increase in the release of 260 nm absorbing material. A study investigating the effects of the EOs of oregano and rosemary on *Pseudomonas fluorescens* found that cell material was released into the growth medium immediately after contact with either EO singly or in combination (53). Electron microscopy of exposed cells revealed alteration in the cell wall structure, rupture of the plasma membrane, shrinking of the cells, condensation of the cytoplasmic content, and leakage of the intracellular material with a 2 h contact time (53). Confocal scanning laser microscopy revealed increased cell membrane permeability, resulting in cell death after exposure times of only 15 min (53). These studies indicate that EOs and components are able to cause macromolecular permeability in a variety of bacteria.

Uptake of Substances

The cell membrane helps cells regulate what enters and exits the cell. When ions are no longer being regulated, it indicates that at the very least small pores have formed in the cell membrane. When larger molecules, such as propidium iodide (PI) or *N*-phenyl-L-napthylamine (NPN), enter the cell without regulation it indicates much larger pores have formed in the membrane and a much higher probability of cell death. Helander et al. (24) examined the uptake of NPN by *E. coli* and *S. typhimurium* after exposure to thymol, carvacrol, (+)-carvone, and *trans*-cinnamaldehyde. Thymol and carvacrol significantly increased the uptake of NPN by both bacteria, while (+)-carvone and *trans*-cinnamaldehyde did not allow uptake. These findings demonstrate that (+)-carvone and *trans*-cinnamaldehyde are unable to form pores large enough for NPN, unlike thymol and carvacrol. *Trans*-cinnamaldehyde has a similar minimal inhibitory concentration (MIC) to carvacrol and thymol, according to Helander's study, but it does not function as a large pore former like carvacrol or thymol. Therefore, there must be another mode of action for *trans*-cinnamaldehyde. Fisher and Phillips (54) also investigated NPN uptake by *Enterococcus faecium* and *Enterococcus faecalis* after exposure to a citrus oil blend. They found that the oil blend was able to increase the NPN uptake over twofold, indicating that the blend is able to cause large pore formation in the bacteria. They also examined the cells using TEM and reported morphological changes in the cells including a loss of distinction of the membrane after being in contact with either the EO or its vapor. Cells that had been in direct contact with the EO appeared to have vacuoles which the authors speculated contained the EO within them. Nearly 100% of *E. coli* cells exhibited increased PI uptake after exposure to tea tree oil, while only around 10% of *S. aureus* cells expressed increased PI uptake. (35). Cox's results indicate that there is a possible difference in the effects of tea tree oil on Gram-negative and Gram-positive bacteria. Similarly, Bouhdid et al. (40) determined that cinnamon EO treatment made *P. aeruginosa* much more susceptible, in terms of PI uptake, than *S. aureus*. Fitzgerald et al. (37) exposed *E. coli*, *L. plantarum*, and *L. innocua* to vanillin and measured subsequent PI uptake; *E. coli* exhibited membrane damage after 15 and 60 min of exposure, but appeared to recover overnight, as the percentage of membrane damage decreased from that seen after 60 min. However, *L. plantarum* exhibited slight damage after 15 and 60 min, but rather than recover overnight as *E. coli* did, damage increased (37). *L. innocua* showed little susceptibility to vanillin. Fitzgerald's results indicate that vanillin does not have a Gram-negative or Gram-positive bias, such as observed with tea tree oil or cinnamon EO, although further studies with tea tree oil and cinnamon EO need to be carried out to determine if they are more effective at large pore formation in Gram-negative bacteria. Based on these studies, large pore formation appears to be a mode of action employed by various EOs against a range of bacteria.

Effects on Membrane Potential

Membrane potential is used by the cell to perform actions necessary for life, such as synthesis of enzymes, nucleic acids, polysaccharides, and other cell components, for cell maintenance and repair of damage, for motility, and for numerous other processes (55), and decrease in this membrane potential is indicative of damage to the cell membrane. Bouhdid et al. (40) used bis-oxonol dye to stain depolarized *P. aeruginosa* and *S. aureus* cells. They found that cinnamon EO at MIC levels was able to decrease the membrane potential of *P. aeruginosa*, but not *S. aureus*. Using 3,3′-dipropylthiacarbocyanide iodide ($DiSC_35$) to monitor membrane potential, Veldhuizen et al. (56) exposed *S. aureus* cells to carvacrol, *o*-cresol, or 2-amino-*p*-cymene at MIC concentrations which were all found to decrease the membrane potential of the cells within seconds of contact. Ultee et al. (28) also employed $DiSC_35$ to look at the disruption of membrane potential of *B. cereus* by carvacrol and cymene. Carvacrol was seen to immediately decrease the membrane potential at concentrations above 0.037 ml/l, while cymene was able to decrease the membrane potential to a lesser extent at a maximum concentration of 0.067 ml/l. Cymene lacks the hydroxyl group that is present on carvacrol, indicating that the hydroxyl group plays an important role in the effect of carvacrol on the membrane potential. Fisher and Phillips (54) also monitored membrane potential with $DiSC_35$ in *E. faecalis* and *E. faecium* after exposure to a 1:1 blend (20.0 ml/l each) of orange and bergamot EOs. They found that the blend was able to dissipate the membrane potential within seconds of contact with the cells. These studies show that when an EO affects the membrane potential of a cell it is an almost immediate reaction. Loss of membrane potential is adverse to cell survival, but could be a consequence of membrane disruption in the case of carvacrol.

Effects on ATP: Leakage from Cells and Usage by Cells

Another target for research on the mode of action of EOs has been to examine the levels of ATP both inside and outside bacterial cells. Ultee et al. (28) determined that cymene, a plant aromatic compound found in cumin and thyme, was unable to cause ATP levels to rise in the extracellular environment or decrease in the intracellular environment. However, carvacrol was able to eliminate the internal ATP of *B. cereus* cells within 20 min of contact at a concentration of 0.150 ml/l (34). Fisher and Phillips (54) utilized an EO blend consisting of a 1:1 mixture of sweet orange and bergamot to treat *E. faecalis* and *E. faecium* and determined that the blend was able to completely dissipate internal ATP in within 10 min of contact. Oussalah et al. (51) examined the effects of Spanish oregano, Chinese cinnamon, and savory EO on the ATP of *E. coli* O157:H7 and *L. monocytogenes*. Savory EO was able to increase extracellular ATP levels in both bacteria, while Spanish oregano was only able to increase extracellular ATP in *E. coli* O157:H7 and Chinese cinnamon was not able to increase extracellular ATP in either organism. Helander et al. (24) looked at the effects of carvacrol, thymol, (+)-carvone, and *trans*-cinnamaldehyde on the ATP of *E. coli* cells. Carvacrol and thymol were both found to decrease intracellular ATP over a 20-min period, and slightly increase external ATP, but (+)-carvone and *trans*-cinnamaldehyde did not affect the ATP of the cells, internally or externally. Fitzgerald et al. (37) looked at the effect of vanillin and carvacrol on ATP of *E. coli*, *L. plantarum*, and *L. innocua*. Vanillin was found to be ineffective at reducing intracellular ATP or increasing extracellular ATP in any bacteria. Carvacrol was very effective at decreasing all bacteria's internal ATP, while only increasing external ATP in *E. coli* and *L. innocua*. The increase in extracellular ATP concentration in the presence of some EOs is of course due to intracellular ATP release, most likely as a consequence of envelope damage induced by the oils.

Some EOs and components, such as cinnamaldehyde, directly target the production of ATP in the cell. Gill and Holley (57) investigated ATP generation in *Lactobacillus sakei* and *L. monocytogenes*. Both bacteria were treated with eugenol, and *L. monocytogenes* was additionally treated with cinnamaldehyde. Eugenol was found to inhibit ATP production but was unable to decrease intracellular ATP. Cinnamaldehyde was found to both inhibit production of ATP and decrease intracellular ATP. These results were determined by adding the EOs to the bacteria before or after the addition of 0.25% glucose to energize the cell. Gill and Holley (57) propose that the mode of action for eugenol relies on inhibiting the cell from using glucose due to its effectiveness when added prior to glucose, but not when added after glucose. Cinnamaldehyde reduced ATP levels when added either prior to or after glucose, which led Gill and Holley (57) to hypothesize that there may be more than one plausible mode of action. Eugenol, carvacrol, and cinnamaldehyde have been found to inhibit the membrane-bound ATPase activity of some bacteria. There are several enzymes with

ATPase activity that are associated with bacterial membranes, including one that is involved in ATP generation and cellular pH regulation (58). Gill and Holley (59) hypothesized that ATPase inhibition plays a significant role in reducing the growth rate of pathogens at sublethal concentrations of the EO.

Effects on pH Gradient

The ability to maintain a pH gradient is necessary for cell survival and thus studying the internal pH or the pH gradient helps to determine if a cell has been severely damaged. Oussalah et al. (51) and Lambert et al. (22) both examined the internal pH of bacteria exposed to EOs. Oussalah et al. (51) found that Spanish oregano, Chinese cinnamon, and Savory EOs were effective at decreasing the internal pH of *E. coli* O157:H7 and *L. monocytogenes*. Lambert et al. (22) determined that oregano EO increased the rate of change in internal pH for *S. aureus* compared with an untreated control, indicating a lack of ability by the cell to maintain the pH gradient. Sikkema et al. (58) tested liposomes that had been reconstituted with beef heart mitochondrial cytochrome c oxidase, in order to give them a proton motive force, with various cyclic hydrocarbons (benzene, toluene, ethylbenzene, *o*-xylene, and others) and found that all of them dissipated the pH gradient at concentrations related to their membrane partition coefficient. Fisher and Phillips (54) employed their 1:1 blend of orange and bergamot EOs (20.0 ml/l of each) to determine that the blend was able to completely eliminate the pH gradients of *E. faecium* and *E. faecalis*. Fitzgerald et al. (37) treated *L. plantarum* with vanillin and determined that 15.2 ml/l of vanillin was able to dissipate the pH gradient. Ultee et al. (28, 34) ascertained that 0.15 ml/l carvacrol completely dissipated the pH gradient across the cytoplasmic membrane of *B. cereus*, while 0.268 ml/l of cymene was ineffective. These studies indicate that many oils act to disrupt the membrane in such a way as to make the cell unable to maintain a pH gradient which is essential for generation of a proton motive force, and thus life.

Effect on Respiration

Respiration is an integral part of aerobic metabolism with the potential to be a target for antimicrobial EOs, and several researchers have examined the effects of EOs on respiration to help elicit their mode of action. Reduction of 5-cyano-2,3-ditolyl tetrazolium chloride (CTC) is an indication of respiratory enzyme activity; Bouhdid et al. (40) determined that in the presence of cinnamon EO <6% of *P. aeruginosa* cells were able to reduce CTC after a 30-min exposure to the MIC of the oil (1.25 ml/l). However, *S. aureus* was found to be more resistant as approximately 10% of the cells were able to reduce CTC after 60 min of exposure to the MIC (1.25 ml/l) and 1.5× MIC (1.87 ml/l) of the oil. Cox et al. (26) examined the oxygen consumption of *E. coli* and *S. aureus* in the presence of tea tree oil at different concentrations; 5.0 ml/l of tea tree oil reduced the oxygen consumption of *E. coli* by 100% and 10.0 ml/l reduced the oxygen consumption of *S. aureus* by 60%. Fitzgerald et al. (37) determined oxygen consumption in *L. innocua* and *E. coli* when exposed to various concentrations of vanillin (0–6.09 ml/l) and discovered that oxygen consumption was reduced by 19 and 52% in *E. coli* and *L. innocua*, respectively, when exposed to 6.09 ml/l of vanillin. These results indicate that some EOs disrupt the ability of bacterial cells to perform oxidation reduction reactions and could be a potential mode of action for the oil.

Effect on Quorum Sensing

Cell-to-cell communication among bacteria [quorum sensing (QS)] is accomplished using small signaling molecules produced by the bacteria and is utilized by the bacteria to evaluate their external environment and their internal physiological status (60). The signaling molecules are in general known as autoinducers; the Gram-negative bacteria use acyl homoserine lactones, whereas the Gram-positive bacteria use modified oligopeptides as signaling molecules (61). QS is involved in biofilm production, motility, swarming, stress resistance, and virulence (61). Researchers have begun to target QS as a means to reduce antimicrobial resistance and food spoilage (62). Additionally, QS is thought to allow pathogens to minimize host immune responses by delaying the production of virulence factors until a large enough bacterial population is present to overwhelm host defense mechanisms and establish infection (63).

Khan et al. (64) screened 21 EOs for anti-QS activity using biosensor strains, *Chromobacterium violaceum* CV12472 and CVO26. They determined that clove oil demonstrated the most anti-QS activity on both wild and mutant strains followed in activity by cinnamon, lavender, and peppermint oils. The effect of clove oil on pigment production, which is QS controlled, was found to be concentration dependent. At sub-MICs of clove oil, there was a 78.4% reduction of pigment production compared with the control and up to a 78% reduction in swarming motility over the control (64). Szabo et al. (65) performed similar studies with a wider range of EOs and established that rose, geranium, lavender, and rosemary oils were the most potent QS inhibitors of the compounds they tested. Eucalyptus and citrus oils moderately reduced pigment production by CV026, while chamomile, orange, and juniper oils were ineffective. Alvarez et al. (66) researched the use of oregano EO in edible films and the effect on QS as well as the antibacterial activity against several pathogens. Pectin films incorporated with 36.10 and 25.90 ml/l of oregano EO inhibited growth of *E. coli* O157:H7, *Salmonella* Cholerasuis, *S. aureus*, and *L. monocytogenes*. All concentrations of oregano EO (0.015, 0.0312, 0.0625, and 0.125 ml/l) and pectin-EO films (15.70, 25.90, and 36.10 ml/l) showed a significant anti-QS activity. They also determined that the pectin-EO films reduced total coliforms, yeast, and molds on shrimp and cucumber slices stored at 4°C for 15 days. Thus, EOs could be used to explicitly target QS in a novel antimicrobial strategy.

Effect of Compound Structure on Antimicrobial Activity

Many researchers have examined the structures of EOs themselves to seek to determine what allows these compounds to affect the various cellular activities of bacteria. Sikkema et al. (58) examined how biological membranes react to cyclic hydrocarbons and determined that the hydrocarbons accumulate in the interior of the membrane causing it to swell. The amount to which a particular hydrocarbon can accumulate in the membrane was found to be directly related to its membrane partition coefficient. Sikkema et al. (58) proposed that the accumulation of these compounds in the membrane result in changes to the membrane structure and function, thus leading to inhibition or cell death.

Carvacrol is an EO that has been shown to have high antibacterial activity and therefore it has been the focus or benchmark for many studies, some of which have studied what it is about the structure of carvacrol that makes it antimicrobial. Carvacrol is a cyclic hydrocarbon which, according to Sikkema et al. (58), allows it to accumulate in the membrane. It also has a hydroxyl group on the ring, which Ultee et al. (28) have proposed gives carvacrol its activity. Ultee et al. (28) also studied thymol, menthol, carvacrol methyl ether, and cymene in addition to carvacrol. These compounds possess similar structures to carvacrol that only differ in one or two ways. Thymol has the same chemical formula as carvacrol, but the hydroxyl group is in the meta position rather than the ortho position. Menthol lacks the benzene ring and instead has a cyclic hexane ring. Carvacrol methyl ether has the hydroxyl group replaced with a methyl ether group. Finally, cymene completely lacks a hydroxyl group. Ultee et al. (28) noted that cymene and carvacrol methyl ether lacked any antibacterial activity. Menthol showed slight inhibitory activity at a concentration of 0.320 ml/l for up to 5 h, but after 24 h, the bacteria had rebounded to levels seen with only a 0.016 ml/l concentration of menthol, which showed no inhibition of the bacteria. Thymol showed a very similar pattern of activity to that of carvacrol, with concentrations above 0.113 ml/l completely inhibitory to the bacteria (28).

Veldhuizen et al. (56) achieved similar results when they examined *o*-cresol, 3-isoporpylphenol, 2-amino-*p*-cymene, *p*-cymene, and 3,4-dimethylcumene in comparison to carvacrol. They found that *p*-cymene and 3,4-methylcumene exhibited no antibacterial activity. In 3,4-methylcumene, there is a methyl group in the place that the hydroxyl group of carvacrol occupies, indicating that the hydroxyl group is an important component of the antibacterial activity. The compound 3-isopropylphenol, which lacks the methyl group on the ring, was found to have an MIC approximately 1.5 times that of carvacrol, while *o*-cresol, which lacks the isopropyl group of carvacrol, was found to have an MIC approximately two times that of carvacrol. The MIC of these two carvacrol-related compounds indicates that the R groups do play a small role in the antibacterial activity of carvacrol, though not as much as the hydroxyl group. The compound 2-amino-*p*-cymene has an amino group in the same position as the hydroxyl group of carvacrol, but the rest of the structure remains the same. The MICs of 2-amino-*p*-cymene were approximately 0.450–0.60 ml/l higher than that of carvacrol and had the highest MIC of all antibacterially active compounds tested. Since 2-amino-*p*-cymene shows antibacterial activity, it seems that the hydroxyl group is not essential for antimicrobial activity, although it appears to enhance activity considerably.

Ben Arfa et al. (67) also examined how the structure of carvacrol affects its antibacterial activity. They compared carvacrol with carvacrol methyl ether, carvacrol acetate, eugenol, and menthol. Carvacrol methyl ether and carvacrol acetate were not found to display any antibacterial activity; both of these compounds have substitutions at the hydroxyl group of carvacrol respective of their names, indicating that these groups cannot convey the same activity as the hydroxyl group of carvacrol. Eugenol, which is another aromatic compound like carvacrol, has a hydroxyl group and an ether group which are para and ortho, respectively, to a three-carbon chain that ends in a double bond. Eugenol was found to exhibit a lower antibacterial activity than carvacrol, but was not inactive like carvacrol acetate and carvacrol methyl ether. Ben Arfa et al. (67) only determined MICs for their compounds, so it is difficult to say if the antibacterial action of eugenol is the same as carvacrol, although it can be said that not all antibacterial EO compounds must have a structure similar to that of carvacrol in order to possess activity. Similar to Ultee et al. (28), Ben Arfa et al. (67) found menthol to possess very little antibacterial activity, which supports the theory that the benzene ring is important for antibacterial activity, but only for those compounds that possess a hydroxyl group or an amino group, as was the case with 2-amino-*p*-cymene in the study by Veldhuizen et al. (56).

Gill and Holley (57) studied the two aromatic compounds eugenol and *trans*-cinnamaldehyde. Both compounds were found to exhibit antibacterial activity, although eugenol had a lower MIC. *Trans*-cinnamaldehyde, which contains an aromatic ring with a three-carbon aldehyde chain containing a double bond at the second position, was able to decrease internal ATP of energized cells and inhibit ATP increases of non-energized cells of *L. monocytogenes*. Eugenol, which was described earlier, was able to inhibit ATP increases of non-energized cells, but was unable to reduce ATP levels of energized cells. Their results indicate that *trans*-cinnamaldehyde could be acting via membrane disruption without the need of the carvacrol hydroxyl group. It is difficult to compare carvacrol and *trans*-cinnamaldehyde since they were not used in the same study, but if one extrapolates the results from Gill and Holley (57) and Ben Arfa et al. (67), one can make the assumption that *trans*-cinnamaldehyde has lower antibacterial activity than carvacrol. This is due to the fact that *trans*-cinnamaldehyde was found to have lower antibacterial activity than eugenol and that eugenol was found to have lower antibacterial activity than carvacrol. Therefore, *trans*-cinnamaldehyde probably causes membrane disruption to a lesser extent than carvacrol due to its lack of a hydroxyl group. Bouhdid et al. (40) examined cinnamon EO, which is mainly composed of *trans*-cinnamaldehyde, and found that the EO caused leakage of potassium ions from *P. aeruginosa* and *S. aureus*, which furthers the idea that *trans*-cinnamaldehyde is a membrane disruptor. Helander et al. (24), however, found that *trans*-cinnamaldehyde was unable to induce ATP leakage. This contradictory result is most likely due to the concentration difference used in the two studies; Helander et al. (24) used 0.264 ml/l, whereas Gill and Holley (57) used 5.29 ml/l.

Conclusion

Several plant-derived EOs are effective as natural alternatives to synthetic food additives, particularly as antimicrobial agents. One of the main actions of EOs is to affect the permeability of cell membranes leading to loss of cellular components or influx of other substances into the cell. New studies on the effects of EOs on the QS systems of foodborne and other pathogens offer an opportunity for the development of natural food antimicrobials that could not only be bactericidal but could also lessen pathogenic effects.

References

1. Deans SG, Ritchie G. Antibacterial properties of plant essential oils. *Int J Food Microbiol* (1987) **5**:165–80. doi:10.1016/0168-1605(87)90034-1
2. Hammer KA, Carson CF, Riley TV. Antimicrobial activity of essential oils and other plant extracts. *J Appl Microbiol* (1999) **86**:985–90. doi:10.1046/j.1365-2672.1999.00780.x
3. Sánchez E, García S, Heredia N. Extracts of edible and medicinal plants damage membranes of *Vibrio cholerae*. *Appl Environ Microbiol* (2010) **76**:6888–94. doi:10.1128/AEM.03052-09
4. Fraenkel GS. The raison d'etre of secondary plant substances. *Science* (1959) **129**:1466–70. doi:10.1126/science.129.3361.1466
5. Tajkarimi MM, Ibrahim SA, Cliver DO. Antimicrobial herb and spice compounds in food. *Food Control* (2010) **21**:1199–218. doi:10.1016/j.foodcont.2010.02.003
6. Boyle W. Spices and essential oils as preservatives. *Am Perfum Essent Oil Rev* (1955) **66**:25–8.
7. Kalemba D, Matla M, Smetek A. Antimicrobial activities of essential oils. *Dietary Phytochemicals and Microbes*. Berlin: Springer (2012). p. 157–83.
8. Lee SH, Lillehoj HS, Lillehoj EP, Cho SM, Park DW, Hong YH, et al. Immunomodulatory properties of dietary plum on coccidiosis. *Comp Immunol Microbiol Infect Dis* (2008) **31**:389–402. doi:10.1016/j.cimid.2007.06.005
9. Lillehoj HS, Kim DK, Bravo DM, Lee SH. Effects of dietary plant-derived phytonutrients on the genome-wide profiles and coccidiosis resistance in the broiler chickens. *BMC Proc* (2011) **5**(Suppl 4):S34. doi:10.1186/1753-6561-5-S4-S34
10. Mathlouthi N, Bouzaienne T, Oueslati I, Recoquillay F, Hamdi M, Urdaci M, et al. Use of rosemary, oregano, and a commercial blend of essential oils in broiler chickens: *in vitro* antimicrobial activities and effects on growth performance. *J Anim Sci* (2012) **90**:813–23. doi:10.2527/jas.2010-3646
11. Betancourt L, Rodriguez F, Phandanouvong V, Ariza-Nieto C, Hume M, Nisbet D, et al. Effect of *Origanum* chemotypes on broiler intestinal bacteria. *Poult Sci* (2014) **93**:2526–35. doi:10.3382/ps.2014-03944
12. Alali WQ, Hofacre CL, Mathis GF, Faltys G. Effect of essential oil compound on shedding and colonization of *Salmonella enterica* serovar Heidelberg in broilers. *Poult Sci* (2013) **92**:836–41. doi:10.3382/ps.2012-02783
13. Cerisuelo A, Marin C, Sanchez-Vizcaino F, Gomez EA, de la Fuente JM, Duran R, et al. The impact of a specific blend of essential oil components and sodium butyrate in feed on growth performance and *Salmonella* counts in experimentally challenged broilers. *Poult Sci* (2014) **93**:599–606. doi:10.3382/ps.2013-03528
14. Ricke SC, Rivera Calo J, Kaldhone P. *Salmonella* control in food production: current issues and perspectives in the United States. In: Ricke SC, Donaldson JR, Phillips CA, editors. *Food Safety Emerging Issues, Technologies and Systems*. London: Academic Press (2015). p. 107–33.
15. Benchaar C, Chaves AV, Fraser GR, Wang Y, Beauchemin KA, McAllister TA. Effects of essential oils and their components on *in vitro* rumen microbial fermentation. *Can J Anim Sci* (2007) **87**:413–9. doi:10.1111/j.1439-0396.2011.01236.x
16. Callaway TR, Carroll JA, Arthington JD, Pratt C, Edrington TS, Anderson RC, et al. Citrus products decrease growth of *E. coli* O157:H7 and *Salmonella typhimurium* in pure culture and in fermentation with mixed ruminal microorganisms *in vitro*. *Foodborne Pathog Dis* (2008) **5**:621–7. doi:10.1089/fpd.2008.0088
17. Callaway TR, Carroll JA, Arthington JD, Edrington TS, Anderson RC, Rossman ML, et al. Orange peel products can reduce *Salmonella* populations in ruminants. *Foodborne Pathog Dis* (2011) **8**:1071–5. doi:10.1089/fpd.2011.0867
18. Schifferstein HNJ, Ophuis PAMO. Health-related determinants of organic food consumption in the Netherlands. *Food Qual Prefer* (1998) **9**:119–33. doi:10.1016/S0950-3293(97)00044-X
19. Williams PRD, Hammitt JK. Perceived risks of conventional and organic produce: pesticides, pathogens, and natural toxins. *Risk Anal* (2001) **21**:319–30. doi:10.1111/0272-4332.212114
20. Williams P, Stirling E, Keynes N. Food fears: a national survey on the attitudes of Australian adults about the safety and quality of food. *Asia Pac J Clin Nutr* (2004) **13**:32–9.
21. Dorman HJD, Deans SG. Antimicrobial agents from plants: antibacterial activity of plant volatile oils. *J Appl Microbiol* (2000) **88**:308–16. doi:10.1046/j.1365-2672.2000.00969.x
22. Lambert RJW, Skandamis PN, Coote PJ, Nychas GJE. A study of the minimum inhibitory concentration and mode of action of oregano essential oil, thymol and carvacrol. *J Appl Microbiol* (2001) **91**:453–62. doi:10.1046/j.1365-2672.2001.01428.x
23. Turgis M, Han J, Caillet S, Lacroix M. Antimicrobial activity of mustard essential oil against *Escherichia coli* O157:H7 and *Salmonella typhi*. *Food Control* (2009) **20**:1073–9. doi:10.1016/j.foodcont.2009.02.001
24. Helander IM, Alakomi HL, Latva-Kala K, Mattila-Sandholm T, Pol I, Smid EJ, et al. Characterization of the action of selected essential oil components on gram-negative bacteria. *J Agric Food Chem* (1998) **46**:3590–5. doi:10.1021/jf980154m
25. Cox SD, Gustafson JE, Mann CM, Markham JL, Liew YC, Hartland RP. Tea tree oil causes K+ leakage and inhibits respiration in *Escherichia coli*. *Lett Appl Microbiol* (1998) **26**:355–8. doi:10.1046/j.1472-765X.1998.00348.x
26. Cox SD, Mann CM, Markham JL, Bell HC, Gustafson JE, Warmington JR. The mode of antimicrobial action of the essential oil of *Melaleuca alternifolia* (tea tree oil). *J Appl Microbiol* (2000) **88**:170–5. doi:10.1046/j.1365-2672.2000.00943.x
27. Ultee A, Kets EPW, Alberda M, Hoekstra FA, Smid EJ. Adaptation of the food-borne pathogen *Bacillus cereus* to carvacrol. *Arch Microbiol* (2000) **174**:233–8. doi:10.1007/s002030000199
28. Ultee A, Bennik MHJ, Moezelarr R. The phenolic hydroxyl group of carvacrol is essential for action against the food-borne pathogen *Bacillus cereus*. *Appl Environ Microbiol* (2002) **68**:1561–8. doi:10.1128/AEM.68.4.1561-1568.2002
29. Nazzaro F, Fratianni F, De Martino L, Coppola R, De Feo V. Effect of essential oils on pathogenic bacteria. *Pharmaceuticals* (2013) **6**:1451–74. doi:10.3390/ph6121451
30. Nikaido H. Prevention of drug access to bacterial targets: permeability barriers and active efflux. *Science* (1994) **264**:382–8. doi:10.1126/science.8153625
31. Nikaido H. Molecular basis of bacterial outer membrane permeability revisited. *Microbiol Mol Biol Rev* (2003) **67**:593–656. doi:10.1128/MMBR.67.4.593-656.2003
32. Trombetta D, Castelli F, Sarpietro MG, Venuti V, Cristani M, Daniele C, et al. Mechanisms of antibacterial action of three monoterpenes. *Antimicrob Agents Chemother* (2005) **49**:2474–8. doi:10.1128/AAC.49.6.2474-2478.2005
33. Plesiat P, Nikaido H. Outer membranes of Gram-negative bacteria are permeable to steroid probes. *Molec Microbiol* (1992) **6**:1323–33. doi:10.1111/j.1365-2958.1992.tb00853.x
34. Ultee A, Kets EPW, Smid EJ. Mechanisms of action of carvacrol on the food-borne pathogens *Bacillus cereus*. *Appl Environ Microbiol* (1999) **65**:4606–10.
35. Cox SD, Mann CM, Markham JL, Gustafson JE, Warmington JR, Wyllie SG. Determining the antimicrobial actions of tea tree oil. *Molecules* (2001) **6**:87–91. doi:10.3390/60100087
36. Walsh SE, Maillard JY, Russell AD, Catrenich CE, Charbonneau DL, Bartolo RG. Activity and mechanisms of action of selected biocidal agents on gram-positive and -negative bacteria. *J Appl Microbiol* (2003) **94**:240–7. doi:10.1046/j.1365-2672.2003.01825.x
37. Fitzgerald DJ, Stratford M, Gasson MJ, Ueckert J, Bos A, Narbad A. Mode of antimicrobial action of vanillin against *Escherichia coli*, *Lactobacillus plantarum* and *Listeria innocua*. *J Appl Microbiol* (2004) **97**:104–13. doi:10.1111/j.1365-2672.2004.02275.x
38. Inoue Y, Shiraishi A, Hada T, Hirose K, Hamashima H, Shimada J. The antibacterial effects of terpene alcohols on *Staphylococcus aureus* and their mode of action. *FEMS Microbiol Lett* (2004) **237**:325–31. doi:10.1016/j.femsle.2004.06.049
39. Togashi N, Inoue Y, Hamashima H, Takano A. Effects of two terpene alcohols on the antibacterial activity and the mode of action of farnesol against *Staphylococcus aureus*. *Molecules* (2008) **13**:3069–76. doi:10.3390/molecules13123069
40. Bouhdid S, Abrini J, Amensour M, Zhiri A, Espuny MJ, Manresa A. Functional and ultrastructural changes in *Pseudomonas aeruginosa* and *Staphylococcus aureus* cells induced by *Cinnamomum verum* essential oil. *J Appl Microbiol* (2010) **109**:1139–49. doi:10.1111/j.1365-2672.2010.04740.x
41. Arrebola ML, Navarro MC, Jiménez J, Ocaña FA. Yield and composition of the essential oil of *Thymus serpylloides* subsp. serpylloides. *Phytochemistry* (1994) **36**:67–72. doi:10.1016/S0031-9422(00)97014-6
42. Lagouri V, Blekas G, Tsimidou M, Kokkini S, Boskou D. Composition and antioxidant activity of essential oils from oregano plants grown wild in Greece. *Eur Food Res Technol* (1993) **197**:20–3. doi:10.1007/BF01202694

43. Bouhdid S, Abrini J, Zhiri A, Espuny MJ, Manresa A. Investigation of functional and morphological changes in *Pseudomonas aeruginosa* and *Staphylococcus aureus* cells induced by *Origanum compactum* essential oil. *J Appl Microbiol* (2009) **106**:1558–68. doi:10.1111/j.1365-2672.2008.04124.x
44. Bajpai VK, Sharma A, Baek KH. Antibacterial mode of action of Ginkgo biloba leaf essential oil: effect on morphology and membrane permeability. *Bangladesh J Pharmacol* (2015) **10**:337–50. doi:10.3329/bjp.v10i2.22546
45. De Clerck LS, Bridts CH, Mertens AM, Moens MM, Stevens WJ. Use of fluorescent dyes in the determination of adherence of human leucocytes to endothelial cells and the effect of fluorochromes on cellular function. *J Immunol Methods* (1994) **172**:115–24. doi:10.1016/0022-1759(94)90384-0
46. Veal DA, Deere D, Ferrari B, Piper J, Attfield PV. Fluorescence staining and flow cytometry for monitoring microbial cells. *J Immunol Methods* (2000) **243**:191–210. doi:10.1016/S0022-1759(00)00234-9
47. Nguefack J, Budde BB, Jakobsen M. Five essential oils from aromatic plants of Cameroon: their antibacterial activity and ability to permeabilize the cytoplasmic membrane of *Listeria innocua* examined by flow cytometry. *Lett Appl Microbiol* (2004) **39**:395–400. doi:10.1111/j.1472-765X.2004.01587.x
48. Xu J, Zhou F, Ji BP, Pei RS, Xu N. The antibacterial mechanism of carvacrol and thymol against *Escherichia coli*. *Lett Appl Microbiol* (2008) **47**:174–9. doi:10.1111/j.1472-765X.2008.02407.x
49. Ifesan BOT, Joycharat N, Voravuthikunchai SP. The mode of antistaphylococcal action of *Eleutherine americana*. *FEMS Immunol Med Microbiol* (2009) **57**:193–201. doi:10.1111/j.1574-695X.2009.00599.x
50. Carson CF, Mee BJ, Riley TV. Mechanism of action of *Melaleuca alternifolia* (tea tree) oil on *Staphylococcus aureus* determined by time-kill, lysis, leakage, and salt tolerance assays and electron microscopy. *Antimicrob Agents Chemother* (2002) **46**:1914–20. doi:10.1128/AAC.46.6.1914-1920.2002
51. Oussalah M, Caillet S, Lacroix M. Mechanism of action of Spanish oregano, Chinese cinnamon, and savory essential oils against cell membranes and walls of *Escherichia coli* O157:H7 and *Listeria monocytogenes*. *J Food Prot* (2006) **69**:1046–55.
52. Oussalah M, Caillet S, Saucier L, Lacroix M. Inhibitory effects of selected plant essential oils on the growth of four pathogenic bacteria: *E. coli* O157:H7, *Salmonella typhimurium*, *Staphylococcus aureus* and *Listeria monocytogenes*. *Food Control* (2007) **18**:414–20. doi:10.1016/j.foodcont.2005.11.009
53. De Souza EL, De Azeredo GA, De Sousa JP, De Figueiredo RCBQ, Stamford TLM. Cytotoxic effects of *Origanum vulgare* L. and *Rosmarinus officinalis* L. essential oils alone and combined at sublethal amounts on *Pseudomonas fluorescens* in a vegetable broth. *J Food Safety* (2013) **33**:163–71. doi:10.1111/jfs.12036
54. Fisher K, Phillips C. The mechanism of action of a citrus oil blend against *Enterococcus faecium* and *Enterococcus faecalis*. *J Appl Microbiol* (2009) **106**:1343–9. doi:10.1111/j.1365-2672.2008.04102.x
55. Ohmizo C, Yata M, Katsu T. Bacterial cytoplasmic membrane permeability assay using ion-selective electrodes. *J Microbiol Methods* (2004) **59**:173–9. doi:10.1016/j.mimet.2004.06.008
56. Veldhuizen EJA, Tjeerdsma-van Bokhoven JLM, Zweijtzer C, Burt SA, Haagsman HP. Structural requirements for the antimicrobial activity of carvacrol. *J Agric Food Chem* (2006) **54**:1874–9. doi:10.1021/jf052564y
57. Gill AO, Holley RA. Mechanisms of bactericidal action of cinnamaldehyde against *Listeria monocytogenes* and of eugenol against *L. monocytogenes* and *Lactobacillus sakei*. *Appl Environ Microbiol* (2004) **70**:5750–5. doi:10.1128/AEM.70.10.5750-5755.2004
58. Sikkema J, de Bont JAM, Poolman B. Interactions of cyclic hydrocarbons with biological membranes. *J Biol Chem* (1994) **269**:8022–8.
59. Gill AO, Holley RA. Disruption of *E. coli*, *Listeria monocytogenes* and *Lactobacillus sakei* cellular membranes by plant oil aromatics. *Int J Food Microbiol* (2006) **108**:1–9. doi:10.1016/j.ijfoodmicro.2005.10.009
60. Miller MB, Bassler BL. Quorum sensing in bacteria. *Annu Rev Microbiol* (2001) **55**:165–99. doi:10.1146/annurev.micro.55.1.165
61. Kjelleberg S, Molin S. Is there a role for quorum sensing signals in bacterial biofilms? *Curr Opin Microbiol* (2002) **5**:254–8. doi:10.1016/S1369-5274(02)00325-9
62. March J, Bentley W. Quorum sensing and bacterial cross-talk in biotechnology. *Curr Opin Biotechnol* (2004) **15**:495–502. doi:10.1016/j.copbio.2004.08.013
63. Deep A, Chaudhary U, Gupta V. Quorum sensing and bacterial pathogenicity: from molecules to disease. *J Lab Physicians* (2011) **3**:4–11. doi:10.4103/0974-2727.78553
64. Khan MSA, Zahin M, Hasan S, Husain FM, Ahmad I. Inhibition of quorum sensing regulated bacterial functions by plant essential oils with special reference to clove oil. *Lett Appl Microbiol* (2009) **49**:354–60. doi:10.1111/j.1472-765X.2009.02666.x
65. Szabo MA, Varga GZ, Hohmann J, Schelz Z, Szegedi E, Amaral L, et al. Inhibition of quorum-sensing signals by essential oils. *Phytother Res* (2010) **24**:782–6. doi:10.1002/ptr.3010
66. Alvarez MV, Ortega-Ramirez LA, Gutierrez-Pacheco MM, Bernal-Mercado AT, Rodriguez-Garcia I, Gonzalez-Aguilar GA, et al. Oregano essential oil-pectin edible films as anti-quorum sensing and food antimicrobial agents. *Front Microbiol* (2014) **5**:699. doi:10.3389/fmicb.2014.00699
67. Ben Arfa A, Combes S, Preziosi-Belloy L, Gontard N, Chalier P. Antimicrobial activities of carvacrol related to its chemical structure. *Lett Appl Microbiol* (2006) **43**:149–54. doi:10.1111/j.1472-765X.2006.01938.x

Conflict of Interest Statement: The authors declare that this review was prepared in the absence of any commercial or financial relationships that could be construed as a potential conflict of interest.

Chromium propionate enhances adipogenic differentiation of bovine intramuscular adipocytes

*Rebecca J. Tokach[1], Flavio R. B. Ribeiro[1], Ki Yong Chung[2], Whitney Rounds[3] and Bradley J. Johnson[1]**

[1] Department of Animal and Food Sciences, Texas Tech University, Lubbock, TX, USA, [2] Hanwoo Research Institute, National Institute of Animal Science, Rural Development Administration, Kangwon, South Korea, [3] Kemin Animal Nutrition and Health North America, Des Moines, IA, USA

In vitro experiments were performed to determine the effects of increasing concentrations of chromium propionate (CrPro) on mRNA and protein abundance of different enzymes and receptors. Intramuscular (IM) and subcutaneous (SC) preadipocytes and bovine satellite cells were isolated from the longissimus muscle to determine the effect of treatment on glucose transporter type 4 (GLUT4) and peroxisome proliferator-activated receptor γ mRNA and GLUT4 protein abundance. Preadipocyte cultures were treated with differentiation media plus either sodium propionate or different concentrations of CrPro for 96, 120, and 144 h before harvest. This study indicated that adipogenesis of the bovine IM adipocytes were more sensitive to the treatment of CrPro as compared to SC adipocytes. Enhancement of adenosine monophosphate-activated protein kinase and GLUT4 mRNA by CrPro treatment may enhance glucose uptake in IM adipocytes. CrPro decreased GLUT4 protein levels in muscle cell cultures suggesting that those cells have increased efficiency of glucose uptake due to exposure to increased levels of CrPro. In contrast, each of the two adipogenic lines had opposing responses to the CrPro. It appeared that CrPro had the most stimulative effect of GLUT4 response in the IM adipocytes as compared to SC adipocytes. These findings indicated opportunities to potentially augment marbling in beef cattle fed CrPro during the finishing phase.

Keywords: beef cattle, chromium, GLUT4, marbling

Edited by:
Minoru Tanaka,
Nippon Veterinary and Life Science University, Japan

Reviewed by:
Takeshi Ohkubo,
Ibaraki University, Japan
Sungkwonk Park,
Sejong University, South Korea

Correspondence:
Bradley J. Johnson,
Box 42141, Lubbock, TX, USA
bradley.johnson@ttu.edu

Introduction

It has been generally accepted that chromium (Cr) potentiates the effects of insulin (1). Chromium, included in the diet as KemTRACE®$_{\text{brand}}$ Chromium Propionate 0.04% (KT Cr), has improved the performance of beef cattle. These improvements have been expressed as additional body weight gain, better feed efficiency, lower morbidity, and mortality (2–4). Initial results from studies with feeder cattle suggest that feeding KT Cr also has positive effects on immune response, cytokines, and acute phase response of cattle to stress (5). The potential effects of improved glucose metabolism on carcass characteristics have shown mixed results (2, 4). The effect of chromium propionate (CrPro) on bovine muscle, intramuscular (IM) adipose, and subcutaneous (SC) adipose tissue development is unknown. This research was conducted to further investigate the effects of CrPro on enhancing adipogenic differentiation of bovine muscle derived cells, IM, and SC adipocytes.

Materials and Methods

Preadipocyte and Satellite Cell Isolation From Tissues

Bovine muscle satellite cells (BSC) and preadipocytes were isolated from four 16-month-old British × Continental crossbred steers. Cattle were harvested by captive bolt followed by exsanguination. All experimental procedures were approved by the Texas Tech University Institutional Animal Care and Use Committee, and performed at the Texas Tech University Beef Cattle Research Center. Immediately after hide removal, a section of the longissimus muscle was removed from between the fifth and eighth thoracic ribs and transported to the cell culture laboratory. The following procedures were conducted in a sterile field under a tissue culture hood. For BSC isolation, connective and adipose tissues were removed from the muscle sample (**Figure 1**). The muscle sample was passed through a sterile meat grinder. The ground muscle was incubated with 0.1% pronase (Calbiochem, La Jolla, CA, USA) in Earl's Balanced Salt Solution (Sigma, St. Louis, MO, USA) for 1 h at 37°C with mixing every 10 min. The mixture was centrifuged at 1,500 × *g* for 4 min at room temperature following incubation. The pellet that was formed during centrifugation was suspended in phosphate buffered saline (PBS; Invitrogen, Grand Island, NY, USA; 140 mM NaCl, 1 mM KH_2PO_4, 3 mM KCl, 8 mM Na_2HPO_4), and the suspension was centrifuged at 500 × *g* at 20°C for 10 min. The supernatant was collected and centrifuged at 1,500 × *g* for 10 min at 20°C to pellet the mononucleated cells. Two additional PBS washes and differential centrifugations were conducted before the resulting mononucleated cell preparation was suspended in cold (4°C) Dulbecco's Modified Eagle Medium (DMEM; Invitrogen) containing 10% fetal bovine serum (FBS; Invitrogen) and 10% (vol/vol) dimethylsulfoxide (Sigma, St. Louis, MO). Cells were stored frozen in liquid nitrogen for future use.

The IM and SC adipose tissues were separated from the muscle, finely minced, and placed in separate containers containing isolation buffer, which consisted of DMEM, collagenase (Sigma, St. Louis, MO, USA), and bovine serum albumin (BSA; Sigma St. Louis, MO, USA). The containers were then incubated in a shaking incubator for 40 min at 38°C. Following incubation, the isolation buffers containing the IM or SC adipose tissue samples were passed through sterilized nylon mesh. Samples were then centrifuged for 5 min at 1,500 rpm. Supernatant was removed and the cell pellet was suspended in 20 mL of warm (37°C) DMEM containing 10% FBS. The centrifugation step was repeated two additional times before the resulting cell pellet was suspended in cold (4°C) DMEM containing 10% FBS and 10% (vol/vol) dimethylsulfoxide. Cells were stored frozen in liquid nitrogen for future use.

Differentiation of BSC and Preadipocyte Cultures

Bovine satellite cells and the IM and SC preadipocyte cultures were plated in DMEM containing 10% FBS. Bovine satellite cell cultures were rinsed with DMEM with 10% FBS at 24 and 72 h of incubation. At 120 h of incubation, the BSCs were treated with differentiation media containing 3% horse serum (Sigma, St. Louis, MO, USA), 1.5 µg/mL of BSA-linoleic acid, and one of five treatments. The treatments for the BSC were as follows: (1) control, (2) 0.1 µM CrPro (Kemin Animal Nutrition and Health North America, Des Moines, IA, USA), (3) 1 µM CrPro, (4) 10 µM CrPro, (5) 10 µM sodium propionate (NaPro; Sigma, St. Louis, MO, USA). Chromium for this study was prepared from KemTRACE®$_{brand}$ CrPro base (lot # 1006101421), assayed to contain 8.59% Cr. A 100 µM solution was prepared from the above base and was utilized in this *in vitro* study.

Intramuscular and SC preadipocyte cultures were incubated until cells reached approximately 100% confluence. When 100%

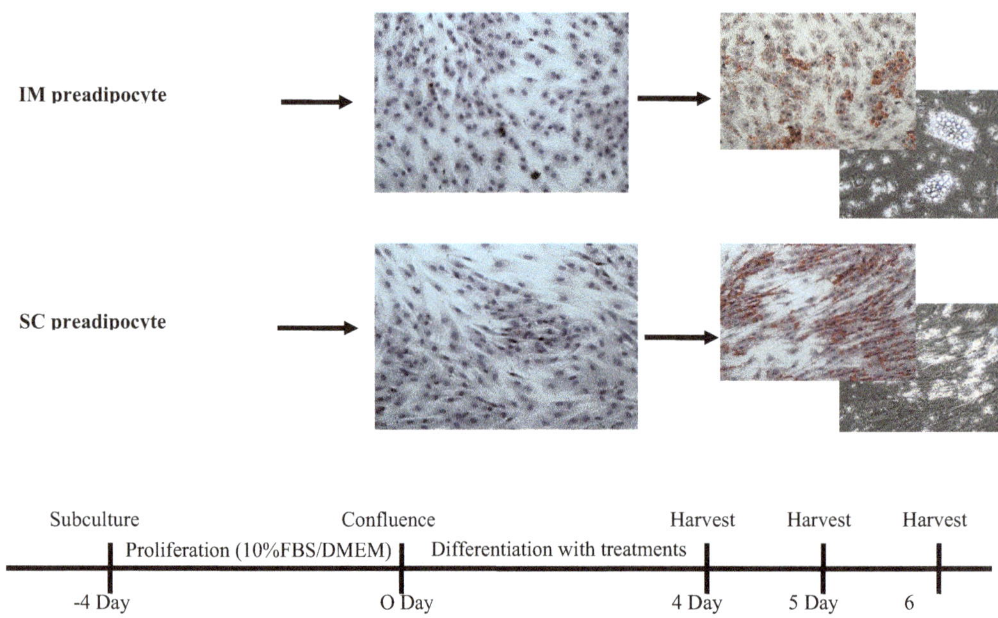

FIGURE 1 | Time frames of bovine intramuscular (IM) and subcutaneous (SC) preadipocyte differentiation in primary cell culture. These intramuscular and subcutaneous adipocytes showed different patterns of accumulated lipid droplets. FBS, fetal bovine serum; DMEM, Dulbecco's modified eagle medium.

confluence was achieved, cultures were rinsed three times with serum-free DMEM and DMEM containing 5% FBS plus treatments were added for 96, 120, or 144 h. The treatments for IM and SC preadipocyte cultures were as follows: (1) control, (2) 1 μM CrPro, (3) differentiation media, (4) differentiation media + 0.1 μM CrPro, (5) differentiation media + 1 μM CrPro, (6) differentiation media + 10 μM CrPro, and (7) differentiation media + 10 μM NaPro. The differentiation media used in treatments 3–7 consisted of 10 μM ciglitizone (Sigma, St. Louis, MO, USA), 100 μM oleic acid (Sigma, St. Louis, MO, USA), 1 μM dexamethasone (Sigma, St. Louis, MO, USA), and 10 μM insulin (Sigma, St. Louis, MO, USA). Oil-Red-O and hematoxylin staining were used to confirm the accumulation of lipid droplets in differentiated BSC and IM and SC preadipocyte cultures. The cells were fixed with 10% neutral buffer formalin. After fixation, the cultures were stained with 0.5% Oil-Red-O solution in darkness. Following Oil-Red-O staining, cultures were stained with Harris' hematoxylin for 30 min in darkness. Cell cultures were mounted in 60% propylene glycol and stored for analysis. IM and SC adipocytes were identified by the presence of lipid droplets in the cytosol, which were changed to a red color by Oil-red-O staining, and hematoxylin staining, which stained the nuclei of cells, was used to identify the multinucleated myotubes of differentiated muscle cells.

Real-Time Quantitative-PCR

RNA from cultured BSC and preadipocytes (IM and SC) were isolated with 500 μL of ice-cold buffer containing TRI reagent (Sigma, St. Louis, MO, USA). Concentration of RNA was determined by absorbance at 260 nm. Real-time quantitative-PCR (RTQ-PCR) was used to measure the quantity of glucose transporter type 4 (GLUT4), CCAAT/enhancer-binding protein β (C/EBPβ), peroxisome proliferator-activated receptor γ (PPARγ), stearoyl-CoA desaturase (SCD), and G protein coupled receptor 43 (GPR43) mRNA relative to the quantity of ribosomal protein subunit 9 (RPS9) mRNA in total RNA isolated from BSC and preadipocyte cultures. The quantity of adenosine monophosphate-activated protein kinase (AMPKα), GLUT4, myosin heavy chain (MHC)-I, MHC-IIa, and MHC-IIX, β1-adernergic receptor (AR), and β2-AR relative mRNA was measured relative to the quantity of RPS9 in total RNA isolated from the bovine satellite cells. Assays were performed in the GeneAmp 7900H Sequence Detection System (Applied Biosystems) using thermal cycling parameters recommended by the manufacturer (40 cycles of 15 s at 95°C and 1 min at 60°C). The endogenous RPS9 mRNA control was used to normalize the expression of GLUT4, PPARγ, C/EBPβ, SCD, and GPR43.

Western Blotting

Protein from cultured BSC and preadipocytes (IM and SC) was isolated with 200 μL of ice-cold buffer containing M-PER (Fisher Scientific, Fair Lawn, NJ, USA), protein inhibitor (Roche, Indianapolis, IN, USA), and 2 mM Na_3VO_4 (Fisher Scientific). Cell homogenates were mixed with an equal volume of 2× standard SDS sample loading buffer (Invitrogen) and loaded onto gels. Gradient gels (10–20%) were used for SDS-PAGE separation of proteins. Membranes were incubated overnight at 4°C with primary antibodies (Abcam, Cambridge, MA, USA) at a dilution of 1:1,000 in TBS-Tween. Membranes were then incubated with horseradish peroxidase-conjugated secondary antibodies at 1:2,000 dilution for 2 h. After three 10-min washes, membranes were visualized using enhanced chemiluminescent substrate (ECL) Western blotting reagents (Amersham Bioscience, Piscataway, NJ, USA) and exposure to film (MR, Kodak, Rochester, NY, USA). Density of bands was quantified using Imager Scanner II and ImageQuant TL software. To reduce the variation between blots, tissue lysates of both groups were run in a single gel. Band density was normalized according to the glyceraldehyde 3-phosphate dehydrogenase (GAPDH) content.

Statistical Analysis

Data were analyzed as a complete randomized block design using the Mixed procedure (PROC MIXED) of SAS (SAS Institute, Cary, NC, USA). Differences between control and treatment were determined using the least significant difference procedure. Means were considered significantly different at $P < 0.05$.

Results

The first experiment used RTQ-PCR analysis of IM and SC adipocytes to examine the effect of a 96 h-treatment of CrPro on preadipocyte differentiation. RTQ-PCR analysis of IM cells revealed that 10 μM CrPro increased AMPKα, PPARγ mRNA, and GLUT 4 abundance compared to all other treatments (**Figure 2**).

These data indicated that the highest dose of CrPro (10 μM) enhanced IM preadipocyte differentiation as evidenced by the increased PPARγ mRNA levels whereas the SC preadipocytes were non-responsive to CrPro in regards to PPARγ concentrations. SC adipocytes treated with 10 μM CrPro had an increased AMPKα mRNA abundance compared to 0.1 and 1 μM CrPro treatments, but did not differ from the differentiated control cultures (**Figure 2**). To verify that these differences between IM and SC adipocytes were a result of Cr and not its carrier, propionate (Pro), a second experiment was conducted with additional treatments.

In the second experiment, an addition of a 10 μM NaPro treatment helped to verify that the effects previously seen were due to the addition of elemental Cr rather than an effect of Pro. Furthermore, IM and SC adipocytes were differentiated with their respective treatments for 96, 120, or 144 h to observe potential time course effects throughout differentiation. Morphological analysis of these cells revealed that primary cultures of preadipocytes treated with the adipogenic differentiation cocktail accumulated lipid droplets in the cell cytosol after 96 h (**Figure 1**). Lipid droplets in the IM and SC preadipocyte cultures increased in a dose-dependent manner when treated with CrPro compared to the control and NaPro treatments (**Figure 3**). However, our qualitative data suggest that a higher dose of Cr may be required to activate lipid filling of IM adipocytes as compared to SC adipocytes as indicated in **Figure 4**. Morphological analysis for BSC (muscle cells) revealed that treatment of CrPro appeared to increase abundance and diameter of myotubes compared to the control and NaPro-treated cultures (**Figure 3**). These data would indicate a positive effect on skeletal muscle hypertrophy (size of

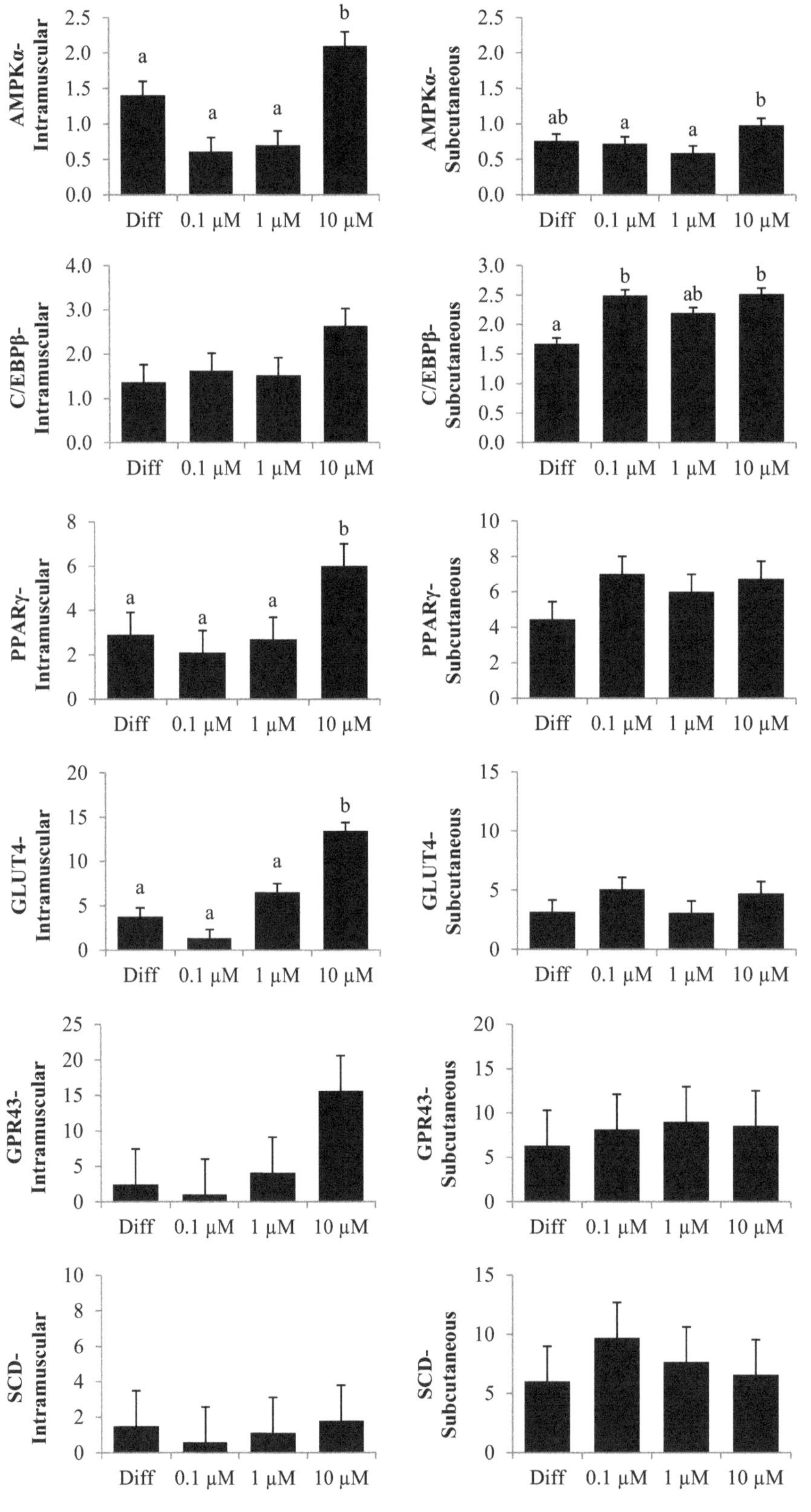

FIGURE 2 | The effect of dose-dependent treatment of chromium propionate (CrPro) on mRNA abundance of key genes regulating differentiation in intramuscular (IM; left) and subcutaneous (SC; right) adipocytes at 96 h post treatment. Chromium propionate regulated mRNA levels of adenosine monophosphate-activated protein kinase (AMPKα), CCAAT/enhancer-binding protein β (C/EBPβ), glucose transporter type 4 (GLUT4), G protein coupled receptor 43 (GPR43), peroxisome proliferator-activated receptor γ (PPARγ), and stearoyl-CoA desaturase (SCD) in the IM and SC adipocytes cultures in a dose-dependent fashion. Assays per treatment, $n = 3$. Treatments with different superscripts differ at $P < 0.05$.

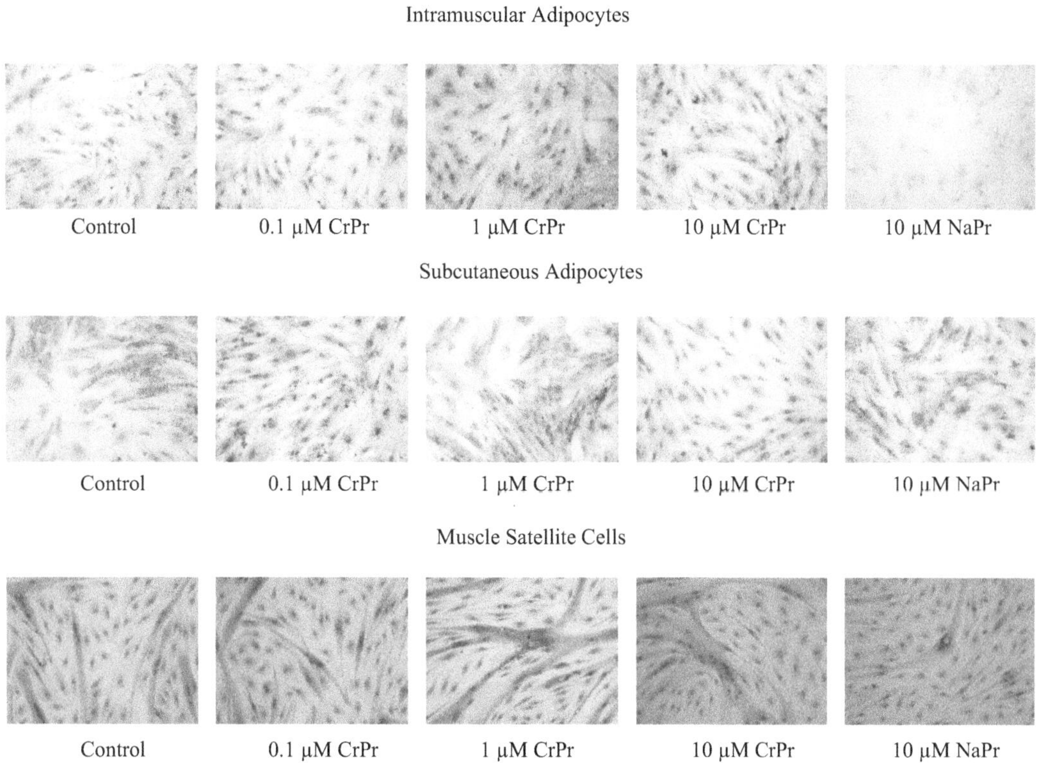

FIGURE 3 | Morphological analysis of dose-dependent treatment of chromium propionate (CrPro) in intramuscular (IM), subcutaneous (SC) adipocyte, and satellite cell cultures at 96 h post treatment. Lipid droplets were stained with Oil-Red-O and nuclei were stained with hematoxylin. Increasing Cr dose on IM adipocytes increases lipid droplet numbers. Lipid droplets increase in SC adipocytes up to 1 μM CrPr. Increasing Cr dose in muscle satellite cells results in increasing muscle fiber size and number.

myotubes) and differentiation (extent and number of myotubes) caused by CrPro addition to these primary cultures of muscle satellite cells.

No difference was detected between differentiation media and CrPro-treated adipocytes and in AMPKα mRNA abundance for either the IM or SC adipocytes at 96, 120, or 144 h (**Figures 4** and **5**). At 144 h in SC cultures, adipocytes treated with differentiation media plus 0.1 or 1 μM CrPro had a greater PPARγ mRNA abundance ($P < 0.01$) compared to adipocytes treated with differentiation media (**Figure 5**). However, the highest dose was not different from negative control. Again, these data indicated that a lower dose of CrPro may stimulate differentiation of SC preadipocytes while IM preadipocytes require a higher dose. The relative abundance of GLUT 4 mRNA at 144 h was not different between differentiation media and CrPro-treated cultures in either IM or SC adipocytes (**Figures 4** and **5**). Additionally, there was no effect on GPR43, and SCD mRNA relative abundance due to CrPro addition in either IM or SC adipocytes at 144 h (**Figures 4** and **5**). However, there was increased ($P < 0.01$) PPARγ mRNA relative abundance when differentiation media was added to the cultures, which indicated that cells underwent normal differentiation in our culture system. In SC adipocytes treated with CrPro or NaPro, no significant differences in GLUT4 protein were detected (**Figure 6**). However, 0.1 μM CrPro treatment tended ($P = 0.10$) to increase the GLUT4 protein level in IM adipocytes compared to NaPro treatment (**Figure 6**).

In the third experiment, BSCs were used to determine the effect of chromium on muscle cells. No differences ($P > 0.10$) in mRNA relative abundance were observed when CrPro or NaPro treatments were added to the media for AMPKα, GLUT 4, MHC I, MHC-IIa, MHC-IIx, β1-AR, and β2-AR expression (**Figure 7**). However, Western blot analysis of BSC indicated that the protein abundance of GLUT4 relative to GAPDH significantly decreased ($P < 0.01$) in a dose-dependent manner as increased concentrations of chromium were added to the BSC culture media (**Figure 8**). These data are very interesting and suggest a potential negative feedback mechanism on GLUT4 protein due to enhanced efficiency of glucose uptake regulated by Cr in a muscle cell culture system.

Discussion

The results from this study indicated that the treatment of cells with CrPro altered mRNA levels of adipogenic and metabolic markers, as well as inducing morphological changes in bovine muscle cells and preadipocytes. Chromium addition had divergent effects in the three different cell types. In IM adipocytes, the NaPro treatment had less lipid droplets compared to the differentiation treatment indicating that chromium itself enhances adipocyte differentiation rather than propionate. Oil-red-O stained images of these treatments indicated that multilocular lipid droplets accumulated in IM preadipocytes compared to the

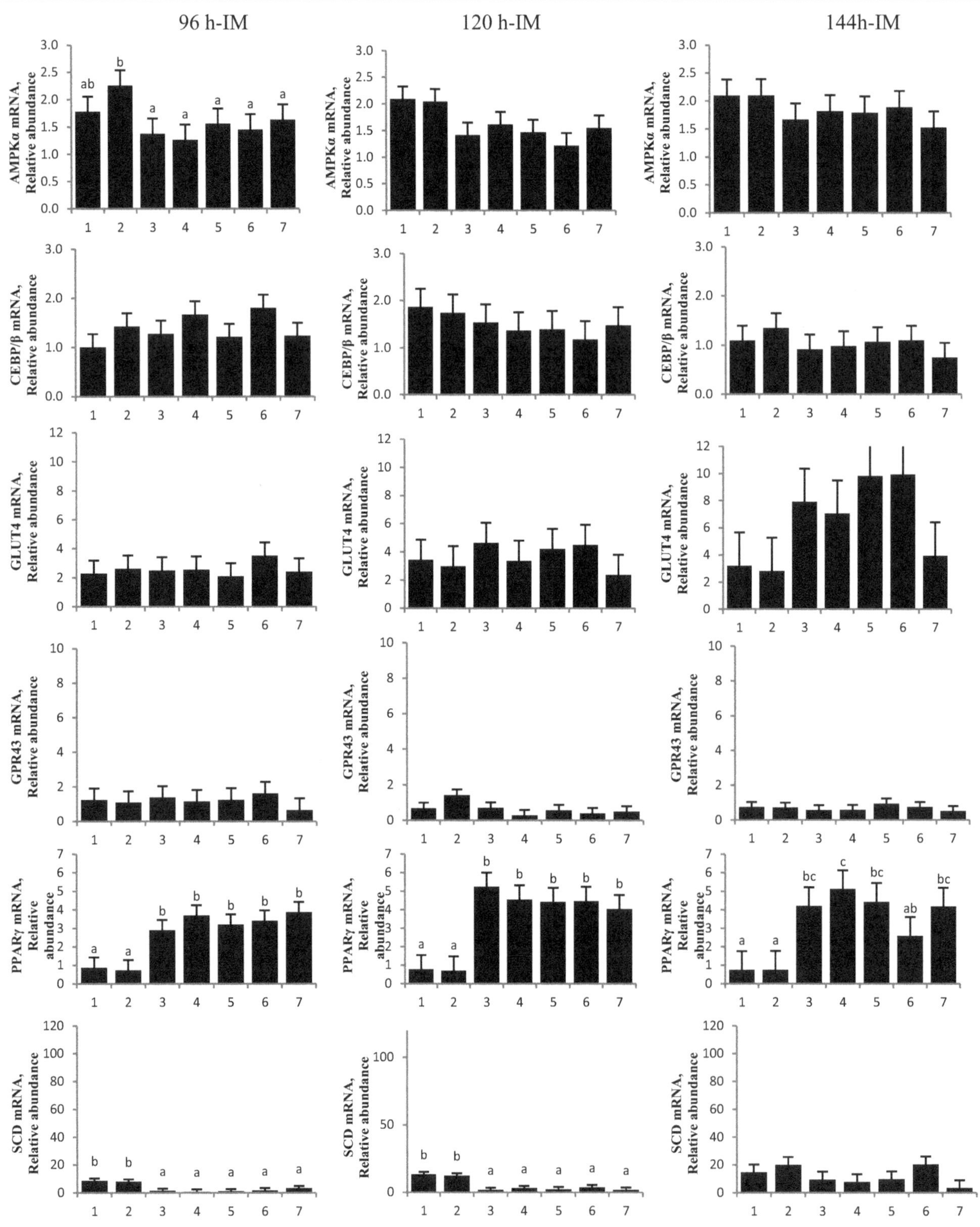

FIGURE 4 | Chromium propionate (CrPro) regulated mRNA levels of adenosine monophosphate-activated protein kinase (AMPKα), CCAAT/enhancer-binding protein β (C/EBPβ), glucose transporter type 4 (GLUT4), G protein coupled receptor 43 (GPR43), peroxisome proliferator-activated receptor γ (PPARγ), and stearoyl-CoA desaturase (SCD) in the intramuscular (IM) adipocytes cultures. Treatments: (1) 5% fetal bovine serum/Dulbecco's Modified Eagle Medium (FBS/DMEM; Cont); (2) Cont + 1 μM CrPro; (3) differentiation media (Diff; 5% FBS/DMEM, 10 μg/mL insulin, 1.0 μg/mL dexamethasone, 10 μM ciglitizone, 100 μM oleic acid; Diff); (4) Diff + 0.1 μM CrPro; (5) Diff + 1 μM CrPro; (6) Diff + 10 μMCrPro; (7) Diff + 10 μM NaPro. [abc]Within time period, treatments with different superscripts differ ($P < 0.05$).

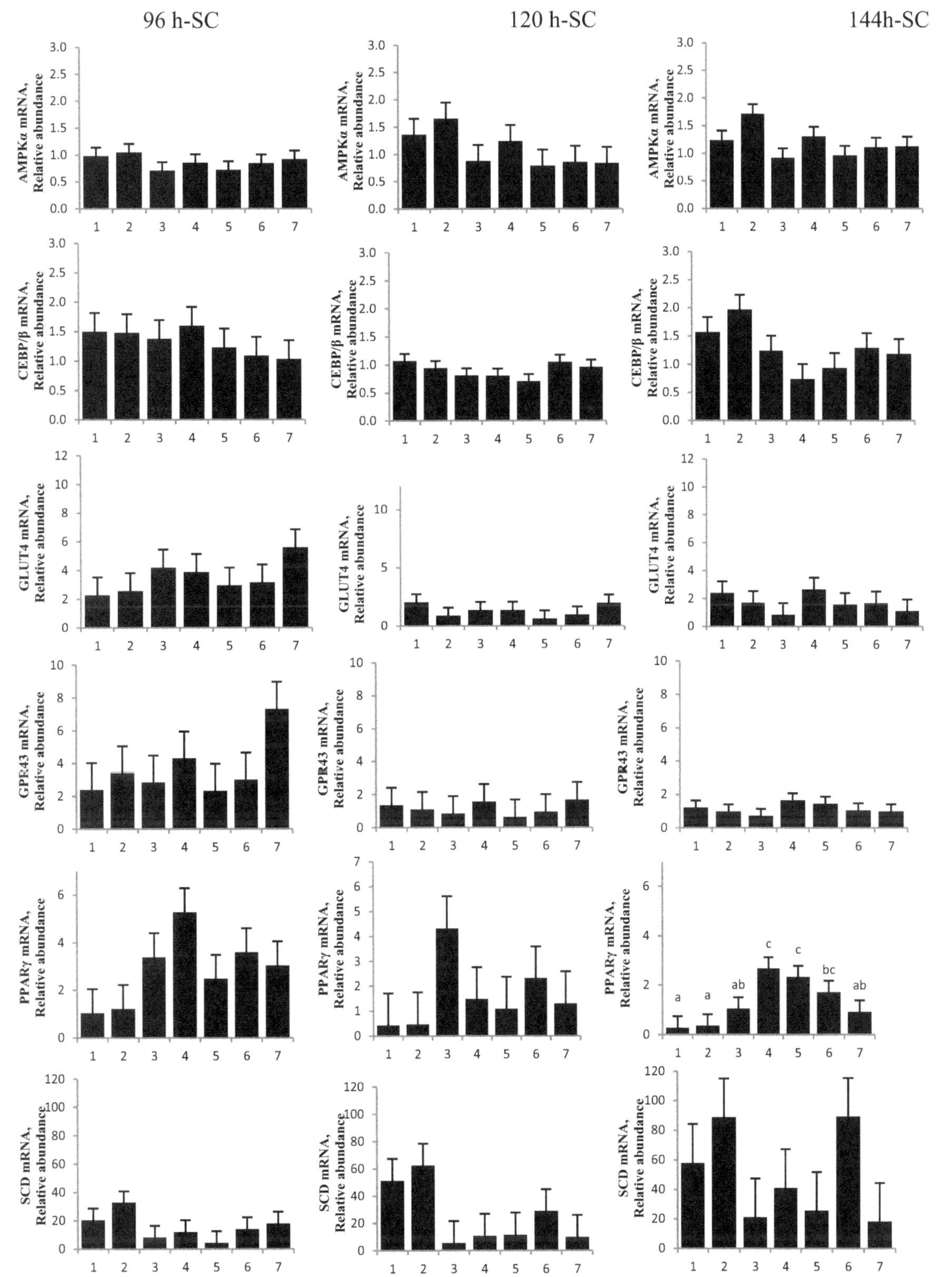

FIGURE 5 | Chromium propionate (CrPro) regulated mRNA levels of adenosine monophosphate-activated protein kinase (AMPKα), CCAAT/enhancer-binding protein β (C/EBPβ), glucose transporter type 4 (GLUT4), G protein coupled receptor 43 (GPR43), peroxisome proliferator-activated receptor γ (PPARγ), and stearoyl-CoA desaturase (SCD) in the subcutaneous (SC) adipocytes cultures. Treatments: (1) 5% fetal bovine serum/Dulbecco's Modified Eagle Medium (FBS/DMEM; Cont); (2) Cont + 1 μM CrPro; (3) differentiation media (Diff; 5% FBS/DMEM, 10 μg/mL insulin, 1.0 μg/mL dexamethasone, 10 μM ciglitizone, 100 μM oleic acid; Diff); (4) Diff + 0.1 μM CrPro; (5) Diff + 1 μM CrPro; (6) Diff + 10 μMCrPro; (7) Diff + 10 μM NaPro. ^{abc}Within time period, treatments with different superscripts differ ($P < 0.05$).

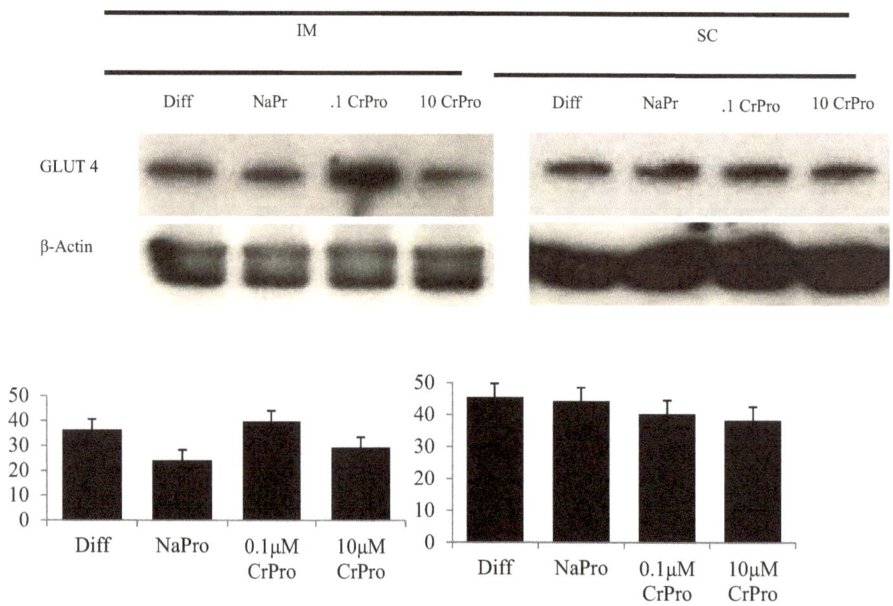

FIGURE 6 | Effects differentiation media (Diff), chromium propionate (CrPro), and sodium propionate (NaPro) on glucose transporter type 4 (GLUT4) protein abundance (*n* = 3). Protein was isolated from bovine intramuscular and subcutaneous adipocytes after 96 h of treatment, and protein abundance was determined through western blot analysis. Bars represent the standard error of the difference between the treatment means.

unilocular lipid droplets that accumulated in the SC preadipocytes at 96 h. The different distribution of lipid droplets indicates a basic morphological difference between IM and SC adipocytes and shows that the cell culture model was accurate in distinguishing the two cell types. Smith and Crouse demonstrated that IM and SC adipose tissues had metabolic differences (6). They also showed that the proportion of carbon provided by glucose for bovine adipocyte development decreased from 65% in IM adipose tissue and from 22% in SC adipose tissue. These findings suggested that glucose is a more important source for IM adipose development than SC adipose development. In contrast, acetate is a more important source for SC adipose tissue development than for IM adipose tissue development. The morphological differences between IM and SC adipocytes may be regulated by these metabolic differences. In IM adipoctyes, the number of lipid droplets increased as the dose of CrPro was increased. Interestingly, in SC adipocytes, the number of lipid droplets also increased as the dose of CrPro was increased up to 1 μM CrPro. However, SC adipocytes treated with 10 μM CrPro had less lipid droplets that SC adipocytes treated with 1 μM CrPro. This suggests that in SC adipocytes, CrPro concentration above 1 μM CrPro may begin to have a negative effect on adipocyte development. The data also suggested that a higher dose is required in IM preadipocyte to get maximal glucose uptake in these cells. The GLUT4 data supported this concept due to an apparent positive effect of CrPro on Glut4 protein in IM preadipocytes but no effect in SC preadipocytes. Taken together, these data indicated that IM adipocytes are more sensitive to Cr from a glucose regulation standpoint as compared to SC adipocytes. Biologically, this makes sense since IM cells require glucose as the energy substrate whereas SC adipocytes can synthesize lipids from acetate (6).

Adipogenic markers, such as PPARγ, were also differentially expressed for IM compared to SC adipocytes. Peroxisome proliferator-activated receptor γ is involved in gene regulation and its transcriptional activity is stimulated by insulin (7). The upregulation of PPARγ that results from this stimulation can increase the cellular uptake of fatty acids and enhance adipocyte development (8). In the first experiment, treatment with 10 μM CrPro upregulated PPARγ mRNA expression in IM adipocytes at 96 h compared to all other treatments. This mirrored the morphological changes seen in the IM adipocytes where an increasing dosage of CrPro resulted in an increase in lipid droplet number. In the second experiment, 0.1 and 1 μM CrPro-treated SC adipocytes had a higher PPARγ mRNA expression than the differentiated control SC adipocytes at 144 h. However, at 144 h in the SC adipocytes, the 10 μM CrPro-treated samples were not different from controls in PPARγ mRNA expression. Again, this mirrored the morphological changes observed in SC adipocytes. In the SC adipocytes, an increasing dose of CrPro, up to 1 μM, is beneficial to lipid droplet number. However, CrPro treatment in excess of 1 μM appears to cause a decline in lipid droplet number and as a result, could hinder adipocyte development. Together, these effects of CrPro on PPARγ and lipid droplet number suggested that higher concentrations of CrPro may be used to enhance IM adipocyte development without augmenting SC adipocyte development.

Adenosine monophosphate-activated protein kinase α, which regulates cellular energy balance, is an important enzyme in regulating lipid metabolism not only in adipocytes but also in BSC. Activation of AMPKα in muscle and adipose tissue triggers metabolic changes, such as the switch from storing to consuming fats and carbohydrates. Phosphorylation of AMPKα has been shown to be positively correlated with GLUT4 activity, which regulates glucose entry into muscle and adipose tissue (9). In

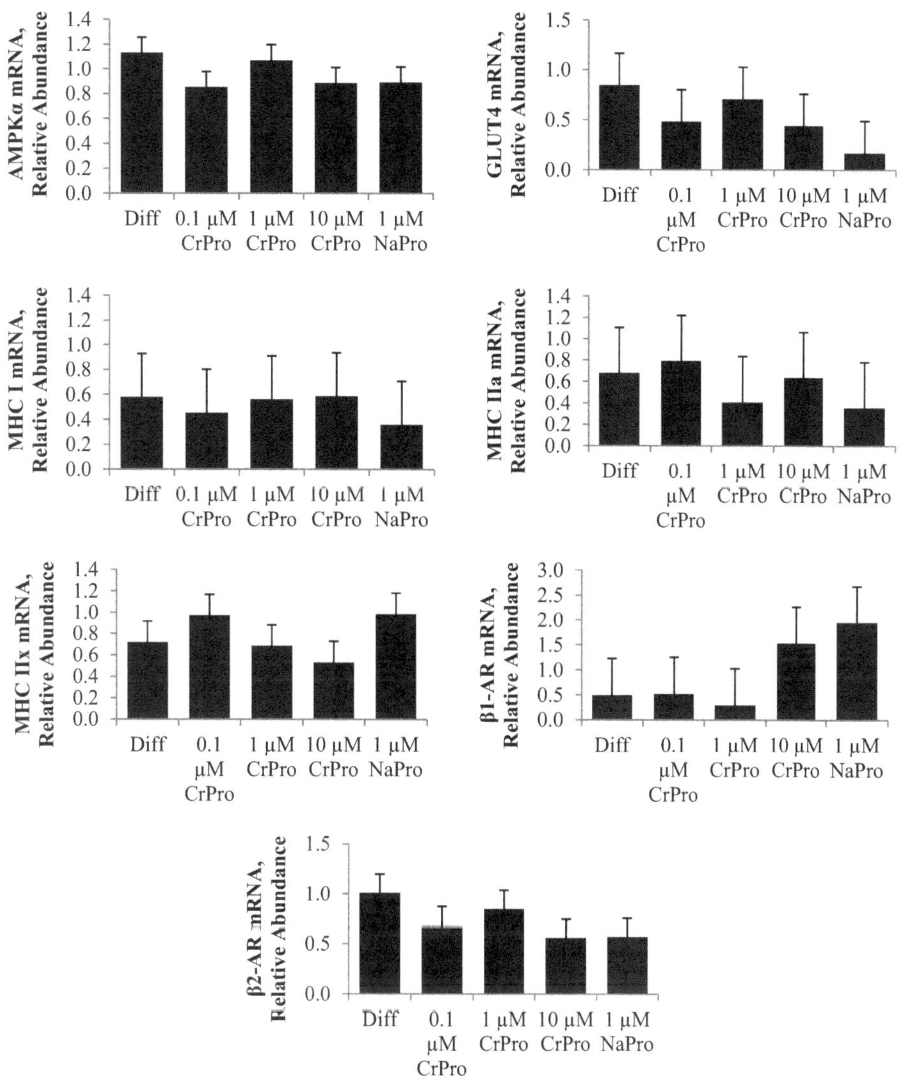

FIGURE 7 | Effect of differentiation media (Diff), chromium propionate (CrPro), and sodium propionate (NaPro) on adenosine monophosphate-activated protein kinase (AMPKα), glucose transporter type 4 (GLUT4), myosin heavy chain (MHC)-I, MHC-IIa, and MHC-IIX, β1-adernergic receptor (AR), and β2-AR mRNA levels in bovine satellite cells ($n = 3$). Bars represent the standard error of the difference between the treatment means. There was no effect ($P > 0.10$) of treatment on the mRNA expression of AMPKα, GLUT4, MHC I, MHC-IIa, MHC-IIx, β1-AR, or β2-AR.

experiment 1 at 96 h, relative AMPKα mRNA levels isolated from IM adipocyte increased with the 10 μM CrPro treatment but were not different from differentiated controls in SC adipocytes. This indicated that the level of AMPKα can be regulated by treatment with CrPro. These data suggest that enhancement of AMPKα by CrPro treatment may improve glucose uptake in IM adipocytes.

In the third experiment, a comparison of the BSC micrographs of 0.1 μM CrPro to either 1 or 10 μM CrPro revealed that there was a qualitative effect of CrPro on BSC cultures. The BSC cultures treated with CrPro appeared to have a greater myotube number and diameter compared to the control cultures. The difference in myotube size may be a result of increased energy or glucose uptake by those cultures, resulting in larger myotubes. *In vivo*, these differences would be manifested as changes in postnatal muscle hypertrophy. Again, this would be positive to muscle growth, especially during the feeding of a beta-adrenergic agonist, the last part of the feeding period. This combination of larger myotubes and the decreased GLUT4/GAPDH protein ratio may suggest that CrPro is causing muscle tissue to be much more efficient at glucose uptake, so the cell actually needs less GLUT4 to take up the same amount of glucose. Since increased myotube number and diameter were still detected, the glucose transporters may be also more efficient with treatment of CrPro. This would explain why mRNA did not change and protein abundance decreased, but morphological effects were still observed. However, the IM preadipocytes normally need to compete with skeletal muscle for glucose in ruminants. Our data indicated that CrPro actually stimulated GLUT4 in those cells in means to more effectively compete with skeletal muscle tissue for glucose. In fact, our dose titration work suggested that higher the dose, the more effect on glucose

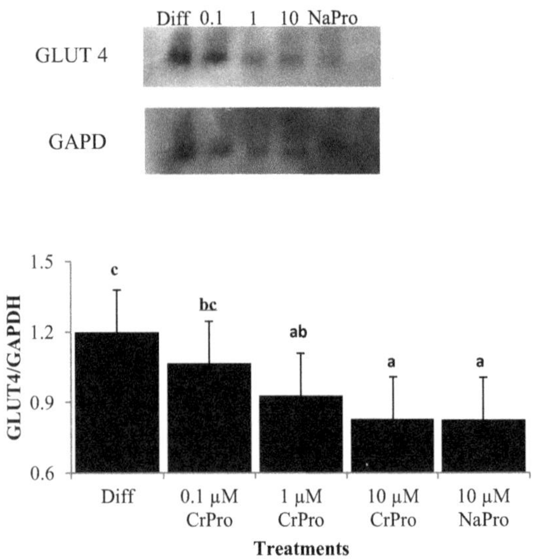

FIGURE 8 | Effect of differentiation media (Diff), chromium propionate (CrPro), and sodium propionate (NaPro) on glucose transporter type 4 (GLUT4)/glyceraldehyde 3-phosphate dehydrogenase (GAPDH) protein abundance ($n = 4$). Protein was isolated from bovine satellite cells after 72 h of treatment and protein abundance was determined through western blot analysis. Bars shown represent the standard error of the difference between the treatment means. Bars with different letters differ ($P < 0.01$).

metabolism and lipid filling in IM preadipocytes. In contrast, CrPro had little effect on glucose transport in SC preadipocytes. This makes sense since they do not require glucose to synthesize lipids and can rely on acetate.

Chromium, a trace mineral required for insulin action, regulated mode of action of insulin signaling and has been shown to induce glucose absorbance in the muscle and adipocytes (10). Chromium Pro and Cr methionine have also been reported to inducing glucose uptake and feed intake (11). This study indicated that a dose-dependent Cr supplementation increased glucose level, decreased insulin, and non-esterified fatty acids in the serum. Recent data indicated that pharmacological doses of Cr appear to increased insulin sensitivity in rodent study and the mode of action of Cr could serve in a regulation of second messenger in animals (12). These data also indicated that transferrin is a major agent as physiological Cr transport in bloodstream. The receptor-specific regulation of transferrin is sensitive to insulin and it results in a stimulation of inorganic second messenger in plasma membrane. Therefore, CrPro likely induces glucose utilization through insulin signaling for growing cattle. Our data indicated that a time-dependent treatment of CrPro increased GLUT4 levels in IM adipocyte cultures. These GLUT4 data indicated that treatment of CrPro may be regulating the early phase of IM adipocyte differentiation. The level of GLUT4 was steadily increased in both IM and SC adipocytes during the late phase of adipocyte differentiation. However, bovine satellite cells treated with CrPro in this study showed no effect on GLUT4 mRNA expression and had decreased GLUT4/GAPDH protein ratio in a dose-dependent fashion. The variation in these results between adipocytes and muscle satellite cells indicated that CrPro has differential effects on different tissues. In essence, the CrPro decreased GLUT4 protein levels in muscle cell cultures (**Figure 8**) indicating that those cells have increased efficiency of glucose uptake due to exposure to increased levels of CrPro. In contrast, each of the two adipogenic lines had opposing responses to the CrPro. It appeared that CrPro had the most stimulative effect of GLUT4 response in the IM adipocytes as compared to SC adipocytes. This suggests opportunities to potentially augment marbling in beef cattle fed elevated levels of CrPro during the finishing period. In addition, skeletal muscle growth could be further enhanced in cattle being fed both a beta-adrenergic agonist and CrPro the last 20–40 days on feed.

Funding

Supported in part by funding from Kemin Animal Nutrition and Health North America, Des Moines, IA 50317 and partially supported by "Cooperative Research Program for Agriculture Science & Technology Development (PJ00941401)" RDA, Republic of Korea. The Gordon W. Davis Regent's Chair in Meat and Muscle Biology Endowment at Texas Tech University provided funding to support this research.

References

1. National Research Council. *The Role of Chromium in Animal Nutrition*. Washington, DC: National Academy Press (1997).
2. Barajas R, Espino MA, Cervantes BJ, Rounds W, Valdez F, Velazquez EA, et al. *Chromium Propionate Supplementation On Feedlot Performance and Carcass Characteristics of Bulls. Kemin Internal Document TD-11-00059*. Des Moines, IA: Kemin Industries (2011).
3. Bernhard BC, Rounds W, Rathmann RJ, Johnson BJ. *Effects of Chromium Propionate Supplementation on Feedlot Performance During the Receiving Period of Stressed Beef Cattle. AB-11-00003* Des Moines, IA: Kemin Industries (2011).
4. Rounds W, Barajas R, Valdez F. *Influence of Chromium Propionate Supplement0061tion On Immunity, Feedlot Performance and Carcass Characteristics of Brahman Cross Bull Calves. Kemin Internal Document WP-09-00082*. Des Moines, IA: Kemin Industries (2009).
5. Burdick NC, Bernhard BC, Carroll JA, Dailey JW, Rathmann RJ, Johnson BJ. Chromium supplementation enhances the acute phase response of steers to a lipopolysaccharide (LPS) challenge. Abstract. *J Anim Sci* (2011) **89**(E-Suppl):2. doi:10.1177/1753425911428964
6. Smith SB, Crouse JD. Relative contributions of acetate, lactate, and glucose to lipogenesis in bovine intramuscular and subcutaneous adipose tissue. *J Nutr* (1984) **114**:792–800.
7. Loviscach M, Rehman N, Carter L, Mudaliar S, Mohadeen P, Ciaraldi TP, et al. Distribution of peroxisome proliferator-activated receptors (PPARs) in human skeletal muscle and adipose tissue: relation to insulin action. *Diabetologia* (2000) **43**:304–11. doi:10.1007/s001250050048
8. Motojima K, Passilly P, Peters JM, Gonzalez FJ, Latruffe N. Expression of putative fatty acid transporter genes are regulated by peroxisome proliferator-activated receptor î± and î³ activators in a tissue- and inducer-specific manner. *J Biol Chem* (1998) **273**:16710–4. doi:10.1074/jbc.273.27.16710
9. Zheng D, Maclean PS, Pohnert SC, Knight JB, Olson AL, Winder WW, et al. Regulation of muscle GLUT-4 transcription by AMP-activated protein kinase. *J Appl Physiol* (2001) **91**:1073–83.
10. Vincent JB. The biochemistry of chromium. *J Nutr* (2000) **130**:715–8.
11. Summer JM, Valdez F, McNamara JP. Effects of chromium propionate on response to an intravenous glucose tolerance test in growing Holstein heifers. *J Dairy Sci* (2007) **90**:3467–74. doi:10.3168/jds.2006-623

12. Vincent JB. Is the pharmacological mode of action of chromium(III) as a second messenger? *Biol Trace Elem Res* (2015) **166**:7–12. doi:10.1007/s12011-015-0231-9

Conflict of Interest Statement: The authors declare that the research was conducted in the absence of any commercial or financial relationships that could be construed as a potential conflict of interest.

21

Hydrothermally Treated Chitosan Hydrogel Loaded with Copper and Zinc Particles as a Potential Micronutrient-Based Antimicrobial Feed Additive

Parthiban Rajasekaran[1] *and Swadeshmukul Santra*[1,2,3,4]*

[1] NanoScience Technology Center, University of Central Florida, Orlando, FL, USA, [2] Department of Chemistry, University of Central Florida, Orlando, FL, USA, [3] Department of Materials Science and Engineering, University of Central Florida, Orlando, FL, USA, [4] Burnett School of Biomedical Sciences, University of Central Florida, Orlando, FL, USA

Edited by:
Stephen Brent Smith,
Texas A&M University, USA

Reviewed by:
Erminio Trevisi,
Università Cattolica del Sacro Cuore,
Italy
Barry Bradford,
Kansas State University, USA

***Correspondence:**
Swadeshmukul Santra
ssantra@mail.ucf.edu

Large-scale use of antibiotics in food animal farms as growth promoters is considered as one of the driving factors behind increasing incidence of microbial resistance. Several alternatives are under investigation to reduce the amount of total antibiotics used in order to avoid any potential transmission of drug resistant microbes to humans through food chain. Copper sulfate and zinc oxide salts are used as feed supplement as they exhibit antimicrobial properties in addition to being micronutrients. However, higher dosage of copper and zinc (often needed for growth promoting effect) to animals is not advisable because of potential environmental toxicity arising from excreta. Innovative strategies are needed to utilize the complete potential of trace minerals as growth promoting feed supplements. To this end, we describe here the development and preliminary characterization of hydrothermally treated chitosan as a delivery vehicle for copper and zinc nanoparticles that could act as a micronutrient-based antimicrobial feed supplement. Material characterization studies showed that hydrothermal treatment makes a chitosan hydrogel that rearranged to capture the copper and zinc metal particles. Systemic antimicrobial assays showed that this chitosan biopolymer matrix embedded with copper (57.6 μg/ml) and zinc (800 μg/ml) reduced the load of model gut bacteria (target organisms of growth promoting antibiotics), such as *Escherichia coli*, *Enterococcus faecalis*, *Staphylococcus aureus*, and *Lactobacillus fermentum* under *in vitro* conditions. Particularly, the chitosan/copper/zinc hydrogel exhibited significantly higher antimicrobial effect against *L. fermentum*, one of the primary targets of antibiotic growth promoters. Additionally, the chitosan matrix ameliorated the cytotoxicity levels of metal supplements when screened against a murine macrophage cell line RAW 264.7 and in TE-71, a murine thymic epithelial cell line. In this proof-of-concept study, we show that by using chitosan as a delivery platform, micronutrient-based metal feed additives could be used to minimize the undesirable levels of microbial population without causing significant cytotoxic effect under *in vitro* conditions. These findings provide the platform for further studies in target animal models to quantify the required physiological concentrations of copper and zinc when delivered via a chitosan hydrogel platform to elicit a growth promoting effect without causing any toxicity.

Keywords: chitosan, copper, zinc, antimicrobial feed additive, antimicrobial resistance, micronutrient

INTRODUCTION

The World Health Organization recently cautioned that antimicrobial resistance amongst infectious agents has reached alarming levels and that it could turn the twenty-first century into a time where common wound injuries can become lethal infections (1). Over use and unregulated use of antibiotics in the past six decades has created a selection pressure for drug resistant microbes (2, 3). Particularly, food animal production facilities, such as cattle, swine, chicken, and fish farms, use subtherapeutic levels of antibiotics as antimicrobial growth promoters (AGPs) in tons scale in developing countries and some developed countries including United States (3, 4). AGPs are used for various benefits including high feed conversion ratio, control of zoonotic infections, and for prevention of herd infections among closely housed animals in intensive farm animal production facilities (5, 6). Various alternatives, such as antimicrobial peptides, recombinant enzymes, plant extracts, and heavy metals, such as copper and zinc salts, are used as growth promoting feed supplements to reduce the usage on classical antibiotics (7).

Copper and zinc are essential micronutrient minerals that play important roles in physiological processes at lower concentrations and so the National Research Council (NRC) recommends them as minor feed supplements in cattle and swine production (8). However, when used at elevated levels as feed additive, copper in the form of copper sulfate ($CuSO_4$) and zinc in the form of zinc oxide (ZnO) have shown to produce a growth promoting effect via reduction of fermentation loss of energy by altering the gut microbiome (9). Higher feeding levels of copper and zinc also have shown to suppress gut pathogens, thereby, posing themselves as a potential substitute for traditional antibiotics in industrial food animal production facilities (8). Despite these advantages, extended and frequent administration of such high doses of copper and zinc salts (**Table 1**) would predispose gut microbes to develop resistance not only against these metals but also to traditional antibiotics that share similar microbe killing mechanisms (10). Further, higher levels of copper and zinc in the animal excretory wastes may pose serious threat to the soil microbial diversity and the surrounding ecosystem. Thus, developing a strategy that can considerably reduce the frequency of administration of copper and zinc in feed, yet maintaining the growth beneficial effect would be a viable alternative. One such strategy would be to increase the gastric retention time of the supplied minerals by embedding the metallic salts in a biocompatible polymer that has affinity for the gastro intestinal tract.

Chitosan is one such biopolymer that consists of long chains of N-acetyl-D-glucosamine molecules and has been investigated extensively for its potential as an animal feed additive in poultry, swine (13, 14) and also in cattle (15, 16). Chitosan and its oligosaccharide derivatives have been shown to promote body weight gain of poultry and swine by enhancing nutrient digestibility, increasing villus height and villus/crypt ratio in the illea and jejuna (13, 14). Additionally, chitosan microparticles have been shown to reduce the shedding of pathogenic *Escherichia coli* strain O157:H7 from the intestinal tract of cattle when supplemented with feed (15). Though, the differences in effect if any, on the gastrointestinal health is not currently available, nevertheless, chitosan appears to be a viable feed additive for ruminants (16) as much as it for monogastric animals (13). Copper-loaded chitosan nanoparticles have been shown to possess beneficial effect on the intestinal health of weaned piglets (14). Similarly, a chitosan–zinc chelate was shown to improve intestinal structure in weaned piglets (17). In all these studies, chitosan was used as either a chelating agent or as an encapsulating micro or nanoparticle for either copper or zinc salt individually. All these strategies would not provide a significant advantage in terms of gastric retention time over the current practice of feeding a salt mixture. Also, uniform loading of both metals in a chelate or inside an encapsulated particle is challenging.

We recently demonstrated that hydrothermal (HT) treatment of chitosan results in depolymerization of chitosan into shorter chain polymers with increased functional groups availability for loading high amounts of antimicrobial copper and similar metals (18). Furthermore, highly depolymerized chitosan possesses exceptional muco-adhesive property owing to the presence of high net positive charge provided by the amine group in the linear polysaccharide matrix (13). We also showed that the increased functional groups after HT treatment help in enhancing the dispersibility of chitosan in water, thus significantly potentiating the usefulness as a feed additive by overcoming the bottleneck of insolubility (18). By taking advantage of the above-mentioned merits, herein, we developed a chitosan hydrogel matrix that is loaded with both copper and zinc metal nanoparticles that can be used as a potential micronutrient-based antimicrobial feed additive. In this proof-of-concept manuscript, we demonstrate the antimicrobial ability of this chitosan–metal composite by screening against model organisms for gut bacteria that are targets of conventional antibiotic growth promoters. We also show how loading of copper and zinc together in a chitosan hydrogel matrix minimized the cytotoxic effects of the metals on eukaryotic cells (model for host tissues). We infer that this report will be the foundation for our future studies that will examine this novel material for its growth promoting effects involving target animals.

TABLE 1 | Current levels of copper and zinc usage as feed additives in food animal farms (references for the values in parenthesis next to the numbers).

Daily feed (kg/day)	Copper (mg/kg diet)	Zinc (mg/kg diet)
Cattle (5.5–10)	10 (8)	30 (8)
Swine (1–2)	100–250 (11)	2000–3000 (11)
Poultry (0.1–0.2)	4–8 (12)	30–60 (12)

MATERIALS AND METHODS

Synthesis of Chitosan–Metal Composites

One pot HT method of making water-dispersible chitosan–metal composite hydrogel was performed as described earlier (18). Briefly, low molecular weight chitosan (Sigma-Aldrich, St. Louis, MO, USA) was dissolved in 1% HCl at 10 mg/ml and HT depolymerization was done inside a preheated Lindeberg/Blue M oven (Thermoelectron Corporation) at 150°C for 90 min. Copper sulfate (10 mg/ml) (CQ concepts Inc, Ringwood, IL, USA) and zinc nitrate (100 mg/ml) were added to the chitosan right after HT

TABLE 2 | Various samples and their abbreviations that were used in this experiment.

Sample name	Contents
HTChitosan	Hydrothermal treated chitosan (in 1% HCl)
HTCh-RTCuZn	Copper sulfate and zinc nitrate at room temperature mixed with HT chitosan
RTCuZn	Mixture of copper sulfate and zinc nitrate in 1% HCl with no HT treatment (no chitosan)
HTCh-RTCu	Copper sulfate mixed with HT chitosan
HTCh-RTZn	Zinc nitrate mixed with HT chitosan

treatment. After overnight stirring, the pH was raised to 7.4 (by adding 1 N NaOH solution) before material characterization, cytotoxic, and antimicrobial studies. The abbreviated code names of the various samples that were used in this experiment and their corresponding contents are provided in **Table 2**.

Scanning Electron Microscopy

A Zeiss ULTRA-55 FEG SEM was used to study the gross morphological characteristics of the chitosan–metal complex. The liquid samples were spin coated (2000 rpm) on boron-doped silicon wafers (Nova electronic materials) and the images were acquired at 5 kV.

High-Resolution Transmission Electron Microscopy

Carbon-filmed gold grids (400 square mesh) (Catalog # CF-400-Au, Electron Microscopy Sciences, Hatfield, PA, USA) were used for preparing samples where the materials were dip coated and air dried at room temperature before they were analyzed in a FEI Tecnai F30 microscope at the Material Characterization Facility (MCF) at the University of Central Florida. An electron beam intensity of 100 kV was used for studying all the materials.

Bacterial Growth Media and Conditions

The growth inhibition effect of the chitosan–metal composites was tested against a range of microorganisms that acted as model organisms for gut microflora of livestock gastrointestinal tract. *E. coli* (ATCC 8739) and *Staphylococcus aureus* (ATCC 25923) were grown in tryptic soy media (Sigma-Aldrich). *Enterococcus faecalis* (ATCC 29212) was grown in brain heart infusion (BHI) media (BD Biosciences). *Lactobacillus fermentum* (ATCC 9338) was grown in MRS medium (BD Biosciences). All incubations were done at 37°C.

Antimicrobial Assays

Initial screening for determining the most effective metallic concentration was performed using a microplate alamar blue assay (MABA) as described elsewhere (18). The MABA assay was used as a substitute for broth microdilution assay to determine minimal inhibitory concentration (MIC) to circumvent the interference of the chitosan hydrogel in light absorbance. Briefly, the chitosan–metal hydrogel were added in triplicates for each concentration considered in a flat bottom 96-well plate. The volume of the sample hydrogel was kept at 20 μl in the final volume of 200 μl in each well. As per clinical and laboratory standards institute (CLSI) requirements, for all the bacterial species, a culture concentration of 0.5 McFarland standards was used as a starter culture and from which 1×10^5 CFU/well (final concentration 5×10^5 CFU/ml) was added. A classical antibiotic kanamycin (50 μg/ml) was used as positive control for killing. After 24 h of incubation at 37°C, 10 μl of alamar blue dye (Molecular probes, Eugene, OR, USA) was added to each well. The plate was then kept back in the incubator for one more hour before the absorbance was measured at both 570 and 600 nm for each well. The reduction of the dye in percentage (correlates to metabolically viable bacteria) value was calculated by using the formula as suggested by the manufacturer. The motivation behind choosing these specific concentrations of metals (copper and zinc) in these assays was to ascertain the difference in antimicrobial activity against gut microbes between the traditional method (no chitosan) and using chitosan hydrogel matrix as a delivery system.

Bacterial Killing Assay

The absolute values of the reduction in bacterial numbers after treatment with various concentrations of chitosan–metal composite were determined using bacterial killing assay (CFU assay). The protocol used in the MABA assay was followed for this assay for treatment of bacteria with samples but at the end of 24 h incubation, serial dilutions of the bacteria from each well were made in phosphate-buffered saline and plated on corresponding agar plates. The colonies were counted after overnight incubation and expressed in logarithmic scale.

Cytotoxicity Experiments

To determine any potential cytotoxicity effects of the newly synthesized chitosan–metal hydrogel, RAW 264.7 murine macrophage and TE-71 mouse thymic epithelial cell lines were treated with various concentrations (6.25, 12.5, 25, and 50 μg/ml of metallic zinc concentration) of the hydrogel. These numbers were selected to identify the specific concentration where there is a difference in cytotoxicity levels between the samples that contained chitosan and those that did not. (The RAW 264.7 macrophages were a kind gift from Dr. J. Manuel Perez at University of Central Florida.) After 24 h of incubation at 37°C in the presence of 5% CO_2, the media containing hydrogel were removed and fresh media [DMEM (Corning, 10-090-CV) complete media containing 10% fetal calf serum and 1% antibiotic and antimycotic] were added to avoid any interference from the material during measurement of fluorescence. Then, to each well in the 96-well flat bottom plates, 20 μl of alamar blue reagent was added. After 3 h of incubation with the alamar blue reagent, the contents of the plates were transferred to black 96-well plate (Costar 3916, Corning life Sciences) and were read for fluorescence (590 nm) in a TECAN infinite M200PRO plate reader. Triplicate wells were used for each sample and the wells containing only the macrophages and media (no samples added) were used as growth control. The percentage viability of cells in the chitosan–metal samples treated wells were deduced by normalizing the viable cells percentage in the growth control wells.

Statistical Analysis

To determine the statistical significance of the difference between treated samples and their corresponding controls in antimicrobial and cytotoxicity experiments, ANOVA and Tukey's honestly significant difference methods were used. For all experiments, $P < 0.05$ was considered significant.

RESULTS

HT-Treated Chitosan Hydrogel Rearranges to Capture Copper and Zinc Nanoparticles

The scanning electron microscopy (SEM) image of the chitosan–metal hydrogel showed that the copper and zinc nanoparticles (of size <5 nm) were uniformly distributed throughout the HT chitosan matrix background (**Figures 1D,E**). Adding copper (**Figure 1A**) and zinc (**Figure 1B**) either individually or together (**Figures 1D,E**) did not affect the distribution characteristics of the metal nanoparticles. The control samples and the metal salt mixture (**Figure 1C**) did not appear to possess any specific morphological features (no chitosan) suggesting that it was a salt mixture. However, in the presence of chitosan, the metal particles can be seen as rounded nanostructures embedded in a hydrogel matrix of chitosan in respective samples (1A–1E). Using dynamic light scattering technique, a polydispersity index of 1.0 was observed for the chitosan–metal hydrogel that verified the finding that they were a hydrogel and not individual particles (data not shown).

Multiple Forms and Oxidation States of Metal Salts were Embedded in the Chitosan Hydrogel

Using selective area electron diffraction (SAED) on the high-resolution transmission electron microscopy (HRTEM) images, the lattice spacing of the metal nanocrystallites (**Figure 2**) were analyzed to determine the form and oxidation states of the metals in the hydrogel. The different forms and oxidation states of the metals were determined by the measuring the "*d*" spacing in the SAED pattern (inset of **Figure 2**). The metals in the hydrogel composite were present as metallic copper, copper oxides (CuO and Cu_2O), copper chloride, copper zinc alloy, metallic zinc, zinc oxide, zinc nitrate, and zinc chloride (**Figure 2**). HRTEM analysis also showed that the size of the metal nanoparticles embedded in the chitosan hydrogel was in the range of 5 nm (indicated by arrows in **Figure 2**).

HT Chitosan Significantly Enhances the Antimicrobial Efficacy of Metals Against the Fermenter Group Bacteria *L. fermentum*

In both MABA and CFU assay, the chitosan hydrogel loaded with copper and zinc salts showed an enhanced killing effect (>99.99%) on *L. fermentum* (**Figures 3** and **4**) at metallic zinc concentrations of 400 and 800 μg/ml when compared to the salt mixture at same concentrations, where it inhibited bacterial growth by only 42.4 and 56.6%, respectively. The corresponding copper and chitosan concentrations were 28.8 and 57.6 μg/ml. The chitosan

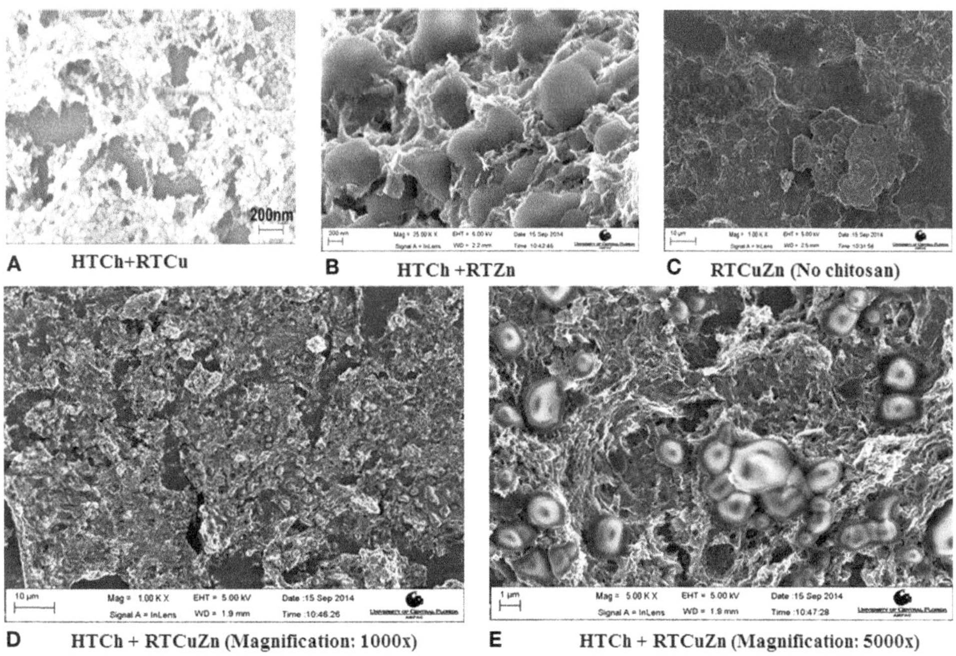

FIGURE 1 | SEM images of chitosan–metal hydrogel. SEM images showing metal particles (round shaped) embedded uniformly on to a chitosan matrix background **(A,B,D,E)** when compared to the sample that have no chitosan **(C)** which appeared to be a mixture of salt solution with no specific morphological features. The chitosan appears in **(A–E)** as a mesh (3-D structure) where the metal particles (rounded structures of ~1–2 μm in diameter) are embedded in between the hydrogel matrix.

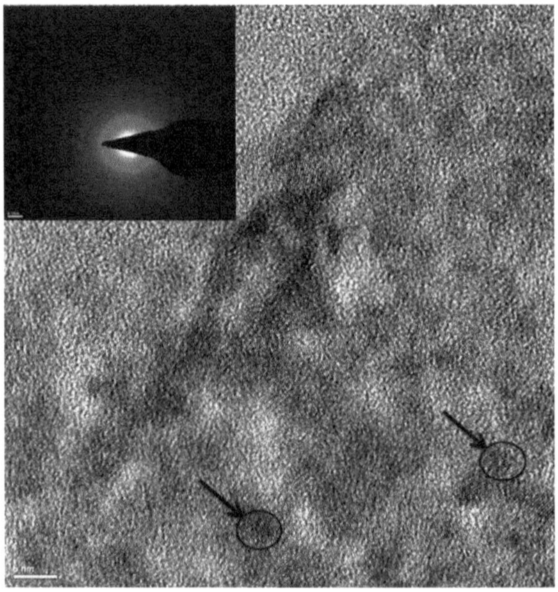

FIGURE 2 | TEM image of HTCh + RTCuZn. Under a transmission electron microscope, the rounded metal particles appear as crystalline structures (indicated by arrows and circles) embedded on an amorphous chitosan hydrogel matrix. Inset picture showing the lattice spacing of the metal crystallites (indicated by arrows in the pictures). The "*d*" spacing (identified by measuring the diameter of the white rings in the inset picture) measured using the inset picture suggested that the metal crystallites were in multiple salt forms and oxidation states. The size of the metal crystallite particles was at 5 nm in diameter (indicated by arrows and circles).

hydrogel appeared to be superior in specifically reducing the *L. fermentum* of bacteria compared to the salt mixture (no chitosan).

Chitosan Hydrogel Did Not Affect the Antimicrobial Effect of Metal Salts on the Opportunistic Pathogen Load

For this study, we used *E. coli*, *S. aureus*, and *E. faecalis* as representative organisms of zoonotic and opportunistic pathogens. At 800 μg/ml of metallic zinc (**Figures 3** and **4**), there was complete inhibition of growth of *S. aureus* (>99.99% reduction of bacteria), while there was a 1.24 log reduction of *E. coli* growth (94.95% reduction of bacteria) by HTCh-RTCuZn. At 800 μg/ml, the metallic zinc containing chitosan–metal hydrogel reduced the load of *E. faecalis* only by 0.61 logs (75.55% reduction), whereas RTCuZn (no chitosan) reduced the load by 90.91%. Also, the salt mixture completely inhibited (>99.99%) growth of *S. aureus* even at 300 μg/ml concentrations. Although not significantly, the growth inhibitory effect of salt mixture was lower in *E. coli* (91.58% reduction) at 800 μg/ml of metallic zinc when compared to HTCh-RTCuZn (94.95%).

HT Chitosan Matrix Minimized the Cytotoxicity Effects of Antimicrobial Metal Salts

The murine macrophage cell line RAW 264.7 (immune cell) and the murine thymic epithelial cell line TE-71 (structural cell) were used to screen for any cytotoxic effect caused by chitosan–metal hydrogel. In case of RAW264.7 cells, only about 5% cells treated with HT chitosan–metal hydrogel were killed, whereas cells treated with just the mixture of copper and zinc salts (with no chitosan) exhibited significant reduction in viable cell numbers (92% of cells killed) at a metallic zinc concentration of 50 μg/ml (**Figure 5A**). Though at lower metallic concentration ($\leq$25 μg/ml), the cytotoxicity levels were not significantly different between the samples. In TE-71 epithelial cells, the metals were more toxic and started killing cells at metallic zinc concentrations as low as 25 μg/ml, whereas at the same concentration (25 μg/ml), the chitosan-containing samples were not toxic to the cells (**Figure 5B**). The HT-chitosan matrix appears to be protective against metal derived cytotoxicity in two different cell lines (structural and immune cells) at least until the concentration of 25 μg/ml of metallic zinc.

DISCUSSION

Commercially feasible potential alternatives are in greater need to reduce the total amount of classical antibiotics that are used as AGPs in food animal production facilities (19, 20). Metals, such as copper and zinc, are already used as salt feed supplements in cattle, swine, and chicken farms owing to their antimicrobial and growth promoting properties (10, 11, 21). In this report, we showed that a hydrothermally treated chitosan hydrogel loaded with copper and zinc metal particles have a growth inhibitory effect on both the "fermenters" group of gastric flora and the "opportunistic pathogen" group; target microbes of the antibiotics that are used as growth promoting feed supplements in animal farms (6). This study also showed that by using chitosan hydrogel matrix, any potential cytotoxic effect of the metals salts on the host tissue can be minimized.

In our previously published studies, we showed that HT treatment generates water-dispersible chitosan, a property that would allow for uniform mixing of chitosan with the animal feed in industrial scale livestock farms (18). The other advantage of HT treatment is that it increased the availability of functional groups that in turn allowed for embedding high amounts of copper (18) and zinc in a chitosan hydrogel matrix (**Figures 1A–E**). Also, we showed earlier that one of the advantages of hydrothermally treated chitosan was that it could alter the oxidation states of metals that were bound in them (18). Hydrogel formation after addition of metal salts to chitosan would allow for formation of a coating on the intestinal tract when fed as a feed additive that in turn would facilitate a larger surface area of metal nanoparticles interacting with gut microbiome. Moreover, the presence of metal nanoparticles in multiple oxidation states and forms (**Figure 2**) would provide the advantage of having multiple modes of killing gut microbes (22, 23); it would significantly reduce the possibility of development of resistance among microbes to these metals. This property in particular is superior over the current method of feeding copper sulfate and zinc oxide salts as they have been indicated in microbial resistance development (10). Multiple oxidation states of metals were not shown in earlier studies that used chitosan as either an encapsulating nanoparticle (14) or as a chelating material (17), suggesting the advantage of HT treatment over

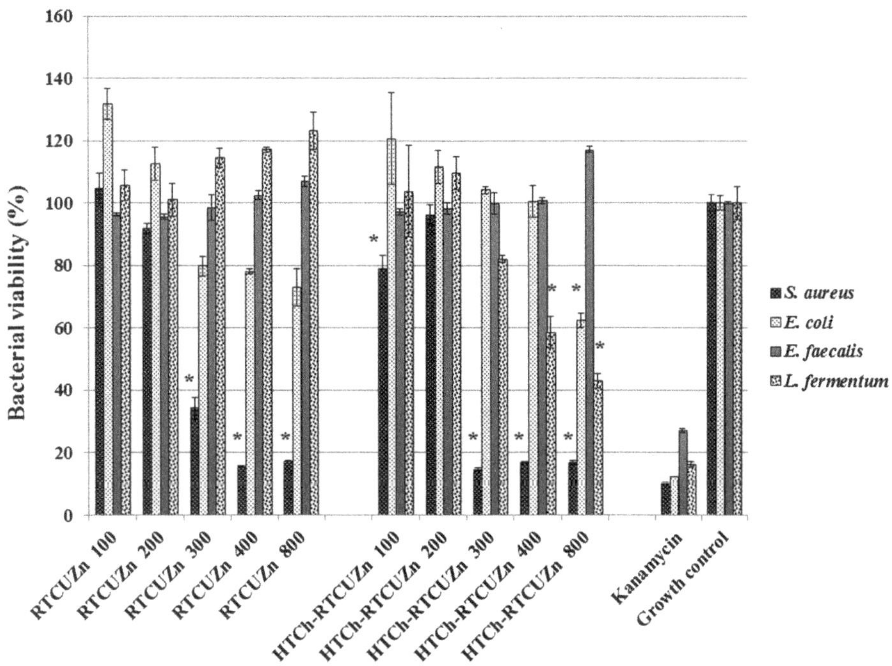

FIGURE 3 | Microplate alamar blue assay (MABA). Sample name explanation: RTCuZn – mixture of copper sulfate and zinc nitrate in 1% HCl with no HT treatment (no chitosan); HTCh-RTCuZ – copper sulfate and zinc nitrate at room temperature mixed with HT chitosan. HTCh-RTCuZn exhibited superior bacterial killing effect at 800 μg/ml of metallic zinc concentration when screened against all the four model gut bacteria. The numbers in the sample labels represent metallic zinc concentration at 100, 200, 300, 400, and 800 μg/ml. The corresponding chitosan and copper concentrations in those samples are 7.2, 14.4, 21.6, 28.8, and 57.6 μg/ml, respectively. Kanamycin (50 μg/ml) was used as control for bacterial killing. MABA was used as a substitute for broth microdilution assay to screen for effective concentration. The absorbance values of all the test samples were normalized for control samples, i.e., the percentage of viable cells in the growth control is considered as the actual bacterial numbers after 24 h of incubation when there were no antimicrobials added. Higher percentage (than control samples) noticed in some samples corresponds to higher metabolic activity in those samples and the actual number of bacteria is presented in **Figure 4**. The alamar blue dye undergoes extinction (at a very slow rate) when exposed to light and ambient temperature in the absence of any reducing agent, such as bacteria, and that is observed (~10–20%) in the kanamycin-labeled columns though there were no viable bacteria in there as expressed in **Figure 4**. [* indicates significant difference between the treatment and respective growth control groups ($P < 0.05$)].

other methodologies for delivering transition metals for eliciting antimicrobial effect.

One of the functions of AGPs is to minimize the load of fermenting bacteria in the gut of the food animals such that minimal or no glucose and/or energy is lost via fermentation that can be converted into muscle weight otherwise. Particularly, *Lactobacillus* species of bacteria have been indicated as one of the primary targets of AGPs because they produce bile salt hydrolase, which has shown to have a negative impact on host animal digestion and absorption of nutrients (5). In this study, we used the strain, *L. fermentum* as a representative organism of *Lactobacillus* species to screen for antimicrobial effect of our chitosan–metal hydrogel (**Figures 3** and **4**). The presence of chitosan enhanced the antimicrobial effect of the metal salts significantly on *L. fermentum* as HTCh-RTCuZn completely inhibited the growth at zinc concentrations of 300 μg/ml while RTCuZn (salts alone without chitosan) did not significantly inhibit the bacterial growth even at the same metallic zinc concentrations. The antimicrobial part of this study used both a metabolic activity based assay (alamar blue assay) and viability count (CFU) assay to cross-verify the effect on the microbes, since metabolic activity may not always correlate with the total number of viable bacteria. For example, in case of *E. coli* treated with HTCh-RTCuZn 800 sample, the dye reduction was statistically significant (**Figure 3**) but, when the viability of the bacteria was counted on a CFU assay (**Figure 4**), there was not a significant reduction in the viable bacterial count in the treated sample when compared to the growth control.

Another function of AGPs is to reduce the load of opportunistic and zoonotic pathogens group in the gut microbiome so that the animal's immune system spends less energy on fighting these microbes. In this study, the chitosan–metal hydrogel reduced the representative model opportunistic pathogen load at comparable levels to the salt mixture suggesting minimal interference from chitosan on the antimicrobial effect of the metals (**Figures 3** and **4**). The advantage of optimal reduction in bacterial load and not a complete elimination of *E. coli*, *S. aureus*, and *E. faecalis* was that it would not significantly alter the balance between commensal beneficial gut microbes. The level of copper in these experiments is lower (57.6 μg/ml) than that of our previous findings (18) where it required about 100–150 μg/ml of metallic copper to exhibit a bacterial killing effect when copper was used alone with chitosan (18). A combination of copper and zinc provided an additive effect where only half the amount of either metal is required to elicit a similar antimicrobial effect that of the case in which the metals were used alone. Also, previous publications have shown that chitosan by themselves

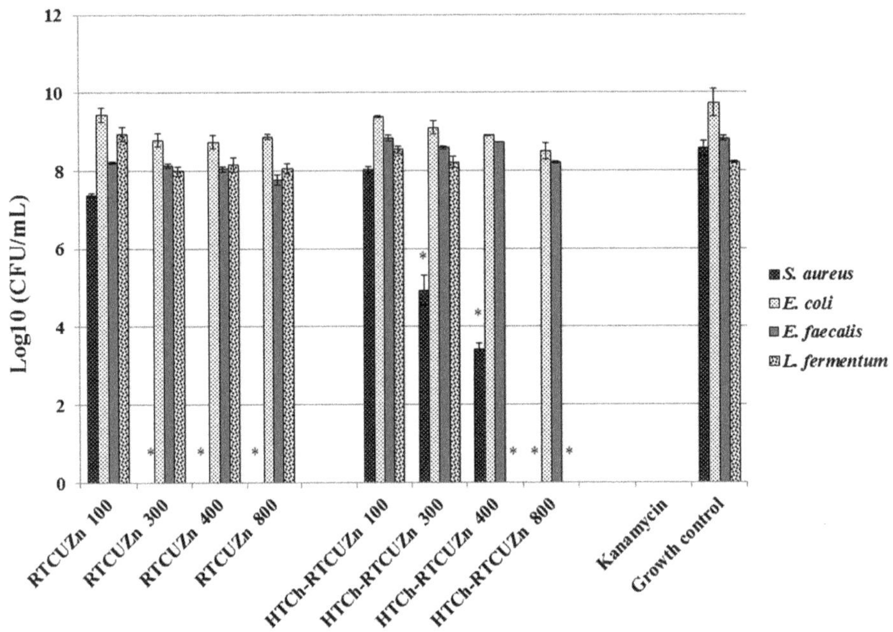

FIGURE 4 | Colony-forming unit (CFU) assay. Absolute bacterial numbers in logarithmic scale after treatment with either HTCh-RTCuZn or RTCuZn for 24 h. Sample name explanation: RTCuZn – mixture of copper sulfate and zinc nitrate in 1% HCl with no HT treatment (no chitosan); HTCh-RTCuZ – copper sulfate and zinc nitrate at room temperature mixed with HT chitosan. The numbers in the sample labels represent metallic zinc concentration at 100, 300, 400, and 800 μg/ml. The corresponding chitosan and copper concentrations are 7.2, 21.6, 28.8, and 57.6 μg/ml, respectively. At 800 μg/ml of metallic zinc concentration, the reduction in bacterial load in the samples treated with HTCh-RTCuZn was >99.99% in *S. aureus* and *L. fermentum* compared to their corresponding growth control group. In *E. coli*, the percentage reduction was 94.95% and in *E. faecalis* the reduction was 75.55%. Kanamycin (50 μg/ml) was used as control for killing. [* indicates significant difference between the treatment and respective growth control groups ($P < 0.05$)].

as microspheres were able to reduce *E. coli* shedding in feces of cattle (15); so we can speculate that the presence of chitosan has added to the cumulative antimicrobial effect. Additionally, Gram-negative organisms (*E. coli* and *E. faecalis*) were killed at higher concentrations (800 μg/ml of metallic zinc) while Gram-positive organisms were killed at lower concentrations (400 μg/ml of metallic zinc) suggesting a cell wall targeting activity of our chitosan–metal hydrogel (**Figures 3** and **4**) though we do not know the exact mechanism of killing yet. Though the concentrations considered were able to provide enhanced antimicrobial effect under *in vitro* conditions in a 96-well plate, further studies in target animals only would unveil the actual concentrations that would be good enough to elicit a growth promoting effect. Additionally, the difference between monogastric animals and ruminants in terms of the diversity of their gut microbial communities would also influence the effective concentration levels in target animals.

The HTCh-RTCuZn significantly reduced the cytotoxic effects of the metallic salts on two different types of eukaryotic cells (**Figure 5**). In both a phagocytic cell line (RAW264.7 macrophages) and in a structural cell line (TE-71 thymic epithelial cells), presence of chitosan appears to have provided a protective effect against toxicity of metals (**Figure 5**). The rationale behind the selected concentrations in cytotoxicity experiments (different from antibacterial assays) was to more closely resemble the (ratio of epithelial cell numbers to metallic concentration) actual animal gut microenvironment. When the same concentrations (100–800 μg/ml of metallic zinc) considered in antimicrobial studies were used, all the samples (with and without chitosan) exhibited significant cytotoxicity in a 96-well plate (data not shown). The cytotoxicity exhibited at those concentrations was understandable considering the low number of macrophages/epithelial cells that were exposed per microgram of metal in a smaller surface area/volume. HT-chitosan alone did not exhibit significant cytotoxicity (at least until 28.8 μg/ml). The toxicity to cell lines was primarily caused by the zinc concentration as the material containing HTCh-RTCu (HT chitosan embedded with copper alone) exhibited reduced toxicity (concentrations adjusted to reflect the copper concentration in the corresponding HTCh-RTCuZn samples) when compared to cells treated with HTCh-RTZn (at 50 μg/ml) (**Figure 5**). Therefore, we can deduce that at higher metallic concentrations (used for growth promoting effect), embedding the copper and zinc in a HT treated chitosan matrix would reduce cytotoxicity to host animal cells. Since the HTCh-RTCuZn material exhibits significantly reduced cytotoxicity, we can speculate that when used as an antimicrobial feed additive in animals, it will elicit minimal or no inflammatory reaction that will in turn help in higher feed conversion ratio. Follow-up publication of this project will include optimization of synthesis protocol by altering the chitosan hydrolyzing components in preparing this chitosan–metal hydrogel and subsequent assessment of cytokine and other immunological responses in relevant eukaryotic cell lines. Further studies involving target animal models will include NRC recommended levels of minerals to accurately quantify the growth promoting effect of chitosan hydrogel-aided delivery of metals.

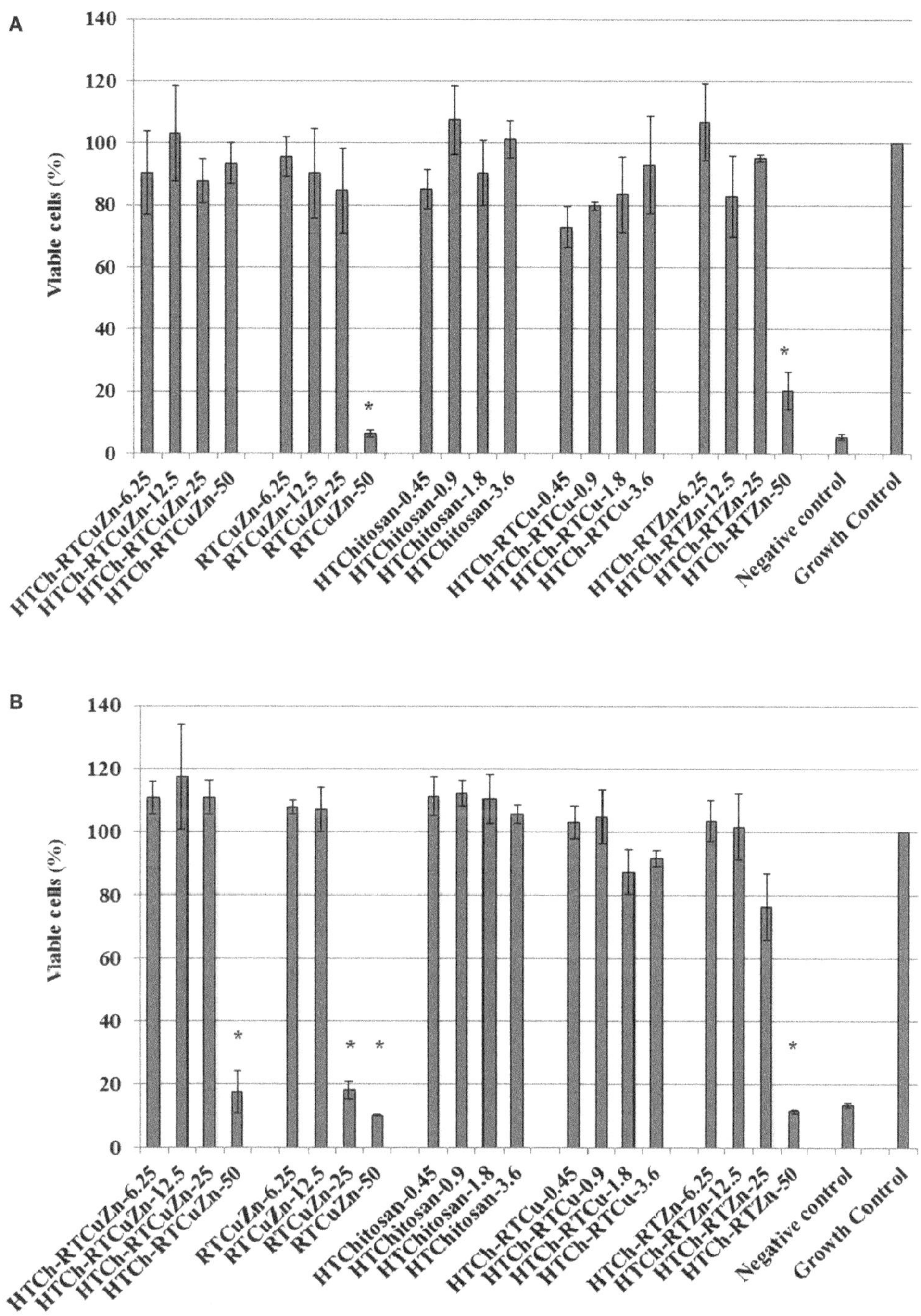

FIGURE 5 | Cytotoxicity assay: cytotoxicity assay results showing the viability percentage of RAW 264.7 macrophages (A) and TE-71 thymic epithelial cell lines (B) after treatment with various chitosan hydrogel containing metal samples for 24 h. Sample name explanation: RTCuZn – mixture of copper sulfate and zinc nitrate in 1% HCl with no HT treatment (no chitosan); HTCh-RTCuZ – copper sulfate and zinc nitrate at room temperature mixed with HT chitosan; HTChitosan – hydrothermal treated chitosan (in 1% HCl); HTCh-RTCu – copper sulfate mixed with HT chitosan; HTCh-RTZn – zinc nitrate mixed with HT chitosan. **(A)** In RAW 264.7 macrophage, at 50 μg/ml of metallic zinc concentration, HT chitosan appears to provide protective effect to macrophages, thereby reducing any potential toxicity caused by higher concentration of metallic salts. **(B)** In case of TE-71 epithelial cells, the metals were toxic at 25 μg/ml, while the chitosan ameliorated the toxicity at the same concentration in the HTCh-RTCuZn sample. The numbers in sample labels corresponds to metallic zinc concentration in samples containing zinc. In samples containing copper, the numbers in sample labels indicate the metallic copper concentration and in HTChitosan, the numbers correspond to chitosan concentration. (The copper and chitosan concentrations were chosen to match those concentrations present in the zinc containing samples). Autoclaved water was used as control for killing cells and labeled as negative control. The growth of the cells in all the samples was normalized for the growth control wells and the viability was expressed as percentage growth compared to growth control wells. [* indicates significant difference between the treatment and growth control groups ($P < 0.05$)].

AUTHOR CONTRIBUTIONS

PR conceived and designed the study, collected data, performed critical analysis and interpretation of data, and wrote the manuscript. Also accepts to be accountable for all aspects of this work. SS helped in conception and design of the study, critical analysis, interpretation of data, and editing the manuscript.

FUNDING

This study was partially supported by United States Department of Agriculture-National Institute of Food and Agriculture (USDA-NIFA) Grant # 2015-70016-23010, Citrus Research and Development Foundation, Inc. Grants # 544, 328 and 907 and the United States National Science Foundation NSF-CBET # 1159500.

REFERENCES

1. World Health Organization. *Antimicrobial Resistance: Global Report on Surveillance*. Geneva: World Health Organization (2014). Available from: http://www.who.int/drugresistance/documents/surveillancereport/en/
2. Van Boeckel TP, Gandra S, Ashok A, Caudron Q, Grenfell BT, Levin SA, et al. Global antibiotic consumption 2000 to 2010: an analysis of national pharmaceutical sales data. *Lancet Infect Dis* (2014) **14**(8):742–50. doi:10.1016/S1473-3099(14)70780-7
3. Marshall BM, Levy SB. Food animals and antimicrobials: impacts on human health. *Clin Microbiol Rev* (2011) **24**(4):718–33. doi:10.1128/CMR.00002-11
4. Wegener HC. Antibiotics in animal feed and their role in resistance development. *Curr Opin Microbiol* (2003) **6**(5):439–45. doi:10.1016/j.mib.2003.09.009
5. Lin J. Antibiotic growth promoters enhance animal production by targeting intestinal bile salt hydrolase and its producers. *Front Microbiol* (2014) **5**:33. doi:10.3389/fmicb.2014.00033
6. Gaskins HR, Collier CT, Anderson DB. Antibiotics as growth promotants: mode of action. *Anim Biotechnol* (2002) **13**(1):29–42. doi:10.1081/ABIO-120005768
7. Thacker PA. Alternatives to antibiotics as growth promoters for use in swine production: a review. *J Anim Sci Biotechnol* (2013) **4**(1):35. doi:10.1186/2049-1891-4-35
8. Jacob ME, Fox JT, Nagaraja TG, Drouillard JS, Amachawadi RG, Narayanan SK. Effects of feeding elevated concentrations of copper and zinc on the antimicrobial susceptibilities of fecal bacteria in feedlot cattle. *Foodborne Pathog Dis* (2010) **7**(6):643–8. doi:10.1089/fpd.2009.0401
9. Hojberg O, Canibe N, Poulsen HD, Hedemann MS, Jensen BB. Influence of dietary zinc oxide and copper sulfate on the gastrointestinal ecosystem in newly weaned piglets. *Appl Environ Microbiol* (2005) **71**(5):2267–77. doi:10.1128/AEM.71.5.2267-2277.2005
10. Yazdankhah S, Rudi K, Bernhoft A. Zinc and copper in animal feed – development of resistance and co-resistance to antimicrobial agents in bacteria of animal origin. *Microb Ecol Health Dis* (2014) **25**:25862. doi:10.3402/mehd.v25.25862
11. Jacela JY, DeRouchey JM, Tokach MD, Goodband RD, Nelssen JL, Renter DG, et al. Feed additives for swine: fact sheets – high dietary levels of copper and zinc for young pigs, and phytase. *J Swine Health Prod* (2010) **18**(2):87–9.
12. Norwegian Scientific Committee for Food Safety. Zinc and copper in pig and poultry production – fate and effects in the food chain and the environment. *Feed PoA* (2014). Available from: http://www.english.vkm.no/eway/default.aspx?pid=278&trg=Content_6444&Main_6359=6582:0:31,2567&Content_6444=6393:2023463::0:6596:1:::0:0
13. Swiatkiewicz S, Swiatkiewicz M, Arczewska-Wlosek A, Jozefiak D. Chitosan and its oligosaccharide derivatives (chito-oligosaccharides) as feed supplements in poultry and swine nutrition. *J Anim Physiol Anim Nutr* (2015) **99**(1):1–12. doi:10.1111/jpn.12222
14. Wang MQ, Du YJ, Wang C, Tao WJ, He YD, Li H. Effects of copper-loaded chitosan nanoparticles on intestinal microflora and morphology in weaned piglets. *Biol Trace Elem Res* (2012) **149**(2):184–9. doi:10.1007/s12011-012-9410-0
15. Jeong KC, Kang MY, Kang J, Baumler DJ, Kaspar CW. Reduction of *Escherichia coli* O157:H7 shedding in cattle by addition of chitosan microparticles to feed. *Appl Environ Microbiol* (2011) **77**(8):2611–6. doi:10.1128/AEM.02587-10
16. Henry DD, Ruiz-Moreno M, Ciriaco FM, Kohmann M, Mercadante VR, Lamb GC, et al. Effects of chitosan on nutrient digestibility, methane emissions, and in vitro fermentation in beef cattle. *J Anim Sci* (2015) **93**(7):3539–50. doi:10.2527/jas.2014-8844
17. Han XY, Ma YF, Lv MY, Wu ZP, Qian LC. Chitosan-zinc chelate improves intestinal structure and mucosal function and decreases apoptosis in ileal mucosal epithelial cells in weaned pigs. *Br J Nutr* (2014) **111**(8):1405–11. doi:10.1017/S0007114513004042
18. Basumallick S, Rajasekaran P, Tetard L, Santra S. Hydrothermally derived water-dispersible mixed valence copper-chitosan nanocomposite as exceptionally potent antimicrobial agent. *J Nanopart Res* (2014) **16**(10):2675. doi:10.1007/s11051-014-2675-9
19. Seal BS, Lillehoj HS, Donovan DM, Gay CG. Alternatives to antibiotics: a symposium on the challenges and solutions for animal production. *Anim Health Res Rev* (2013) **14**(1):78–87. doi:10.1017/S1466252313000030
20. Diarra MS, Malouin F. Antibiotics in Canadian poultry productions and anticipated alternatives. *Front Microbiol* (2014) **5**:282. doi:10.3389/fmicb.2014.00282
21. Perez VG, Waguespack AM, Bidner TD, Southern LL, Fakler TM, Ward TL, et al. Additivity of effects from dietary copper and zinc on growth performance and fecal microbiota of pigs after weaning. *J Anim Sci* (2011) **89**(2):414–25. doi:10.2527/jas.2010-2839
22. Young M, Santra S. Copper (Cu)-silica nanocomposite containing valence-engineered Cu: a new strategy for improving the antimicrobial efficacy of Cu biocides. *J Agric Food Chem* (2014) **62**(26):6043–52. doi:10.1021/jf502350w
23. Dupont CL, Grass G, Rensing C. Copper toxicity and the origin of bacterial resistance – new insights and applications. *Metallomics* (2011) **3**(11):1109–18. doi:10.1039/c1mt00107h

Conflict of Interest Statement: The authors declare that the research was conducted in the absence of any commercial or financial relationships that could be construed as a potential conflict of interest.

22

Regulation of the Intestinal Barrier Function by Host Defense Peptides

*Kelsy Robinson[1], Zhuo Deng[1], Yongqing Hou[2] and Guolong Zhang[1,2]**

[1] *Department of Animal Science, Oklahoma State University, Stillwater, OK, USA,* [2] *Hubei Key Laboratory of Animal Nutrition and Feed Science, Wuhan Polytechnic University, Wuhan, China*

Intestinal barrier function is achieved primarily through regulating the synthesis of mucins and tight junction (TJ) proteins, which are critical for maintaining optimal gut health and animal performance. An aberrant expression of TJ proteins results in increased paracellular permeability, leading to intestinal and systemic disorders. As an essential component of innate immunity, host defense peptides (HDPs) play a critical role in mucosal defense. Besides broad-spectrum antimicrobial activities, HDPs promotes inflammation resolution, endotoxin neutralization, wound healing, and the development of adaptive immune response. Accumulating evidence has also indicated an emerging role of HDPs in barrier function and intestinal homeostasis. HDP deficiency in the intestinal tract is associated with barrier dysfunction and dysbiosis. Several HDPs were recently shown to enhance mucosal barrier function by directly inducing the expression of multiple mucins and TJ proteins. Consistently, dietary supplementation of HDPs often leads to an improvement in intestinal morphology, production performance, and feed efficiency in livestock animals. This review summarizes current advances on the regulation of epithelial integrity and homeostasis by HDPs. Major signaling pathways mediating HDP-induced mucin and TJ protein synthesis are also discussed. As an alternative strategy to antibiotics, supplementation of exogenous HDPs or modulation of endogenous HDP synthesis may have potential to improve intestinal barrier function and animal health and productivity.

Keywords: host defense peptides, barrier function, tight junction, gut health, innate immunity

Edited by:
Michael Kogut, USDA – Agricultural Research Service, USA

Reviewed by:
Kenneth James Genovese, USDA – Agricultural Research Service, USA
Ryan Arsenault, University of Delaware, USA
Matthew Jon Sylte, USDA – Agricultural Research Service, USA

***Correspondence:**
Guolong Zhang
zguolon@okstate.edu

INTRODUCTION

The gastrointestinal (GI) tract is lined by a single layer of epithelial cells that serve to facilitate digestion and absorption of nutrients and also act as a barrier to invading microorganisms, toxins, and dietary antigens. Intestinal barrier function is achieved through coating of the epithelial cells with a

Abbreviations: aPKC, atypical protein kinase C; CCR2, CC chemokine receptor 2; CD, Crohn's disease; DSS, dextran sulfate sodium; EGF, epidermal growth factor; EGFR, EGF receptor; ERK, extracellular signal-regulated kinase; ETEC, enterotoxigenic *E. coli*; GI, gastrointestinal; GSK-3, glycogen synthase kinase 3; GUK, guanylate kinase; HBD, human β-defensin; HDPs, host defense peptides; JAM, junction adhesion molecule; LPS, lipopolysaccharides; MAMPs, microbe-associated molecular patterns; MAPK, mitogen-activated protein kinase; MBD, mouse β-defensin; MLCK, myosin light chain kinase; MUC, mucin; P2X7, P2X purinergic receptor 7; PAMPs, pathogen-associated molecular patterns; PBD, porcine β-defensin; PDZ, post-synaptic density 95, disk-large, and zonula occludens; PI3K, phosphatidylinositol-3-kinase; PKA, protein kinase A; PKC, protein kinase C; PRRs, pattern recognition receptors; SEA, sea urchin sperm protein, enterokinase and agrin; TACE, TNF-α-converting enzyme; TEER, transepithelial electrical resistance; TGF, transforming growth factor; TJ, tight junction; TR, tandem repeat; UC, ulcerative colitis; VWF, von Willebrand factor domain, ZO, zonula occludens.

mucus layer and the formation of a selectively permeable barrier across and between epithelial cells (1). The mucus layer consists primarily of mucin glycoproteins that are secreted by goblet cells, functioning as a physical barrier between the luminal contents and the host and also to facilitate nutrient digestion and absorption (2). However, the primary barrier function of the GI tract resides with epithelial cells, which transport water, ions, and macromolecules through either of two routes, i.e., the transcellular and paracellular pathways (1, 3, 4). The transcellular pathway refers to the movement of small molecules through epithelial cells either by active or passive transport, whereas the paracellular pathway refers to the diffusion of water, macromolecules, and immune cells between epithelial cells. In the presence of intact epithelial cells, the paracellular pathway dictates the intestinal permeability and is regulated by inter-epithelial connections known as tight junctions (TJs) (1, 3, 4).

Maintenance of mucin and TJ assembly ensures proper absorption and transport of nutrients, water, and electrolytes, while shielding the host from pathogens, toxins, intestinal microbiota, and dietary antigens. Disruption of the mucus layer and TJ complex, on the other hand, results in an increase in intestinal permeability, followed by heightened bacterial translocation, inflammation, and possibly the onset of various enteric and systemic disorders (1, 3, 4). In livestock production, impaired intestinal barrier function leads to reduced animal health and growth performance (5, 6). Therefore, it is critically important to understand how the intestinal barrier function is maintained and regulated in order to achieve optimal animal health and productivity.

Host defense peptides (HDPs), also known as antimicrobial peptides, are an important component of the animal innate immune system, and a majority of HDPs are expressed on mucosal surfaces, including the GI tract (7, 8). With potent antimicrobial and immunomodulatory activities, HDPs exert a pleiotropic effect on innate adaptive immune responses (9–11). Recent research has further shed light on the direct involvement of epithelial HDPs in regulating intestinal mucin and TJ protein expression and microbiota composition. The focus of this review is to summarize the latest advances regarding the emerging role of HDPs in maintaining intestinal barrier and homeostasis with a goal of exploring HDP-based therapies to improve gut health and performance of food-producing animals.

HOST DEFENSE PEPTIDES: A CRITICAL COMPONENT OF INNATE IMMUNITY

A variety of HDPs with direct antimicrobial activities are produced by host cells in response to infections. Among them are several major families found in vertebrate species such as defensins, cathelicidins, the S100 family, the RNase A superfamily, regenerating islet-derived III (REGIII) C-type lectins, and peptidoglycan-recognition proteins (12, 13). Defensins are primarily identified by three conserved disulfide bridges that form several antiparallel β-sheets due to the presence of multiple cysteine residues (14). Based on the spacing pattern of six cysteines, vertebrate defensins are further categorized into three subfamilies, including α-, β-, and θ-defensins. While β-defensins are present in all vertebrate animals, α-defensins are found in most but not all mammals, and θ-defensins only exist in primates (14). Cathelicidins are structurally recognized by the highly conserved cathelin domain found in the precursor that is cleaved off to release the biologically active peptides adopting a variety of structures such as α-helix (15).

The S100 family proteins are 9–14 kDa in mass containing two highly conserved Ca^{2+}-binding EF-hand domains that are separated by four α-helical domains with a variable C-terminal region (16, 17). The RNase A superfamily are characterized by the presence of 6–8 conserved cysteines forming distinct disulfide bridges, together with two invariantly spaced histidines and a lysine (18, 19). The REGIII family proteins are a group of soluble C-type lectins with a conserved carbohydrate-recognition domain that binds to sugars in a Ca^{2+}-dependent manner (20). Peptidoglycan-recognition proteins constitute a family of phylogenetically conserved host defense molecules with a PGRP domain that binds to bacterial peptidoglycans through specific interactions with the muramyl-tripeptide fragments (21).

Expression of HDPs

Six α-defensins (22) and a minimum of 39 β-defensins (23) have been reported in humans. The genomes of cattle and pigs encode at least 57 and 29 β-defensin genes, respectively (24, 25), while the chicken genome harbors a total of 14 β-defensin genes (26, 27), with no α-defensins being found in cattle, pigs, or chickens. All β-defensin genes are located in tandem in a single genomic region in the chicken (26) and are expanded to 4–5 different clusters in humans, cattle, and pigs (23–25). Interestingly, all human α-defensin genes form a single cluster within a β-defensin gene cluster (22), suggesting that α-defensins likely diverged from β-defensins. While four human α-defensins (HNP1–4) are abundantly present in neutrophil granules, the other two α-defensins (HD5 and HD6) are specific to Paneth cells in the crypts of the human small intestinal tract (14). On the other hand, a majority of β-defensins are expressed in a wide range of cell types, particularly the epithelial cells lining the skin, GI, respiratory, and urogenital tracts of all livestock species as well as humans (14).

A single cathelicidin known as LL-37, CAMP, or hCAP-18 is present in humans (28) and four cathelicidins are reported in chickens (29, 30). In cattle and pigs, 10 and 11 cathelicidins have been identified, respectively (31, 32). All cathelicidin genes are located in a syntenic chromosomal region in vertebrate species. Expressions of cathelicidins are widespread with abundant presence in neutrophil granules as well as various epithelial mucosal surfaces of cattle, pigs, and humans. Four chicken cathelicidins are similarly expressed in a broad range of tissues as well as in heterophils (29, 30, 33, 34), which are equivalent to neutrophils in mammals. Additionally, chicken cathelicidin-B1 is highly expressed in M cells of the bursa of Fabricius (30), a type of specialized epithelial cells involved primarily in antigen transportation from the intestinal lumen to submucosal immune cells (35).

The S100 family members have been found in all vertebrates (17). A total of 21 S100 proteins are present in humans, with 17 members clustered in the same 2-Mb region on chromosome

1q21 (17). The tissue expression pattern of S100 proteins is unique and isoform specific (16). For example, S100A7 (also known as psoriasin) isolated initially from the skin of psoriatic patients is mainly expressed in the skin and breast tissues, whereas the heterodimer S100A8/S100A9, or calgranulin A/B, is expressed in keratinocytes, neutrophils, monocytes, and macrophages.

Biological Functions of HDPs

Host defense peptides are an integral part of the innate immune system. Historically, HDPs are known for their ability to function as natural antibiotics with broad-spectrum antimicrobial activities against Gram-negative and Gram-positive bacteria, fungi, viruses, protozoa, and even cancerous cells (7, 36). Human LL-37 and α- and β-defensins are all capable of killing a broad spectrum of pathogens (7, 36). All four chicken cathelicidins have been demonstrated to be active at low micromolar concentrations against both Gram-positive and Gram-negative bacteria, including antibiotic-resistant strains (29, 30, 37–39). Several chicken β-defensins are also potent against a range of human and zoonotic pathogens (40–42). Similarly, β-defensins and cathelicidins in the cattle and pigs are broadly active against multiple pathogens as well (32).

Because of the cationic and amphipathic properties associated with a majority of HDPs, they kill bacteria primarily through disruption of cell membranes and/or interaction with intracellular macromolecules (43). A net positive charge allows HDPs to bind to negatively charged phospholipid groups on the bacterial membrane through electrostatic interactions. The amphipathic nature of HDPs facilitates their insertion into target cellular membranes allowing them to disrupt its integrity. Multiple models of membrane disruption, such as "barrel-stave", "carpet," or "toroidal-pore" models, have been proposed (43). Intracellularly, certain HDPs are also capable of inhibiting protein, DNA and RNA synthesis, or binding to specific targets (43). Because of their primary membrane-lytic activities, HDPs are generally equally active among drug-resistant and -susceptible pathogens. It is conceivably more difficult for pathogens to develop resistance to HDPs, although certain bacteria have developed mechanisms to resist their action in order to infect and colonize the hosts (44). It appears that commensal bacteria are generally resistant to the action of the constitutively expressed HDPs, but sensitive to certain inducibly expressed HDPs in the human intestinal tract (45). However, the mechanism by which commensal and probiotic bacteria show a reduced sensitivity to HDPs remains elusive.

Besides their antimicrobial activity, HDPs are involved in the modulation of innate and adaptive immune responses (10, 11) (**Figure 1**). Many human HDPs have been shown to promote the recruitment of neutrophils or monocytes and suppress proinflammatory response. Human HDPs also induce the differentiation and activation of macrophages and dendritic cells. Additionally, human cathelicidin LL-37 facilitates the resolution of inflammation by promoting re-epithelialization and wound healing as well as autophagy and apoptosis (10, 11). Three chicken cathelicidins known as fowlicidin 1–3 bind to bacterial lipopolysaccharides (LPS) directly with a strong capacity to neutralize LPS-induced production of inflammatory cytokines in macrophage cells (37–39). Furthermore, chicken fowlicidin-1 is chemotactic to neutrophils, but not monocytes or lymphocytes (46). Fowlicidin-1 also activates macrophages by inducing modest synthesis of inflammatory cytokines and chemokines and further potentiates the antibody response if co-administered with a model antigen (ovalbumin) in mice (46). Importantly, a single application of fowlicidin-1 is not only able to protect animals from an established infection (47) but also to prevent the disease beyond a 2- to 4-day window (46) in a murine model of methicillin-resistant *Staphylococcus aureus* (MRSA) infection (46).

Among 14 bovine β-defensins examined, three (BNBD3, BNBD9, and EBD) are chemotactic to immature monocyte-derived dendritic cells (48). Porcine cathelicidin PR-39 is also capable of inhibiting phagocyte NADPH oxidase activity and attenuating myocardial ischemia–reperfusion injury (49) by blocking the assembly of the enzyme complex through binding to p47phox, a cytosolic component of the NADPH oxidase (50). PR-39 accelerates wound repair by inducing syndecans (51). Furthermore, PR-39 facilitates angiogenesis and formation of functional blood vessels by inhibiting the ubiquitin–proteasome-dependent degradation of hypoxia-inducible factor (HIF)-1α (52). Several porcine cathelicidins also help with the update of bacterial DNA and subsequent activation of dendritic cells (53). HDPs with potent antimicrobial activity and the ability to modulate innate and adaptive immunity are, therefore, being actively exploited as novel antibiotics.

Additionally, recent emerging evidence has highlighted the beneficial effect of HDPs on mucosal barrier permeability by directly regulating mucin and TJ protein expression and shaping microbiota composition. This emerging role of HDPs in intestinal barrier function and homeostasis will be the focus of this review.

MUCUS LAYER: A LAYER OF INTIMATE PROTECTION FOR MUCOSAL SURFACE

An intact mucus layer that is composed primarily of secreted mucins plays a critical role in maintaining the intestinal barrier function (54, 55). Mucins are large, highly glycosylated proteins ranging from 0.5 to 20 MDa. Synthesized and released by goblet cells, mucins function to coat the mucosal surface to facilitate the passage of substances, maintain proper cell hydration, act as a permeable barrier for the exchange of gas and nutrients, and also protect the epithelial cells from invading pathogens and toxins (54, 55). Structurally, a hallmark of all mucin protein backbones is the presence of 1–5 tandem repeat (TR) domains, which consist of an excessive number of identical or nearly identical TR sequences rich in serine, threonine, and proline residues (56) (**Figure 2**). The TR domain is heavily glycosylated because of attachment of oligosaccharides to serine and threonine through *O*-linked glycosylation, giving rise to 50–80% glycans in mass. Saturated sugar coating is beneficial to increase the water-holding capacity and the resistance of mucins to proteolytic cleavage.

In humans, the mucin family consists of up to 20 members, including both secreted and membrane-bound forms. Secreted mucins form homo-oligomeric, gel-like structures constituting the mucosal layer, while the membrane-bound mucins are part

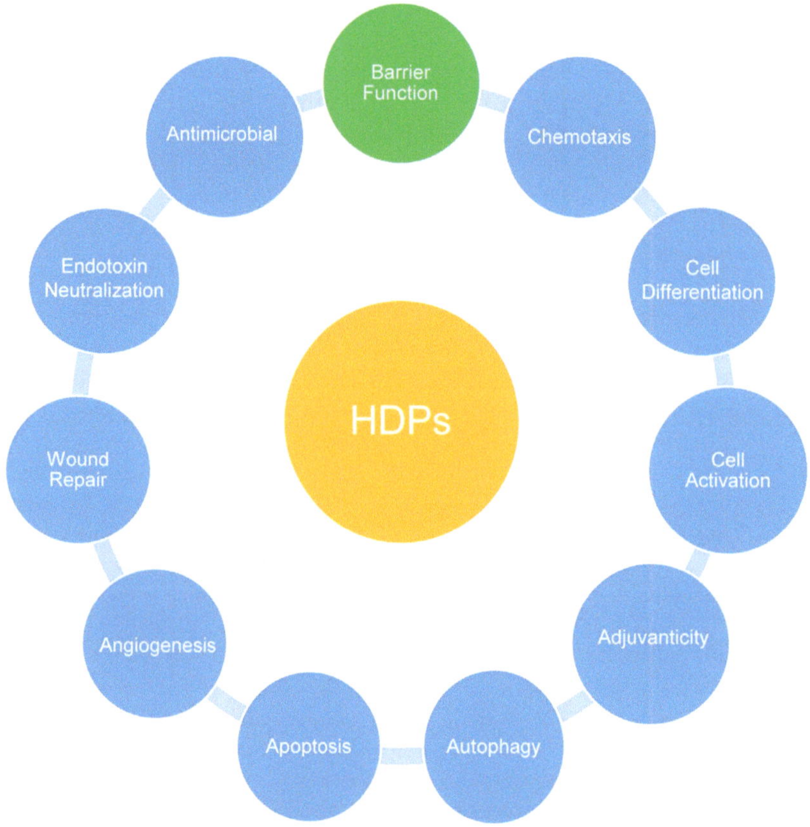

FIGURE 1 | Multifunctional roles of host defense peptides (HDPs). Besides direct antimicrobial activities, HDPs actively participate in systemic and mucosal epithelial defense by modulating a range of host innate and adaptive immune responses as indicated. Recent accumulating evidence has highlighted a direct involvement of HDPs in improving intestinal and epidermal barrier function.

of the epithelial glycocalyx that are involved in cell signaling and interactions with the environment without forming gel or oligomerization (57). Secreted human mucins include MUC2, -5AC, -5B, -6, -7, and -19, and the transmembrane mucins consist of MUC1, -3, -4, -12, -13, -15, -16, -17, and -20 (54, 55). Structurally, most secreted mucins are unique in the presence of multiple von Willebrand factor (VWF) domains and a C-terminal cysteine-knot domain, while a majority of membrane-bound mucins specifically consist of a transmembrane domain, a cytoplasmic tail, 1–2 epidermal growth factor (EGF)-like domains, and a sea urchin sperm protein, enterokinase, and agrin (SEA) domain (56, 58) (**Figure 2**). The VWF domains and cysteine-knot domain of secreted mucins are responsible for formation of higher-order structures through oligomerization, while the EGF-like and SEA domains of membrane-bound mucins mediate signaling transduction and cleavage of the extracellular portion of mucins, respectively (58). Among all secreted mucins, MUC2 is the most abundant in the human small intestine and colon, and MUC5AC is predominant in the stomach. Structurally, similar mucins have been found in most other vertebrate species, including cattle, pigs, and chickens (59–62).

The mucus layer formed by secreted mucins varies in composition along the GI tract. The stomach and large intestine consist of two distinct mucus layers: a "loose" outer layer and a "thick" inner layer (2). The inner layer closest to epithelial cells is densely packed and holds firmly to the cells. The inner mucus layer is largely free of bacteria, providing a sterile protective environment for the epithelium. The outer mucus layer is much more soluble due to proteolytic cleavages that allow the mucus layer to expand without disrupting mucin polymers. This outer layer provides a habitat for commensal bacteria to bind via specific adhesins and to thrive via breaking down the mucin glycans as a food source. Specificity of bacteria for different glycans is speculated to be important for developing species-specific microbiota (2).

Altered expression or glycosylation of mucins is often associated with intestinal barrier dysfunction (57). For example, Muc2 deficiency in mice causes increased permeability, gross bleeding, spontaneous development of inflammation in the GI tract, as well as severe growth retardation (63, 64). Muc1- or Muc2-deficient mice become more prone to infections with *Campylobacter jejuni*, *Helicobacter pylori*, *Salmonella enterica* serovar Typhimurium, and *Citrobacter rodentium* (64–67). Moreover, mice lacking the enzyme, β1,3-*N*-acetylglucosaminyltransferase that synthesizes *O*-glycans on mucins, exhibit a thinner mucus layer showing an enhanced susceptibility to enteric bacterial infections (67) and dextran sodium sulfate (DSS)-induced colitis (68). Additionally,

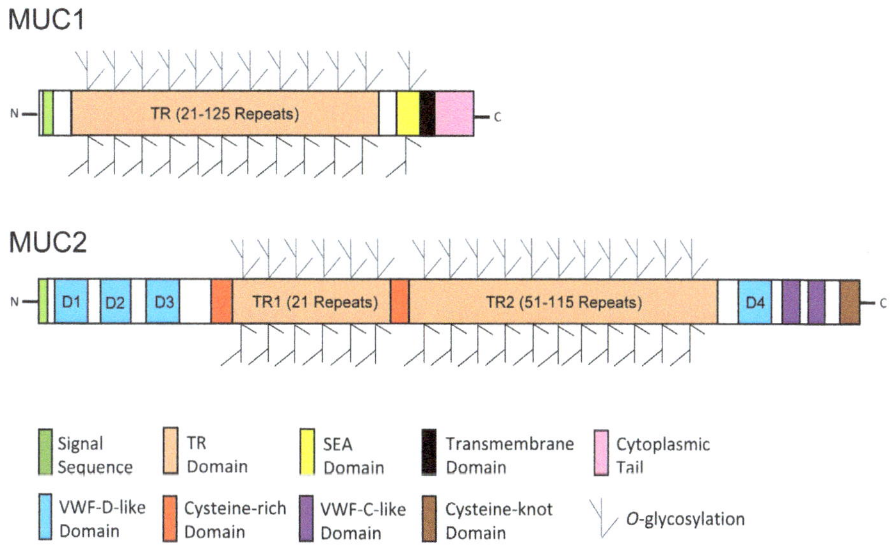

FIGURE 2 | Schematic diagrams of glycosylated mucin monomers. Representative membrane-bound and secreted mucins are exemplified by mucin 1 (MUC1) and MUC2, respectively. The protein backbone of mucins is characterized by the presence of an excessive number of tandem repeat (TR) sequences. Mucins are heavily *O*-glycosylated through enriched threonine and serine residues in the TR domain. A transmembrane domain, a cytoplasmic tail, and a sea urchin sperm protein, enterokinase, and agrin (SEA) domain are unique to most membrane-bound mucins, whereas the presence of several von Willebrand factor (VWF) domains and a C-terminal cysteine-knot domain is specific to a majority of secreted mucins. The diagrams were modified primarily from reference (56).

significantly reduced expressions of multiple mucins such as MUC1, MUC3, MUC4, and MUC5B are observed in ileal mucosa of Crohn's disease (CD) patients (69), although the expression changes of mucins are less clear in ulcerative colitis (UC) patients (70).

TIGHT JUNCTIONS: GATE GUARDS FOR BORDER PROTECTION

The intestinal epithelium is made up of several different cell types organized into crypts and villi. These include intestinal epithelial stem cells, enterocytes, and secretory cells, such as Paneth, goblet, and enteroendocrine cells (71). Intestinal stem cells give rise to all other epithelial cell types, while enterocytes primarily function in nutrient absorption with the ability to synthesize and release HDPs and mucins. Paneth and goblet cells are major producers of HDPs and mucins, respectively, while enteroendocrine cells have a primary role of secreting numerous hormones that act as regulators of digestive function (71). All intestinal epithelial cells are linked at lateral membranes through formation of three major types of junctional complexes, i.e., TJs, adherens junctions, and desmosomes (1, 3, 72). Collectively, they form a virtually impermeable seal to the paracellular space. Besides the barrier function, these junctional complexes maintain cell polarity by separating the apical from basolateral membranes. TJs are multi-protein complexes located at the most apical end of the lateral membrane. The TJ assembly is composed of both transmembrane and cytoplasmic plaque proteins that interact directly with the cytoskeleton (**Figure 3**). Among all three major junctional complexes, only TJs have the ability to control the selective paracellular permeability for ions, water, and other small molecules (1, 3, 72). Therefore, TJs are the major determinant of mucosal epithelial permeability.

Tight Junction Structures

Among the proteins involved in TJ assembly, claudins, occludin, junctional adhesion molecules (JAM), and tricellulin are the major transmembrane proteins that constitute a selective paracellular barrier, whereas zonula occludens (ZO) and cingulin are the main cytoplasmic plaque proteins located at the peripheral membrane (1, 3, 72). All TJ proteins are highly conserved in vertebrate species. Claudins are a large family of small proteins of 21–34 kDa that make up the backbone of the TJ structure, with at least 26 members reported in humans (73). Remarkably, each claudin shows a unique tissue expression pattern with varied levels of expression in different segments of the GI tract. Occludin (65 kDa) was the first transmembrane TJ protein identified (74), with no homologs being found (75). On the other hand, the JAM family is comprised of three classical members (JAM-1, -2, and -3) and four related molecules (JAM-4, JAM-L, CAR, and ESAM) at ~40 kDa each (76). Tricellulin is a 64-kDa protein located preferentially at tricellular junctions, although it is also present in bicellular junctions (77). Tricellulin shares 32% identity in the amino acid sequence with the C-terminal tail of occludin. ZO proteins belong to the family of membrane-associated guanylate kinase (GUK) homologs that include three members, i.e., ZO-1 (~220 kDa), ZO-2 (~160 kDa), and ZO-3 (~130 kDa) (78), whereas cingulin is an ~140-kDa protein that links ZO proteins to the actin cytoskeleton (79).

Claudins, occludin, and tricellulin are all membrane proteins with four transmembrane domains, one intracellular and two

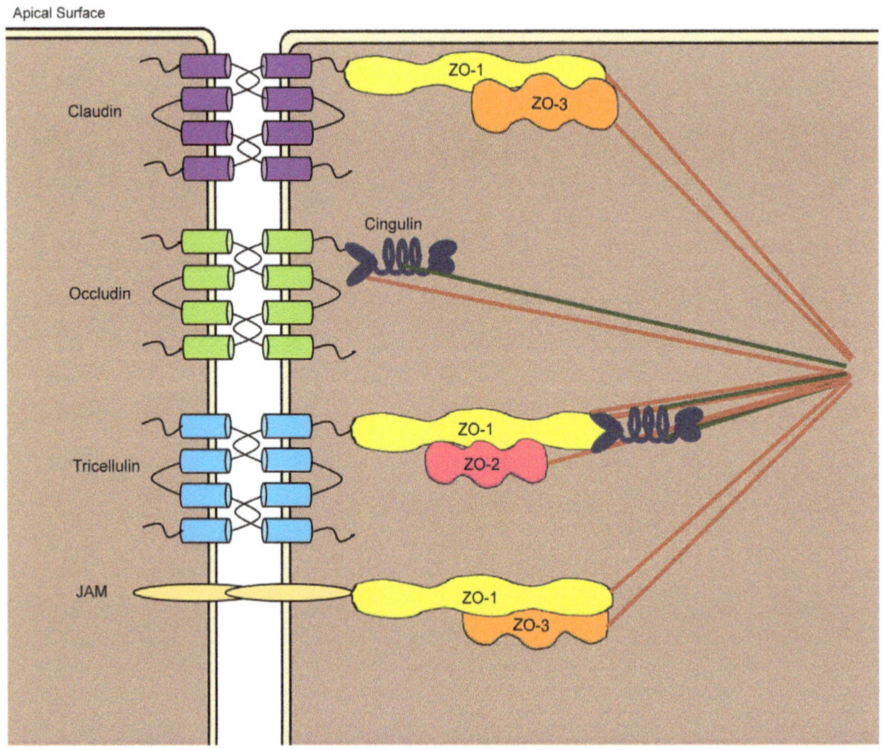

FIGURE 3 | Schematic drawing of tight junction structures at the apicolateral membranes of the paracellular space. Tight junctions are comprised of transmembrane proteins such as claudins, occludin, junctional adhesion molecules (JAM), and tricellulin as well as cytoplasmic plaque proteins such as three zonula occludens (ZO) proteins and cingulin. Claudins, occludin, and tricellulin consist of four transmembrane domains, while JAMs have a single transmembrane domain. Through largely homophilic interactions, neighboring cells are sealed at the apicolateral region. Cytoplasmic proteins link the tight junction assembly to the cytoskeleton to control the opening of paracellular pores.

extracellular loops, and two cytoplasmic tails, whereas the JAM proteins are single-pass transmembrane proteins consisting of two extracellular immunoglobulin (Ig)-like domains, a single transmembrane domain, and a short intercellular C-terminal tail (72) (**Figure 4**). While the N-terminal tail is generally short, the longer C-terminal tail of claudins consists of a post-synaptic density 95, disk-large, and zonula occludens (PDZ)-binding motif that interacts with the first PDZ domain of ZO-1 (73). The crystal structure of claudins as exemplified by mouse claudin-15 indicates that the four transmembrane segments form a tight four-helix bundle with parts of the two extracellular loops forming a "palm-shaped" structure (80). A model for the architecture of claudin-formed TJ strands in the membrane has been proposed based on the results of crosslinking experiments and electron microscopy (81). In this model, claudins show an antiparallel, double-layer arrangement (**Figures 5A,B**). The association of claudin double layers in neighboring lateral membranes results in the formation of multiple extracellular β-barrel-like pores parallel with the membrane plane to allow the passage of ions through the paracellular space (**Figure 5C**).

As for occludin, its two extracellular loops mediate homophilic interactions and permeability to macromolecules. The occludin–ELL domain in the C-terminal tail of occludin is responsible for interacting with the GUK domain of ZO proteins, while the N-terminal tail lacks a defined function (75) (**Figure 4**). In comparison with claudins and occludin, tricellulin consists of two long tails, with the C-terminal tail containing an occludin–ELL domain that is likely to interact with the GUK domain of ZO proteins (82). JAM proteins also contain a cytoplasmic tail with a PDZ-binding motif that interacts with the third PDZ domain of ZO-1 (83) (**Figure 4**). The extracellular Ig-like domains of JAM proteins are responsible for homophilic and heterophilic interactions.

The cytoplasmic ZO proteins contain three PDZ domains, a Src homology-3 (SH3) domain, and a GUK domain (78). As stated above, ZO-1 directly interacts with claudins, ZO-2, and JAM-1 through the first, second, and third PDZ domain, respectively. The GUK domain of ZO proteins is known to associate with occludin, while the C-terminal actin-binding region is responsible for bridging with actin, raising the possibility of forming a large protein complex through simultaneous interactions of many TJ proteins with ZO-1 (78). Cingulin is another intracellular plaque protein that is predicted to form a homodimer with globular head and tail at both ends connected by a coiled-coil "rod" domain in the central region. The head of cingulin is known to bind to ZO proteins and the coiled-coil domain interacts with myosin (79). The interactions between the TJ protein complex and cytoskeleton are critical in maintaining and regulating the TJ

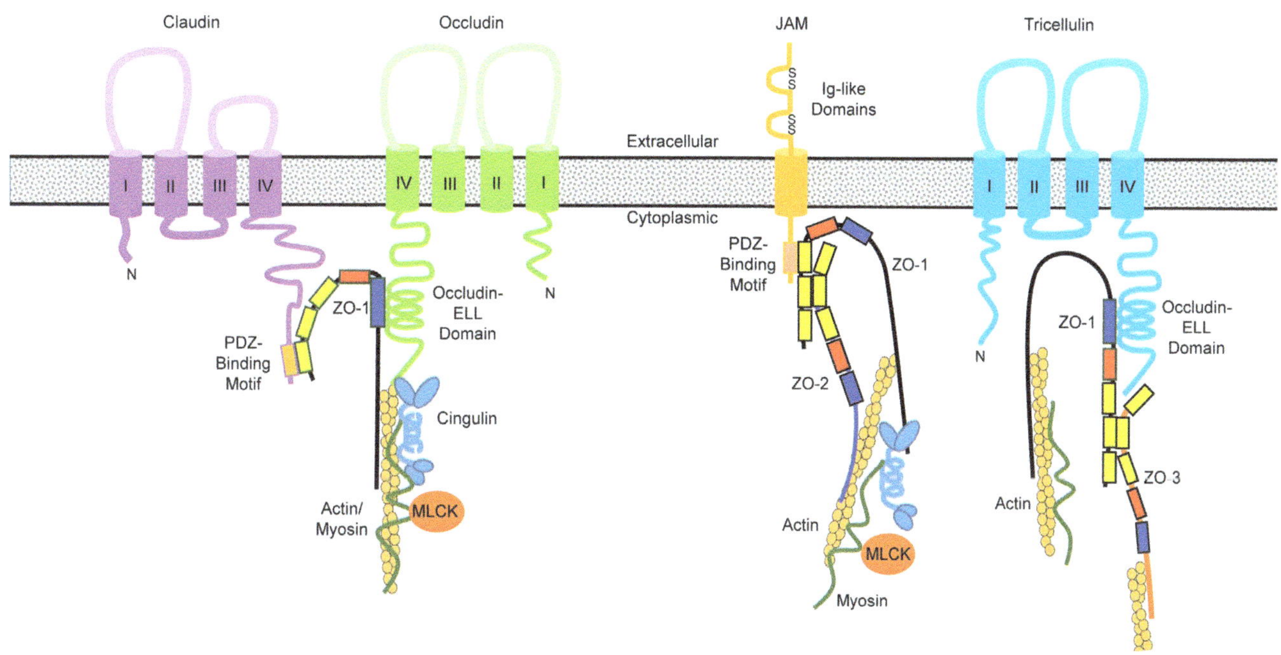

FIGURE 4 | Domain structures of primary tight junction proteins and their interactions. Claudins consist of four transmembrane domains with a PDZ-binding motif at the C-terminal tail, which interacts with the first PDZ domain (in yellow) of zonula occludens (ZO)-1. The GUK domain (in blue) of ZO-1 binds to the occludin–ELL domain at the C-terminal tail of occludin and possibly tricellulin as well. Junctional adhesion molecules (JAM) contain a single transmembrane domain, two immunoglobulin (Ig)-like domains in the extracellular region, and a PDZ-binding motif at the C-terminal tail that interacts with the third PDZ domain of ZO-1. ZO molecules form heterodimers through interactions at their second PDZ domain. The C-terminal segment of ZO proteins binds directly to actin filaments as well as the globular head of cingulin that interacts with myosin through its rod domain. The globular head of cingulin also binds to the C-terminal occludin and actin filaments. Phosphorylation of myosin light chain by myosin light chain kinase (MLCK) will cause contraction of the perijunctional actomyosin ring and opening of the tight junction channels.

structure and function, as the mucosal permeability is regulated heavily by the phosphorylation status of myosin light chain, which can be modified by the kinases such as myosin light chain kinase (MLCK) (72, 73) (**Figure 4**).

Tight Junctions' Function in Selective Permeability

Tight junctions are distributed at the apical surface of epithelial and endothelial cells throughout the body in vertebrate animals, including the skin, GI, respiratory, and urogenital tracts as well as the blood vessels (72). TJs are the major determinant of mucosal barrier permeability. Ions, water, and macromolecules pass TJs through either of the two major types of pores. The non-restrictive pathway, also known as the "leak" pathway, allows the transport of macromolecules through large pores with no charge selectivity, while the restrictive or "pore" pathway is only permeable to small ions through pores of ~4 Å in radius with charge selectivity (1, 3, 4). Claudins are mainly responsible for the "pore" pathway, and the two extracellular loops work as an "electrostatic selective filter" to select the size and charge for small pores (**Figure 5**). The charge selectivity of individual claudins is determined by the net charge of the amino acid residues in the first extracellular loop. For example, claudin-1 is selective for anions, while claudin-2 prefers cations. In the intestinal tract, claudin-1, -3, -4, -5, -8, -9, -11, and -14 decrease paracellular permeability and are regarded as barrier-forming claudins, while claudin-2, -7, -12, and -15 are to increase permeability and generally referred as pore-forming claudins (72, 73).

The non-restrictive "leak" pathway is primarily dependent on occludin as evidenced by an increase in paracellular flux of macromolecules without a noticeable effect on transepithelial electrical resistance (TEER) both *in vitro* and *in vivo* after occludin knock-down (84). JAM proteins also enhance the TJ function by decreasing permeability and facilitating the assembly of occludin to the TJ complex (83). In addition, JAMs can regulate the paracellular barrier for the transmigration of leukocytes from the blood vessel to inflamed sites in response to inflammation (76). It is noteworthy that paracellular water permeability is mainly dictated by claudin-2.

Modulation of Paracellular Permeability

A number of agents such as cytokines, growth factors, pathogens, probiotics, nutrients, and phytochemicals have been found to impact TJ permeability and mucosal barrier functions through transcriptional regulation and posttranslational modification of TJ proteins (72, 73). Increased expressions of barrier-forming claudins, occludin, and JAM proteins are commonly associated with reduced paracellular permeability and improved barrier function, whereas an elevation in the expression of pore-forming claudins often leads to barrier dysfunction. For example,

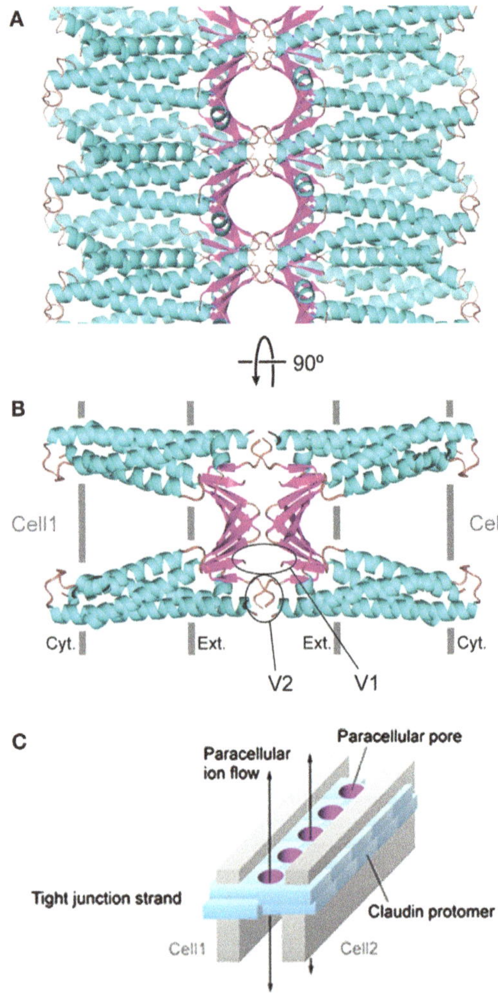

FIGURE 5 | A model of paracellular claudin-based tight junction channels. Putative β-barrel-like channels are formed by the extracellular domains (in magenta) of double-layered claudins, whose transmembrane helices are depicted in cyan. The tight junction complex is shown in parallel **(A)** and perpendicular **(B)** views, respectively, from the apical surface of the cells. **(C)** A schematic drawing of claudin-based tight junction channels. The paracellular pores are colored in magenta and double-layered claudins are represented by cyan blocks. Two gray plates indicate two neighboring cell membranes, and the arrows indicate the directions of ions passing through the tight junction channels. The graphs are adopted from the open-access reference (81).

transforming growth factor (TGF)-β enhances barrier integrity of intestinal epithelial cells by augmenting claudin-1 and -4 expression, while IL-1β, IL-6, and TNF-α increase intestinal cell permeability by increasing claudin-2 expression and/or reducing occludin and ZO-1 expression (72).

Tight junction barrier integrity is also affected by post-translational modifications of transmembrane and cytoplasmic proteins and associated regulatory proteins. Phosphorylation, glycosylation, and/or ubiquitination of the TJ proteins have a profound impact on barrier permeability. For example, claudin-1 is phosphorylated by atypical protein kinase C (aPKC), protein kinase A (PKA), and mitogen-activated protein kinases (MAPK) and dephosphorylated by protein phosphatase 2A (72, 73). Phosphorylation of claudins generally promotes their assembly into the TJ, whereas dephosphorylation often results in the dissociation of claudins from the TJ (72, 73). Similarly, phosphorylation of occludin enhances the barrier function, while dephosphorylation delays the TJ assembly resulting in barrier dysfunction (72, 75).

Besides those proteins involved directly in the TJ assembly, paracellular permeability is also heavily influenced by actin–myosin filaments that are linked to the TJ proteins. It is well known that up-regulation of MLCK is linked to an increase in the TJ permeability by catalyzing the phosphorylation of myosin light chain, which in turn induces the contraction of actin–myosin filaments and opening of the TJ barrier (85). Both IL-1β and TNF-α are strong inducers of the MLCK gene transcription and activation, resulting increased myosin light chain phosphorylation and TJ barrier permeability (86, 87).

The expression and posttranslational modifications of TJ proteins are influenced by a complicated network of signaling pathways that intertwine with each other. Activation of nuclear factor (NF)-κB signaling by pathogens, pathogen-associated molecular patterns (PAMPs), and proinflammatory cytokines often causes an increase in intestinal epithelial permeability through induction of pore-forming claudin-2 and suppression of barrier-forming claudins such as claudin-1, -3, -4, -5, -7, and -8. On the other hand, activation of TGF-β/SMAD and PPAR-α/γ signaling are generally barrier protective by enhancing claudin-1 and -4 expressions while downregulating claudin-2 (73).

Implication of Tight Junction Dysfunction in Disease Pathogenesis

The intestinal barrier helps to maintain homeostasis between gut microbiota and the immune system. TJ dysfunction is associated with many enteric disorders such as CD, UC, and celiac disease (3, 72). In CD patients, the expressions of barrier-forming claudin-3, -5, -8, occludin, and JAM-1 are decreased, while pore-forming claudin-2 is significantly increased; and in UC patients, a down-regulation of claudin-1, -4, and JAM-1, and up-regulation of claudin-2, is observed (3, 72). Moreover, increased MLCK expression and activity are evident in both CD and UC patients (85). These factors collectively exacerbate the intestinal paracellular permeability leading to a "leaky gut syndrome." However, many of these clinical conditions are also accompanied with increase synthesis of proinflammatory cytokines, which are known to cause barrier dysfunction. Thus, it is difficult to determine whether barrier dysfunction is a cause or effect of many of these diseases.

Several enteric pathogens such as *Vibrio cholera*, enteropathic *Escherichia coli*, *Clostridium perfringens* are known to cause diarrhea mainly through disruption of the intestinal barrier function by secretion of exotoxins (72). For example, claudin-3 and -4 are receptors for *C. perfringens* enterotoxin, and the binding of enterotoxin to the extracellular loops of claudins causes internalization of claudins and disintegration of the TJ assembly (88). Early weaning (<3 weeks of age) is known to impair the development of intestinal barrier functions of pigs leading to more pronounced diarrhea (89), and was recently found to lead to reduced expressions of occludin, claudin-1, and ZO-1 in the jejunum (90).

REGULATION OF TIGHT JUNCTION AND MUCIN PRODUCTION BY HOST DEFENSE PEPTIDES

Association of HDP Expression with Barrier Dysfunction

Along with decreased TJ protein expression, aberrant HDP expression is common in CD and UC patients (91). The expression of Paneth cell α-defensins (HD5 and HD6) is significantly reduced in ileal CD patients, but unaffected in colonic CD patients Z (92). Instead, a reduced expression of HBD-1 and HBD-2 is observed in colonic CD (93). Moreover, induction of cathelicidin LL-37 and HBD-2, -3, and -4 is also reduced in colonic CD relative to healthy subjects (94–97). This lack of HDP induction in CD patients is thought to play a key role in CD pathogenesis as it indicates a lack of intestinal immune response. A deficiency in HD5 and HD6 synthesis is even more pronounced in patients carrying a mutation in the intracellular NOD2 receptor (98), which is expressed by Paneth cells. Consistently, NOD2-knockout mice show a diminished expression of Paneth cell α-defensins known as cryptdins in mice (99). In contrast to CD patients, UC patients display unchanged HD5 and HD6 expressions (92), while LL-37, HBD-2, -3, and -4 are upregulated (94–97). A thin or even absent mucus layer is evident in UC intestinal segments, which causes intestinal inflammation due to direct adhesion and invasion of bacteria to mucosal epithelial cells. Although UC patients produce HDPs, these peptides are not retained in the intestinal tract. Perhaps the most convincing evidence linking the positive role of HDPs in barrier function comes from the studies with cathelicidin (CRAMP)-deficient mice. These mice show delayed recovery of barrier permeability in response to acute disruption of epidermal barrier, albeit with subtle barrier abnormalities in the epidermis (100). Collectively, these lines of evidence suggest a direct impact of HDPs on intestinal barrier function and homeostasis.

Transcriptional Regulation of Mucins and TJ Proteins by HDPs

Accumulating pieces of evidence suggest a direct involvement of HDPs in regulating the synthesis of mucins and TJ proteins in the intestinal tract. HBD-2 upregulates MUC2, MUC3, but not MUC1 or MUC5AC in human HT-29 colonic epithelial cells (101). MUC2 expression is also enhanced in human Caco-2 colonic epithelial cells in response to HBD-2 (101), and upregulated MUC2 in turn promotes HBD-2 expression (102), suggestive of a positive feedback mechanism between MUC2 and HBD-2. LL-37 also enhances MUC1, MUC2, and MUC3 expressions in HT-29 cells (103, 104) and MUC3 expression only in Caco-2 cells (104). Buforin II, a 21-amino acid HDP isolated from the stomach of an Asian toad (*Bufo bufo garagriozans*), improves intestinal barrier function in weaned piglets challenged with three enterotoxigenic *E. coli* (ETEC) strains (105). Oral administration (twice daily) of buforin II leads to an increase in claudin-1, occludin, and ZO-1 expression in the jejunal segments of *E. coli*-challenged piglets (105). Importantly, buforin II also improves intestinal morphology and growth performance and reduced bacterial shedding in fecal swabs (105). Additionally, administration of a banded krait HDP known as cathelicidin-BF induces ZO-1 expression in the jejunum of healthy mice and also restores LPS-mediated impairment of ZO-1 and intestinal barrier function (106). Furthermore, porcine β-defensin-2 (PBD-2) is capable of restoring the expression of MUC1, MUC2, claudin-1, ZO-1, and ZO-2 as well as the barrier integrity of the colon of DSS-treated mice (107).

Besides direct regulation of the intestinal paracellular permeability, several HDPs also positively influence the barrier effect of the respiratory tract and the skin. LL-37 induces MUC5AC in human NCI-H292 airway epithelial cells (108). LL-37, HBD-3, and S100A7/psoriasin are all able to augment the expression of TJ proteins in human skin keratinocytes (109–111). HBD-3 induces the expressions of all 14 claudins examined, but not occludin or ZO 1–3 in human keratinocytes (110). Similarly, LL-37 dose-dependently enhances the expressions of 11 claudins and occludin in skin keratinocytes, but not JAM 1–3 or ZO 1–3 (109). S100A7 also promotes the expressions of multiple claudins and occludin, but not JAM 1–3 or ZO 1–3 in human keratinocytes (111). Multiple signaling pathways are involved in HDP-induced barrier protein synthesis as detailed below.

MOLECULAR MECHANISMS OF HDP REGULATION OF BARRIER FUNCTIONS

A number of extracellular and intracellular receptors have been reported to be responsible for a range of physiological functions of cathelicidins and defensins in humans and mice. LL-37 and the mouse ortholog (CRAMP) are ligands for P2X purinergic receptor 7 (P2X7), formyl peptide receptor-like (FPRL) 1/2, glyceraldehyde 3-phosphate dehydrogenase, and sequestosome-1/p62, whereas several human and mouse β-defensins bind to CC chemokine receptor 2 (CCR2), CCR6, CXC chemokine receptor 2 (CXCR2), and toll-like receptor 1/2/4 (112, 113). The receptors and signaling pathways by which HDPs induce the expression of mucins and TJ proteins have been studied, but remain elusive in most cases. It is worth noting that, although most published mechanistic studies were based on skin keratinocytes, the following overall conclusions are believed to be applicable to intestinal epithelia as well: (1) HDPs vary greatly in their ability to modulate barrier function, albeit with structural similarities, (2) mucins and TJ proteins are differentially regulated by HDPs, (3) multiple signaling pathways are employed by the same HDP, and (4) receptors appear to be differentially engaged in mediating the induction of mucins and TJ proteins by different HDPs. The current findings are summarized below.

Signaling Mechanisms of HDP-Mediated Mucin Induction

LL-37-induced MUC5AC expression in lung epithelial cells appears to be mediated mainly through transactivation of the EGF receptor (EGFR) (108), although EGFR is not a direct receptor for LL-37 (**Figure 6A**). Initially, LL-37

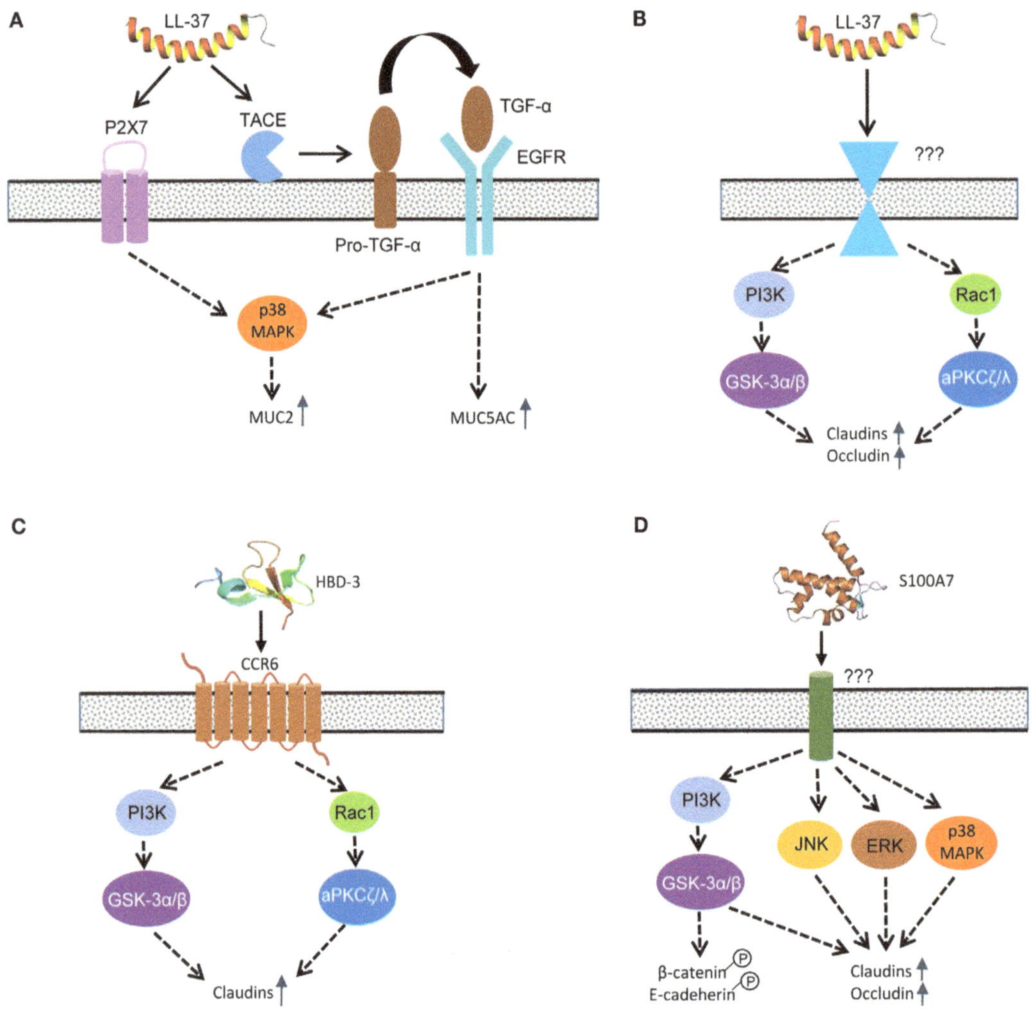

FIGURE 6 | Host defense peptide-mediated signaling pathways to induce mucins and tight junction proteins in epidermal and intestinal epithelial cells. (A) LL-37 primarily utilizes purinergic receptor P2X7 and transactivates EGFR to mediate MUC2 and MUC5AC induction. **(B)** LL-37 induces the synthesis of multiple claudins and occludin in skin keratinocytes mainly through PI3K-GSK-3α/β and Rac1-aPKCζ/λ pathways; however, the receptor that mediates the effect is currently unknown. **(C)** HBD-3 mainly engages CCR6 to induce claudin synthesis in skin keratinocytes through the PI3K-GSK-3α/β and Rac1-aPKCζ/λ pathways. **(D)** S100A7 enhances the synthesis of claudins and occludin through PI3K-GSK-3α/β and three canonical MAPK pathways. S100A7 also triggers phosphorylation of β-catenin and E-cadherin to enhance the adherens junction. A solid arrow indicates a direct effect, whereas a dashed arrow refers to an indirect action. It is noted that cross-talks among different signaling pathways likely exist, but they have not been reported.

triggers the activation of TNF-α-converting enzyme, which in turn cleaves the membrane-bound form of TGF-α, but not heparin binding-EGF. Released TGF-α subsequently interacts with and phosphorylates its receptor, EGFR, which induces MUC5AC gene expression through activation of multiple signaling pathways (108). For LL-37 to induce MUC2 and MUC3 expression in human intestinal epithelial cells, both EGFR and P2X7, but not G-protein-coupled receptors, are involved (104). HBD-2-induced mucin expression in human intestinal epithelial cells is shown to be partially mediated through CCR6 (101). The p38 MAPK, but not extracellular signal-regulated kinase (ERK) or PI3K, is involved in mediating P2X7- and EGFR-activation of MUC2 production in human Caco-2 cells (104).

LL-37-Mediated TJ Protein Induction

Rac1, aPKCζ/λ, glycogen synthase kinase (GSK)-3α/β, and PI3K are all phosphorylated and activated in human skin keratinocytes in response to LL-37, and blockage of any enzyme with a specific inhibitor results in a substantial reduction in the TEER and a significant increase in the permeability to FITC-dextran (109) (**Figure 6B**). Rac1 is a small GTPase that functions upstream of aPKCζ/λ as part of the Par3/Par6/aPKCζ/λ polarity complex, which in turn phosphorylates the C-terminal domain of occludin (114) or JAM-1 (115), promoting its assembly into the TJ complex and enhancing the barrier function (116). GSK-3α/β is involved in a number of signaling pathways (117) and is required for induction of occludin and claudin-1 in intestinal and kidney epithelial cells (118). Consistently, LL-37 triggers phosphorylation and activation of GSK-3α/β at Tyr 216 and Tyr 279 in human keratinocytes at 1–2 h after exposure, leading to the improvement of epidermal barrier function (109).

PI3K functions upstream of GSK-3, and the PI3K signaling cascade has been implicated in both the degradation and stimulation of TJ barrier function depending on the stimulating agent (119). PI3K is quickly phosphorylated within 30 min in human keratinocytes upon stimulation with LL-37 (109). In intestinal cells, PI3K plays a key role in directing proper occludin localization and subsequent tightening of epithelial barrier function in response to prostaglandins (120). Inhibition of PI3K in porcine ischemia-injured ileal mucosa attenuates the ability of prostaglandin to recover proper barrier function. In rat Con8 mammary epithelial cells, glucocorticoid recruits Ras and the p85 subunit of PI3K to the TJ complex and increases barrier function (121). However, the specific cellular receptor(s) mediating LL-37-induced TJ protein expression remain unknown and warrant further investigation.

HBD-3-Mediated TJ Protein Induction

Although HBD-2 is capable of inducing mucin expression (101), only HBD-3 triggers the synthesis of multiple TJ proteins (110). CCR6 has been shown to be primarily responsible for HBD-3-induced enhancement of barrier integrity in epidermis (110). Similar to LL-37, HBD-3 is also capable of phosphorylating and activating Rac1, aPKCζ/λ, PI3K, and GSK-3α/β in similar kinetics in human skin keratinocytes (110) (**Figure 6C**). Of note, toll-like receptors, PKA, and MAPK pathways are not involved in mediating HBD-3-induced barrier function improvement (110). Although HBD-1, HBD-2, and HBD-4 fail to alter the epidermal permeability, they also have weak activities in activating Rac1, aPKC, GSK-3, and PI3K (110), suggesting those pathways may not be solely devoted to the TJ functions. It is important to note that, although similar in the tertiary structure, only HBD-3, but not HBD-1, -2 or -4, has the ability to trigger the induction of TJ proteins (115).

S100A7-Mediated TJ Protein Induction

The role of GSK-3α/β and MAPK in human epidermal barrier function mediated by S100A7 has been studied (111) (**Figure 6D**). GSK-3α/β is phosphorylated and activated at Tyr 216 and Tyr 279 within 30 min following exposure of human keratinocytes to S100A7/psoriasin. Specific inhibition of GSK-3 activation abolishes induction of claudins and epidermal TEER by S100A7 (111). Because β-catenin is regulated directly by GSK-3 (117), S100A7 is revealed to phosphorylate and activate β-catenin, which is vital to the assembly of adherens junctions. E-cadherin, another essential component of the adherens junction complex, is also phosphorylated by S100A7 (111), suggesting that, besides the TJs, S100A7 also improves the assembly of adherens junctions.

The MAPK pathway includes three canonical signaling cascades that consist of ERK, c-Jun N-terminal kinase (JNK), and p38 (122). Collectively, they are critical to many important physiological processes ranging from cell division and differentiation to stress and immune responses. Unlike HBD-3, S100A7 is capable of activating all three canonical MAPK cascades (111). ERK is quickly phosphorylated in 2 min in human skin keratinocytes following exposure to S100A7, while JNK and p38 MAPK are also phosphorylated in 30 min. Inhibition of individual MAPK signaling cascades leads to a substantial reduction in claudin induction and epidermal TEER (111), implying that all three major MAPK pathways are required. However, the involvement of any specific receptors or other signaling pathways remains to be studied.

ROLE OF HDPs IN INTESTINAL MUCOSAL HOMEOSTASIS, IMMUNE DEFENSE, AND GROWTH PERFORMANCE

One of the major functions of the intestinal epithelium is to act as a barrier against the invasion of microorganisms. This task is especially difficult considering that the intestinal mucosa is colonized by over 1013 microorganisms (123), with the majority being commensal bacteria that are beneficial to the host through their ability to improve digestion, absorption, and vitamin synthesis while also limiting pathogen growth (124). The two most dominant bacterial phyla present in the intestinal tract of humans and mice are Gram-negative Bacteriodetes and Gram-positive Firmicutes, which together comprise about 70–80% of the total bacteria present (125). Commensal bacteria are vital to the development of normal intestinal morphology and immune system (126, 127). While commensal bacteria are beneficial to the host under homeostatic conditions, a state of dysbiosis, or imbalance of the microbial community, leads to inflammation and disturbed epithelial homeostasis. This is particularly seen in the CD patients in which the host immune system displays increased activation against commensal microbiota.

The intestinal epithelium continuously monitors resident microbes through interactions between pattern recognition receptors (PRRs) and microbe-associated molecular patterns (MAMPs). Activation of PRRs stimulates the synthesis and release of HDPs and mucins from intestinal cells (126, 127). A large amount of HDPs secreted from Paneth cells and enterocytes are retained in the mucus layer to create a strong barrier against bacterial invasion (128). Studies with HDP-knockout and -transgenic mice have illuminated the role of HDPs in intestinal homeostasis and immune defense. Knockout of the mouse cathelicidin CRAMP gene causes exaggerated colitis in the colon of mice, and the disease symptoms are further exacerbated following DSS treatment (129). Adoptive transfer of bone marrow cells from the wild-type mice to CRAMP-knockout mice alleviates DSS-induced colitis (129). Mice carrying the transgene for HD5 show an augmented ability to fight off orally challenged *S. enterica* serovar Typhimurium (130). Conversely, matrix metalloproteinase 7 (MMP7)-knockout mice with a deficiency in producing biologically active enteric defensins display reduced capacity to clear enteric pathogens (131). Furthermore, a comparison between those two complementary mouse models has revealed dramatic defensin-dependent reciprocal shifts in the intestinal bacterial composition. In comparison with wild-type mice, Firmicutes are reduced and Bacteriodes are increased in small intestine of HD5-transgenic mice, while the opposite is true with MMP7-deficient mice (125, 132). Moreover, overexpression of HD5 in mice causes a significant loss of segmented filamentous bacteria in the distal small intestine and a reduced presence of Th17 cells in the lamina propria (132), suggesting clearly that enteric HDPs represent a critical factor in shaping the microbiota composition and inflammatory status of the GI tract.

Multiple studies have highlighted the beneficial effects of direct feeding of HDPs on growth, intestinal morphology, and immune status in pigs (133, 134). Dietary supplementation of an *E. coli*-producing bacteriocin, colicin E1, significantly improved weight gain and feed efficiency of ETEC-challenged weanling pigs in a 4-day trial, relative to the control pigs (135). Colicin E1 inclusion also reduced the *E. coli* titers in both the fecal and ileal samples as well as the incidence and severity of diarrhea (135). Moreover, the expression levels of proinflammatory cytokines (IL-1β and TNF-α) were reduced in the ileum of pigs in response to colicin E1 feeding (135). Similarly, feeding a recombinant silkworm HDP, cecropin A/D, improved growth and feed efficiency and reduced diarrhea incidence in ETEC-challenged weanling pigs, without an obvious impact on intestinal morphology or nitrogen/energy utilization over a period of 6 days (136). Dietary inclusion of a recombinant fusion HDP derived from bovine lactoferrin also enhanced growth performance and decreased the incidence of diarrhea in ETEC-challenged piglets over a 21-day period (137). Across five different commercial farms, feeding a mixture of four recombinant HDPs, including lactoferrin, cecropin, defensin, and plectasin resulted in an enhancement of growth and feed efficiency and a reduction in diarrhea incidence in normally reared weanling pigs (138). Parallel to the studies above, supplementation of a synthetic HDP (AMP-A3 or P5) improved nutrient digestibility, intestinal morphology, and growth performance of normally reared weanling pigs in a 4-week trial, without affecting serum concentrations of IgA, IgG, or IgM (139, 140). Additionally, AMP-A3 and P5 appeared to reduce the titers of potentially harmful *Clostridium* spp. and coliforms in the ileum, cecum, and feces (140). Feeding a combination of two HDPs and a probiotic yeast led to an improvement in intestinal morphology and feed efficiency of piglets challenged with deoxynivalenol, a mycotoxin commonly found in grains (141, 142). In most trials above, HDPs performed indistinguishably with in-feed antibiotics in promoting growth, feed efficiency, and intestinal morphology (133).

The beneficial effects of direct feeding of HDPs are not limited to pigs. Supplementation of AMP-A3 to broiler chickens resulted in an increase in weight gain and feed efficiency over control birds, which was comparable to the birds fed avilamycin, an in-feed antibiotic (143). Intestinal morphology was also improved in broilers as measured by increased villus heights and villus height:crypt depth ratios in the small intestine (143). Similar to the results in pigs, broilers also displayed an improvement in nutrient utilization and a reduction in *Clostridium* spp. and coliforms in the intestinal tract (143). Supplementation of a yeast broth containing recombinant cecropin A/D improved intestinal morphology and nutrient utilization, with a tendency to enhance growth performance of broiler chickens in a 4-week trial (144). Cecropin A/D inclusion also reduced the total aerobic bacterial counts in both the jejunal and cecal contents of 42-day-old chickens (144). Collectively, these animal results have suggested the beneficial effects of HDP feeding, justifying dietary supplementation of HDPs as an antibiotic-alternative strategy in growth promotion and disease control.

However, because of HDP's proneness to enzymatic degradation and high production costs with either the synthetic or recombinant form, it may not be biologically efficient and economically effective for direct supplementation of HDPs in animal diets. Recently, several classes of small-molecule compounds, such as butyrate, have been found to induce HDP synthesis and enhance bacterial clearance in humans, chickens, pigs, and cattle without triggering inflammatory response (145–151). Dietary supplementation of these simple HDP-inducing compounds or their combinations may prove to be an alternative, cost-effective approach to antibiotics for livestock applications (152). However, the efficacy of these HDP-inducing compounds in promoting growth, intestinal health, and microbiota balance is yet to be demonstrated in animal trials.

CONCLUDING REMARKS

A comprehensive understanding of intestinal barrier function and its regulation is paramount to ensuring the sustainability of the food animal industry because disruption of the barrier results in disease states and decreased production efficiency (6). With potent antimicrobial and immunomodulatory properties, HDPs are further revealed to hold a new capacity to directly regulate barrier function. Aberrant synthesis of epithelial HDPs often leads to barrier dysfunction, and the diseases with impaired barrier integrity are commonly associated with reduced HDP synthesis, raising the possibility of treating barrier dysfunction with HDPs. However, a number of questions remain before HDP-based therapies can be devised for augmentation of intestinal barrier function, animal health, and production efficiency.

On the one hand, several structurally diverse HDPs (e.g., cathelicidins, defensins, and S100A7) have a similar ability to induce the expression of mucins and TJ proteins in both epidermal and intestinal epithelial cells. On the other hand, certain structurally similar HDPs (e.g., HBD-3 vs. HBD-1, -2, and -4) behave quite differently in their capacity to induce TJ proteins. Only HBD-3, but not other HBDs, has the capacity to enhance the barrier effect (110). Structure–activity relationship studies of HDPs may reveal whether there is an optimal physicochemical or structural feature for maximal induction of mucins and TJ proteins.

A number of different extracellular and intracellular receptors have been identified for human HDPs to mediate different physiological functions. However, the identities of the receptors utilized by different classes of HDPs to regulate paracellular permeability remain largely unclear in most cases. There are a number of questions on the signaling mechanisms of HDP-mediated barrier function that need to be answered. For example, what are the major receptors involved in HDP-induced synthesis of mucins and TJ proteins in humans? Do the same set of receptors that are utilized by human HDPs work similarly in the livestock species? Are there any new, unidentified receptors specific for regulation of barrier function? Besides the Rac1-aPKC, PI3K-GSK-3, and MAPK pathways, what are other major signaling pathways that mediate the barrier effect? How do these pathways cross-talk with each other? What are those major transcription factors that are required for induction of different mucin and TJ proteins? How and whether are mucins and TJ proteins differentially regulated? Do epithelial cells on epidermis, GI, respiratory, and genitourinary tracts engage in different receptors and signaling pathways?

Besides the abundance of TJ proteins, both posttranslational modifications of TJ proteins and the status of associated actomyosin ring have a strong impact on barrier permeability. Many agents are shown to alter the barrier function through phosphorylation of certain TJ proteins or through activation of MLCK, which in turn phosphorylates myosin light chain and causes contraction of the perijunctional actomyosin ring and opening of the paracellular pores. It will be important to examine whether and how HDPs influence posttranslational modifications of TJ proteins as well as the transcription and activity of MLCK.

Nevertheless, it is exciting to reveal a direct involvement of HDPs in barrier function and the potential of HDPs in enhancing gut health and animal performance. Additional studies along this line may someday turn the HDP-based therapies into reality. Although administration of synthetic peptides may be feasible in human medicine, it is cost-prohibitive in the livestock industry. Supplementation of exogenous recombinant HDPs or dietary compounds with the capacity to induce the synthesis of HDPs in the GI tract has emerged as a cost-effective strategy in antimicrobial therapy and may have potential to replace antibiotics in food animal production.

ACKNOWLEDGMENTS

This work was supported in part by Oklahoma Center for the Advancement of Science and Technology grants (AR12.2-077, HR12-051, and AR15.049), Oklahoma State University Cowboy Technologies Business Development Program grant, and Oklahoma Agricultural Experiment Station project H-2811. KR was supported by a USDA-NIFA National Needs Fellowship grant (2013-38420-20500).

REFERENCES

1. Turner JR. Intestinal mucosal barrier function in health and disease. *Nat Rev Immunol* (2009) **9**:799–809. doi:10.1038/nri2653
2. Johansson ME, Sjovall H, Hansson GC. The gastrointestinal mucus system in health and disease. *Nat Rev Gastroenterol Hepatol* (2013) **10**:352–61. doi:10.1038/nrgastro.2013.35
3. Groschwitz KR, Hogan SP. Intestinal barrier function: molecular regulation and disease pathogenesis. *J Allergy Clin Immunol* (2009) **124**:3–20; quiz 1–2. doi:10.1016/j.jaci.2009.05.038
4. Rescigno M. The intestinal epithelial barrier in the control of homeostasis and immunity. *Trends Immunol* (2011) **32**:256–64. doi:10.1016/j.it.2011.04.003
5. Liu D, Guo Y, Wang Z, Yuan J. Exogenous lysozyme influences *Clostridium perfringens* colonization and intestinal barrier function in broiler chickens. *Avian Pathol* (2010) **39**:17–24. doi:10.1080/03079450903447404
6. Mani V, Weber TE, Baumgard LH, Gabler NK. Growth and development symposium: endotoxin, inflammation, and intestinal function in livestock. *J Anim Sci* (2012) **90**:1452–65. doi:10.2527/jas.2011-4627
7. Zasloff M. Antimicrobial peptides of multicellular organisms. *Nature* (2002) **415**:389–95. doi:10.1038/415389a
8. Brogden KA, Ackermann M, McCray PB Jr, Tack BF. Antimicrobial peptides in animals and their role in host defences. *Int J Antimicrob Agents* (2003) **22**:465–78. doi:10.1016/S0924-8579(03)00180-8
9. Hancock RE, Nijnik A, Philpott DJ. Modulating immunity as a therapy for bacterial infections. *Nat Rev Microbiol* (2012) **10**:243–54. doi:10.1038/nrmicro2745
10. Hilchie AL, Wuerth K, Hancock RE. Immune modulation by multifaceted cationic host defense (antimicrobial) peptides. *Nat Chem Biol* (2013) **9**:761–8. doi:10.1038/nchembio.1393
11. Mansour SC, Pena OM, Hancock RE. Host defense peptides: front-line immunomodulators. *Trends Immunol* (2014) **35**:443–50. doi:10.1016/j.it.2014.07.004
12. Kolls JK, McCray PB Jr, Chan YR. Cytokine-mediated regulation of antimicrobial proteins. *Nat Rev Immunol* (2008) **8**:829–35. doi:10.1038/nri2433
13. Gallo RL, Hooper LV. Epithelial antimicrobial defence of the skin and intestine. *Nat Rev Immunol* (2012) **12**:503–16. doi:10.1038/nri3228
14. Selsted ME, Ouellette AJ. Mammalian defensins in the antimicrobial immune response. *Nat Immunol* (2005) **6**:551–7. doi:10.1038/ni1206
15. Zanetti M. Cathelicidins, multifunctional peptides of the innate immunity. *J Leukoc Biol* (2004) **75**:39–48. doi:10.1189/jlb.0403147
16. Donato R, Cannon BR, Sorci G, Riuzzi F, Hsu K, Weber DJ, et al. Functions of s100 proteins. *Curr Mol Med* (2013) **13**:24–57. doi:10.2174/15665240113 07010024
17. Bresnick AR, Weber DJ, Zimmer DB. S100 proteins in cancer. *Nat Rev Cancer* (2015) **15**:96–109. doi:10.1038/nrc3893
18. Rosenberg HF. Rnase a ribonucleases and host defense: an evolving story. *J Leukoc Biol* (2008) **83**:1079–87. doi:10.1189/jlb.1107725
19. Simanski M, Koten B, Schroder JM, Glaser R, Harder J. Antimicrobial RNAses in cutaneous defense. *J Innate Immun* (2012) **4**:241–7. doi:10.1159/000335029
20. Santaolalla R, Abreu MT. Innate immunity in the small intestine. *Curr Opin Gastroenterol* (2012) **28**:124–9. doi:10.1097/MOG.0b013e3283506559
21. Royet J, Gupta D, Dziarski R. Peptidoglycan recognition proteins: modulators of the microbiome and inflammation. *Nat Rev Immunol* (2011) **11**:837–51. doi:10.1038/nri3089
22. Patil A, Hughes AL, Zhang G. Rapid evolution and diversification of mammalian alpha-defensins as revealed by comparative analysis of rodent and primate genes. *Physiol Genomics* (2004) **20**:1–11. doi:10.1152/physiolgenomics.00150.2004
23. Patil AA, Cai Y, Sang Y, Blecha F, Zhang G. Cross-species analysis of the mammalian beta-defensin gene family: presence of syntenic gene clusters and preferential expression in the male reproductive tract. *Physiol Genomics* (2005) **23**:5–17. doi:10.1152/physiolgenomics.00104.2005
24. Meade KG, Cormican P, Narciandi F, Lloyd A, O'Farrelly C. Bovine beta-defensin gene family: opportunities to improve animal health? *Physiol Genomics* (2014) **46**:17–28. doi:10.1152/physiolgenomics.00085.2013
25. Choi MK, Le MT, Nguyen DT, Choi H, Kim W, Kim JH, et al. Genome-level identification, gene expression, and comparative analysis of porcine ss-defensin genes. *BMC Genet* (2012) **13**:98. doi:10.1186/1471-2156-13-98
26. Xiao Y, Hughes AL, Ando J, Matsuda Y, Cheng JF, Skinner-Noble D, et al. A genome-wide screen identifies a single beta-defensin gene cluster in the chicken: implications for the origin and evolution of mammalian defensins. *BMC Genomics* (2004) **5**:56. doi:10.1186/1471-2164-5-56
27. Lynn DJ, Higgs R, Lloyd AT, O'farrelly C, Herve-Grepinet V, Nys Y, et al. Avian beta-defensin nomenclature: a community proposed update. *Immunol Lett* (2007) **110**:86–9. doi:10.1016/j.imlet.2007.03.007
28. Gudmundsson GH, Agerberth B, Odeberg J, Bergman T, Olsson B, Salcedo R. The human gene fall39 and processing of the cathelin precursor to the antibacterial peptide ll-37 in granulocytes. *Eur J Biochem* (1996) **238**:325–32. doi:10.1111/j.1432-1033.1996.0325z.x
29. Xiao Y, Cai Y, Bommineni YR, Fernando SC, Prakash O, Gilliland SE, et al. Identification and functional characterization of three chicken cathelicidins with potent antimicrobial activity. *J Biol Chem* (2006) **281**:2858–67. doi:10.1074/jbc.M507180200
30. Goitsuka R, Chen CL, Benyon L, Asano Y, Kitamura D, Cooper MD. Chicken cathelicidin-b1, an antimicrobial guardian at the mucosal m cell gateway. *Proc Natl Acad Sci U S A* (2007) **104**:15063–8. doi:10.1073/pnas.0707037104

31. Whelehan CJ, Barry-Reidy A, Meade KG, Eckersall PD, Chapwanya A, Narciandi F, et al. Characterisation and expression profile of the bovine cathelicidin gene repertoire in mammary tissue. *BMC Genomics* (2014) **15**:128. doi:10.1186/1471-2164-15-128
32. Sang Y, Blecha F. Porcine host defense peptides: expanding repertoire and functions. *Dev Comp Immunol* (2009) **33**:334–43. doi:10.1016/j.dci.2008.05.006
33. Lynn DJ, Higgs R, Gaines S, Tierney J, James T, Lloyd AT, et al. Bioinformatic discovery and initial characterisation of nine novel antimicrobial peptide genes in the chicken. *Immunogenetics* (2004) **56**:170–7. doi:10.1007/s00251-004-0675-0
34. Van Dijk A, Veldhuizen EJ, Van Asten AJ, Haagsman HP. Cmap27, a novel chicken cathelicidin-like antimicrobial protein. *Vet Immunol Immunopathol* (2005) **106**:321–7. doi:10.1016/j.vetimm.2005.03.003
35. Mabbott NA, Donaldson DS, Ohno H, Williams IR, Mahajan A. Microfold (m) cells: important immunosurveillance posts in the intestinal epithelium. *Mucosal Immunol* (2013) **6**:666–77. doi:10.1038/mi.2013.30
36. Wang G. Human antimicrobial peptides and proteins. *Pharmaceuticals (Basel)* (2014) **7**:545–94. doi:10.3390/ph7050545
37. Xiao Y, Dai H, Bommineni YR, Soulages JL, Gong YX, Prakash O, et al. Structure-activity relationships of fowlicidin-1, a cathelicidin antimicrobial peptide in chicken. *FEBS J* (2006) **273**:2581–93. doi:10.1111/j.1742-4658.2006.05261.x
38. Bommineni YR, Dai H, Gong YX, Soulages JL, Fernando SC, Desilva U, et al. Fowlicidin-3 is an alpha-helical cationic host defense peptide with potent antibacterial and lipopolysaccharide-neutralizing activities. *FEBS J* (2007) **274**:418–28. doi:10.1111/j.1742-4658.2006.05589.x
39. Xiao Y, Herrera AI, Bommineni YR, Soulages JL, Prakash O, Zhang G. The central kink region of fowlicidin-2, an alpha-helical host defense peptide, is critically involved in bacterial killing and endotoxin neutralization. *J Innate Immun* (2009) **1**:268–80. doi:10.1159/000174822
40. Van Dijk A, Veldhuizen EJ, Haagsman HP. Avian defensins. *Vet Immunol Immunopathol* (2008) **124**:1–18. doi:10.1016/j.vetimm.2007.12.006
41. Cuperus T, Coorens M, Van Dijk A, Haagsman HP. Avian host defense peptides. *Dev Comp Immunol* (2013) **41**:352–69. doi:10.1016/j.dci.2013.04.019
42. Zhang G, Sunkara LT. Avian antimicrobial host defense peptides: from biology to therapeutic applications. *Pharmaceuticals (Basel)* (2014) **7**:220–47. doi:10.3390/ph7030220
43. Brogden KA. Antimicrobial peptides: pore formers or metabolic inhibitors in bacteria? *Nat Rev Microbiol* (2005) **3**:238–50. doi:10.1038/nrmicro1098
44. Peschel A, Sahl HG. The co-evolution of host cationic antimicrobial peptides and microbial resistance. *Nat Rev Microbiol* (2006) **4**:529–36. doi:10.1038/nrmicro1441
45. Nuding S, Zabel LT, Enders C, Porter E, Fellermann K, Wehkamp J, et al. Antibacterial activity of human defensins on anaerobic intestinal bacterial species: a major role of hbd-3. *Microbes Infect* (2009) **11**:384–93. doi:10.1016/j.micinf.2009.01.001
46. Bommineni YR, Pham GH, Sunkara LT, Achanta M, Zhang G. Immune regulatory activities of fowlicidin-1, a cathelicidin host defense peptide. *Mol Immunol* (2014) **59**:55–63. doi:10.1016/j.molimm.2014.01.004
47. Bommineni YR, Achanta M, Alexander J, Sunkara LT, Ritchey JW, Zhang G. A fowlicidin-1 analog protects mice from lethal infections induced by methicillin-resistant *Staphylococcus aureus*. *Peptides* (2010) **31**:1225–30. doi:10.1016/j.peptides.2010.03.037
48. Mackenzie-Dyck S, Attah-Poku S, Juillard V, Babiuk LA, Van Drunen Littel-Van Den Hurk S. The synthetic peptides bovine enteric beta-defensin (ebd), bovine neutrophil beta-defensin (bnbd) 9 and bnbd 3 are chemotactic for immature bovine dendritic cells. *Vet Immunol Immunopathol* (2011) **143**:87–107. doi:10.1016/j.vetimm.2011.06.028
49. Ikeda Y, Young LH, Scalia R, Ross CR, Lefer AM. Pr-39, a proline/arginine-rich antimicrobial peptide, exerts cardioprotective effects in myocardial ischemia-reperfusion. *Cardiovasc Res* (2001) **49**:69–77. doi:10.1016/S0008-6363(00)00226-1
50. Shi J, Ross CR, Leto TL, Blecha F. Pr-39, a proline-rich antibacterial peptide that inhibits phagocyte nadph oxidase activity by binding to src homology 3 domains of p47 phox. *Proc Natl Acad Sci U S A* (1996) **93**:6014–8. doi:10.1073/pnas.93.12.6014
51. Gallo RL, Ono M, Povsic T, Page C, Eriksson E, Klagsbrun M, et al. Syndecans, cell surface heparan sulfate proteoglycans, are induced by a proline-rich antimicrobial peptide from wounds. *Proc Natl Acad Sci U S A* (1994) **91**:11035–9. doi:10.1073/pnas.91.23.11035
52. Li J, Post M, Volk R, Gao Y, Li M, Metais C, et al. Pr39, a peptide regulator of angiogenesis. *Nat Med* (2000) **6**:49–55. doi:10.1038/71527
53. Baumann A, Demoulins T, Python S, Summerfield A. Porcine cathelicidins efficiently complex and deliver nucleic acids to plasmacytoid dendritic cells and can thereby mediate bacteria-induced ifn-alpha responses. *J Immunol* (2014) **193**:364–71. doi:10.4049/jimmunol.1303219
54. Corfield AP. Mucins: a biologically relevant glycan barrier in mucosal protection. *Biochim Biophys Acta* (2015) **1850**:236–52. doi:10.1016/j.bbagen.2014.05.003
55. Linden SK, Sutton P, Karlsson NG, Korolik V, McGuckin MA. Mucins in the mucosal barrier to infection. *Mucosal Immunol* (2008) **1**:183–97. doi:10.1038/mi.2008.5
56. Rose MC, Voynow JA. Respiratory tract mucin genes and mucin glycoproteins in health and disease. *Physiol Rev* (2006) **86**:245–78. doi:10.1152/physrev.00010.2005
57. Etzold S, Juge N. Structural insights into bacterial recognition of intestinal mucins. *Curr Opin Struct Biol* (2014) **28**:23–31. doi:10.1016/j.sbi.2014.07.002
58. Hollingsworth MA, Swanson BJ. Mucins in cancer: protection and control of the cell surface. *Nat Rev Cancer* (2004) **4**:45–60. doi:10.1038/nrc1251
59. Hoorens PR, Rinaldi M, Li RW, Goddeeris B, Claerebout E, Vercruysse J, et al. Genome wide analysis of the bovine mucin genes and their gastrointestinal transcription profile. *BMC Genomics* (2011) **12**:140. doi:10.1186/1471-2164-12-140
60. Kim CH, Oh Y, Ha Y, Ahn Q, Kim SH, Cho KD, et al. Expression of mucins in the mucosal surface of small intestines in 1 week-old pigs. *J Vet Med Sci* (2010) **72**:245–7. doi:10.1292/jvms.09-0308
61. Kim CH, Lee K, Han K, Oh Y, Kim D, Seo HW, et al. Expression of mucins on the mucosal surface of lungs of 4-week-old pigs. *Vet Res Commun* (2011) **35**:255–60. doi:10.1007/s11259-011-9465-y
62. Lang T, Hansson GC, Samuelsson T. An inventory of mucin genes in the chicken genome shows that the mucin domain of Muc13 is encoded by multiple exons and that ovomucin is part of a locus of related gel-forming mucins. *BMC Genomics* (2006) **7**:197. doi:10.1186/1471-2164-7-197
63. Van Der Sluis M, De Koning BA, De Bruijn AC, Velcich A, Meijerink JP, Van Goudoever JB, et al. Muc2-deficient mice spontaneously develop colitis, indicating that Muc2 is critical for colonic protection. *Gastroenterology* (2006) **131**:117–29. doi:10.1053/j.gastro.2006.04.020
64. Bergstrom KS, Kissoon-Singh V, Gibson DL, Ma C, Montero M, Sham HP, et al. Muc2 protects against lethal infectious colitis by disassociating pathogenic and commensal bacteria from the colonic mucosa. *PLoS Pathog* (2010) **6**:e1000902. doi:10.1371/journal.ppat.1000902
65. McAuley JL, Linden SK, Png CW, King RM, Pennington HL, Gendler SJ, et al. Muc1 cell surface mucin is a critical element of the mucosal barrier to infection. *J Clin Invest* (2007) **117**:2313–24. doi:10.1172/JCI26705
66. McGuckin MA, Every AL, Skene CD, Linden SK, Chionh YT, Swierczak A, et al. Muc1 mucin limits both *Helicobacter pylori* colonization of the murine gastric mucosa and associated gastritis. *Gastroenterology* (2007) **133**:1210–8. doi:10.1053/j.gastro.2007.07.003
67. Zarepour M, Bhullar K, Montero M, Ma C, Huang T, Velcich A, et al. The mucin muc2 limits pathogen burdens and epithelial barrier dysfunction during *Salmonella enterica* serovar typhimurium colitis. *Infect Immun* (2013) **81**:3672–83. doi:10.1128/IAI.00854-13
68. An G, Wei B, Xia B, McDaniel JM, Ju T, Cummings RD, et al. Increased susceptibility to colitis and colorectal tumors in mice lacking core 3-derived O-glycans. *J Exp Med* (2007) **204**:1417–29. doi:10.1084/jem.20061929
69. Buisine MP, Desreumaux P, Debailleul V, Gambiez L, Geboes K, Ectors N, et al. Abnormalities in mucin gene expression in Crohn's disease. *Inflamm Bowel Dis* (1999) **5**:24–32. doi:10.1002/ibd.3780050105
70. Corfield AP, Carroll D, Myerscough N, Probert CS. Mucins in the gastrointestinal tract in health and disease. *Front Biosci* (2001) **6**:D1321–57. doi:10.2741/Corfield
71. Peterson LW, Artis D. Intestinal epithelial cells: regulators of barrier function and immune homeostasis. *Nat Rev Immunol* (2014) **14**:141–53. doi:10.1038/nri3608
72. Suzuki T. Regulation of intestinal epithelial permeability by tight junctions. *Cell Mol Life Sci* (2013) **70**:631–59. doi:10.1007/s00018-012-1070-x

73. Gunzel D, Yu AS. Claudins and the modulation of tight junction permeability. *Physiol Rev* (2013) **93**:525–69. doi:10.1152/physrev.00019.2012
74. Furuse M, Hirase T, Itoh M, Nagafuchi A, Yonemura S, Tsukita S, et al. Occludin: a novel integral membrane protein localizing at tight junctions. *J Cell Biol* (1993) **123**:1777–88. doi:10.1083/jcb.123.6.1777
75. Cummins PM. Occludin: one protein, many forms. *Mol Cell Biol* (2012) **32**:242–50. doi:10.1128/MCB.06029-11
76. Luissint AC, Nusrat A, Parkos CA. JAM-related proteins in mucosal homeostasis and inflammation. *Semin Immunopathol* (2014) **36**:211–26. doi:10.1007/s00281-014-0421-0
77. Kojima T, Ninomiya T, Konno T, Kohno T, Taniguchi M, Sawada N. Expression of tricellulin in epithelial cells and non-epithelial cells. *Histol Histopathol* (2013) **28**:1383–92. doi:10.14670/HH-28.1383
78. Herve JC, Derangeon M, Sarrouilhe D, Bourmeyster N. Influence of the scaffolding protein zonula occludens (ZOs) on membrane channels. *Biochim Biophys Acta* (2014) **1838**:595–604. doi:10.1016/j.bbamem.2013.07.006
79. Citi S, Pulimeno P, Paschoud S. Cingulin, paracingulin, and plekha7: signaling and cytoskeletal adaptors at the apical junctional complex. *Ann N Y Acad Sci* (2012) **1257**:125–32. doi:10.1111/j.1749-6632.2012.06506.x
80. Suzuki H, Nishizawa T, Tani K, Yamazaki Y, Tamura A, Ishitani R, et al. Crystal structure of a claudin provides insight into the architecture of tight junctions. *Science* (2014) **344**:304–7. doi:10.1126/science.1248571
81. Suzuki H, Tani K, Tamura A, Tsukita S, Fujiyoshi Y. Model for the architecture of claudin-based paracellular ion channels through tight junctions. *J Mol Biol* (2015) **427**:291–7. doi:10.1016/j.jmb.2014.10.020
82. Mariano C, Sasaki H, Brites D, Brito MA. A look at tricellulin and its role in tight junction formation and maintenance. *Eur J Cell Biol* (2011) **90**:787–96. doi:10.1016/j.ejcb.2011.06.005
83. Ebnet K, Suzuki A, Ohno S, Vestweber D. Junctional adhesion molecules (JAMs): more molecules with dual functions? *J Cell Sci* (2004) **117**:19–29. doi:10.1242/jcs.00930
84. Al-Sadi R, Khatib K, Guo S, Ye D, Youssef M, Ma T. Occludin regulates macromolecule flux across the intestinal epithelial tight junction barrier. *Am J Physiol Gastrointest Liver Physiol* (2011) **300**:G1054–64. doi:10.1152/ajpgi.00055.2011
85. Cunningham KE, Turner JR. Myosin light chain kinase: pulling the strings of epithelial tight junction function. *Ann N Y Acad Sci* (2012) **1258**:34–42. doi:10.1111/j.1749-6632.2012.06526.x
86. Ye D, Ma I, Ma TY. Molecular mechanism of tumor necrosis factor-alpha modulation of intestinal epithelial tight junction barrier. *Am J Physiol Gastrointest Liver Physiol* (2006) **290**:G496–504. doi:10.1152/ajpgi.00318.2005
87. Al-Sadi R, Ye D, Dokladny K, Ma TY. Mechanism of IL-1beta-induced increase in intestinal epithelial tight junction permeability. *J Immunol* (2008) **180**:5653–61. doi:10.4049/jimmunol.180.8.5653
88. Sonoda N, Furuse M, Sasaki H, Yonemura S, Katahira J, Horiguchi Y, et al. *Clostridium perfringens* enterotoxin fragment removes specific claudins from tight junction strands: evidence for direct involvement of claudins in tight junction barrier. *J Cell Biol* (1999) **147**:195–204. doi:10.1083/jcb.147.1.195
89. Smith F, Clark JE, Overman BL, Tozel CC, Huang JH, Rivier JE, et al. Early weaning stress impairs development of mucosal barrier function in the porcine intestine. *Am J Physiol Gastrointest Liver Physiol* (2010) **298**:G352–63. doi:10.1152/ajpgi.00081.2009
90. Hu CH, Xiao K, Luan ZS, Song J. Early weaning increases intestinal permeability, alters expression of cytokine and tight junction proteins, and activates mitogen-activated protein kinases in pigs. *J Anim Sci* (2013) **91**:1094–101. doi:10.2527/jas.2012-5796
91. Antoni L, Nuding S, Wehkamp J, Stange EF. Intestinal barrier in inflammatory bowel disease. *World J Gastroenterol* (2014) **20**:1165–79. doi:10.3748/wjg.v20.i5.1165
92. Wehkamp J, Salzman NH, Porter E, Nuding S, Weichenthal M, Petras RE, et al. Reduced paneth cell alpha-defensins in ileal crohn's disease. *Proc Natl Acad Sci U S A* (2005) **102**:18129–34. doi:10.1073/pnas.0505256102
93. Peyrin-Biroulet L, Beisner J, Wang G, Nuding S, Oommen ST, Kelly D, et al. Peroxisome proliferator-activated receptor gamma activation is required for maintenance of innate antimicrobial immunity in the colon. *Proc Natl Acad Sci U S A* (2010) **107**:8772–7. doi:10.1073/pnas.0905745107
94. Wehkamp J, Fellermann K, Herrlinger KR, Baxmann S, Schmidt K, Schwind B, et al. Human beta-defensin 2 but not beta-defensin 1 is expressed preferentially in colonic mucosa of inflammatory bowel disease. *Eur J Gastroenterol Hepatol* (2002) **14**:745–52. doi:10.1097/00042737-200207000-00006
95. Wehkamp J, Harder J, Weichenthal M, Mueller O, Herrlinger KR, Fellermann K, et al. Inducible and constitutive beta-defensins are differentially expressed in Crohn's disease and ulcerative colitis. *Inflamm Bowel Dis* (2003) **9**:215–23. doi:10.1097/00054725-200307000-00001
96. Fahlgren A, Hammarstrom S, Danielsson A, Hammarstrom ML. Beta-defensin-3 and -4 in intestinal epithelial cells display increased mRNA expression in ulcerative colitis. *Clin Exp Immunol* (2004) **137**:379–85. doi:10.1111/j.1365-2249.2004.02543.x
97. Schauber J, Rieger D, Weiler F, Wehkamp J, Eck M, Fellermann K, et al. Heterogeneous expression of human cathelicidin hCAP18/ll-37 in inflammatory bowel diseases. *Eur J Gastroenterol Hepatol* (2006) **18**:615–21. doi:10.1097/00042737-200606000-00007
98. Wehkamp J, Harder J, Weichenthal M, Schwab M, Schaffeler E, Schlee M, et al. Nod2 (card15) mutations in Crohn's disease are associated with diminished mucosal alpha-defensin expression. *Gut* (2004) **53**:1658–64. doi:10.1136/gut.2003.032805
99. Kobayashi KS, Chamaillard M, Ogura Y, Henegariu O, Inohara N, Nunez G, et al. Nod2-dependent regulation of innate and adaptive immunity in the intestinal tract. *Science* (2005) **307**:731–4. doi:10.1126/science.1104911
100. Aberg KM, Man MQ, Gallo RL, Ganz T, Crumrine D, Brown BE, et al. Co-regulation and interdependence of the mammalian epidermal permeability and antimicrobial barriers. *J Invest Dermatol* (2008) **128**:917–25. doi:10.1038/sj.jid.5701099
101. Otte JM, Werner I, Brand S, Chromik AM, Schmitz F, Kleine M, et al. Human beta defensin 2 promotes intestinal wound healing in vitro. *J Cell Biochem* (2008) **104**:2286–97. doi:10.1002/jcb.21787
102. Cobo ER, Kissoon-Singh V, Moreau F, Chadee K. Colonic muc2 mucin regulates the expression and antimicrobial activity of beta-defensin 2. *Mucosal Immunol* (2015) **8**(6):1360–72. doi:10.1038/mi.2015.27
103. Tai EK, Wong HP, Lam EK, Wu WK, Yu L, Koo MW, et al. Cathelicidin stimulates colonic mucus synthesis by up-regulating Muc1 and Muc2 expression through a mitogen-activated protein kinase pathway. *J Cell Biochem* (2008) **104**:251–8. doi:10.1002/jcb.21615
104. Otte JM, Zdebik AE, Brand S, Chromik AM, Strauss S, Schmitz F, et al. Effects of the cathelicidin LL-37 on intestinal epithelial barrier integrity. *Regul Pept* (2009) **156**:104–17. doi:10.1016/j.regpep.2009.03.009
105. Tang ZR, Deng H, Zhang XL, Zen Y, Xiao DF, Sun WZ, et al. Effects of orally administering the antimicrobial peptide buforin II on small intestinal mucosal membrane integrity, the expression of tight junction proteins and protective factors in weaned piglets challenged by enterotoxigenic *Escherichia coli*. *Anim Feed Sci Technol* (2013) **186**:177–85. doi:10.1016/j.anifeedsci.2013.10.012
106. Song D, Zong X, Zhang H, Wang T, Yi H, Luan C, et al. Antimicrobial peptide cathelicidin-BF prevents intestinal barrier dysfunction in a mouse model of endotoxemia. *Int Immunopharmacol* (2015) **25**:141–7. doi:10.1016/j.intimp.2015.01.017
107. Han F, Zhang H, Xia X, Xiong H, Song D, Zong X, et al. Porcine beta-defensin 2 attenuates inflammation and mucosal lesions in dextran sodium sulfate-induced colitis. *J Immunol* (2015) **194**:1882–93. doi:10.4049/jimmunol.1402300
108. Zhang Y, Zhu M, Yang Z, Pan X, Jiang Y, Sun C, et al. The human cathelicidin LL-37 induces muc5ac mucin production by airway epithelial cells via TACE-TGF-alpha-EGFR pathway. *Exp Lung Res* (2014) **40**:333–42. doi:10.3109/01902148.2014.926434
109. Akiyama T, Niyonsaba F, Kiatsurayanon C, Nguyen TT, Ushio H, Fujimura T, et al. The human cathelicidin LL-37 host defense peptide upregulates tight junction-related proteins and increases human epidermal keratinocyte barrier function. *J Innate Immun* (2014) **6**:739–53. doi:10.1159/000362789
110. Kiatsurayanon C, Niyonsaba F, Smithrithee R, Akiyama T, Ushio H, Hara M, et al. Host defense (antimicrobial) peptide, human beta-defensin-3, improves the function of the epithelial tight-junction barrier in human keratinocytes. *J Invest Dermatol* (2014) **134**:2163–73. doi:10.1038/jid.2014.143
111. Hattori F, Kiatsurayanon C, Okumura K, Ogawa H, Ikeda S, Okamoto K, et al. The antimicrobial protein S100a7/psoriasin enhances the expression of keratinocyte differentiation markers and strengthens the skin's tight junction barrier. *Br J Dermatol* (2014) **171**:742–53. doi:10.1111/bjd.13125

112. Choi KY, Chow LN, Mookherjee N. Cationic host defence peptides: multifaceted role in immune modulation and inflammation. *J Innate Immun* (2012) **4**:361–70. doi:10.1159/000336630
113. Erridge C. Endogenous ligands of TLR2 and TLR4: agonists or assistants? *J Leukoc Biol* (2010) **87**:989–99. doi:10.1189/jlb.1209775
114. Iitaka D, Moodley S, Shimizu H, Bai XH, Liu M. PKCdelta-iPLA2-PGE2-PPARgamma signaling cascade mediates TNF-alpha induced claudin 1 expression in human lung carcinoma cells. *Cell Signal* (2015) **27**:568–77. doi:10.1016/j.cellsig.2014.12.015
115. Iden S, Misselwitz S, Peddibhotla SS, Tuncay H, Rehder D, Gerke V, et al. aPKC phosphorylates JAM-A at Ser285 to promote cell contact maturation and tight junction formation. *J Cell Biol* (2012) **196**:623–39. doi:10.1083/jcb.201104143
116. Suzuki A, Ishiyama C, Hashiba K, Shimizu M, Ebnet K, Ohno S. aPKC kinase activity is required for the asymmetric differentiation of the premature junctional complex during epithelial cell polarization. *J Cell Sci* (2002) **115**:3565–73. doi:10.1242/jcs.00032
117. Beurel E, Michalek SM, Jope RS. Innate and adaptive immune responses regulated by glycogen synthase kinase-3 (GSK3). *Trends Immunol* (2010) **31**:24–31. doi:10.1016/j.it.2009.09.007
118. Severson EA, Kwon M, Hilgarth RS, Parkos CA, Nusrat A. Glycogen synthase kinase 3 (GSK-3) influences epithelial barrier function by regulating occludin, claudin-1 and e-cadherin expression. *Biochem Biophys Res Commun* (2010) **397**:592–7. doi:10.1016/j.bbrc.2010.05.164
119. González-Mariscal L, Tapia R, Chamorro D. Crosstalk of tight junction components with signaling pathways. *Biochim Biophys Acta* (2008) **1778**:729–56. doi:10.1016/j.bbamem.2007.08.018
120. Little D, Dean RA, Young KM, McKane SA, Martin LD, Jones SL, et al. PI3K signaling is required for prostaglandin-induced mucosal recovery in ischemia-injured porcine ileum. *Am J Physiol Gastrointest Liver Physiol* (2003) **284**:G46–56. doi:10.1152/ajpgi.00121.2002
121. Woo PL, Ching D, Guan Y, Firestone GL. Requirement for ras and phosphatidylinositol 3-kinase signaling uncouples the glucocorticoid-induced junctional organization and transepithelial electrical resistance in mammary tumor cells. *J Biol Chem* (1999) **274**:32818–28. doi:10.1074/jbc.274.46.32818
122. Su B, Karin M. Mitogen-activated protein kinase cascades and regulation of gene expression. *Curr Opin Immunol* (1996) **8**:402–11. doi:10.1016/S0952-7915(96)80131-2
123. Lozupone CA, Stombaugh JI, Gordon JI, Jansson JK, Knight R. Diversity, stability and resilience of the human gut microbiota. *Nature* (2012) **489**:220–30. doi:10.1038/nature11550
124. Saulnier DM, Kolida S, Gibson GR. Microbiology of the human intestinal tract and approaches for its dietary modulation. *Curr Pharm Des* (2009) **15**:1403–14. doi:10.2174/138161209788168128
125. Salzman NH. Paneth cell defensins and the regulation of the microbiome: detente at mucosal surfaces. *Gut Microbes* (2010) **1**:401–6. doi:10.4161/gmic.1.6.14076
126. McDermott AJ, Huffnagle GB. The microbiome and regulation of mucosal immunity. *Immunology* (2014) **142**:24–31. doi:10.1111/imm.12231
127. Kabat AM, Srinivasan N, Maloy KJ. Modulation of immune development and function by intestinal microbiota. *Trends Immunol* (2014) **35**:507–17. doi:10.1016/j.it.2014.07.010
128. Ostaff MJ, Stange EF, Wehkamp J. Antimicrobial peptides and gut microbiota in homeostasis and pathology. *EMBO Mol Med* (2013) **5**:1465–83. doi:10.1002/emmm.201201773
129. Koon HW, Shih DQ, Chen J, Bakirtzi K, Hing TC, Law I, et al. Cathelicidin signaling via the toll-like receptor protects against colitis in mice. *Gastroenterology* (2011) **141**(1852–63):e1–3. doi:10.1053/j.gastro.2011.06.079
130. Salzman NH, Ghosh D, Huttner KM, Paterson Y, Bevins CL. Protection against enteric salmonellosis in transgenic mice expressing a human intestinal defensin. *Nature* (2003) **422**:522–6. doi:10.1038/nature01520
131. Wilson CL, Ouellette AJ, Satchell DP, Ayabe T, Lopez-Boado YS, Stratman JL, et al. Regulation of intestinal alpha-defensin activation by the metalloproteinase matrilysin in innate host defense. *Science* (1999) **286**:113–7. doi:10.1126/science.286.5437.113
132. Salzman NH, Hung K, Haribhai D, Chu H, Karlsson-Sjoberg J, Amir E, et al. Enteric defensins are essential regulators of intestinal microbial ecology. *Nat Immunol* (2010) **11**:76–83. doi:10.1038/ni.1825
133. Xiao H, Shao F, Wu M, Ren W, Xiong X, Tan B, et al. The application of antimicrobial peptides as growth and health promoters for swine. *J Anim Sci Biotechnol* (2015) **6**:19. doi:10.1186/s40104-015-0018-z
134. Wang S, Thacker PA, Watford M, Qiao S. Functions of antimicrobial peptides in gut homeostasis. *Curr Protein Pept Sci* (2015) **16**:582–91. doi:10.2174/1389203716666150630135847
135. Cutler SA, Lonergan SM, Cornick N, Johnson AK, Stahl CH. Dietary inclusion of colicin E1 is effective in preventing postweaning diarrhea caused by F18-positive *Escherichia coli* in pigs. *Antimicrob Agents Chemother* (2007) **51**:3830–5. doi:10.1128/AAC.00360-07
136. Wu S, Zhang F, Huang Z, Liu H, Xie C, Zhang J, et al. Effects of the antimicrobial peptide cecropin ad on performance and intestinal health in weaned piglets challenged with *Escherichia coli*. *Peptides* (2012) **35**:225–30. doi:10.1016/j.peptides.2012.03.030
137. Tang XS, Fatufe AA, Yin YL, Tang ZR, Wang SP, Liu ZQ, et al. Dietary supplementation with recombinant lactoferrampin-lactoferricin improves growth performance and affects serum parameters in piglets. *J Anim Vet Adv* (2012) **11**:2548–55. doi:10.3923/javaa.2012.2548.2555
138. Xiong X, Yang HS, Li L, Wang YF, Huang RL, Li FN, et al. Effects of antimicrobial peptides in nursery diets on growth performance of pigs reared on five different farms. *Livest Sci* (2014) **167**:206–10. doi:10.1016/j.livsci.2014.04.024
139. Yoon JH, Ingale SL, Kim JS, Kim KH, Lohakare J, Park YK, et al. Effects of dietary supplementation with antimicrobial peptide-P5 on growth performance, apparent total tract digestibility, faecal and intestinal microflora and intestinal morphology of weanling pigs. *J Sci Food Agric* (2013) **93**:587–92. doi:10.1002/jsfa.5840
140. Yoon JH, Ingale SL, Kim JS, Kim KH, Lee SH, Park YK, et al. Effects of dietary supplementation of synthetic antimicrobial peptide-A3 and P5 on growth performance, apparent total tract digestibility of nutrients, fecal and intestinal microflora and intestinal morphology in weanling pigs. *Livest Sci* (2014) **159**:53–60. doi:10.1016/j.livsci.2013.10.025
141. Xiao H, Wu MM, Tan BE, Yin YL, Li TJ, Xiao DF, et al. Effects of composite antimicrobial peptides in weanling piglets challenged with deoxynivalenol: I. Growth performance, immune function, and antioxidation capacity. *J Anim Sci* (2013) **91**:4772–80. doi:10.2527/jas.2013-6426
142. Xiao H, Tan BE, Wu MM, Yin YL, Li TJ, Yuan DX, et al. Effects of composite antimicrobial peptides in weanling piglets challenged with deoxynivalenol: II. Intestinal morphology and function. *J Anim Sci* (2013) **91**:4750–6. doi:10.2527/jas.2013-6427
143. Choi SC, Ingale SL, Kim JS, Park YK, Kwon IK, Chae BJ. An antimicrobial peptide-A3: effects on growth performance, nutrient retention, intestinal and faecal microflora and intestinal morphology of broilers. *Br Poult Sci* (2013) **54**:738–46. doi:10.1080/00071668.2013.838746
144. Wen LF, He JG. Dose-response effects of an antimicrobial peptide, a cecropin hybrid, on growth performance, nutrient utilisation, bacterial counts in the digesta and intestinal morphology in broilers. *Br J Nutr* (2012) **108**:1756–63. doi:10.1017/S0007114511007240
145. Schauber J, Svanholm C, Termen S, Iffland K, Menzel T, Scheppach W, et al. Expression of the cathelicidin LL-37 is modulated by short chain fatty acids in colonocytes: relevance of signalling pathways. *Gut* (2003) **52**:735–41. doi:10.1136/gut.52.5.735
146. Raqib R, Sarker P, Bergman P, Ara G, Lindh M, Sack DA, et al. Improved outcome in shigellosis associated with butyrate induction of an endogenous peptide antibiotic. *Proc Natl Acad Sci U S A* (2006) **103**:9178–83. doi:10.1073/pnas.0602888103
147. Ochoa-Zarzosa A, Villarreal-Fernandez E, Cano-Camacho H, Lopez-Meza JE. Sodium butyrate inhibits *Staphylococcus aureus* internalization in bovine mammary epithelial cells and induces the expression of antimicrobial peptide genes. *Microb Pathog* (2009) **47**:1–7. doi:10.1016/j.micpath.2009.04.006
148. Sunkara LT, Achanta M, Schreiber NB, Bommineni YR, Dai G, Jiang W, et al. Butyrate enhances disease resistance of chickens by inducing antimicrobial host defense peptide gene expression. *PLoS One* (2011) **6**:e27225. doi:10.1371/journal.pone.0027225
149. Sunkara LT, Jiang W, Zhang G. Modulation of antimicrobial host defense peptide gene expression by free fatty acids. *PLoS One* (2012) **7**:e49558. doi:10.1371/journal.pone.0049558

150. Zeng X, Sunkara LT, Jiang W, Bible M, Carter S, Ma X, et al. Induction of porcine host defense peptide gene expression by short-chain fatty acids and their analogs. *PLoS One* (2013) **8**:e72922. doi:10.1371/journal.pone.0072922
151. Sunkara LT, Zeng X, Curtis AR, Zhang G. Cyclic AMP synergizes with butyrate in promoting beta-defensin 9 expression in chickens. *Mol Immunol* (2014) **57**:171–80. doi:10.1016/j.molimm.2013.09.003
152. Lyu W, Curtis AR, Sunkara LT, Zhang G. Transcriptional regulation of antimicrobial host defense peptides. *Curr Protein Pept Sci* (2015) **16**:672–9. doi:10.2174/1389203716666150630133432

Conflict of Interest Statement: The authors declare that the research was conducted in the absence of any commercial or financial relationships that could be construed as a potential conflict of interest.

23

Immunometabolism and the kinome peptide array: a new perspective and tool for the study of gut health

Ryan J. Arsenault[1] and Michael H. Kogut[2]*

[1] *Department of Animal and Food Sciences, University of Delaware, Newark, DE, USA,* [2] *United States Department of Agriculture, Agricultural Research Service, Southern Plains Agricultural Research Center, College Station, TX, USA*

Immunometabolism is a relatively new research perspective, focusing on both metabolism and immunology and the cross-talk between these biological processes. Immunometabolism can be considered from two perspectives; 1) the role that immune cells play in organ metabolism and metabolic disease, and 2) the metabolic processes that occur within immune cells and how they affect overall immunity. The gut may be the prototypical organ of immunometabolism. The gut is the site of nutrient absorption and is a major, if not the major, immune organ. We also describe the integration of kinomics and the species-specific peptide array to the study of the gut. This unique immunometabolic tool combined with the unique immunometabolic nature of the gut provides significant research potential to many animal health applications.

Keywords: immunometabolism, gut health, kinome, immunity, metabolism, animal agriculture

Edited by:
Carl James Yeoman, Montana State University, USA

Reviewed by:
Franck Carbonero, University of Arkansas, USA
Isis Kanevsky-Mullarky, Virginia Tech, USA
Lindsey Eve Hulbert, Kansas State University, USA

****Correspondence:***
Ryan J. Arsenault
rja@udel.edu

IMMUNOMETABOLISM

The interface of the immune system and metabolism is an emerging field of study. Relatively recently, immunity and metabolism were treated as distinct processes carried out by an organism. Immunity was focused on the recognition and resistance to a pathogen and involved its own set of cells and tissue activities. Metabolism was solely the chemical processes that provided the energy to carry out the various functions of the organism; this included immune functions, but metabolism was simply the source of energy for the immune system.

The perspective linking immunity and metabolism is styled as immunometabolism. Immunometabolism can be considered from two sides: 1) the role of immune cells in metabolism in organs and the effects on whole organism metabolism or 2) the role of metabolic pathways in immune cells and the effect on broader immunity (1). Early studies in immunometabolism from the first perspective involved human health concerns related to obesity, diabetes, and metabolic disorder (2). Excessive fat deposition can lead to an innate immune inflammatory response. Chronic low-grade inflammation has been linked to metabolic diseases, such as type 2 diabetes, fatty liver disease, and atherosclerosis. Studies typifying the second perspective involved the role of some of the classic metabolic energy sensors and energy switches, such as the signaling proteins AKT1–3, AMPK, mTOR, and LKB1; these were shown to be linked to CD8+ T cell (3) and other immune cell functions. From there, links between metabolism, immunity, and host response to infectious disease grew.

Within animal agriculture, a consideration of immunometabolism in animal production has been ongoing, though not coined as such. It has been clear to poultry producers that a focus solely on maximizing animal growth can be detrimental to immune potential, while an innate immune response has negative consequences on growth (4). Integrating metabolism and immunity provides a research avenue for the ultimate goal of maximizing growth and animal production without having a negative impact on animal health and immunity. Our own research has shown the nearly innumerable links between cellular signaling proteins classically characterized as members of either the immune or metabolic functional groups (5). Due to these links, we feel that an integrated immunometabolic approach is worth considering for anyone researching animal production from either a nutrition/metabolism or immunity/disease perspective. Below, we describe some research categories that fall under the immunometabolism umbrella and their relevance to animal agriculture.

Growth/Immunity Balance

A significant avenue of research combining immunity and metabolism in animal production was how mounting an immune response affected energy levels and the transfer of energy from growth to immunity (4). Research into the energy consequences of immunity is relatively advanced in animal science. It has been well understood for many decades that an animal that initiates an innate immune/inflammatory response will likely grow slower and have worse feed conversion (6, 7). It is thought that one mode of action of growth-promoting antibiotics given to food animals is a general reduction in inflammation. Indeed, it has been argued that the anti-inflammatory effects of growth-promoting antibiotics are even more important than their reduction/elimination of disease-causing pathogens (8). In human medicine, disease early in life has been linked to ultimate growth potential. Less incidence of disease as infants results in greater growth and ultimate height in adulthood (9).

Obesity, Inflammation, Immunity, and Metabolism

With growing research into obesity and associated ailments, including metabolic syndrome, diabetes, and heart disease, a new perspective on the interaction of immunity and metabolism emerged (10). It was found that chronic low-level inflammation was a symptom of obesity (11); this inflammation could lead to diseases like diabetes, among other ailments.

In the animal science field, feed-induced inflammation has been a concern. Certain feed ingredients can lead to an inflammatory gut response; examples include non-digestible components of wheat and rye in chickens (12) and soybean meal in fish (13, 14). Even an excess of feed can lead to changes in immune response (15). One current animal feed strategy involves adding enzymes to break down certain indigestible and/or inflammatory feed components in the gut, with the aim to reduce immune response and redirect this energy to growth (16). A current feed trend involves trying to find natural additives that enhance the animal's resistance to disease, either by influencing the host immune response or the gut microbiota. Caution must be exercised when evaluating these feed additives; robust scientific methodology must be used to determine efficacy and understand the mechanism of action.

In dairy cattle, the transition period immediately before and after calving is an important immunometabolic period. During this time, a dairy cow's immune functions are impaired, as the mobilization of lipids causes susceptibility to both metabolic and infectious disease (17). This increase in fatty acids (FAs) in the blood can lead to uncontrolled inflammation and oxidative stress. The dysfunction in the inflammatory response, due to the free FAs increase, is the link between metabolism and immunity during the calving period.

In poultry, there has been a significant amount of research into nutrition's effects on immunity (18) and the use of pre- and probiotic feed ingredients to improve growth and disease resistance (19–21). However, the literature is limited on the immunometabolism link between stress or disease and production issues. The links between disease and production issues are certainly there, and poultry production problems ranging from lameness (22) to muscle fat deposition (23) have been explored.

As discussed in the following section, the study of immunometabolism now incorporates the metabolic pathway changes in immune effector cells, such as macrophages and T-cells that lead to changes in their activation or immune activity. A promising new avenue of research is the targeting of metabolic machinery and metabolic pathways of immune cells as an alternative means of modulating the immune response.

Intracellular Immunometabolism Interactions

The recent expansion of the immunometabolism field involves characterizing the direct intracellular pathway links between metabolism and immunity (1, 24). Research is focusing on signaling molecules that integrate both metabolic energy sensing and immune response signals; some examples include mTOR, AMPK, and sirtuins. The protein synthesis pathway is regulated by mTOR and is also involved in T-cell fate (25), determining whether the cell becomes an effector T-cell or a regulatory T-cell (3). AMPK is an energy sensor that monitors the ratio of AMP:ATP, altering anabolic and catabolic processes; it is also involved in innate immune response and has a direct link to mTOR (26). Evidence also points to metabolic-induced epigenetic reprograming of immune pathways via the sirtuins (27). The past perspective of separating immunity and metabolism meant a focus on targeting immune pathways in infectious disease and metabolism pathways for growth/metabolic disorders. With an integrated approach, we can broaden our potential targets for disease intervention and our understanding of how metabolic processes can influence health.

Oxidative Phosphorylation, Glycolysis, Warburg Effect, and Immune Response

Studies of the metabolism of immune cells have shown that metabolic processes determine immune function. In dendritic cells and macrophages, the switch from oxidative phosphorylation (OXPHOS) to aerobic glycolysis, which can be triggered by immune ligands like LPS, leads to profound immune activity changes (24). These changes include a release of proinflammatory cytokines, an increase in cell migration, and the utilization of OXPHOS machinery (28, 29) for the production of immune effectors such as nitric oxide (NO) and reactive oxygen species (ROS) (30, 31). In fact, without the change to aerobic glycolysis initiated by immune ligands, the electron transport chain proteins in the mitochondria would not be available to generate these potent antibacterial molecules. The change in metabolism when immune cells are activated has been described as akin to the Warburg effect in cancerous cells, leading to aerobic glycolysis-fueled proliferation and activity (32).

T-Cells and Metabolism

In T-cells, the metabolic processes that are activated can help determine the ultimate function of the cell. Effector T-cells undergo active glycolysis, utilizing this energy to carry out immune activities and proliferate. Quiescent T-cells rely on glycolysis, the citric acid cycle, and OXPHOS (1). Memory T cell metabolism is biased toward free FA metabolism, and the proliferative machinery is turned off. This gives memory T-cells a lower metabolic rate and a longer life span, allowing them to survive and circulate longer than effector T-cells (33).

IMMUNOMETABOLISM AND THE GUT

The gut is the prototypical organ for considering immunity and metabolism as an integrated whole. The gastrointestinal system is the site of significant food breakdown and nutrient absorption, and it is the largest lymphoid organ in the body secreting the most antibodies in humans (34) and animals (35).

In the production of food animals, the gut is a major focus. Effective and efficient nutrient absorption is the first and major step in cost-effective animal production. With the gut as the site of nutrient absorption, any defect in the ability to extract nutrients from feed can have a profound impact on growth and disease susceptibility. In addition, feed efficiency is of critical importance to animal producers, as higher feed efficiency increases the amount of commodity produced and reduces costs. Any increases in feed efficiency from an animal perspective must take place in the gut.

The gut is a major, if not the major, immune organ. It is the main mucosal immune site, and a majority of a body's immune tissue and immunoglobulin producing cells are found in the gut. Infections of the gastrointestinal tract can have huge implications on animal health, gut function, meat contamination, and the spread of disease. A large proportion of disease-causing microbes in food animals enter the host via the gut (36). Manipulation of the gut is a multi-billion dollar target for animal industry products, including prebiotics, probiotics, antibiotics, anti-parasitics, feed enzymes, and feed additives, among others. Many of the pathogens that are considered a food safety concern originate or reside in the animal gut. A proper understanding of the gut can lead to more efficient animal production, less disease, and safer food.

The microbiome, the central component of gut physiology, should be considered in any discussion of the gut and immunometabolism. The microbiome is a key nutritional/metabolic component of the gut, as gut microbes break down otherwise indigestible components of food, providing absorbable and further digestible metabolites (37). The microbiome is an immune component of the gut, as the resident microbes are competitors for pathogens that enter the gut (37, 38). Adding microbes or altering the ratio of microbe species in the animal gut to competitively exclude pathogens is undergoing a significant amount of research and development. The commensal microbes are also critical to proper stimulation and development of the neonatal immune system and help the gut immune system to maintain a balance between tolerance and active immune response (38, 39).

IMMUNOMETABOLISM AND THE KINOME PEPTIDE ARRAY

Species-Specific Peptide Arrays for Kinome Analysis

Peptide arrays have become a productive, high-throughput method of studying the active kinome, the kinase complement of a cell or tissue (40). The principle involves immobilized kinase-target peptide sequences printed on a glass array. Exposing the array to lysate containing active kinases, from gut tissue, for example, results in peptide phosphorylation and can generate a visual signal of substrate–enzyme phosphorylation. By comparing the relative signal of experimental cell or tissue samples, one can identify changes in signal transduction pathways and phosphorylation-regulated events.

It is often the case that new, high-throughput methodologies are designed for the standard laboratory species, mice, and rats, or for work with human samples. This was also the case with the kinome peptide arrays. Through extensive research and development, a methodology for designing and using species-specific kinome arrays was developed (41–43). The use of this technology in agricultural species has been reviewed extensively elsewhere (44) and has been used to design peptide arrays to study important biological questions in a number of agriculturally important species, including bovine (45) and poultry (46).

Immunometabolism Array

Not only are the peptide arrays designed to be species-specific but also they can be process-specific. The initial species-specific arrays were designed to study the innate immune response and contained numerous signaling pathways intermediates involved in this response, such as toll-like receptor (TLR) signaling members, inflammatory intermediates, and others (45). Subsequently, in order to study the metabolic consequences of stress responses, a metabolic peptide array was designed. This array incorporated protein, carbohydrate, and FA metabolic signaling intermediates as well as key energy regulating proteins (23, 47). We have conducted numerous studies on the physiology and host–pathogen interactions in agricultural species using the species-specific peptide arrays. Our analysis of these data showed that the metabolism and immune processes may be distinctions without differences, in that they are two integrated parts of a single cellular process (5). It became clear how much protein–protein interaction there was in the pathways represented on each array. This level of interaction was the impetus for our design of an immunometabolic, species-specific peptide array for both poultry (chicken and turkey) and cattle. This latest generation of species-specific peptide arrays provides an integrated immunometabolic approach to studying kinome response (5). These large arrays, representing approximately 1,000 individual peptides, have been designed to cover the entire network of immunometabolism, including innate and adaptive immunity, protein, carbohydrate, and FA metabolism, as well as hormone and stress response. This integrated peptide array will allow for the study of both the immune and metabolic consequences of an environmental condition, disease, treatment, additive or intervention, and the interactions between them.

In the realm of animal agriculture, nutrition/metabolism and immune performance have been two fields that have been converging for many years. Producers, veterinarians, and animal scientists have come to understand that a sole focus on growth can often come at the expense of health and disease susceptibility, and a strong response to disease can have significant effects on growth. With a tool that can study both metabolism and immunity simultaneously, these two areas of animal science no longer have to be at odds. We can study nutrition and observe effects on immune responses or, conversely, study disease and see how this may effect growth. Our group has already published data that show that *Salmonella* infection of chicken can have effects on the fat deposition and carbohydrate metabolism in peripheral muscle (23). The results indicated that the dysbiosis caused by the *Salmonella* in the gut effected metabolic processes in the skeletal muscle. We are currently working on projects to in which we hope to show an immunometabolic response to infectious diseases and feed-induced inflammation of the gut. This represents only a small fraction of the research potential of this approach.

CONCLUSION

The search for antibiotic alternatives in animal production has renewed the research focus on gut health. It seems likely that any effective alternative will center in the gut. Immunometabolism has expanded from the study of chronic, low-level inflammation, and obesity to a full research perspective, encompassing a variety of fields. The adaption of kinomics to animal agriculture is a relatively recent development and has provided valuable insight into animal biology. Integrating gut health, immunometabolism, and kinomics have significant potential in animal production/health, feed additive development, drug discovery, reproduction, and disease research. Here, we have described this new perspective in gut health and animal production research and a useful tool to carry it out.

REFERENCES

1. Pearce EL, Pearce EJ. Metabolic pathways in immune cell activation and quiescence. *Immunity* (2013) **38**:633–43. doi:10.1016/j.immuni.2013.04.005
2. Ferrante AW. Macrophages, fat, and the emergence of immunometabolism. *J Clin Invest* (2013) **123**:4992–3. doi:10.1172/JCI73658
3. Chi H. Regulation and function of mTOR signalling in T cell fate decisions. *Nat Rev Immunol* (2012) **12**:325–38. doi:10.1038/nri3198
4. Klasing KC. Nutrition and the immune system. *Br Poult Sci* (2007) **48**:525–37. doi:10.1080/00071660701671336
5. Arsenault RJ, Trost B, Kogut MH. A comparison of the chicken and Turkey proteomes and phosphoproteomes in the development of poultry-specific immuno-metabolism kinome peptide arrays. *Vet Infect Dis* (2014) **1**:22. doi:10.3389/fvets.2014.00022
6. Klasing KC. Nutritional aspects of leukocytic cytokines. *J Nutr* (1988) **118**:1436–46.
7. Klasing KC, Korver DR. Leukocytic cytokines regulate growth rate and composition following activation of the immune system. *J Anim Sci* (1997) **75**:58–67. doi:10.2134/animalsci1997.75Supplement_258x
8. Niewold TA. The nonantibiotic anti-inflammatory effect of antimicrobial growth promoters, the real mode of action? A Hypothesis. *Poult Sci* (2007) **86**:605–9. doi:10.1093/ps/86.4.605
9. Bozzoli C, Deaton A, Quintana-Domeque C. Adult height and childhood disease. *Demography* (2009) **46**:647–69. doi:10.1353/dem.0.0079
10. Mathis D, Shoelson SE. Immunometabolism: an emerging frontier. *Nat Rev Immunol* (2011) **11**:81–3. doi:10.1038/nri2922
11. Xu H, Barnes GT, Yang Q, Tan G, Yang D, Chou CJ, et al. Chronic inflammation in fat plays a crucial role in the development of obesity-related insulin resistance. *J Clin Invest* (2003) **112**:1821–30. doi:10.1172/JCI200319451
12. Teirlynck E, Bjerrum L, Eeckhaut V, Huygebaert G, Pasmans F, Haesebrouck F, et al. The cereal type in feed influences gut wall morphology and intestinal immune cell infiltration in broiler chickens. *Br J Nutr* (2009) **102**:1453–61. doi:10.1017/S0007114509990407
13. Urán PA, Gonçalves AA, Taverne-Thiele JJ, Schrama JW, Verreth JAJ, Rombout JHWM. Soybean meal induces intestinal inflammation in common carp (Cyprinus carpio L.). *Fish Shellfish Immunol* (2008) **25**:751–60. doi:10.1016/j.fsi.2008.02.013
14. Bakke-McKellep AM, Press CM, Baeverfjord G, Krogdahl Å, Landsverk T. Changes in immune and enzyme histochemical phenotypes of cells in the intestinal mucosa of Atlantic salmon, Salmo salar L., with soybean meal-induced enteritis. *J Fish Dis* (2000) **23**:115–27. doi:10.1046/j.1365-2761.2000.00218.x
15. Klasing KC. Influence of acute feed deprivation or excess feed intake on immunocompetence of broiler chicks. *Poult Sci* (1988) **67**:626–34. doi:10.3382/ps.0670626
16. Choct M. Enzymes for the feed industry: past, present and future. *Worlds Poult Sci J* (2006) **62**:5–16. doi:10.1079/WPS200480
17. Sordillo LM, Raphael W. Significance of metabolic stress, lipid mobilization, and inflammation on transition cow disorders. *Vet Clin North Am Food Anim Pract* (2013) **29**:267–78. doi:10.1016/j.cvfa.2013.03.002
18. Korver DR. Implications of changing immune function through nutrition in poultry. *Anim Feed Sci Technol* (2012) **173**:54–64. doi:10.1016/j.anifeedsci.2011.12.019
19. Patterson JA, Burkholder KM. Application of prebiotics and probiotics in poultry production. *Poult Sci* (2003) **82**:627–31. doi:10.1093/ps/82.4.627
20. Griggs JP, Jacob JP. Alternatives to antibiotics for organic poultry production. *J Appl Poult Res* (2005) **14**:750–6. doi:10.1093/japr/14.4.750
21. Hume ME. Historic perspective: prebiotics, probiotics, and other alternatives to antibiotics. *Poult Sci* (2011) **90**:2663–9. doi:10.3382/ps.2010-01030
22. Kogut MH. The gut microbiota and host innate immunity: regulators of host metabolism and metabolic diseases in poultry? *J Appl Poult Res* (2013) **22**:637–46. doi:10.3382/japr.2013-00741
23. Arsenault RJ, Napper S, Kogut MH. *Salmonella enterica* Typhimurium infection causes metabolic changes in chicken muscle involving AMPK, fatty acid and insulin/mTOR signaling. *Vet Res* (2013) **44**:35. doi:10.1186/1297-9716-44-35
24. Kelly B, O'Neill LA. Metabolic reprogramming in macrophages and dendritic cells in innate immunity. *Cell Res* (2015) **25**:771–84. doi:10.1038/cr.2015.68
25. Pollizzi KN, Powell JD. Regulation of T cells by mTOR: the known knowns and the known unknowns. *Trends Immunol* (2015) **36**(1):13–20. doi:10.1016/j.it.2014.11.005
26. O'Neill LAJ, Hardie DG. Metabolism of inflammation limited by AMPK and pseudo-starvation. *Nature* (2013) **493**:346–55. doi:10.1038/nature11862
27. Preyat N, Leo O. Sirtuin deacylases: a molecular link between metabolism and immunity. *J Leukoc Biol* (2013) **93**:669–80. doi:10.1189/jlb.1112557
28. Krawczyk CM, Holowka T, Sun J, Blagih J, Amiel E, DeBerardinis RJ, et al. Toll-like receptor–induced changes in glycolytic metabolism regulate dendritic cell activation. *Blood* (2010) **115**:4742–9. doi:10.1182/blood-2009-10-249540
29. Rodríguez-Prados J-C, Través PG, Cuenca J, Rico D, Aragonés J, Martín-Sanz P, et al. Substrate fate in activated macrophages: a comparison between innate, classic, and alternative activation. *J Immunol* (2010) **185**:605–14. doi:10.4049/jimmunol.0901698
30. Everts B, Amiel E, van der Windt GJW, Freitas TC, Chott R, Yarasheski KE, et al. Commitment to glycolysis sustains survival of NO-producing inflammatory dendritic cells. *Blood* (2012) **120**:1422–31. doi:10.1182/blood-2012-03-419747
31. West AP, Brodsky IE, Rahner C, Woo DK, Erdjument-Bromage H, Tempst P, et al. TLR signalling augments macrophage bactericidal activity through mitochondrial ROS. *Nature* (2011) **472**:476–80. doi:10.1038/nature09973
32. Palsson-McDermott EM, O'Neill LAJ. The Warburg effect then and now: from cancer to inflammatory diseases. *Bioessays* (2013) **35**(11):965–73. doi:10.1002/bies.201300084

33. van der Windt GJW, Everts B, Chang C-H, Curtis JD, Freitas TC, Amiel E, et al. Mitochondrial respiratory capacity is a critical regulator of CD8+ T Cell memory development. *Immunity* (2012) **36**:68–78. doi:10.1016/j.immuni.2011.12.007
34. Mayer L. Mucosal immunity and gastrointestinal antigen processing. *J Pediatr Gastroenterol Nutr* (2000) **30**:S4–12. doi:10.1097/00005176-200001001-00002
35. Burkey TE, Skjolaas KA, Minton JE. Board-invited review: porcine mucosal immunity of the gastrointestinal tract. *J Anim Sci* (2009) **87**:1493–501. doi:10.2527/jas.2008-1330
36. Barrington GM, Gay JM, Evermann JF. Biosecurity for neonatal gastrointestinal diseases. *Vet Clin North Am Food Anim Pract* (2002) **18**:7–34. doi:10.1016/S0749-0720(02)00005-1
37. Pflughoeft KJ, Versalovic J. Human microbiome in health and disease. *Annu Rev Pathol Mech Dis* (2012) **7**:99–122. doi:10.1146/annurev-pathol-011811-132421
38. Hooper LV, Littman DR, Macpherson AJ. Interactions between the microbiota and the immune system. *Science* (2012) **336**:1268–73. doi:10.1126/science.1223490
39. Taschuk R, Griebel PJ. Commensal microbiome effects on mucosal immune system development in the ruminant gastrointestinal tract. *Anim Health Res Rev* (2012) **13**:129–41. doi:10.1017/S1466252312000096
40. Arsenault R, Griebel P, Napper S. Peptide arrays for kinome analysis: new opportunities and remaining challenges. *Proteomics* (2011) **11**:4595–609. doi:10.1002/pmic.201100296
41. Jalal S, Arsenault R, Potter AA, Babiuk LA, Griebel PJ, Napper S. Genome to kinome: species-specific peptide arrays for kinome analysis. *Sci Signal* (2009) **2**:l1–1. doi:10.1126/scisignal.254pl1
42. Li Y, Arsenault RJ, Trost B, Slind J, Griebel PJ, Napper S, et al. A systematic approach for analysis of peptide array kinome data. *Sci Signal* (2012) **5**:l2–2. doi:10.1126/scisignal.2002429
43. Trost B, Arsenault R, Griebel P, Napper S, Kusalik A. Dapple: a pipeline for the homology-based prediction of phosphorylation sites. *Bioinformatics* (2013) **29**:1693–5. doi:10.1093/bioinformatics/btt265
44. Daigle J, Van Wyk B, Trost B, Scruten E, Arsenault R, Kusalik A, et al. Peptide arrays for kinome analysis of livestock species. *Vet Infect Dis* (2014) **1**:4. doi:10.3389/fvets.2014.00004
45. Arsenault RJ, Li Y, Maattanen P, Scruten E, Doig K, Potter A, et al. Altered toll-like receptor 9 signaling in *Mycobacterium* avium subsp. paratuberculosis-infected bovine monocytes reveals potential therapeutic targets. *Infect Immun* (2013) **81**:226–37. doi:10.1128/IAI.00785-12
46. Kogut MH, Swaggerty CL, Chiang H-I, Genovese KJ, He H, Zhou H, et al. Critical role of glycogen synthase kinase-3β in regulating the avian heterophil response to *Salmonella enterica* serovar Enteritidis. *Vet Infect Dis* (2014) **1**:10. doi:10.3389/fvets.2014.00010
47. Napper S, Dadgar S, Arsenault RJ, Trost B, Scruten E, Kusalik A, et al. Induction of tissue- and stressor-specific kinomic responses in chickens exposed to hot and cold stresses. *Poult Sci* (2015) **94**(6):1333–45. doi:10.3382/ps/pev046

Conflict of Interest Statement: The authors declare that the research was conducted in the absence of any commercial or financial relationships that could be construed as a potential conflict of interest.

24

The gut microbiome and its potential role in the development and function of newborn calf gastrointestinal tract

*Nilusha Malmuthuge[1], Philip J. Griebel[2,3] and Le Luo Guan[1]**

[1] Department of Agricultural, Food and Nutritional Science, University of Alberta, Edmonton, AB, Canada, [2] Vaccine and Infectious Disease Organization, University of Saskatchewan, Saskatoon, SK, Canada, [3] School of Public Health, University of Saskatchewan, Saskatoon, SK, Canada

A diverse microbial population colonizes the sterile mammalian gastrointestinal tract during and after the birth. There is increasing evidence that this complex microbiome plays a crucial role in the development of the mucosal immune system and influences newborn health. Microbial colonization is a complex process influenced by a two-way interaction between host and microbes and a variety of external factors, including maternal microbiota, birth process, diet, and antibiotics. Following this initial colonization, continuous exposure to host-specific microbes is not only essential for development and maturation of the mucosal immune system but also the nutrition and health of the animal. Thus, it is important to understand host–microbiome interactions within the context of individual animal species and specific management practices. Data is now being generated revealing significant associations between the early microbiome, development of the mucosal immune system, and the growth and health of newborn calves. The current review focuses on recent information and discusses the limitation of current data and the potential challenges to better characterizing key host-specific microbial interactions. We also discuss potential strategies that may be used to manipulate the early microbiome to improve production and health during the time when newborn calves are most susceptible to enteric disease.

Edited by:
Michael Kogut, Agricultural Research Service, United States Department of Agriculture, USA

Reviewed by:
Christi Swaggerty, United States Department of Agriculture, USA
Franck Carbonero, University of Arkansas, USA

***Correspondence:**
Le Luo Guan, 4-16F Agriculture/Forestry Center, Department of Agricultural, Food and Nutritional Science, University of Alberta, Edmonton, AB T6G 2P5, Canada
lguan@ualberta.ca

Keywords: gut microbiota, neonatal ruminants, gut development, mucosal immune system, enteric infections

Introduction

The *in utero* sterile mammalian gastrointestinal tract (GIT) is rapidly colonized by an array of microbiota during and after birth. This process of colonization has been described as a co-evolution due to the two-way interaction between host and microbes (1). Host (luminal pH, food retention time in the gut, and immune defense mechanisms), microbial factors (adhesion, survival mechanisms under oxygen gradient, and mechanisms to obtain nutrients from the host), and external factors, such as maternal microbiota, delivery mode, diet, and antibiotic treatment during early life, all combine to influence gut colonization (2–4). The initial colonizers (*Streptococcus* and *Enterococcus*) utilize available oxygen in the gut and create the anaerobic environment required for strict anaerobic gut residents, such as *Bifidobacterium* and *Bacteroides* (2, 5, 6). *Bifidobacterium* and *Bacteroides* are two of the main gut bacteria present in the majority of human infants (3) that have a beneficial impact on mucosal immune system. The presence of *Bacteroides* in the gut plays a vital role in the development of immunological tolerance to commensal microbiota (7), while the composition of

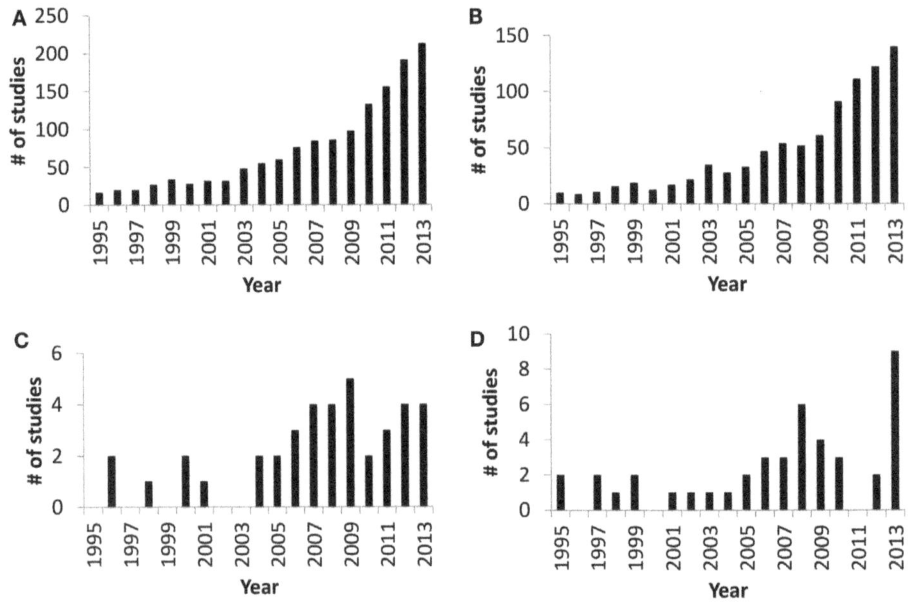

FIGURE 1 | Number of publication entries in Medline (PubMed) trend* from 1995 to 2013. (A) Publication entries searched with query "gut colonization." **(B)** Publication entries searched with query "gut colonization and human." **(C)** Publication entries searched with query "gut colonization and ruminant." **(D)** Publication entries searched with query "rumen colonization." *Medline Trend, URL: http://dan.corlan.net/medline-trend.html.

Bifidobacterium in the infant gut is linked to a reduced incidence of allergy (8). Therefore, neonatal gut colonization is a crucial period for the developing gut and naïve immune system (9, 10) and may have long-term health effects (5). Although research focused on understanding gut colonization of mammals has increased dramatically over the last decade (**Figures 1A,B**), there are still very few studies focused on domestic livestock species, especially ruminants (**Figures 1C,D**). Information is extremely limited on ruminant gut colonization, especially when focusing on the role of the microbiota in the early development of the GIT during the pre-ruminant period. Therefore, the present review builds on the information available for early colonization of the ruminant GIT to identify challenges in understanding the complex interaction between host and microbiome. We also use this information to speculate on possible strategies to engineer the microbiome and improve ruminant health and production.

Gut Microbiota in Ruminants

Gut microbes of ruminants, mainly the rumen microbiota, provide 70% of their daily energy requirement via the fermentation of undigestible dietary substrates (11). Therefore, studies in ruminant gut microbiota have focused mainly on the rumen to understand how this microbiome impacts meat and milk production. Rumen microbiota consists of bacteria, archaea, protozoa, and fungi involved in the fermentation of complex carbohydrates, and their composition is influenced by a number of factors. For example, distinct microbial populations have been identified for the particle-attached, fluid-associated, and tissue-attached fractions of the rumen (12). Rumen microbial composition can also vary significantly depending on the ruminant species, diet, host age, season, and geographic region (13). Bacteria dominate the rumen microbiome and contribute mainly to the production of volatile fatty acids (VFAs) and microbial protein (14). Despite numerous human and mouse studies reporting the importance of early gut microbiota on host health, there are few attempts to understand the role of early gut/rumen colonization on GIT development or host health in neonatal ruminants. Furthermore, rumen/gut development and establishment of the microbiota have always been studied as separate aspects of ruminant biology and there have been few attempts to understand possible interactions between these two events.

Rumen Colonization in Pre-Ruminants

Colonization of pre-ruminant rumen was first studied using light microscopy and Gram-staining to visualize bacteria in the late 1940s (15, 16). In the 1980s, Gerard Fonty started to investigate the establishment of the rumen microbial community in lambs by using culture-dependent approaches and was the first to report age-dependent changes in the appearance of different microbial populations (17). Anaerobic bacteria dominate in the rumen of neonatal ruminants by the second day of life (10^9 CFU/ml of rumen fluid) and the density of cellulolytic bacteria stabilized (10^7 CFU/ml of rumen fluid) within the first week of life (17). This study revealed that the dominant bacterial species in the neonatal lamb rumen was different from those species colonizing the adult rumen. When the establishment of other microbial groups was investigated, their appearance was delayed until after bacteria were established (17). Anaerobic fungi and methanogens appear in the neonatal rumen between 8 and 10 days postpartum (17), while protozoa appear only after 15 days postpartum (18). Furthermore, comparison of conventionalized lambs with conventionally reared lambs suggested that the establishment of protozoa required a well-established bacterial population (18).

The early rumen microbiota consist of bacterial species from *Propionibacterium*, *Clostridium*, *Peptostreptococcus* and *Bifidobacterium* genera, while *Ruminococcus* species dominated the cellulolytic bacterial population (17). Restricted exposure of lambs to their dams or other animals also delayed the establishment of cellulolytic bacteria, when compared to lambs reared in close contact with their dams during the first few weeks of life (19). This observation revealed the important role of early environmental exposure for the establishment of a host-specific microbiota. Fonty and colleagues have also extended their studies to explore the establishment of tissue-attached (epimural) bacteria in the ovine rumen (20). Similar to the fluid-associated community, the complexity of the epimural community and homogeneity among individuals increased with increasing age (20). A recent study revealed, however, that the rumen epimural bacterial community in pre-weaned calves differs significantly from the content-associated community (21). This observation suggests that host–microbial interactions might play an important role in defining these two distinct microbial communities.

Rumen microbiota has a significant impact on pre-ruminant management, especially the weaning process, which depends on rumen development and the ability of the microbiome to ferment complex carbohydrates (22). The presence of VFAs (acetate, propionate, and butyrate) in the rumen plays an important role in rumen development, especially the development of rumen papillae (23). The fermentation of undigestible dietary substrates by rumen microbiota is the major source of VFAs in ruminants (11, 14), and it is generally believed that feeding a solid diet accelerates this process in pre-ruminants (22). Although the establishment of rumen microbiota has long been studied and their importance in the rumen development has been suggested, the mechanisms by which bacteria influence rumen development remain poorly defined. Moreover, culture-based studies can only identify around 10% of the total rumen microbiota, leaving the majority of the microbiome undefined (24).

Recently, enhanced molecular-based technologies, such as next generation sequencing (NGS), provide an excellent platform to identify both culturable and non-culturable microbes as well as characterizing their potential functions (25). It is now possible to generate a comprehensive profile of both microbial diversity and functions and explore potential associations between the microbiome and early rumen development. Using NGS, a comparison of the rumen bacteriome and metagenome in 2-week-old and 6-week-old calves, fed a milk replacer diet, revealed a taxonomically and functionally diverse rumen microbiome in pre-ruminant calves with significant age-dependent changes (26). This study revealed that *Bacteroidetes*, followed by *Firmicutes* and *Proteobacteria*, colonized in the rumen content of pre-weaned calves, which displayed age-dependent variations in their relative abundance. For example, the abundance of *Bacteroidetes* increased from 45.7% at 2 weeks to 74.8% at 6 weeks of age, despite calves receiving the same diet over time. Such age-related differences were more prominent at the bacterial genera level, where the predominant *Prevotella* (33.1%) at 2 weeks was replaced by *Bacteroides* (71.4%) at 6 weeks.

Since the study by Li and colleagues (26), there have been further studies analyzing changes in the composition of the rumen microbial community from birth to weaning. Rumen fluid or content was used as a proxy for the rumen microbiome and 16S rRNA amplicon-based sequencing approaches were used to identify and quantify bacteria (21, 27–29). These studies revealed marked heterogeneity in the rumen bacterial composition of individual animals immediately postpartum, but greater similarity in bacterial composition was observed with increasing age (26–29). There were, however, a number of discrepancies in terms of rumen bacterial composition when comparing among studies. For example, Jami and colleagues (27) reported a higher abundance of *Streptococcus* belonging to the phylum *Firmicutes* in 1–3-day-old calves. In contrast, Rey and colleagues (28) reported a higher abundance of *Proteobacteria* in 2-day-old calves. Furthermore, both Jami et al. (27) and Rey et al. (28) reported a higher abundance of *Bacteroides* in rumen fluid at 2 weeks of life, while Li and colleagues (26) observed a greater abundance of *Prevotella* in rumen content. Targeting different variable regions of 16S rRNA gene (V1/V2 versus V3/V4) for amplicon-based sequencing and differences in the environment, in which these calves were raised, may have influenced the apparent bacterial composition of rumen fluid.

A study comparing content-associated versus epimural bacterial populations in 3-week-old calves revealed that bacterial phylotypes belonging to *Bacteroidetes* (43.8%) and -*Proteobacteria* (25.1%) dominated the epimural community. In contrast, phylotypes from *Bacteroidetes* (54.8%) and *Firmicutes* (29.6%) dominated the rumen content-associated community (21). Using 16S rRNA amplicon-based sequencing, temporal changes in the epimural bacterial community have also been reported in goat kids during the first 10 weeks of life (30). The predominant *Proteobacteria* (>85%) during the first week of life were gradually replaced by an increasing abundance of *Bacteroidetes* (~10%) and *Firmicutes* (>15%) (30). Similar to previous culture-based approaches, these recent studies have confirmed that dynamic changes occur in the rumen bacterial community during early life, with significant differences between the epimural and fluid-associated communities in the pre-weaned rumen.

Associated with the age-dependent changes in rumen microbial composition (**Figure 2**), there are also changes in the activity of the rumen microbiota. These functional changes occur in the absence of dietary changes during the first 6 weeks of life (26). Currently, this is the only study using a metagenomic approach to assess the metabolic potential of pre-ruminant rumen microbiome. Li and colleagues (26) revealed that ATP-binding cassette family transporters are more abundant at 2 weeks than 6 weeks of age but TonB-dependent receptors are more abundant at 6 weeks. Glycoside hydrolases (GH2, GH3, GH42, and GH92), which breakdown complex carbohydrates, were also detected in the pre-ruminant rumen, even when the diet did not contain complex carbohydrates. These observations suggest that early rumen microbiota has the capacity to ferment dietary fiber prior to being exposed to this material. Moreover, a recent study investigating the activity of the early rumen microbiome revealed that VFA production and xylanase and amylase, enzymes that breakdown complex carbohydrates, were active within 2 days postpartum (31). The observed glycoside hydrolase activity, in conjunction with VFA production, reveals establishment of a metabolically

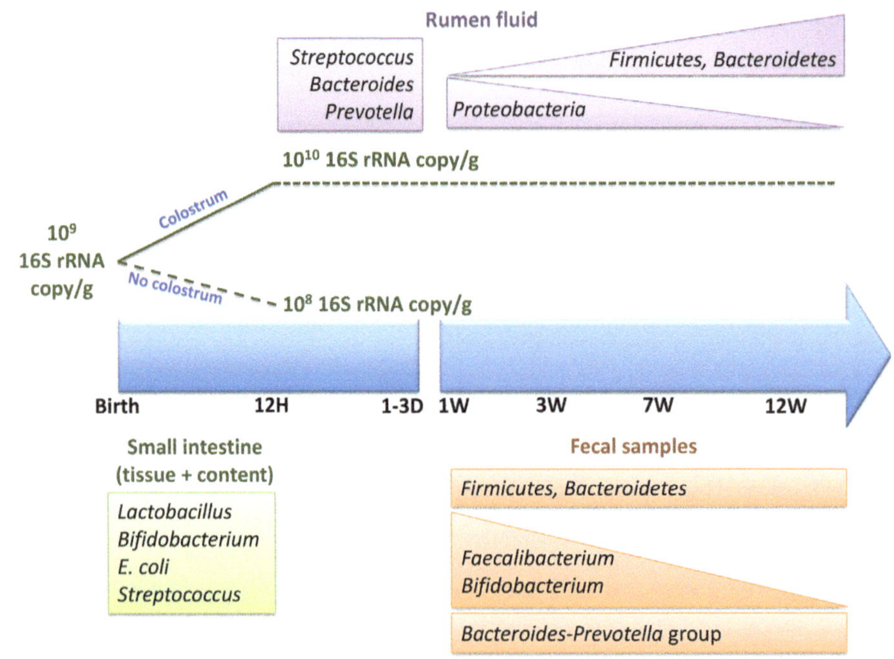

FIGURE 2 | Colonization of neonatal calf rumen/gut, immediately postpartum and within the first 12 weeks of life.

active adult-like microbiome in the neonatal rumen prior to exposure to appropriate dietary substrates. Thus, the establishment of metabolically active microbiome may occur along with the transfer of microbiome from the dam to newborn calf and the colonization of a species-specific microbiome.

Diet is one of the main factors that influences the composition of gut microbiota and may also play an important role in the observed temporal changes of the rumen microbiome in neonatal calves (27, 28). The rumen content of 3-week-old calves fed milk replacer, supplemented with a calf starter ration (20% crude protein, 3% crude fat, and 5.7% crude fiber), contained a similar abundance of *Prevotella* (15.1%) and *Bacteroides* (15.8%) (21). Calves that received milk replacer only, however, displayed a shift in the predominant rumen content-associated bacteria from *Prevotella* to *Bacteroides* (26) within the first 6 weeks of life. Thus, the observed similar abundance of these two bacterial genera in 3-week-old calves fed milk supplemented with calf starter suggests that the age-dependent shift in the dominant bacteria may have been triggered by the dietary supplement that contained fiber. In general, it is believed that the introduction of solid diet plays a key role in promoting the establishment of rumen microbiota as milk bypasses the rumen to enter the abomasum (22). Moreover, pre-weaning diet and feeding methods have been reported to have more pronounced and long-lasting impacts on rumen microbial composition (29, 32, 33). Altering feeding practices during the pre-weaning period were reported to significantly alter methanogen composition after weaning (32) as well as the density of bacteria and protozoa in pre-weaned lambs (33). Therefore, managing pre-weaning feeding may be as important as managing feeding during the weaning period in terms of microbiota establishment as well as development of the microbial fermentation capacity of the rumen.

Currently, characterization of the rumen microbiota is based primarily on the sequencing of DNA, which represents both active and dead microbiota. Therefore, the use of RNA-based metatranscriptome approaches may provide a better understanding of the biological activity of the early rumen microbiome. Understanding the activity of the rumen microbiota may help designing multidisciplinary approaches to engineer the early rumen microbiome with the objective of promoting both rumen development and function that better supports the critical transition that occurs when ruminants are weaned.

Intestinal Tract Colonization in Pre-Ruminants

Early studies on bacterial colonization of the pre-ruminant intestine focused primarily on pathogenic *Escherichia coli* in calves and described the pathogenesis of neonatal diarrhea (34–37). Microscopic imaging revealed that pathogenic *E. coli* preferably attached to and effaced the mucosal epithelium in the ileum and large intestine, but not the duodenum and jejunum of neonatal calves (36). Feeding of probiotic strains isolated from the intestine of calves reduced enteric colonization of pathogenic *E. coli* O157:H7 in pre-weaned calves (38). Furthermore, the administration of *Bifidobacterium* and *Lactobacillus* to newborn calves during the first week of life increased weight gain and the feed conversion ratio, while decreasing diarrhea incidences (39). These effects were most pronounced in pre-weaned calves than weaned calves (39), suggesting the probiotic supplements are more effective when the gut microbiota is being established and less effective when the microbiome has stabilized.

Supplementation of *Lactobacillus* in young calves was also reported to increase the total serum immunoglobulin G concentration (40), providing evidence of a host–microbiome interaction that may influence calf health. More recently, supplementation of newborn calves with prebiotics (galactooligo saccharides) was associated with an increased abundance of *Lactobacillus* and *Bifidobacterium* in the colon of 2-week-old calves (41). However, this effect was less pronounced in 4-week-old calves (41), suggesting that as with probiotics, it may be easier to manipulate the microbiome during the early colonization period (39). In an attempt to reduce antibiotic usage during the pre-weaning period, studies continue to investigate the impact of both probiotics and prebiotics on calf growth and health (42). The full impact of these approaches on gut microbial colonization and composition throughout the pre-ruminant period has yet to be understood and studies are lacking on how altering the gut microbiome may impact mucosal immune defenses in the GIT.

In 1965, Williams Smith used culture-dependent approaches for the first time to study bacterial colonization in the pre-ruminant GIT, beginning immediately postpartum. He reported colonization by *E. coli* and *Streptococcus* in all gut regions (stomach, small intestine, and cecum) of calves within 8 h after birth, while *Lactobacillus* colonization was only observed 1 day after birth. *Lactobacillus* then predominated throughout all regions of the GIT tested within the first week (43). *Bacteroides* were observed only in the cecum and feces after the second day of life (43). The colonization of *Clostridium perfringens*, previously known as *Clostridium welchii*, was also observed in the cecum within 8 h after birth; however, it was not detected in other gut regions until 18 h after birth (43). This study suggested that the newborn GIT was first colonized by facultative anaerobes, which then created the anaerobic conditions required for colonization by obligate anaerobic gut microbiota, such as *Lactobacillus* and *Bacteroides*. A similar evolution of bacterial colonization of the GIT has been reported for other newborn mammals (6).

Subsequent studies have revealed a higher abundance of *Bifidobacterium* and *Lactobacillus* in fecal samples and throughout the GIT of newborn calves (44, 45). A higher abundance of *Bifidobacterium* in 3–7 days old calves was also associated with a lower abundance of *E. coli* (44). More recently, culture-independent approaches have been employed to better understand the diversity and abundance of bacteria throughout the neonatal ruminant GIT (46, 47). RNA-based, sequence-specific rRNA cleavage analysis of bacteria throughout the first 12 weeks postpartum revealed a higher abundance of the *Bacteroides–Prevotella* and *Clostridium coccoides–Eubacterium rectale* groups in the feces of dairy calves (46). *Faecalibacterium* was one of the most abundant bacteria in 1-week-old calves (21.7%), but then declined with increasing calf age (46). *Ruminococcus flavefaciens* and *Fibrobacter*, fibrolytic bacteria, were only observed after 5 weeks postpartum, while *Streptococcus* and *Lactococcus* could not be detected after the fifth week (46). These studies confirmed that there were significant age-dependent changes in the composition of the GIT microbiome and revealed substantial differences between the rumen and lower GIT microbiome.

Regional variations in bacterial phylotypes richness, diversity, density, and composition throughout the GIT of newborn calves have been described, using both culture-dependent and independent approaches (21, 45, 48, 49). When bacterial populations throughout the GIT of 20-week-old calves were analyzed, *Bifidobacterium* and *Lactobacillus* displayed greater survival of stomach passage than coliforms and *E. coli* (45). The density of these beneficial bacteria was high throughout all GIT regions (rumen, abomasum, duodenum, jejunum, cecum, and colon) of the 20-week-old calves (45). Using culture-independent approaches, higher bacterial phylotype richness was observed in the rumen and large intestinal regions than the small intestinal regions of lambs and calves (21, 48, 49). Collado and Sanz (48) reported, however, a similar bacterial richness throughout the GIT, when using a culture-dependent approach. This observation is consistent with there being many more unculturable bacterial species in the rumen and large intestine than the small intestine. A longer retention time, higher availability of nutrients, and reduced scrutiny by the host mucosal immune system have all been suggested to contribute to the increase in bacterial diversity and density in the rumen and large intestine of mammals (1).

When bacterial composition throughout the GIT is explored, the rumen and large intestinal regions consist primarily of *Bacteroidetes* and *Firmicutes*, while >95% of the bacteria in the small intestine contents are composed of *Firmicutes* (21). In contrast, the mucosa-associated bacterial community in the small intestine is composed of primarily *Bacteroidetes*, *Firmicutes*, and *Proteobacteria*, including 17 genera that are unique to this region of the GIT (21). The presence of bacteria unique to the small intestine (21) suggests that fecal sample-based studies do not reveal the true GIT microbiome and may not reveal important regional host–microbial interactions. A recent study in human infants reported similar observations and it was also concluded that feces was not representative of host–microbiota interactions throughout the gut (50).

There is increasing evidence that mucosa-attached microbiota are significantly different from those associated with ingesta and present in the intestinal lumen. Collado and Sanz (48) first studied mucosa-attached bacteria and reported that *Bifidobacterium* and *Lactobacillus* were predominant throughout the GIT (rumen, duodenum, and colon) of calves (9–11 months) and lambs (6–9 months). They did not, however, compare mucosa-associated versus intestinal content communities. Studies by Malmuthuge and colleagues (21, 49) compared mucosa-attached and content-associated bacterial communities throughout the GIT of calves and reported that at 3 weeks of life, distinct mucosa-attached bacterial phylotypes had been established. Furthermore, bacterial richness in mucosa-attached communities, especially in the ileum, was higher than the content-associated community (49). These distinct and richer mucosa-attached bacterial communities were subsequently confirmed by using pyrosequencing of 16S rRNA gene amplicons (21). Although the majority of mucosa-attached bacteria could not be assigned at a genus level, the use of a NGS approach provided a greater understanding of region- (rumen, small intestine, and large intestine) and sample type- (content and mucosa) specific bacteria throughout the GIT of pre-weaned calves (21).

Based on the previously cited studies, it is clear that the composition, diversity, and richness of rumen and intestinal microbiota in pre-weaned ruminants can vary depending on various factors,

TABLE 1 | Factors influencing pre-weaned calf rumen/gut microbiota.

Factor	Study
Age	(17, 26–28, 30, 46, 47, 49)
Diet (colostrum, calf starter)	(28, 29, 32, 33, 46, 51, 52)
Feeding method (suckling, bottle feeding)	(53)
Probiotic, prebiotics	(39, 41)
Exposure to dam	(19, 53)
Sample site	(21, 43, 48, 49)
Sample type (fluid, content, mucosa)	(20, 21, 49)
Host (individuality)	(27)
Infections	(47)

such as age, diet, feeding method, feed additives, sampling location (content, mucosa, and feces), and gut region (rumen, large intestine, and small intestine) (**Table 1**; **Figure 2**). Furthermore, variation in microbial composition among individual animals is higher in young than adult ruminants (27). The high variation in bacterial diversity and density (27, 49) among individual ruminants during early life also suggests that the gut microbiome may be more easily changed at this time of life than in adults. This may explain why probiotics and prebiotics have been reported to have a much greater effect in young animals than older calves (39, 41). Of particular interest are the recent studies conducted by Abecia and colleagues, which revealed long-lasting consequences when dietary interventions were used to manipulate the rumen microbiota in young calves. Thus, a much greater understanding of early gut microbial colonization and the factors influencing establishment of microbiota may provide the basis for rational strategies to manipulate the gut microbiome and improve the growth and health of ruminants throughout the entire production cycle.

Influence of Microbiome on Gut Development and Mucosal Immune Functions

Gut microbiota are essential for the development and differentiation of the intestinal mucosal epithelium as well as the mucosal immune system (54). Most of our knowledge regarding host–microbiome interactions in the GIT has been obtained from a variety of mouse models. Comparisons between gnotobiotic and conventionally reared mice revealed decreased development of the intestinal epithelium and the mucosal immune system in the absence of gut microbiota. Thickness of the mucus barrier is reduced in germfree mice, but administration of microbe-derived lipopolysaccharides and peptidoglycans to the colonic mucosal surface stimulated mucus production and within 40 min restored the thickness of the mucus layer to that of conventional mice (55). This observation supports the conclusion that the gut microbiota is essential for the secretion of intestinal mucus, an important physical barrier throughout the GIT. In addition, the generation rate of epithelial cells in germfree mice is lower than that of the conventionally raised mice (56), revealing the importance of gut microbiota for maintaining intestinal epithelial cells proliferation and ensuring recovery of the mucosal barrier following injuries.

The presence of gut microbiota in mice is also necessary for the development of secondary lymphoid structure, such as Peyer's patches (PPs), mesenteric lymph nodes, and isolated lymphoid follicles (54). The establishment of host-specific microbiota, especially bacterial species belong to phylum *Firmicutes*, is essential for the development of a variety of intestinal immune cells (57). For example, when human microbiota colonized the mouse intestine there were low numbers of $CD4^+$ and $CD8^+$ T cells, and fewer proliferating T cells and dendritic cells when compared to mice colonized with mouse microbiota (57). Interestingly, the immune cell profile of human microbiota colonized mice was similar to that of germfree mice (57), suggesting the presence of a host-specific microbiota is fundamental for mucosal immune system development. Thus, host–microbial interactions in the developing gut of newborn animals must be studied within relevant host species to accurately understand the role of early microbiota on gut development.

In ruminants, development of mucosa-associated lymphoid tissues (MALTs) in the GIT begins *in utero* and there is active proliferation of B cells in lymphoid follicles of the PP in the complete absence of the gut microbiome (58, 59). Furthermore, oral delivery of antigens *in utero* has confirmed that these MALTs are fully functional and can generate specific immune responses with the production of secretory IgA (60). In the absence of an *in utero* infection, however, the appearance of IgG^+ and IgA^+ cells in PPs is delayed until after birth (59). Since immunoglobulin class switching occurs in the germinal centers of PPs (54), this suggests that the full development of germinal centers requires exposure to the gut microbiota. However, information regarding the role of the gut microbiota in the early postnatal development of MALT in ruminants is scarce. There is a single report that preventing exposure of the ileal PPs to gut microbiome results in premature involution of lymphoid follicles in the PPs of newborn lambs (61). However, restoration of the gut microbiome at 4 weeks after birth reversed lymphoid follicle involution in the ileal PPs (61). Thus, the gut microbiome appears to provide critical signals that maintain the production of the pre-immune B cell repertoire. It remains to be determined whether specific microbial species may influence the selection of this immunoglobulin repertoire or if this interaction is restricted to an interaction with innate immune receptors.

The host uses pattern recognition receptors, such as toll-like receptors (TLRs), to recognize the commensal microbiota and maintain intestinal homeostasis (62). Activation of TLR signaling by intestinal tissue invading pathogens generally stimulates inflammatory responses. In contrast, commensal microbiota activation of TLR signaling promotes the production of interleukin 6 and tumor necrosis factor that protect intestinal epithelial cells against injury (62). Therefore, commensal microbial recognition by mucosal TLRs is crucial for the maintenance of intestinal homeostasis and protection of the gut from injuries. The expression of TLRs in the blood of infants (63) was downregulated with increasing age, while memory T cells, such as $CD4^+$ and $CD8^+$, increased in number (63). These changes are consistent with a decrease in innate immune responses that is balanced by an increase in adaptive immune responses with increasing age. Downregulation of innate immune responses with increasing age has been suggested as one mechanism by which the host avoids unnecessary inflammatory responses to commensal microbiota (63). Similar results have been reported when analyzing the intestinal immune system of calves (64, 65). The expression of mucosal TLR genes was downregulated in weaned calves when compared to pre-weaned calves (65). In contrast, total leukocytes including, $CD3^+$, $CD4^+$, and $CD8^+$ T cells, increased in the jejunal and ileal mucosa of calves with increasing age (64). Moreover, a negative correlation was observed between the expression of mucosal TLRs and mucosa-attached bacteria, suggesting a possible link between the gut microbiota and the observed age-related changes in the mucosal immune responses (65). However, the mechanism by which gut microbiome colonization affects this shift of mucosal and systemic immune responses from innate to adaptive remains to be defined. There is, however, emerging evidence that microbial colonization is associated with substantial changes in the transcriptome of the bovine intestine during the first week of life (66). Transcriptome changes occurred at the level of miRNA and significant correlations were identified between the gut microbiome and these transcriptome changes.

Experiments with the mouse model have clearly demonstrated the importance of gut microbiota in the development of both innate and adaptive components of the mucosal immune system as well as development and maintenance of the intestinal epithelial barrier. Increased susceptibility to enteric infections in gnotobiotic and antibiotic treated mice may also be due to the underdeveloped mucosal immune system and epithelial barrier (54). The immunologically naïve neonatal GIT and the colonizing microbiota undergo a rapid co-evolution during early life and these interactions may be crucial in determining the susceptibility of the neonate to enteric infections. Pre-weaned ruminants are highly susceptible to a variety of viral and bacterial enteric infection within the first few weeks of life (67). Therefore, a thorough understanding of early gut microbiota and its role in regulating and directing early development of the mucosal immune system is essential to improving the health of young calves and reducing susceptibility to enteric infections.

The Commensal Microbiome and Enteric Infections in Young Ruminants

Neonatal diarrhea is the major cause of death in pre-weaned calves and accounts for >50% of calf deaths in the dairy industry (67). Establishment of the gut microbiome within the first 7 weeks of life and an association with calf health and growth (neonatal diarrhea, pneumonia, and weight gain) was recently reported (47). Bacterial diversity was lower in calves with pneumonia and neonatal diarrhea when compared to healthy calves (47), suggesting a possible link between gut microbiota and host health. The authors speculate that antibiotic treatment may have been one factor influencing the gut microbiome in pneumonic calves. Furthermore, colonization by enteric pathogens may be responsible for the observed dysbiosis in gut microbiota during neonatal diarrhea (47). Increased fecal bacteria diversity was also associated with increased weight gain in healthy calves, while a high abundance of *Faecalibacterium* during the first week of life was associated with a lower incidence of diarrhea in calves after the fourth week of life (47). Thus, it is difficult to determine if changes in the fecal microbiome were a consequence of prior disease and associated therapeutic interventions or if colonization of the GIT by specific commensal bacteria had a beneficial effect in terms of disease resistance.

Uyeno and colleagues (46) also reported a high abundance of *Faecalibacterium* in the feces of 1-week-old calves and their abundance was higher in the large intestine compared to the small intestine of 3-week-old calves (21). *Faecalibacterium prausnitzii*, one of the main butyrate producers in the large intestine, displayed a negative association with calf diarrhea incidences (47), suggesting the high prevalence of this species during early life may decrease susceptibility to enteric infections. *F. prausnitzii* also plays a pivotal role in maintaining intestinal homeostasis by promoting anti-inflammatory responses and has been shown to decrease in prevalence in patients with inflammatory bowel disease (68). Inflammatory bowel disease was also associated with a reduced prevalence of *Bifidobacterium* (68), suggesting that these two bacterial groups may have important roles in maintaining intestinal homeostasis and preventing enteric infections. Thus, it will be important to further explore the potential role of such beneficial bacteria in the early gut development and their capacity to promote host health.

Poor management of colostrum feeding in newborn calves is one of the main triggers of neonatal calf diarrhea. Feeding calves with highly contaminated (bacteria > 106 CFU/ml, coliform > 103 CFU/ml) and of low quality (IgG < 50 mg/ml) colostrum (69), poor surveillance of calves born at night, and relying on dams to feed colostrum (70) are some of the major risk factors currently contributing to poor neonatal calf health in the North American dairy industry. Although the importance of timed feeding of high quality colostrum for passive transfer of immunity has been well studied (71), the influence of colostrum on gut microbial establishment and susceptibility to enteric infection in young ruminants is not clearly understood. A recent study revealed that feeding colostrum within 1 h postpartum facilitated bacterial colonization of the small intestine within the first 12 h postpartum. Calves-fed colostrum achieved bacterial numbers similar to older calves [10^{10} 16S rRNA gene copy/g of intestinal sample (49)], but significantly fewer bacteria were observed in the intestine of calves deprived of colostrum (52). Furthermore, when comparing to colostrum-deprived calves at 12 h postpartum, there was a significant increase in the prevalence of *Bifidobacterium* and a decreased prevalence of *E. coli* in the mucosa-attached communities of calves fed either heat-treated or fresh colostrum (52). Changes in the abundance of mucosa-attached *Bifidobacterium* and *E. coli* populations were most pronounced when calves were fed heat-treated colostrum versus fresh colostrum (52). Heat treatment (60°C, 60 min) decreases the density of total bacteria including pathogens present in colostrum, which has been suggested to decrease neonatal diarrhea in calves (71). The results from Malmuthuge and colleagues (52), however, suggest that timed feeding of high quality colostrum has a direct effect on bacterial colonization of the bovine small intestine, in particular the mucosa-attached community that is in close contact with the host mucosal immune system. Establishing a bacterial population dominated by beneficial bacteria may suppress colonization of enteropathogens (72) immediately postpartum and provide protection against enteric infections in young ruminants with a naïve immune system. Further investigations are necessary to also understand how a *Bifidobacterium*-dominated early gut microbiome may influence host performances (weight gain, resistance to enteric infections) within the first few weeks and identify the mechanisms by which the commensal microbiome alter both enteric health and general physiology.

Manipulation of the Early Gut Microbiome to Improve Health and Production

Manipulation of gut microbiota by feeding microbes, probiotics, or prebiotics has been widely studied in livestock animals as a strategy to improve production and health through altering rumen fermentation and preventing pathogen colonization (24, 42). Direct-fed microbials have been shown to decrease rumen acidosis in cattle, increase milk production in cows, and decrease fecal shedding of *E. coli* in calves (73). These direct-fed microbials may prevent enteropathogen colonization of the gut by either competing for nutrients, space in the gut environment, or producing antimicrobial substances (73). *Megasphaera elsdenii* modifies ruminal fermentation and decreases ruminal acidosis by utilizing lactic acid produced in the rumen (73). However, most of these outcomes are limited to a relatively short interval following feeding (24) or are effective only in pre-weaned calves (39), suggesting that these manipulations are either temporary or need to be instituted within a defined developmental period. Moreover, it is essential to know how the autochthonous gut microbial population responds to these dietary manipulations and how their compositional changes influence overall gut metabolic and immune functions. It may also be important to determine if developing probiotics or direct-fed microbials, based on *Faecalibacterium* and *Bifidobacterium* that have already been linked to calf health, provides a more effective or long-lasting effect. The establishment of host-specific bacteria is crucial for the development of mucosal immune system, especially for the differentiation and proliferation of T cell populations (57). Thus, there would be substantial value in both isolating and testing bacteria within the same host species that might provide the basis for the developing microbial manipulation techniques.

Conclusion

Interactions between host and gut microbiota have been explored extensively in humans and mice but these investigations are still in their infancy in ruminants (**Figure 1**). However, the studies reviewed to date are generating promising results, describing GIT microbial composition (**Figure 2**) and functions in greater depth and identifying factors that significantly influence microbial establishment. It is also notable that recent results are based primarily on nucleic acid sequencing, which may be limited by sampling location, the type of sample collected, extraction methods, sequencing depth, and the analysis pipeline used. In addition, the taxonomic and functional identification of the rumen/gut microbiome is dependent on existing databases and identified organisms and functions are remaining unclassified at lower taxonomic levels and at the level of protein coding genes. Single cell genome sequencing and more comprehensive databases for the ruminant gut microbiome are vital to understanding their role in host development.

A substantial step forward in being able to explain the role of the gut microbiome in host physiology would be to understand the metabolic capacity of the early microbiome. Metabolic functions of the rumen microbiota appear to be highly redundant, which may be essential to ensure optimum fermentation of ingested substrates. Therefore, isolation of metabolically active rumen microbiota may be important to further our understanding of their roles in monocultures and mixed populations. This information will provide the basis for future strategies designed to manipulate the microbiome and improve both production and health.

Finally, there is a substantial need to develop ruminant animal models that can be used to investigate the effects of controlled changes in the gut microbiome on both host mucosal immunity and host metabolism. The rearing of gnotobiotic calves is limited by large technical and financial barriers and to date studies have been limited to changes in diet or the feeding of pre- or probiotics and subsequent sampling of rumen or fecal microflora. The challenge is to develop animal models that allow us to ask questions regarding microbiome changes within specific regions of the GIT and to analyze local effects on mucosal immune and barrier function. The use of a surgically isolated intestinal segment model in fetal lambs (61) provided an elegant model system to create a localized gnotobiotic environment in the GIT of a developmentally normal animal. A similar model system was developed in newborn calves to study the effects of a persistent enteric bacterial infection (74). Thus, it should now be possible to manipulate local exposure to the microbiome and analyze the effects on neonatal mucosal immune system and barrier development. A critical question to be addressed is whether dysbiosis of the microbiome during colonization of the newborn GIT has long-term effects, both locally in the GIT and systemically, that impacts the health and production of animals. If long-term effects are observed, then it will be important to determine if restoration of the complex microbiome, or specific bacterial species, can effectively reverse the effects of early microbial dysbiosis.

Acknowledgments

The authors appreciate the financial support from Agriculture and Food Council, Alberta Livestock Industry Development Fund, Alberta Milk, Alberta Livestock and Meat Agency Ltd. (Grant number: 2011F129R), and Natural Sciences and Engineering Research Council of Canada (NSERC Discovery Grant). PG is the holder of a Tier I CRC in Neonatal Mucosal Immunology, which is funded by the Canadian Institutes of Health Research (CIHR).

References

1. Van den Abbeele P, Van de Wiele T, Verstraete W, Possemiers S. The host selects mucosal and luminal associations of coevolved gut microorganisms: a novel concept. *FEMS Microbiol Rev* (2011) **35**:681–704. doi:10.1111/j.1574-6976.2011.00270
2. Fanaro S, Chierici R, Guerrini P, Vigi V. Intestinal microflora in early infancy: composition and development. *Acta Paediatr Suppl* (2003) **91**:48–55.
3. Penders J, Thijs C, Vink C, Stelma FF, Snijders B, Kummeling S, et al. Factors influencing the composition of the intestinal microbiota in early infancy. *Pediatrics* (2006) **118**:511–21. doi:10.1542/peds.2005-2824
4. Adlerberth I, Wold AE. Establishment of the gut microbiota in western infants. *Acta Paediatr* (2009) **98**:229–38. doi:10.1111/j.1651-2227.2008.01060
5. Conroy ME, Shi HN, Walker WA. The long-term health effects of neonatal microbial flora. *Curr Opin Allergy Clin Immunol* (2009) **9**:197–201. doi:10.1097/ACI.0b013e32832b3f1d
6. Jost T, Lacroix C, Braegger CP, Chassard C. New insights in gut microbiota establishment in healthy breast fed neonates. *PLoS One* (2012) **7**:e44595. doi:10.1371/journal.pone.0044595
7. Mazmanian SK, Round JL, Kasper DL. A microbial symbiosis factor prevents intestinal inflammatory disease. *Nature* (2008) **453**:620–5. doi:10.1038/nature07008
8. Sjogren YM, Jenmalm MC, Bottcher MF, Bjorksten B, Sverremark-Ekstrom E. Altered early infant gut microbiota in children developing allergy up to 5 years of age. *Clin Exp Allergy* (2009) **39**:518–26. doi:10.1111/j.1365-2222.2008.03156
9. Fouhy F, Guinane CM, Hussey S, Wall R, Ryan CA, Dempsey EM, et al. High-throughput sequencing reveals the incomplete, short-term recovery of infant gut microbiota following parenteral antibiotic treatment with ampicillin and gentamicin. *Antimicrob Agents Chemother* (2012) **56**:5811–20. doi:10.1128/AAC.00789-12
10. Hansen CHF, Nielsen DS, Kverka M, Zakostelska Z, Klimesova K, Hudcovic T, et al. Patterns of early gut colonization shape future immune responses of the host. *PLoS One* (2012) **7**:e34043. doi:10.1371/journal.pone.0034043
11. Yeoman CJ, White BA. Gastrointestinal tract microbiota and probiotics in production animals. *Annu Rev Anim Biosci* (2014) **2**:469–86. doi:10.1146/annurev-animal-022513-114149
12. Cho SJ, Kim H, Yun HD, Cho KM, Shin EC, Lim WJ, et al. 16S rDNA analysis of bacterial diversity in three fractions of cow rumen. *J Microbiol Biotechnol* (2006) **16**:92–101.
13. Tajima K, Aminov RI, Nagamine T, Matsui H, Nakamura M, Benno Y. Diet-dependent shifts in the bacterial population of the rumen revealed with real-time PCR. *Appl Enivorn Microbiol* (2001) **66**:2766–74. doi:10.1128/AEM.67.6.2766-2774.2001
14. Kim M, Morrison M, Yu Z. Status of the phylogenetic diversity census of ruminal microbiomes. *FEMS Microbiol Ecol* (2011) **76**:49–63. doi:10.1111/j.1574-6941.2010.01029
15. Pounden WD, Hibbs JW. The influence of ration and rumen inoculation on the establishment of certain microorganisms in the rumens of young calves. *J Dairy Sci* (1948) **31**:1041–50. doi:10.3168/jds.S0022-0302(48)92296-6
16. Pounden WD, Hibbs JW. The influence of pasture and rumen inoculation on the establishment of certain microorganisms in the rumen of young dairy calves. *J Dairy Sci* (1949) **32**:1025–32. doi:10.3168/jds.S0022-0302(49)92157-8
17. Fonty G, Gouet P, Jounay JP, Senaud J. Establishment of the microflora and anaerobic fungi in the rumen of lambs. *Microbiology* (1987) **133**:1835–43. doi:10.1099/00221287-133-7-1835
18. Fonty G, Senaud J, Jouany JP, Gouet P. Establishment of ciliate protozoa in the rumen of conventional and conventionalized lambs: influence of diet and management conditions. *Can J Microbiol* (1988) **34**:235–41. doi:10.1139/m88-044
19. Fonty G, Gouet P, Nebout JM. Development of the cellulolytic microflora in the rumen of lambs transferred into sterile isolators a few days after birth. *Can J Microbiol* (1989) **35**:416–22. doi:10.1139/m89-064
20. Rieu F, Fonty G, Gaillard B, Gouet P. Electron microscopy study of the bacteria adherent to the rumen wall in young conventional lambs. *Can J Microbiol* (1990) **36**:140–4. doi:10.1139/m90-025
21. Malmuthuge N, Griebel PJ, Guan LL. Taxonomic identification of commensal bacteria associated with the mucosa and digesta throughout the gastrointestinal tracts of pre-weaned calves. *Appl Environ Microbiol* (2014) **80**:2012–28. doi:10.1128/AEM.03864-13
22. Heinrichs J. Rumen development in the dairy calf [abstract]. *Adv Dairy Technol* (2005) **17**:179–87. Abstract retrieved from western Canadian Dairy Seminar 2005 proceedings.
23. Lane BA, Jesse BW. Effect of volatile fatty acid infusion on development of the rumen epithelium in neonatal sheep. *J Dairy Sci* (1997) **80**:740–6. doi:10.3168/jds.S0022-0302(97)75993-9
24. Weimer PJ. Redundancy, resilience, and host specificity of the ruminal microbiota: implications for engineering improved ruminal fermentations. *Front Microbiol* (2015) **6**:296. doi:10.3389/fmicb.2015.00296
25. McCann JC, Wickersham TA, Loor JJ. High-throughput methods redefine the rumen microbiome and its relationship with nutrition and metabolism. *Bioinform Biol Insights* (2014) **8**:109–25. doi:10.4137/BBI.S15389
26. Li RW, Connor EE, Baldwin RL, Sparks ML. Characterization of the rumen microbiota of pre-ruminant calves using metagenomic tools. *Environ Microbiol* (2012) **14**:129–39. doi:10.1111/j.1462-2920.2011.02543
27. Jami E, Israel A, Kotser A, Mizrahi I. Exploring the bovine rumen bacterial community from birth to adulthood. *ISME J* (2013) **7**:1069–79. doi:10.1038/ismej.2013.2
28. Rey M, Enjalbert F, Combes S, Cauquil L, Bouchez O, Monteils V. Establishment of ruminal bacterial community in dairy calves from birth to weaning is sequential. *J Appl Microbiol* (2014) **116**:245–57. doi:10.1111/jam.12405
29. De Barbieri I, Hegarty RS, Silveira C, Gulino LM, Oddy VH, Gilbert RA, et al. Programming rumen bacterial communities in newborn Merino lambs. *Small Rumin Res* (2015) **129**:48–59. doi:10.1016/j.smallrumres.2015.05.015
30. Jiao J, Huang J, Zhou C, Tan Z. Taxonomic identification of ruminal epithelial bacterial diversity during rumen development in goats. *Appl Environ Microbiol* (2015) **81**:3502–9. doi:10.1128/AEM.00203-15
31. Rey M, Enjalbert F, Monteils V. Establishment of ruminal enzymatic activities and fermentation capacity in dairy calves from birth through weaning. *J Dairy Sci* (2012) **95**:1500–12. doi:10.3168/jds.2011-4902
32. Abecia L, Martin-Garcia AI, Martinez-Fernandez G, Newbold CJ, Yanez-Ruiz DR. Nutritional intervention in early life to manipulate rumen microbial colonization and methane output by kid goats postweaning. *J Anim Sci* (2013) **91**:4832–40. doi:10.2527/jas.2012-6142
33. Abecia L, Waddams KE, Martinez-Fernandez G, Martin-Garcia AI, Ramos-Morales E, Newbold CJ, et al. An antimethanogenic nutritional intervention in early life of ruminants modifies ruminal colonization by archaea. *Archaea* (2014) **2014**:841463. doi:10.1155/2014/841463
34. Chanter N, Hall GA, Bland AP, Hayle AJ, Parsons KR. Dysentery in calves caused by an atypical strain of *Escherichia coli* (S102-9). *Vet Microbiol* (1984) **12**:241–53. doi:10.1016/0378-1135(86)90053-2
35. Hall GA, Reynold DJ, Chanter N, Morgan JH, Parsons KR, Debney TA, et al. Dysentery caused by *Escherichia coli* (S102-9) in calves: natural and experimental disease. *Vet Pathol* (1985) **22**:156–63. doi:10.1177/030098588502200210
36. Moxley RA, Francis DH. Natural and experimental infection with an attaching and effacing strain of *Escherichia coli* in calves. *Infect Immunol* (1986) **53**:336–49.
37. Janke BH, Francis DH, Collins JE, Libal MC, Zeman DH, Johnson DD. Attaching and effacing *Escherichia coli* infections in calves, pigs, lambs, and dogs. *J Vet Diagn Invest* (1989) **1**:6–11. doi:10.1177/104063878900100104
38. Zhao T, Doyle MP, Harmon BG, Brown CA, Mueller POE, Parks AH. Reduction of carriage of enterohemorrhagic *Escherichia coli* O157:H7 in cattle by inoculation with probiotic bacteria. *J Clin Microbiol* (1998) **36**:641–7.
39. Abe F, Ishibashi N, Shimamura S. Effect of administration of bifidobacteria and lactic acid bacteria to newborn calves and piglets. *J Dairy Sci* (1995) **73**:2838–46. doi:10.3168/jds.S0022-0302(95)76914-4
40. Al-Saiady MY. Effect of probiotic bacteria on immunoglobulin G concentration and other blood components of newborn calves. *J Anim Vet Adv* (2010) **9**:604–9. doi:10.3923/java.2010.604.609
41. Marquez CJ. *Calf Intestinal Health: Assessment and Dietary Interventions for its Improvement*. PhD thesis, University of Illinois at Urbana-Champaign, Champaign, IL (2014).
42. Uyeno Y, Shigemori S, Shimosato T. Effect of probiotics/prebiotics on cattle health and productivity. *Microbes Environ* (2015) **30**:126–32. doi:10.1264/jsme2.ME14176
43. Smith HW. The development of the flora of the alimentary tract in young animals. *J Pathol Bacteriol* (1965) **90**:495–513. doi:10.1002/path.1700900218

44. Rada V, Vlkov E, Nevoral J, Trojanov I. Comparison of bacterial flora and enzymatic activity in faeces of infants and calves. *FEMS Microbiol Lett* (2006) **258**:25–8. doi:10.1111/j.1574-6968.2006.00207
45. Vlkova E, Nevoral J, Rada V. Distribution of bifidobacteria in the gastrointestinal tract of calves. *Folia Microbiol* (2006) **51**:325–8. doi:10.1007/BF02931825
46. Uyeno Y, Sekiguchi Y, Kamagata Y. rRNA-based analysis to monitor succession of fecal bacterial communities of Holstein calves. *Lett Appl Microbiol* (2010) **51**:570–7. doi:10.1111/j.1472-765X.2010.02937
47. Oikonomou G, Teixeira AG, Foditsch C, Bichalho ML, Machado VS, Bicalho RC. Fecal microbial diversity in pre-weaned dairy calves as described by pyrosequencing of metagenomic 16S rDNA. Associations of *Faecalibacterium* species with health and growth. *PLOS One* (2013) **8**:e63157. doi:10.1371/journal.pone.0063157
48. Collado MC, Sanz Y. Quantification of mucosa-adhered microbiota of lambs and calves by the use of culture methods and fluorescent in situ hybridization coupled with flow cytometry techniques. *Vet Microbiol* (2007) **121**:299–306. doi:10.1016/j.vetmic.2006.12.006
49. Malmuthuge N, Li M, Chen Y, Fries P, Griebel PJ, Baurhoo B, et al. Distinct commensal bacteria associated with ingesta and mucosal epithelium in the gastrointestinal tracts of calves and chickens. *FEMS Microbiol Ecol* (2012) **79**:337–47. doi:10.1111/j.1574-6941.2011.01220
50. Romano-Keeler J, Moore DJ, Wang C, Brucker RM, Fonnesbeck C, Slaughter JC, et al. Early life establishment of site-specific microbial communities in the gut. *Gut Microbes* (2014) **5**:192–201. doi:10.4161/gmic.28442
51. Malmuthuge N, Li M, Goonewardene LA, Guan LL. Effect of calf starter feeding on gut microbial diversity and expression of genes involved in host immune responses and tight junctions in dairy calves during weaning transition. *J Dairy Sci* (2013) **96**:3189–200. doi:10.3168/jds.2012-6200
52. Malmuthuge N, Chen Y, Liang G, Goonewardane LA, Guan LL. Heat-treated colostrum feeding promotes beneficial bacteria colonization in the small intestine of neonatal calves. *J Dairy Sci* (2015) (in press). doi:10.3168/jds.2015-9607
53. Abecia L, Ramos-Morales E, Martinez-Fernandez G, Arco A, Martin-Garcia AI, Newbold CJ, et al. Feeding management in early life influences microbial colonization and fermentation in the rumen of newborn goat kids. *Anim Prod Sci* (2014) **54**:1449–54. doi:10.1071/AN14337
54. Sommer F, Backhed F. The gut microbiota – masters of host development and physiology. *Nat Rev Micorbiol* (2013) **11**:227–38. doi:10.1038/nrmicro2974
55. Petersson J, Schreiber O, Hansson GC, Gendler SJ, Velcich A, Lundberg JO, et al. Importance and regulation of the colonic mucus barrier in a mouse model of colitis. *Am J Physiol Gastrointest Liver Physiol* (2011) **300**:G327–33. doi:10.1152/ajpgi.00422.2010
56. Nowacki MR. Cell proliferation in colonic crypts of germ-free and conventional mice – preliminary report. *Folia Histochem Cytobiol* (1993) **31**: 77–81.
57. Chung H, Pamp SJ, Hill JA, Surana NK, Edelman SM, Troy EB, et al. Gut immune maturation depends on colonization with a host-specific microbiota. *Cell* (2012) **149**:1578–93. doi:10.1016/j.cell.2012.04.037
58. Griebel PJ, Hein WR. Expanding the role of Peyer's patches in B-cell ontogeny. *Immunol Today* (1996) **17**:30–8. doi:10.1016/0167-5699(96)80566-4
59. Yasuda M, Fujino M, Nasu T, Murakami T. Histological studies on the ontogeny of bovine gut-associated lymphoid tissue: appearance of T cells and development of IgG+ and IgA+ cells in lymphoid follicles. *Dev Comp Immunol* (2004) **28**:357–69. doi:10.1016/j.dci.2003.09.013
60. Gerdts V, Babiuk LA, van Drunen Littel-van den Hurk S, Griebel PJ. Fetal immunization by a DNA vaccine delivered orally into the amniotic fluid. *Nat Med* (2000) **6**:929–32. doi:10.1038/78699
61. Reynolds JD, Morris B. The effect of antigen on the development of Peyer's patches in sheep. *Eur J Immunol* (1984) **14**:1–6. doi:10.1002/eji.1830140102
62. Rakoff-Nahoum S, Paglino J, Eslami-Varzaneh F, Edberg S, Medzhitov R. Recognition of commensal microflora by toll-like receptors is required for intestinal homeostasis. *Cell* (2004) **118**:229–41. doi:10.1016/j.cell.2004.07.002
63. Teran R, Mitre E, Vaca M, Erazo S, Oviedo G, Hubner MP, et al. Immune system development during early childhood in tropical Latin America: evidence for the age-dependent down regulation of the innate immune response. *Clin Immunol* (2011) **138**:299–310. doi:10.1016/j.clim.2010.12.011
64. Fries P, Popwych YI, Guan LL, Griebel PJ. Age-related changes in the distribution and frequency of myeloid and T cell populations in the small intestine of calves. *Cell Immunol* (2011) **271**:428–37. doi:10.1016/j.cellimm.2011.08.012
65. Malmuthuge N, Fries P, Griebel PJ, Guan LL. Regional and age dependent changes in gene expression of toll-like receptors and key antimicrobial defence molecules throughout the gastrointestinal tract of dairy calves. *Vet Immunol Immunopathol* (2012) **146**:18–26. doi:10.1016/j.vetimm.2012.01.010
66. Liang G, Bao H, McFadden T, Stothard P, Griebel PJ, Guan LL. Potential regulatory role of microRNAs in the development of bovine gastrointestinal tract during early life. *PLoS One* (2014) **9**:e92592. doi:10.1371/journal.pone.0092592
67. Uetake K. Newborn calf welfare: a review focusing on mortality rates. *Anim Sci J* (2013) **84**:101–5. doi:10.1111/asj.12019
68. Sokol H, Seksik P, Furet JP, Fermisse O, Nion-Larmurier I, Beaugerie L, et al. Low counts of *Faecalibacterium prausnitzii* in colitis microbiota. *Inflamm Bowel Dis* (2009) **15**:1183–9. doi:10.1002/ibd.20903
69. Morrill KM, Conrad E, Lago A, Campbell J, Quigley J, Tyler H. Nationwide evaluation of quality and composition of colostrum on dairy farms in the United States. *J Dairy Sci* (2012) **95**:3997–4005. doi:10.3168/jds.2011-5174
70. Vasseur E, Borderas F, Cue RI, Lefebvre D, Pellerin D, Rushen J, et al. A survey of dairy calf management practices in Canada that affect animal welfare. *J Dairy Sci* (2010) **93**:1307–15. doi:10.3168/jds.2009-2429
71. Godden SM, Smolenski DJ, Donahue M, Oakes JM, Bey R, Wells S, et al. Heat-treated colostrum and reduced morbidity in preweaned dairy calves: results of a randomized trial and examination of mechanisms of effectiveness. *J Dairy Sci* (2012) **95**:4029–40. doi:10.3168/jds.2011-5275
72. Fukuda S, Toh H, Hase K, Oshima K, Nakanishi Y, Yoshimura K, et al. Bifidobacteria can protect from enteropathogenic infection through production of acetate. *Nature* (2011) **469**:543–7. doi:10.1038/nature09646
73. Krehbiel CR, Rust SR, Zhang G, Gilliland SE. Bacterial direct-fed microbials in ruminant diets: performance response and mode of action. *J Anim Sci* (2003) **81**:E120–32.
74. Charavaryamath C, Gonzalez-Cano P, Fries P, Gomis S, Doig K, Scruten E, et al. Host responses to persistent *Mycobacterium avium* subspecies *paratuberculosis* infection in surgically isolated bovine ileal segments. *Clin Vaccine Immunol* (2013) **20**:156–65. doi:10.1128/CVI.00496-12

Conflict of Interest Statement: The authors declare that the research was conducted in the absence of any commercial or financial relationships that could be construed as a potential conflict of interest.

25

Evaluation of Gastrointestinal Leakage in Multiple Enteric Inflammation Models in Chickens

*Vivek A. Kuttappan, Eduardo A. Vicuña, Juan D. Latorre, Amanda D. Wolfenden, Guillermo I. Téllez, Billy M. Hargis and Lisa R. Bielke**

Department of Poultry Science, University of Arkansas, Fayetteville, AR, USA

Edited by:
Ryan Arsenault, University of Delaware, USA

Reviewed by:
Wolfgang Ludwig Köster, University of Saskatchewan, Canada
Bernd Kaspers, University of Munich, Germany

***Correspondence:**
Lisa R. Bielke
bielke.1@osu.edu

Enteric inflammation models can help researchers' study methods to improve health and performance and evaluate various growth promoters and dietary formulations targeted to improve performance in poultry. Oral administration of fluorescein isothiocyanate-dextran (FITC-d; 3–5 kDa) and its pericellular mucosal epithelial leakage are an established marker to evaluate enteric inflammation in multiple species. The present study evaluated different methods to induce gut inflammation in poultry based on FITC-d leakage. Four independent experiments were completed with different inflammation treatment groups, and serum FITC-d and/or retention of FITC-d in GI tract were determined. In experiment 1 ($n = 10$ birds/treatment, broilers, processed at 14 days), groups included control (CON), dextran sodium sulfate (DSS; drinking water at 0.75%) and feed restriction (FRS; 24 h before processing). Experiment 2 ($n = 14$ birds/treatment, leghorns, processed at 7 days) included CON, DSS, FRS, and rye-based diet (RBD). In experiments 3 and 4 ($n = 15$ birds/treatment, broilers, processed at 7 days), groups were CON, DSS, high fat diet (HFD), FRS, and RBD. In all experiments, FRS and RBD treatments showed significantly higher serum FITC-d levels compared to the respective CON. This indicates that FRS and RBD results in disruption of the intact barrier of the gastrointestinal tract (GIT), resulting in increased gut permeability. DSS and HFD groups showed elevation of serum FITC-d levels although the magnitude of difference from respective CON was inconsistent between experiments. FRS was the only treatment which consistently showed elevated retention of FITC-d in GIT in all experiments. The results from present studies showed that FRS and RBD, based on serum FITC-d levels, can be robust models to induce gut leakage in birds in different age and species/strains.

Keywords: dextran sodium sulfate, serum FITC-d, rye-based diet, enteric inflammation, feed restriction

INTRODUCTION

It is well known that antibiotic growth promoters (AGP) can improve production performance in birds (1) although the exact mode of action is still not completely understood. According to (2), a major hypothesis about the action of AGP is through the reduction of innate inflammatory response in the gastrointestinal tract (GIT) of birds. Now that the use of AGP is discouraged in food animals, and worldwide, it is time to identify growth promoters which are as effective or even better and at the same time safer than AGP.

In addition to its role in endocrine and paracrine hormones' production, nutrient permeability, water and electrolyte exchange, and digestion, the intestinal mucosa is an important barrier for protecting animals against both commensal and pathogenic microorganisms and other insults (3–5). The intestinal first line of defense is composed of the mucus layer and epithelium (6). It has been proposed that intestinal epithelial cell defenses are essential to prevent inflammation, for example, by offering protection against microbial pathogens and oxidative stresses (7). If the intestinal barrier is damaged and becomes non-selectively permeable, the submucosa and deeper layers will be subjected to continuous exposure to antigenic molecules from food and microorganisms, causing inflammatory conditions (8).

Dextran sodium sulfate (DSS) is a heparin-like polysaccharide (9) which can cause disruption of the epithelial lining in the GIT of poultry (10). In addition, our laboratory has already used the gut inflammation induced with DSS to identify various markers to measure gut health.

Fluorescein isothiocyanate-dextran is an established method to measure paracellular leakage in rodent enteric inflammation models (11–13). Since increased mucosal permeability is the first step in the cascade of enteric inflammation, fluorescein isothiocyanate-dextran (FITC-d) model to identify gut leakage would be an effective way to detect the efficiency of various alternative growth promoters, quite early, and predict their beneficial effect on growth and production performance. Studies in our laboratory thus far have shown that oral administration of FITC-d, its leakage to circulation through disrupted epithelial lining of GIT, and subsequent measurement of FITC-d levels in serum is effective in evaluating gut leakage in birds (14, 15). The main use of this marker is to determine the effect of various growth promoters on gut health in birds.

Although DSS produces enteric inflammation in birds, our previous studies suggest that birds were more sensitive to DSS (10) compared to rodents, and achieving acceptable levels of toxicity and lesions was very narrow. Thus, other methods of induction of mucosal permeability in poultry were tested and compared with the previously established DSS model. Alternatives for DSS were feed restriction (FRS) and dietary models, such as rye-based diet (RBD) and high fat diet (HFD). A major advantage to these alternatives was the reduced risk of toxicity and severe illness to birds. At the same time, these alternatives represented various real-world scenarios which can reduced in production performance in poultry.

Feed restriction has been historically used as a way to maintain appropriate body weight of parent stock in meat-type chickens to reduce lameness and health risks, as well as improve fertility rates (16, 17). However, FRS has also been shown to increase enteric permeability, translocation of enteric bacteria to various organs (14), and could make birds more susceptible to various disease conditions related to translocation of pathogens from the GIT to systemic circulation. In addition, some regions of the world use alternate feed stuffs such as rye in place of corn. But, high levels of non-starch polysaccharides (NSP) in rye result in increased digesta viscosity as well as other associated gut health problems, thereby increasing the chance of necrotic enteritis (18–20). Furthermore, inclusion of higher levels of fat in poultry diet has been a common practice that increases growth rate; however, some of studies in mice have shown that this could also produce enteric health problems (21). Based on these facts, the main objective of the present studies was to compare the effect of DSS, FRS, HFD, and RBD on enteric leakage in chickens, measured using serum FITC-d model.

MATERIALS AND METHODS

Experimental Design

Four independent experiments were conducted, and each used different combinations of diets (**Table 1**), as well as other treatments such as FRS (for 24 h before processing) and DSS (MW 40,000; Alfa Aesar, Ward Hill, MA, USA) administered 0.75% in drinking water for 3 days before processing, as given below. Different diets used in the study were basal, RBD, and HFD, of which all met or exceeded NRC requirements (22). In all experiments, birds were administered FITC-d (MW 3,000–5,000 Da; Sigma-Aldrich Co., St. Louis, MO, USA) by oral gavage, 2.5 h before processing, to determine levels of mucosal leakage by evaluating serum FITC-d and the level of FITC-d retained in different regions of GI tract. Birds were humanely killed by inhalation of carbon

TABLE 1 | Ingredients of the feed formulations used in the study.

	CON[a]	HFD[b]	RBD[c]
Ingredients (%)			
Corn	56.59	53.57	–
Rye	–	–	58.19
Soybean meal	35.74	35.13	31.16
Vegetable oil	3.29	6.60	6.29
Dicalcium phosphate	1.81	1.87	1.79
Calcium carbonate	1.12	0.98	1.05
Salt	0.38	0.52	0.38
DL-Methionine	0.31	0.34	0.35
Vitamin premix[d]	0.20	0.20	0.20
L-Lysine HCL	0.19	0.30	0.22
Choline chloride 60%	0.10	0.20	0.10
Mineral premix[e]	0.10	0.10	0.10
Threonine	0.06	0.16	0.08
Antioxidant[f]	0.02	0.02	0.02
Mold propionic acid	0.05	0.05	0.05
Total	100	100	100
Calculated analysis			
ME (kcal/kg)	3,035	3,191	2,850
CP (%)	21.7	22.1	22.4
Lys (%)	1.32	1.35	1.32
Met (%)	0.63	0.64	0.64
Met + Cys (%)	0.98	0.99	0.98
Thr (%)	0.86	0.91	0.86
Trp (%)	0.25	0.28	0.3
Total calcium (%)	0.9	0.9	0.9
Available phosphorus (%)	0.45	0.45	0.45
Sodium (%)	0.16	0.21	0.16

[a]CON, control.
[b]HFD, high fat diet.
[c]RBD, rye-based diet.
[d]Vitamin premix (per 1,000 kg): vitamin A, 20,000,000 IU; vitamin D3, 6,000,000 IU; vitamin E, 75,000 IU; vitamin K3, 9 g; thiamine, 3 g; riboflavin, 8 g; pantothenic acid, 18 g; niacin, 60 g; pyridoxine, 5 g; folic acid, 2 g; biotin, 0.2 g; cyanocobalamin, 16 mg; and ascorbic acid, 200 g (Nutra Blend LLC, Neosho, MO, USA).
[e]Mineral premix (per 1,000 kg): manganese, 120 g; zinc, 100 g; iron, 120 g; copper, 10–15 g; iodine, 0.7 g; selenium, 0.4 g; and cobalt, 0.2 g (Nutra Blend LLC).
[f]Ethoxyquin.

dioxide gas prior to the collection of blood and GIT samples. All studies were conducted in accordance with protocols approved by the University of Arkansas Institutional Animal Care and Use Committee.

In experiment 1, 30-day-old broiler chicks were randomly assigned to one of the three treatment groups ($n = 10$/group), control (CON), FRS, or DSS. All birds were provided *ad libitum* with the basal diet (**Table 1**) until 13 days. Twenty-four hours prior to the end of the experiment, feed was removed from FRS through the end of the experiment. On day 14, all birds were given an oral gavage of FITC-d (2.2 mg/mL/bird) 2.5 h before they were processed. Blood and tissue samples from duodenum, ileum, and cecum were collected from each bird. Levels of FITC-d in serum and GI tract were determined as explained below.

Day of hatch Leghorns ($n = 56$) was used for experiment 2 and was randomly assigned to CON, DSS, FRS, and RBD ($n - 14$/treatment). In this experiment, all treatment groups except RBD were given basal diet, while RBD was given a RBD (**Table 1**), and feed removed from FRS 24 h prior to end of the experiment. All birds were processed on day 7 after oral gavage with FITC-d (2.2 mg/bird) 2.5 h before processing. Blood and GIT tissue (duodenum and cecum) samples were collected for determination of enteric inflammation.

Experiments 3 and 4 had the same experimental design but were conducted independently. For both experiment, 75-day-old broiler chicks were randomly assigned to CON, DSS, FRS, RBD, or HFD group ($n = 15$ birds/treatment). All groups except RBD and HFD were given basal diet throughout the trail while RBD and HFD were given RBD as well as HFDs, respectively (**Table 1**). As in previous experiments, feed was removed from FRS 24 h prior to the end. On day 7, all birds were given oral gavage with FITC-d (2.2 mg/bird), and serum level and GIT retention (duodenum and cecum) of FITC-d were determined.

Determination of Serum FITC-d Levels

Serum level of FITC-d, a measurement of enteric inflammation and mucosal permeability, was determined as explained by Kuttappan et al. (14). After humane slaughter of birds, femoral artery was severed to collect blood and allowed to clot under room temperature for 3 h. Then, the samples were centrifuged at $500 \times g$ for 15 min, and serum samples were collected. The serum samples were then diluted in phosphate buffer saline (1:1), and fluorescence was measured at 485 nm excitation and 528 nm emission (Synergy HT, multimode microplate reader, BioTek Instruments, Inc., VT, USA). Levels of fluorescence in the samples were converted to respective FITC-d microgram per milliliter of serum based on a calculated standard curve previously obtained from known levels of FITC-d.

Level of FITC-d Retained in Gastrointestinal Tract Tissue

Amount of FITC-d retained in different regions of GI tract were determined using the method suggested by Kuttappan et al. (14) and Vicuña et al. (15). For this, 2.5-cm-long tissue sections were collected from the descending duodenum, ileum immediately proximal to the Meckel's diverticulum, and a single entire cecum (opened at both ends). These samples were cleaned by flushing with Hanks buffered salt solution. After cleaning, samples were gently mopped to remove excess fluid, weighed, and dropped in tubes containing 10 mL Hanks buffer with glutamine (0.3 g/L) and antimicrobial agents (penicillin 100 U/mL, streptomycin 0.01 mg/mL, and amphotericin B 0.25 μg/mL). The tubes were incubated at 42°C for 2 h, and the FITC-d released to the buffer from the tissue was determined and reported as microgram per gram of the respective tissue.

Statistical Analysis

Data were analyzed using ANOVA (SAS 9.3, SAS Institute Inc., Cary, NC, USA) considering individual birds as experimental units for all experiments. Means were separated using Duncan's significant different test at $p < 0.05$. The serum FITC-d data showed occasional, but random outliers, <+2 SD from group mean, which were not representative of the respective groups similar to the reports by Kuttappan et al. (14) and Vicuña et al. (15). It is clear that these outliers were not related to treatments administered; however, the reasons for the occurrence of these erratic outliers are not yet clear. For the present studies, we focused on the effect of treatments, and the noise from these outliers was identified using the empirical or 68–95–99.7 rule and trimmed or truncated (23) at mean ± two SDs (14, 15).

RESULTS

Control levels of FITC-d in serum stayed consistent throughout experiments 1–3 with measured serum FITC-d at 0.18 ± 0.01, 0.18 ± 0.02, and 0.17 ± 0.02 μg/mL, respectively (**Tables 2–4**).

TABLE 2 | Serum FITC-d and FITC-d retentions in GI tract from experiment 1 using 2-week-old broiler birds.

Treatments	Serum FITC-d (μg/mL)	FITC-d retention (microgram per gram of tissue)		
		Duodenum	Ileum	Cecum
CON	$0.18^{c} \pm 0.01$	$0.27^{b} \pm 0.01$	$0.34^{a} \pm 0.02$	$0.37^{b} \pm 0.01$
DSS	$0.29^{b} \pm 0.02$	$0.28^{ab} \pm 0.01$	$0.35^{a} \pm 0.01$	$0.41^{b} \pm 0.01$
FRS	$0.36^{a} \pm 0.02$	$0.29^{a} \pm 0.01$	$0.38^{a} \pm 0.02$	$0.46^{a} \pm 0.02$

a–c Significant ($p < 0.05$) difference within each column.
CON, control (basal diet); DSS, dextran sodium sulfate administered at 0.75% in drinking water; FRS, feed restriction for 24 h before processing; n = 10/treatment.

TABLE 3 | Serum FITC-d and FITC-d retentions in GI tract from experiment 2 using 1-week-old leghorn birds.

Treatments	Serum FITC-d (μg/mL)	FITC-d retention (microgram per gram of tissue)	
		Duodenum	Cecum
CON	$0.18^{c} \pm 0.02$	$3.19^{b} \pm 0.33$	$26.16^{b} \pm 5.00$
DSS	$0.24^{bc} \pm 0.02$	$0.73^{c} \pm 0.24$	$12.64^{b} \pm 2.38$
FRS	$0.37^{a} \pm 0.01$	$5.16^{a} \pm 0.63$	$63.17^{a} \pm 13.84$
RBD	$0.28^{b} \pm 0.02$	$2.51^{b} \pm 0.25$	$25.74^{b} \pm 12.42$

a–c Significant ($p < 0.05$) difference within each column.
CON, control (basal diet); DSS, dextran sodium sulfate administrated at 0.75% in drinking water; FRS, feed restriction for 24 h before processing; RBD, rye-based diet; n = 14/treatment.

TABLE 4 | Serum FITC-d and FITC-d retentions in GI tract from experiments 3 and 4 using 1-week-old broiler birds.

	Serum (μg/mL)		Duodenum (microgram per gram of tissue)		Cecum (microgram per gram of tissue)	
	Experiment 3	**Experiment 4**	**Experiment 3**	**Experiment 4**	**Experiment 3**	**Experiment 4**
CON	$0.17^{c} \pm 0.02$	$0.25^{c} \pm 0.03$	$0.73^{c} \pm 0.16$	$0.48^{b} \pm 0.12$	$22.36^{b} \pm 6.47$	$7.55^{b} \pm 1.61$
DSS	$0.26^{bc} \pm 0.04$	$0.28^{bc} \pm 0.02$	$1.25^{bc} \pm 0.11$	$0.70^{ab} \pm 0.06$	$13.95^{b} \pm 3.73$	$8.65^{b} \pm 1.66$
HFD	$0.29^{abc} \pm 0.02$	$0.29^{bc} \pm 0.01$	$1.35^{bc} \pm 0.18$	$0.77^{ab} \pm 0.18$	$9.68^{b} \pm 1.48$	$5.83^{b} \pm 1.78$
FRS	$0.46^{a} \pm 0.10$	$0.32^{b} \pm 0.03$	$2.13^{a} \pm 0.22$	$1.15^{a} \pm 0.21$	$49.69^{a} \pm 16.42$	$37.33^{a} \pm 11.17$
RBD	$0.44^{ab} \pm 0.08$	$0.38^{a} \pm 0.02$	$1.63^{ab} \pm 0.32$	$1.05^{a} \pm 0.12$	$4.71^{b} \pm 0.90$	$2.59^{b} \pm 0.45$

[a–c]*Significant ($p < 0.05$) difference within each column.*
CON, control (basal diet); DSS, dextran sodium sulfate administrated at 0.75% in drinking water; HFD, high fat diet; FRS, feed restriction for 24 h before processing; RBD, rye-based diet; n = 15/treatment.

Though there was a slight increase noted in experiment 4, at 0.25 ± 0.0 3 μg/mL, significant differences were still noted with FRS and RBD. Levels recovered from the various GIT tissues varied greatly. In experiment 1, serum FITC-d in both treatments was significantly higher than CON, with DSS at 0.29 ± 0.02 μg/mL and FRS at 0.36 ± 0.02 μg/mL, compared to 0.18 ± 0.01 μg/mL (**Table 2**). For FRS, this difference was repeated in experiment 2 with serum FITC-d measured at 0.37 ± 0.01 and 0.18 ± 0.02 μg/mL in CON, but DSS was not significantly higher at only 0.24 ± 0.02 μg/mL (**Table 3**). This experiment included an additional group, RBD, which had serum FITC-d levels higher than CON, but no different than DSS, and lower than FRS at 0.28 ± 0.02 μg/mL. In experiments 3 and 4, only FRS and RBD resulted in greater passage of FITC-d to serum with 0.32 ± 0.03 and 0.38 ± 0.02 μg/mL, respectively, compare to 0.25 ± 0.03 μg/mL in the CON group. Neither DSS nor HFD increased FITC-d levels in serum for those experiments.

Retention of FITC-d in GIT tissue was measured in duodenum, ileum, and cecum in experiment 1 and duodenum and cecum in the other experiments. Differences in retention were noted between FRS and CON groups for duodenum and cecum, but not ileum in the first experiment, though the level of change was not likely biologically significant (**Table 2**). In experiment 2, FRS resulted in higher retention of FITC-d in both duodenal and cecal tissue with levels measured at $5.16^{a} \pm 0.63$ and $63.17^{a} \pm 13.84$ μg/g of tissues, respectively, while DSS levels in the duodenum were lower than CON tissue, this decrease is not consistent with other experiments reported here (**Table 3**). RBD did not result in changes, compared to CON, in retention of FITC-d in either the duodenum or the cecum (**Table 3**).

Duodenal retention of FITC-d was affected by FRS (2.13 ± 0.22 and 1.15 ± 0.21 μg/g) and RBD (1.63 ± 0.32 and 1.05 ± 0.12 μg/g) in experiments 3 and 4, compared to CON (0.73 ± 0.16 and 0.48 ± 0.12 μg/g; **Table 4**). Whereas, in the cecum for experiments 3 and 4, only FRS was different from all other groups with FICT-d retained in tissue, which was 49.69 ± 16.42 and 37.33 ± 11.17 μg/g.

DISCUSSION

Serum FITC-d Levels

Determination of serum FITC-d to evaluate enteric inflammation has long been established marker in murine models (11–13). Results from these studies, conducted on chickens, using DSS-FITC-d model (14) suggest that DSS could have caused the disruption of tight junctions in GI tract, increased mucosal permeability (13, 24), ultimately resulting in increased serum FITC-d levels. In experiment 1, the DSS and FRS groups showed higher ($p < 0.05$) serum FITC-d levels when compared to the respective CON (**Table 2**). This result was in accordance with reports from the studies conducted by Kuttappan et al. (14). Furthermore, FRS group had even higher serum FITC-d level when compared to the respective DSS group (**Table 1**). Kuttappan et al. (14) showed comparable levels of serum FITC-d between the DSS and FRS groups. This could be because of the fact that Kuttappan et al. (14) used an oral gavage with DSS while the present study administered DSS at the level of 0.75% in drinking water. Thus, when DSS was administered as a high dose for a short period of time (14), it could have a greater impact when compared to low dose prolonged period of administration in the present study, though a direct comparison of the two methods was not completed. In addition, Kuttappan et al. (14) used broilers which were 1-week old while the present study used broiler birds which were 2 weeks old. In fact, the results from these two studies suggested that the serum FITC-d could be used as a marker for gut health in birds across different age groups.

In experiment 2, DSS showed elevated serum FITC-d levels when compared to the respective CON group although it was not significant ($p > 0.05$). However, FRS and RBD groups showed significantly ($p < 0.05$) higher serum FITC-d levels when compared to the respective CON group. Kuttappan et al. (14) previously reported that FRS could result in increased serum FITC-d leakage in broilers. Furthermore, van der Hulst et al. (25, 26) reported that starvation in human patients could result in lack of enough glutamine which could lead to increased gut leakage. Additionally, Tellez et al. (20, 27) reported that RBD, in comparison to corn-based diet, resulted in increased serum FITC-d levels and also significantly ($p < 0.05$) higher translocation of enteric bacteria to liver, both in broiler chicks and turkey poults. The present study was completed in leghorns, and these results confirmed that the model for measuring gut health using serum FITC-d is reliable through different species and strains of poultry.

Experiments 3 and 4 compared serum FITC-d in broilers in CON, DSS, HFD, FRS, and RBD (**Table 3**). Similar to experiment 2, DSS showed elevated serum FITC-d levels with CON although, it was not significantly different. HFD resulted in a trend similar to DSS both in experiments 3 and 4.

de Lartigue et al. (21) had reported that HFD in mice could increase intestinal permeability by altering the expression of tight junction proteins, though results in chickens were not as marked as were reported in mice. Consistent with experiment 2, both FRS and RBD showed higher serum FITC-d levels compared to the respective CON. The results from all four experiments in this trial showed that FRS and RBD could cause increased gut leakage in poultry, which are relevant to current poultry practices. FRS, most commonly skip-a-day feeding, is widely used in meat-type poultry breeder stocks to regulate weight gain and maintain fertility. Increased serum FITC-d due to FRS as reported by the present study suggested that FRS in breeders could result in increased gut leakage and could lead to translocation of enteric bacteria to other tissue organs which could result in disease conditions, such as lameness (28). Similarly, attempts to use least cost feed formulation for poultry often includes the incorporation of alternative feed grains, such as wheat and rye in poultry feed, quite often resulting in reduced performance and poor litter conditions (18, 29, 30). Rye contains high levels of NSP, comprised of highly branched arabinoxylans, which are mainly responsible for increased digesta viscosity, reduced activity of digestive enzymes, and reduced intestinal absorption, making birds susceptible to economically significant conditions, such as necrotic enteritis (19, 31, 32). Our laboratory is currently investigating the effect of various probiotics and dietary enzymes in reducing the gut leakage associated with FRS and RBD based on the serum FITC-d marker.

Retention of FITC-d in Gastrointestinal Tract Tissues

Kuttappan et al. (14) suggested that the disruption of epithelial layer in the GIT could result in increased infiltration of FITC-d in the paracellular space between cells on the mucosal surface. In all experiments, FRS showed significantly higher FITC-d levels in duodenum and cecum compared to the respective CON birds (**Tables 2–4**). This was in accordance with the results reported by Kuttappan et al. (14). However, Kuttappan et al. (14) also found that administration of DSS as oral gavage resulted in increased retention of FITC-d in duodenum of broiler chickens when compared to CON, although the cecum did not show any significant difference. With a prolonged administration of low dose DSS (0.75% in drinking water) in the present study, FITC-d did not significantly increase (**Tables 2–4**). Moreover, RBD, which consistently showed elevated serum FITC-d levels, failed to reflect any difference in GIT tissue FITC-d levels with respect to the CON (**Tables 3** and **4**). These data suggest that the retention of FITC-d could be more complex which depends upon factors, such as rate of GI passage, which could be affected by irritation on GIT wall, and viscosity of diet as in the case of rye diet. Thus, level of FITC-d retained in GIT tissue may not be a direct measurement of gut leakage as compared to serum FITC-d levels.

CONCLUSION

The results from present studies showed that FRS and RBD are consistent methods for inducing mucosal leakage that could lead to enteric inflammation in poultry. Serum FITC-d measurement was proven to be a very reliable and non-invasive marker to determine gut leakage in birds across different age and strains. Since the method involves oral administration of FITC-d and subsequent measurement of FITC-d in serum, it could possibly be used in live birds at multiple time points throughout a single experiment. Further studies will be conducted in our laboratory comparing different growth promoters in poultry and their effect on gut leakage under various conditions using serum FITC-d model.

REFERENCES

1. Butaye P, Devriese LA, Haesebrouck F. Antimicrobial growth promoters used in animal feed: effects of less well known antibiotics on gram-positive bacteria. *Clin Microbiol Rev* (2003) **16**:175–88. doi:10.1128/CMR.16.2.175-188.2003
2. Niewold TA. The nonantibiotic anti-inflammatory effect of antimicrobial growth promoters, the real mode of action? A hypothesis. *Poult Sci* (2007) **86**:605–9. doi:10.1093/ps/86.4.605
3. Kitajima S, Takuma S, Morimoto M. Changes in colonic mucosal permeability in mouse colitis induced with dextran sulfate sodium. *Exp Anim* (1999) **48**(3):137–43. doi:10.1538/expanim.48.137
4. Kitajima S, Takuma S, Morimoto M. Histological analysis of murine colitis induced by dextran sulfate sodium of different molecular weights. *Exp Anim* (2000) **49**(1):9–15. doi:10.1538/expanim.49.9
5. Sansonetti PJ. War and peace at mucosal surfaces. *Nat Rev Immunol* (2004) **4**:953–64. doi:10.1038/nri1499
6. Fasina YO, Hoerr FJ, McKee SR, Conner DE. Influence of *Salmonella enterica* serovar Typhimurium infection on intestinal goblet cells and villous morphology in broiler chicks. *Avian Dis* (2010) **54**:841–7. doi:10.1637/9055-090809-Reg.1
7. Kawada M, Arihiro A, Mizoguchi E. Insights from advances in research of chemically induced experimental models of human inflammatory bowel disease. *World J Gastroenterol* (2007) **13**:5581–93. doi:10.3748/wjg.v13.i42.5581
8. Quinteiro-Filho WM, Gomes AVS, Pinheiro ML, Ribeiro A, Ferraz-de-Paula V, Astolfi-Ferreira CS, et al. Heat stress impairs performance and induces intestinal inflammation in broiler chickens infected with *Salmonella* Enteritidis. *Avian Pathol* (2012) **41**(5):421–7. doi:10.1080/03079457.2012.709315
9. Laroui H, Ingersoll SA, Liu HC, Baker MT, Ayyadurai S, Charania MA, et al. Dextran sodium sulfate (DSS) induces colitis in mice by forming nano-lipocomplexes with medium-chain-length fatty acids in the colon. *PLoS One* (2012) **4**:e32084. doi:10.1371/journal.pone.0032084
10. Menconi A, Hernandez-Velasco X, Vicuña EA, Kuttappan VA, Faulkner OB, Tellez G, et al. Histopathological and morphometric changes induced by a dextran sodium sulfate (DSS) model in broilers. *Poult Sci* (2015) **94**:906–11. doi:10.3382/ps/pev054
11. Shah YM, Ma X, Morimura K, Kim I, Gonzalez FJ. Pregnane X receptor activation ameliorates DSS-induced inflammatory bowel disease via inhibition of NF-κB target gene expression. *Am J Physiol Gastrointest Liver Physiol* (2007) **292**:G1114–22. doi:10.1152/ajpgi.00528.2006
12. Brandl K, Rutschmann S, Li X, Du X, Xiao N, Schnabl B, et al. Enhanced sensitivity to DSS colitis caused by a hypomorphic Mbtps1 mutation disrupting the ATF6-driven unfolded protein response. *Proc Natl Acad Sci U S A* (2009) **106**:3300–5. doi:10.1073/pnas.0813036106
13. Yan Y, Kolachala V, Dalmasso G, Nguyen H, Laroui H, Sitaraman SV, et al. Temporal and spatial analysis of clinical and molecular parameters in dextran sodium sulfate induced colitis. *PLoS One* (2009) **4**:e6073. doi:10.1371/journal.pone.0006073
14. Kuttappan VA, Berghman LR, Vicuña EA, Latorre JD, Menconi A, Wolchok JD, et al. Poultry enteric inflammation model with dextran sodium sulfate mediated chemical induction and feed restriction in broilers. *Poult Sci* (2015) **94**:1220–6. doi:10.3382/ps/pev114

15. Vicuña EA, Kuttappan VA, Tellez G, Hernandez-Velasco X, Seeber-Galarza R, Latorre JD, et al. Dose titration of FITC-D for optimal measurement of enteric inflammation in broiler chicks. *Poult Sci* (2015) **94**:1353–9. doi:10.3382/ps/pev111
16. Lee PJW, Gulliver AL, Morris TR. Restricted feeding of broiler breeder pullets during the rearing period and its effect on productivity and breeding. *Br Poult Sci* (1971) **12**:499–510. doi:10.1080/00071667108415905
17. Yu MW, Robinson FE, Robblee AR. Effect of feed allowance during rearing and breeding on female broiler breeders. 1. growth and carcass characteristics. *Poult Sci* (1992) **71**:1739–49. doi:10.3382/ps.0711739
18. Choct M, Hughes RJ, Trimble RP, Angkanaporn K, Annison G. Non-starch polysaccharide-degrading enzymes increase the performance of broiler chickens fed wheat of low apparent metabolizable energy. *J Nutr* (1995) **125**: 485–92.
19. Annett CB, Viste JR, Chirino-Trejo M, Classen HL, Middleton DM, Simko E. Necrotic enteritis: effect of barley, wheat and corn diets on proliferation of *Clostridium perfringens* type A. *Avian Pathol* (2002) **31**:598–601. doi:10.1080/0307945021000024544
20. Tellez G, Latorre JD, Kuttappan VA, Kogut MH, Wolfenden A, Hernandez-Velasco X, et al. Utilization of rye as energy source affects bacterial translocation, intestinal viscosity, microbiota composition, and bone mineralization in broiler chickens. *Front Genet* (2014) **5**:339. doi:10.3389/fgene.2014.00339
21. de Lartigue G, de La Serre CB, Raybould HE. Vagal afferent neurons in high fat diet-induced obesity; intestinal microflora, gut inflammation and cholecystokinin. *Physiol Behav* (2011) **105**:100–5. doi:10.1016/j.physbeh.2011.02.040
22. National Research Council. *Nutrient Requirements of Poultry*. 9th revised ed. Washington, DC: National Academy Press (1994).
23. Ghosh D, Vogt A. Outliers: an evaluation of methodologies. *Joint Statistical Meetings*. San Diego, CA: American Statistical Association (2012). p. 3455–60.
24. Johansson MEV, Gustafsson JK, Sjöberg KE, Petersson J, Holm L, Sjövall H, et al. Bacteria penetrate the inner mucus layer before inflammation in the dextran sulfate colitis model. *PLoS One* (2010) **5**:e12238. doi:10.1371/journal.pone.0012238
25. van der Hulst RR, van Kreel BK, von Meyenfeldt MF, Brummer RJ, Arends JW, Deutz NE, et al. Glutamine and the preservation of gut integrity. *Lancet* (1993) **341**:1363–5. doi:10.1016/0140-6736(93)90939-E
26. van der Hulst RR, Deutz NE, von Meyenfeldt MF, Elbers JM, Stockbrügger RW, Soeters PB. Decrease of mucosal glutamine concentration in the nutritionally depleted patient. *Clin Nutr* (1994) **13**:228–33. doi:10.1016/0261-5614(94)90080-9
27. Tellez G, Latorre JD, Kuttappan VA, Hargis BM, Hernandez-Velasco X. Rye affects bacterial translocation, intestinal viscosity, microbiota composition and bone mineralization in Turkey poults. *PLoS One* (2015) **10**(4):e0122390. doi:10.1371/journal.pone.0122390
28. Wideman RF, Prisby RD. Bone circulatory disturbances in the development of spontaneous bacterial chondronecrosis with osteomyelitis: a translational model for the pathogenesis of femoral head necrosis. *Front Endocrinol* (2013) **3**:183. doi:10.3389/fendo.2012.00183
29. Campbell GL, Campbell LD, Classen HL. Utilisation of rye by chickens: effect of microbial status, diet gamma irradiation and sodium taurocholate supplementation. *Br Poult Sci* (1983) **24**:191–203. doi:10.1080/00071668308416730
30. Fengler AI, Marquardt RR. Water soluble pentosans from rye. I. Isolation, partial purification, and characterization. *Cereal Chem* (1988) **65**:291–7.
31. Hofacre CL. Necrotic enteritis, currently a billion dollar disease: is there anything new on the horizon. In: Lyons TP, Jacques KA, editors. *Proceedings of Alltech's 17th Annual Symposium Science and Technology in the Feed Industry*. Nottingham: Nottingham University Press (2001). p. 79–86.
32. Timbermont L, Lanckriet A, Dewulf J, Nollet N, Schwarzer K, Haesebrouck F, et al. Control of *Clostridium perfringens*-induced necrotic enteritis in broilers by target-released butyric acid, fatty acids and essential oils. *Avian Pathol* (2010) **39**:117–21. doi:10.1080/03079451003610586

Conflict of Interest Statement: The authors declare that the research was conducted in the absence of any commercial or financial relationships that could be construed as a potential conflict of interest.

Salmonella enterica Serovars Enteritidis Infection Alters the Indigenous Microbiota Diversity in Young Layer Chicks

*Khin K. Z. Mon, Perot Saelao, Michelle M. Halstead, Ganrea Chanthavixay, Huai-Chen Chang, Lydia Garas, Elizabeth A. Maga and Huaijun Zhou**

Department of Animal Science, University of California Davis, Davis, CA, USA

Edited by:
Michael Kogut, USDA-ARS, USA

Reviewed by:
Lisa Bielke, Ohio State University, USA
Guillermo Tellez, University of Arkansas, USA

***Correspondence:**
Huaijun Zhou
hzhou@ucdavis.edu

Avian gastrointestinal (GI) tracts are highly populated with a diverse array of microorganisms that share a symbiotic relationship with their hosts and contribute to the overall health and disease state of the intestinal tract. The microbiome of the young chick is easily prone to alteration in its composition by both exogenous and endogenous factors, especially during the early posthatch period. The genetic background of the host and exposure to pathogens can impact the diversity of the microbial profile that consequently contributes to the disease progression in the host. The objective of this study was to profile the composition and structure of the gut microbiota in young chickens from two genetically distinct highly inbred lines. Furthermore, the effect of the *Salmonella* Enteritidis infection on altering the composition makeup of the chicken microbiome was evaluated through the 16S rRNA gene sequencing analysis. One-day-old layer chicks were challenged with *S.* Enteritidis and the host cecal microbiota profile as well as the degree of susceptibility to *Salmonella* infection was examined at 2 and 7 days post infection. Our result indicated that host genotype had a limited effect on resistance to *S.* Enteritidis infection. Alpha diversity, beta diversity, and overall microbiota composition were analyzed for four factors: host genotype, age, treatment, and postinfection time points. *S.* Enteritidis infection in young chicks was found to significantly reduce the overall diversity of the microbiota population with expansion of *Enterobacteriaceae* family. These changes indicated that *Salmonella* colonization in the GI tract of the chickens has a direct effect on altering the natural development of the GI microbiota. The impact of *S.* Enteritidis infection on microbial communities was also more substantial in the late stage of infection. Significant inverse correlation between *Enterobacteriaceae* and *Lachnospiraceae* family in both non-infected and infected groups, suggested possible antagonistic interaction between members of these two taxa, which could potentially influences the overall microbial population in the gut. Our results also revealed that genetic difference between two lines had minimal effect on the establishment of microbiota population. Overall, this study provided preliminary insights into the contributing role of *S.* Enteritidis in influencing the overall makeup of chicken's gut microbiota.

Keywords: ***Salmonella* Enteritidis, chickens, gut microbiota, 16S rRNA, MHC haplotypes**

INTRODUCTION

The avian gastrointestinal (GI) tract is home to complex and diverse bacterial populations that provide many beneficial functions to host, which includes conferring colonization resistance against the invading pathogenic microorganisms. Development of the GI microbiota in chickens occurs immediately after hatching and is influenced by both genetic and external factors like diet and environment (1). Unlike other animals, a newly hatched chick does not have acquired healthy maternal microbiota as they are housed separately from the adult hens immediately after hatch in commercial production (2). Therefore, the GI tract of newly hatched chickens is usually sterile and presents an empty ecological niche that provides easy access for the pathogen to colonize with limited restriction (2). This factor alone makes young chickens highly susceptible to enteric bacterial infections, such as *Salmonella*, which can result in different degrees of disease spectrum from a subclinical carrier state to a high mortality rate depending on the infecting bacterial serovar and host's susceptibility.

Salmonella enterica subsp. *enterica* serovar Enteritidis is a zoonotic enteric pathogen that is most frequently associated with diarrheal disease in humans while chickens serve as asymptotic carrier (3). Consumption of contaminated eggs produced by infected layer hens is one of the leading causes of *Salmonella* food poisoning in humans (4). In chickens, S. Enteritidis can be easily transmitted horizontally via the fecal–oral route as well as vertically via the reproductive tract, which can contaminate the egg (5). Additionally, chickens can also harbor S. Enteritidis asymptomatically and persist throughout their lifespan, which makes the identification of infected chickens and the eradication of the pathogen much more challenging. Young chickens can be exposed to S. Enteritidis through numerous external sources like contaminated feed or environment. The sterile GI tract of the newly hatched chickens also provides ample opportunities for a pathogenic organism like S. Enteritidis to firmly establish its own niche in the gut as early colonizer and potentially further impact the development of the gut microbiota during the disease state. Early exposure to *Salmonella* in young chick could result in two potential alternative outcomes: high mortality rate or persistence of infection in surviving chickens (6). Prolonged persistent infection with S. Enteritidis in the GI tract of chickens throughout their lifespan could alter the development of gut microbiota and have detrimental effect on the overall gut health of the chicken host.

The impact of genetic background on the composition of chicken gut microbiota has been mostly investigated in broilers due to the association of intestinal microbiota with performance of broiler chickens in terms of feed conversion efficiency (7–11). Studies in broiler chickens have indeed shown evidence that host genotype had significant impact on shaping the composition of the gut microbiota (7, 9, 11). Few studies had explored the relationship between the host genotype and its influence on microbiota composition in layer chickens, especially related to disease resistance. The host genetic background plays an important role in the resistance and susceptibility to *Salmonella* infection (12). Several studies have reported that many genes have been found to be associated with *Salmonella* resistance in the chicken (6, 13). One of the key candidate genes, known as major histocompatibility complex (MHC), plays an important role in disease resistance in the chicken (13–20). University of California, Davis (UCD) maintains a number of congenic layer lines differing in MHC B-complex haplotypes. A study by Cotter et al. had previously examined the association of B-complex immunity to S. Enteritidis using 12 congenic lines from UCD, differing in various B-complex haplotypes (13). Results from the study had suggested that chickens from UCD254 (B^{15}/B^{15}) were more susceptible to *Salmonella* infection compared to other lines in term of mortality and morbidity (13). However, underlying mechanism associated with susceptibility to *Salmonella* remains to be elucidated. As microbiota is a significant contributor to disease resistance, two highly inbred line UCD254 (B^{15}/B^{15}) and UCD077 (B^{15}/B^{16}) at UCD were used to examine MHC effect on microbial community in chicken intestinal gut.

The main objective of this study was to examine the impact of host genetic background on influencing early establishment of microbiota in combination with S. Enteritidis infection to determine S. Enteritidis-associated alteration in gut microbiota.

MATERIALS AND METHODS

Experimental Animals

Two genetically distinct, highly inbred layer chickens from line UCD077 and UCD254 were obtained on the day of hatch from UCD's poultry farm. A cloaca swab was performed to ensure all birds were *Salmonella*-free. The chickens were then transferred and housed in the temperature-controlled chambers with *ad libitum* access to water and commercial feed without antibiotic treatment. At 1 day of age, chickens were orally inoculated with 1×10^8 c.f.u of S. Enteritidis TN2 nalidixic acid-resistant strain (kindly provided by Dr. Andreas Baumler) or PBS for the non-infected birds. Dosage of S. Enteritidis was confirmed by serial dilution plating of the inoculum. A total of three replicate trials were conducted. For the duration of the trials, all non-infected chickens were housed together in the concrete floor pen with fresh, wood shaving for bedding material inside the environmental chamber. The infected group of chickens was housed separately in another chamber with the same environmental conditions as the control chamber. At 2 and 7 days postinoculation (DPI), chickens were euthanized by the carbon dioxide asphyxiation to collect spleen and cecal content for further analysis. Similarly, the organs from the same-age counterpart in non-infected group of 3 days old (3 D) and 8 days old (8 D) were also collected. All animal experiments were performed according to the guidelines approved by the Institutional Animal Care and Use Committee at the UCD.

Enumeration of Bacteria in Spleen and Cecal Content

Viable counts of S. Enteritidis were recovered from one of the ceca pouches by squeezing its contents into 10 ml PBS and placing immediately on ice after the collection. The second pouch of ceca was collected on ice and frozen at −20°C for the DNA extraction. The weight of the cecum content was measured prior to spreading serial 10-fold dilutions on Xylose Lysine Tergitol-4 (XLT4) selective agar plates containing tetracycline. Similarly, half of the spleen was weighted and homogenized in 1 ml PBS by using the black rubber end of the sterile plunger from the 2 ml syringe before plating. The plates were then incubated at 37°C for 24 h. Counts of S. Enteritidis were log transformed and expressed as $\log_{10}$ CFU per gram of the cecal content for further statistical analysis.

DNA Extraction and PCR Amplification of 16S rRNA Gene Sequences

Approximately 150 mg of total cecal content was used for DNA isolation by Zymo fecal DNA miniprep (Zymo Research, Irvine, CA, USA) in accordance with the manufacturer's instructions. In brief, bead-beating step was performed using the Bullet Blender Storm 24 (Next Advance Inc., Averill Park, NY, USA) for 5 min at maximum speed setting. Concentration and purity of the extracted DNA was measured on the NanoDrop ND-2000C spectrophotometer (ThermoScientific Inc., USA). All extracted DNA samples were stored at −20°C until further analysis. PCR amplification was performed with F515 (5′NNNNNNNN**GT**GTGCCAGCMGCCGCGGTAA3′) and R806 (5′GGACTACHVGGGTWTCTAAT3′) primers targeting the V4 segment of the bacterial 16S rRNA gene where the forward primer was modified to contain the linker region (GT) for sequencing on the Illumina MiSeq platform and a unique 8 bp barcode sequence (*N*) for each sample (21). PCR conditions were set at initial denaturation for 94°C for 3 min; followed by 35 cycles of 94°C for 45 sec, 50°C for 1 min, 72°C for 1 min 30 s with final extension step at 72°C for 10 min. The PCR reaction contained 12.5 µl 2× GoTaq Green Master Mix (Promega, Madison, WI, USA), 9.5 µl nuclease-free water, 0.5 µl forward and reverse primers, and 2.0 µl DNA. All samples were amplified in triplicate and combined after PCR for the purification. The PCR products were inspected on a 1% agarose gel stained with SYBR safe (Life Technologies, CA, USA) and stored at −20°C. The PCR amplicons were purified with QIAquick PCR Purification kit (Qiagen, Valencia, CA, USA) according to the manufacturer's instruction. The pooled amplicons were then submitted to the University of California, Davis Genome Center, DNA Technology Core Facility for generating 250 paired-end reads on the Illumina MiSeq sequencing platform.

16S rRNA Sequence Data Processing

The Quantitative Insights into Microbial Ecology (QIIME) version 1.9.1 was used to analyze the sequencing data generated from three replicate trials samples (**Table 1**). Raw data were demultiplexed, and quality filtered with QIIME default settings (22). The 250-bp reads were truncated at any site of more than three sequential bases receiving a quality score <Q10 and any read containing ambiguous base calls or barcode/primer errors were discarded as were reads with <75% (of total read length) consecutive high-quality base calls. Similar sequences were clustered together into the operational taxonomic units (OTUs) at 97% identity using QIIME open reference OTU picking against the Greengenes 16S rRNA database (version 13_8) (23).

TABLE 1 | Summary of number of chickens used in each of the replicate trials for 16S rRNA gene sequencing analysis.

Trial	Line	Non-infected (3 D)	S. Enteritidis-infected (2 DPI)	Non-infected (8 D)	S. Enteritidis-infected (7 DPI)
1	UCD077	4	11	0	0
	UCD254	4	21	3	11
2	UCD077	5	8	4	5
	UCD254	5	6	5	5
3	UCD077	5	8	5	5
	UCD254	5	10	5	8

3 D, 3 days old; 8 D, 8 days old; 2 DPI, 2 days post infection; 7 DPI, 7 days post infection.

Microbiota Diversity Analysis

Both alpha and beta diversity metrics were used to analyze micro biome composition. Alpha diversity metrics analysis includes Chao1 index (richness estimate), Shannon's diversity, and Simpson's diversity index. Chao1 richness estimates the total number of species present in the community. The difference between the Shannon and Simpson indices is that the weights of abundant species are accounted differently. Both the abundance and evenness in distribution of species present in the community is included in Shannon index analysis, while only the abundance of species is considered in Simpson indices (24). Microbial community dominated by a few species is considered to exhibit low evenness, while the community where the species abundances are distributed equally within the community are considered as balance community.

Rarefaction curve was constructed based on the observed number of OTUs as function of number of sequences analyzed with QIIME to compare between non-infected and infected groups. Estimates of beta diversity were made using both unweighted UniFrac and weighted UniFrac (25) followed by principal coordinate analysis (PCoA) in QIIME to characterize the microbial population diversity. To analyze the relative abundance of the microbial members at the family level, we identified eight major family groups that adhered to two conditions: classified OTU and population density detectable at more than 2% of the total community in all samples. For OTUs that were unclassified or in low abundances (below 2%), were binned together in others/unknown category. The results from the QIIME were further analyzed with linear discriminate analysis effect size (LEfSe) (26). Then Kruskal–Wallis rank sum test was used to identify significantly differential abundance of the microbiota community between the comparison groups. Differentially distributed microbiome taxa were identified based on Ribosomal Database Project (RDP) that generated LEfSe cladograms for the each category comparison. Cladograms that had statistically significant taxonomic differences between the groups were identified. Significant alpha values of 0.05 and effect size threshold of 2 were used in the LEfSe analysis.

Statistical Analysis

Splenic and cecal bacterial burden recovered from individual chickens between comparison groups were evaluated using unpaired *t*-test by the GraphPad Prism version 6.00 (GraphPad Software, La Jolla, CA, USA, www.graphpad.com). Furthermore, statistically significant differences in alpha diversity metrics were determined by performing Mann–Whitney *U* test with the Prism. Comparisons of relative abundance level of microbial members at the family level between different categories of comparisons that include treatment at different time point of experiment (non-infected at 3 and 8 D vs. *S.* Enteritidis-infected chickens at 2 and 7 DPI, respectively), days post infection (2 vs. 7 DPI), and age (3 vs. 8 D), were evaluated by performing Wilcoxon rank sum test with the JMP statistical software (version 12). To compare the relative abundance of dominant bacteria group at the family level in both non-infected and infected group, correlation coefficients and linear regression were also performed using the JMP.

RESULTS

Effect of MHC Haplotypes on the Degree of Susceptibility to *S.* Enteritidis Infection Between Two Genetically Distinct Inbred Layer Lines

To determine whether the chicken MHC haplotype difference between the two genetic lines has an effect on the resistance or susceptibility to *S.* Enteritidis infection, kinetics of *S.* Enteritidis dissemination into spleen organ was examined to characterize the phenotypic difference between the two genetically distinct inbred lines. Three replicate trials were carried out. There was significant difference in splenic bacterial load detected between the two genetic lines at 2 DPI for the trial 1 ($p < 0.0001$) and combined data of three trials ($p < 0.01$) (Figure S1 in Supplementary Material). *S.* Enteritidis-infected chickens from UCD254 showing significantly higher bacterial burden at 2 DPI than from UCD077. There was no significant difference in splenic bacterial load at 7 DPI for either three individual trials or combined data of three trials.

The intestinal colonization level in the ceca of the two lines was also evaluated. There was no significant difference between two genetic lines in both trials 1 and 2 for both time points except trial 3 at 2 DPI ($p < 0.0001$). *S.* Enteritidis colonization level in cecal was significantly higher for UCD077 than UCD254 (Figure S2 in Supplementary Material). However, combined data from all three trials was significant at 7 DPI ($p < 0.01$) with higher cecal colonization detected in UCD254 than in UCD077 (Figure S2 in Supplementary Material).

MHC Haplotype Effect on Microbiota Composition in Non-Infected and Infected Chickens

A total of 1,773,077 reads were generated from a total of 148 individuals combined from all three trials. Altogether, 15,618 different OTUs were identified from 50 non-infected chickens and 98 *S.* Enteritidis-infected chickens with 64 samples from 2 DPI and 34 samples from 7 DPI. There was no significant difference in alpha diversity metrics between two genetic lines of non-infected chickens at both 3 and 8 D (Figures S3 and S4 in Supplementary Material).

Alpha diversity metrics evaluated between two genetic lines of *S.* Enteritidis-infected chickens showed no significant difference at both days of postinfection periods (2 and 7 DPI) for all indices except for Simpson's diversity in *S.* Enteritidis-infected groups at 7 DPI ($p < 0.05$) (Figures S5 and S6 in Supplementary Material).

Developmental Differences in Cecal Microbiota Composition in Non-Infected Chickens

In general, the results above suggested that there was no significant difference in microbial composition between two genetic lines. Therefore, data from both genetic lines were combined for further analysis. The alpha diversity metrics were compared between the two age groups of non-infected chickens. Both Chao1 richness and Simpson's diversity showed no significant differences between the two age groups (**Figures 1A,B**). However, chickens at 8 days old of age had significantly more diverse microbial community structure in Shannon's index ($p < 0.01$), suggesting a more balance distribution of the species in the community in older chickens than younger birds (**Figure 1C**).

Beta diversity of the two age groups was also compared via unweighted UniFrac distance metric followed by the PCoA analysis (**Figure 2A**). Microbial composition differences between two age groups were significant ($p = 0.001$), but two clusters were not clearly separable ($r = 0.488$) (**Figure 2A**). Furthermore, weighted UniFrac distance metric was also used to compare between the two age groups followed by the PCoA analysis in considering the effect of relative abundance of microorganisms in each age group (**Figure 2B**). ANOSIM analysis showed significant difference in microbial community structure between two age groups ($p = 0.001$) and higher r value of more than 0.5 ($r = 0.5403$) indicated that separation of two groups was significant (**Figure 2B**).

Microbiota compositions between two age groups were further analyzed using the linear discriminant analysis with effect size (LEfSe). Differentially abundant phyla detected in the age groups showed that Proteobacteria phylum was most dominantly present in younger chickens (3 D), while the most abundant phylum was Firmicutes for the older chickens (8 D) (**Figure 3A**). Three differentially represented core major groups at the order level were identified. For 8-day-old chickens, overrepresentation of Clostridiales and underrepresentation of Burkholderiales and Enterobacteriales were found (**Figure 3B**). Relative abundance of microbiota composition differences at eight major families were then compared between the two age groups using a Wilcoxon rank sum test. There was significantly marked decrease in *Clostridiaceae* ($p < 0.0001$), *Peptostreptococcaceae* ($p < 0.0015$), and *Enterobacteriaceae* ($p < 0.0001$) and higher abundance of *Lachnospiraceae* ($p < 0.0001$), and *Ruminococcaceae* ($p < 0.0001$) in older chickens than in young chickens (**Figure 3C**). In addition, the correlation between different members of the gut microbiota was also assessed for eight major families. A strong inverse correlation was observed between the *Enterobacteriaceae* and *Lachnospiraceae* ($r = -0.7881, p < 0.0001$), which suggested potential competition between these two members of the community.

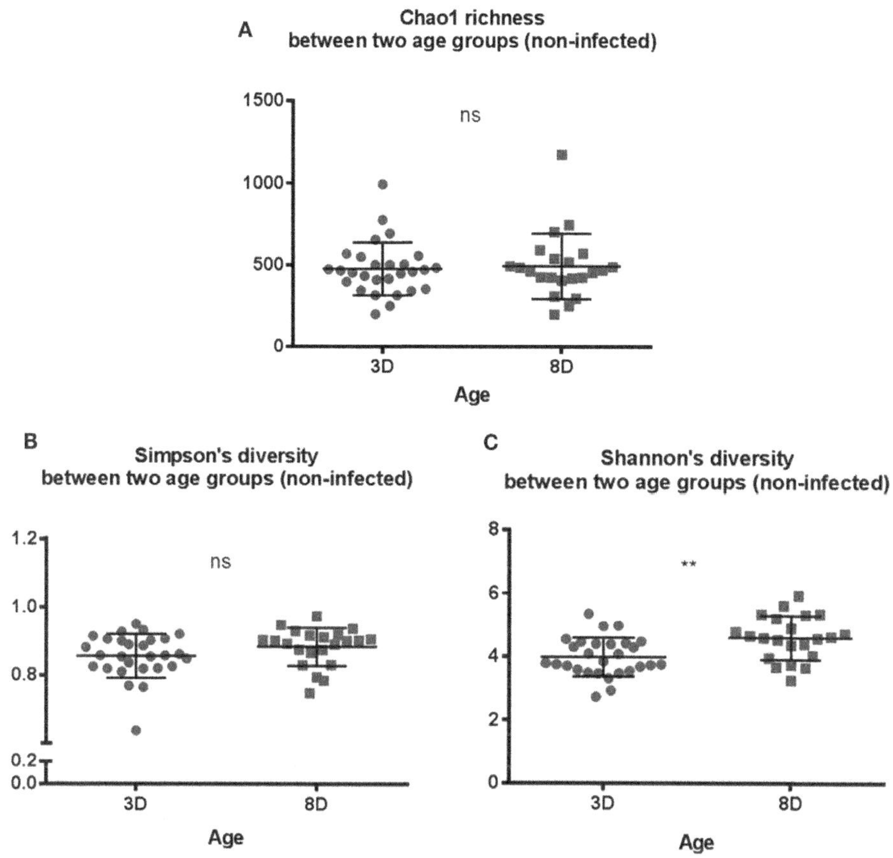

FIGURE 1 | Microbial alpha diversity between two age groups of 3 days old (3 D) and 8 days old (8 D). Alpha diversity metrics of **(A)** Chao1 richness estimate, **(B)** Simpson's diversity, and **(C)** Shannon's diversity index were analyzed. Shannon's diversity index was significantly higher for 8-days-old chicks suggesting that as number of species increases, there is more even distribution of species in the community compared to 3-days-old chicks. All three diversity metrics were evaluated using Mann–Whitney *U* test. $^{**}p$ value < 0.01 and ns = non-significant.

Developmental Differences in Cecal Microbiota Composition in Infected Chickens

To assess whether the microbiota diversity of the infected chickens differed between the two postinfection periods, both alpha and beta diversity indices were analyzed. There was no significant difference in Chao1 richness index (**Figure 4A**). However, both Simpson and Shannon indices showed highly significant difference in microbiota diversity ($p < 0.0001$) with increased diversity at 7 DPI compared to 2 DPI (**Figures 4B,C**). There was no significant difference in PCoA plot of unweighted UniFrac distance ($r = 0.035$, $p = 0.150$) (**Figure 5A**) between two postinfection time points. On the other hand, the weighted UniFrac distance analyzed with PCoA plot showed significant difference between two groups with $p = 0.001$ from ANOSIM analysis, suggesting the relative abundance of dominant taxa contributing to the differences, although the *r* value ($r = 0.414$) did not meet the cut-off threshold of 0.5 defined as two separated microbial community (**Figure 5B**). With LEfSe analysis, the phylum of Proteobacteria was dominated at (2 DPI) while Firmicutes phylum was found to be most abundant at 7 DPI (**Figure 6A**). At 7 DPI, a total of seven core microbiome groups at the order level were identified with enrichment of Erysipelotrichales, Clostridiales, and Lactobacillales (**Figure 6B**). Specifically at the family level, significantly ($p < 0.0001$) highly relative abundant of *Enterococcaceae*, *Lactobacillaceae*, *Clostridiaceae*, *Lachnospiraceae*, *Erysipelotrichaceae*, *Peptostreptococcaceae* ($p = 0.0013$), and *Ruminococcaceae* ($p = 0.0025$), and lower levels of *Enterobacteriaceae* ($p < 0.0001$) were observed at 7 DPI (**Figure 6C**). These findings indicated a slow recovery of microbial diversity in the infected individuals at 7 DPI with significant reduction of the dominant *Enterobacteriaceae* family.

While assessing the microbiota profile of individual chick within the *S.* Enteritidis-infected group, a general trend pattern with an increase in *Enterobacteriaceae* accompanied by either a decrease or absence of *Lachnospiraceae* and *Ruminococcaceae* was found at the family classification level (Figures S7 and S8 in Supplementary Material). Therefore, the inverse correlations in relative abundance of *Enterobacteriaceae* with seven other major family groups were further evaluated. Significant inverse correlations ($p < 0.0001$) were found between *Enterobacteriaceae* and four other bacterial families including *Lachnospiraceae* ($r = -0.7985$), *Erysipelotrichaceae* ($r = -0.7586$), *Ruminococcaceae* ($r = -0.6569$) and *Peptostreptococcaceae* ($r = -0.6105$). Linear regression analysis revealed that the

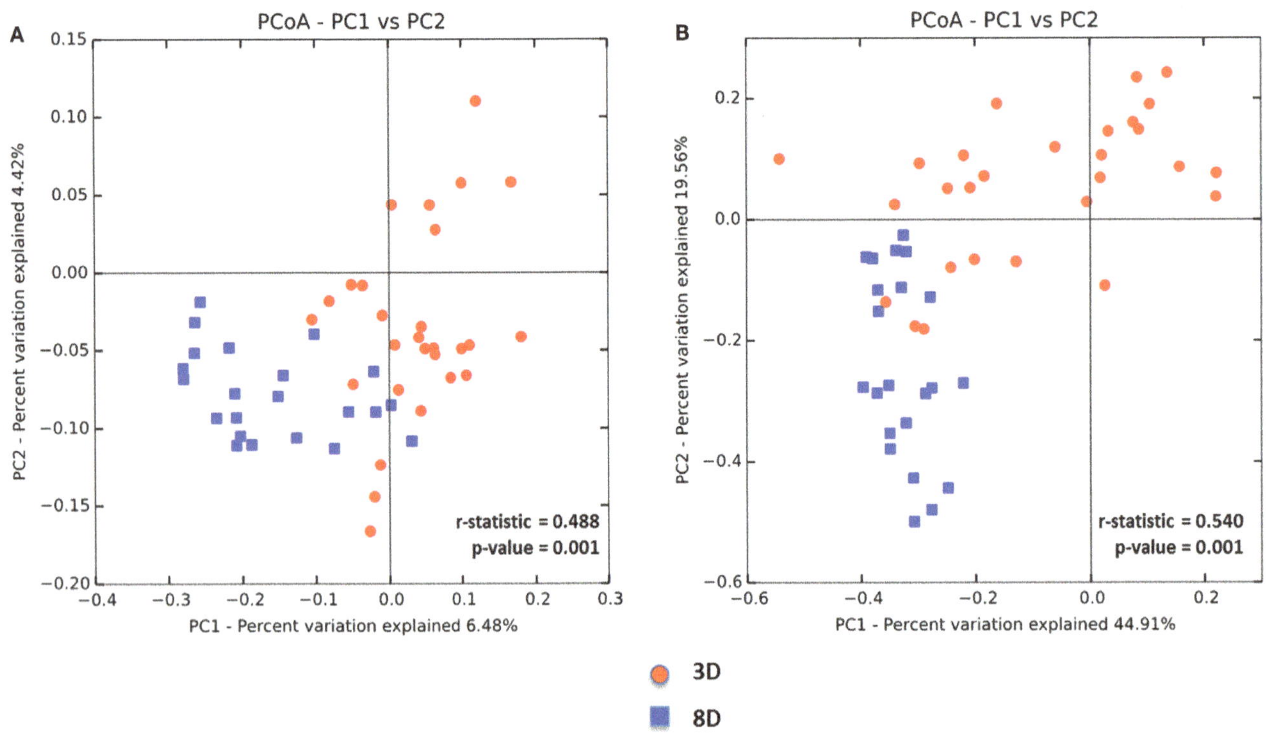

FIGURE 2 | Principal coordinate analysis (PCoA) based on (A) unweighted and (B) weighted UniFrac distances was analyzed for two age groups of non-infected chicks. ANOISM with 999 permutations was used to detect the statistical significant difference between microbial communities of different groups, where both *r* and *p* value is reported. Abbreviations: 3 D, 3 days old; 8 D, 8 days old.

population density of *Enterobacteriaceae* was negatively correlated with other family members of the community (**Figures 7A–D**).

S. Enteritidis-Associated Alteration in Chicken Cecum Microbiota Profile

Microbiota data were also analyzed to examine the effect of S. Enteritidis infection at two different postinfection times of the experiments. With *S.* Enteritidis infection, Chao1 richness showed no differences between the two groups at both postinfection time points (**Figures 8A,D**). Both Simpson and Shannon's diversity indices showed that there was significant reduction in microbiota diversity of the *S.* Enteritidis-infected chickens at 2 DPI compared to non-infected chickens ($p < 0.0001$ and $p < 0.001$, respectively) (**Figures 8B,C**). However, there was no significant difference between non-infected and *S.* Enteritidis-infected groups at 7 DPI for both indices (**Figures 8E,F**). Rarefaction curves highlighted a lower species richness of *S.* Enteritidis-infected groups at both time points compared to non-infected groups (**Figure 9**). Beta diversity was also analyzed to examine differences or similarities in cecal microbiota community composition between non-infected and *S.* Enteritidis-infected groups. PCoA plots based on unweighted UniFrac distance metric showed that there was significant separation in microbial community of non-infected and infected chickens at later postinfection time of 7 DPI ($p = 0.001$, $r = 0.618$) compared to early postinfection time at 2 DPI ($p = 0.032$, $r = 0.089$) (**Figures 10A,B**). With the PCoA plot based on weighted UniFrac distance metric where the relative abundance of OTUs were considered, there was more significant clustering pattern observed between the 8-day-old non-infected chickens and the same-age infected counterparts at 7 DPI ($p = 0.001$, $r = 0.841$) (**Figure 10D**). In contrast, the microbial communities of non-infected and infected groups at early time points (3 D vs. 2 DPI) showed no visible separation between two groups ($r = 0.398$) although the p value $= 0.001$ (**Figure 10C**).

To compare OTUs abundance between two treatment groups that were significantly different, ANOVA test was performed. Abundance of *Lachnospiraceae* family was found to significantly decrease in *S.* Enteritidis-infected group compared to the non-infected group [false discovery rate (FDR) < 0.05]. GI tract of young layer chickens were dominated by two main phyla belonging to Firmicutes and Proteobacteria. With *S.* Enteritidis infection, major phylum level shifted toward increased abundance of Proteobacteria at both time points when compared to non-infected same-age counterpart (Figures S9 and S10 in Supplementary Material). Representative of the bacterial family belonging to *Enterobacteriaceae*, *Erysipelotrichaceae*, *Ruminococcaceae*, *Peptostreptococcaceae*, *Lachnospiraceae*, *Clostridiaceae*, *Lactobacillaceae*, and *Enterococcaceae* dominated in the cecal microbiota of the young layer chickens.

The microbiota compositions of non-infected were compared against the same-age counterparts of chickens in infected groups with LEfSe. The phyla of Actinobacteria and Proteobacteria

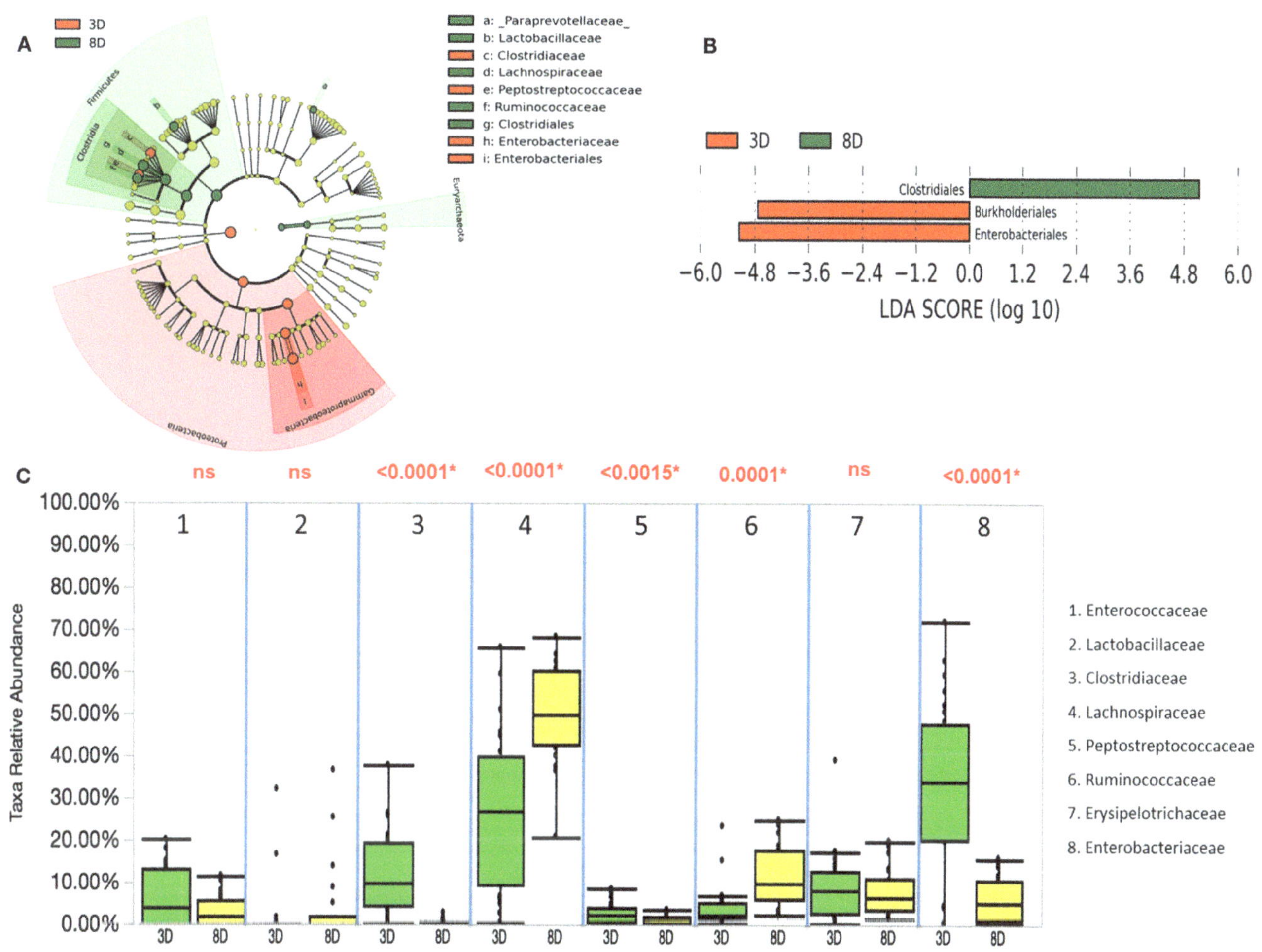

FIGURE 3 | Differential abundances of cecal microbial communities between two age groups. (A) Taxonomic cladogram generated from LefSe analysis showing significant difference in microbiota profile of two age groups, red represented the enriched taxa in 3 days olds' microbial community and green represented the enriched taxa in 8 days olds' microbial community. **(B)** Differently abundant taxa detected with cut-off value of linear discriminant analysis (LDA) score >2.0. Enriched taxa in 8-days-old chicks (green) were indicated with positive LDA score, while taxa enriched in 3-days-old chicks (red) have negative LDA score. **(C)** Comparison of relative abundance levels of cecal microbiota at family level in 3 and 8 days old chicks was evaluated. The boxplot shows the quartiles above and below the median with dark line at center of the box denoting median, black dots showing the outlier. The respective *p* value for each family group is reported using Wilcoxon rank sum test. Abbreviations: 3 D, 3 days old; 8 D, 8 days old.

were significantly enriched in the *S.* Enteritidis-infected groups of 2 DPI, while Firmicutes were significantly enriched in the non-infected group of 3 D (**Figure 11A**). Differentially representation of 11 groups at order level were identified with underrepresentation of four groups and enrichment of seven groups in the *S.* Enteritidis-infected group at 2 DPI (**Figure 11B**). Using a Wilcoxon rank sum test by JMP software, the relative abundance of gut microbes at the family level was compared between the *S.* Enteritidis-infected group of 2 DPI and the non-infected group of 3 D (**Figure 11C**). A marked decrease in *Enterococcaceae* ($p = 0.0092$), *Clostridiaceae* ($p < 0.0001$), *Lachnospiraceae* ($p < 0.0001$), *Peptostreptococcaceae* ($p < 0.0001$), *Ruminococcaceae* ($p = 0.0006$), and *Erysipelotrichaceae* ($p = 0.0025$) was found in the *S.* Enteritidis-infected group. On the other hand, *Enterobacteriaceae* ($p < 0.0001$) were highly abundant in the *S.* Enteritidis-infected group at 2 DPI.

Similarly, both Actinobacteria and Proteobacteria phyla were also enriched in *S.* Enteritidis-infected groups of 7 DPI, while the non-infected group at 8 D showed significant abundance in Firmicutes and Euryarchaeota phyla (**Figure 12A**). A total of six groups at order level were differentially represented with underrepresentation of two groups and overrepresentation of four groups in *S.* Enteritidis-infected group at 7 DPI (**Figure 12B**). Using Wilcoxon rank sum test, higher abundance level of *Enterococcaceae* ($p = 0.0073$), *Clostridiaceae* ($p = 0.0008$), *Peptostreptococcaceae* ($p = 0.0089$), *Erysipelotrichaceae* ($p < 0.0001$), and *Enterobacteriaceae* ($p < 0.0001$) were found in the *S.* Enteritidis-infected group than in the non-infected group at 7 DPI. In contrast, *Lachnospiraceae* ($p < 0.0001$), and *Ruminococcaceae* ($p < 0.0001$) were significantly decreased in the infected group compared to the non-infected same-age counterparts (**Figure 12C**).

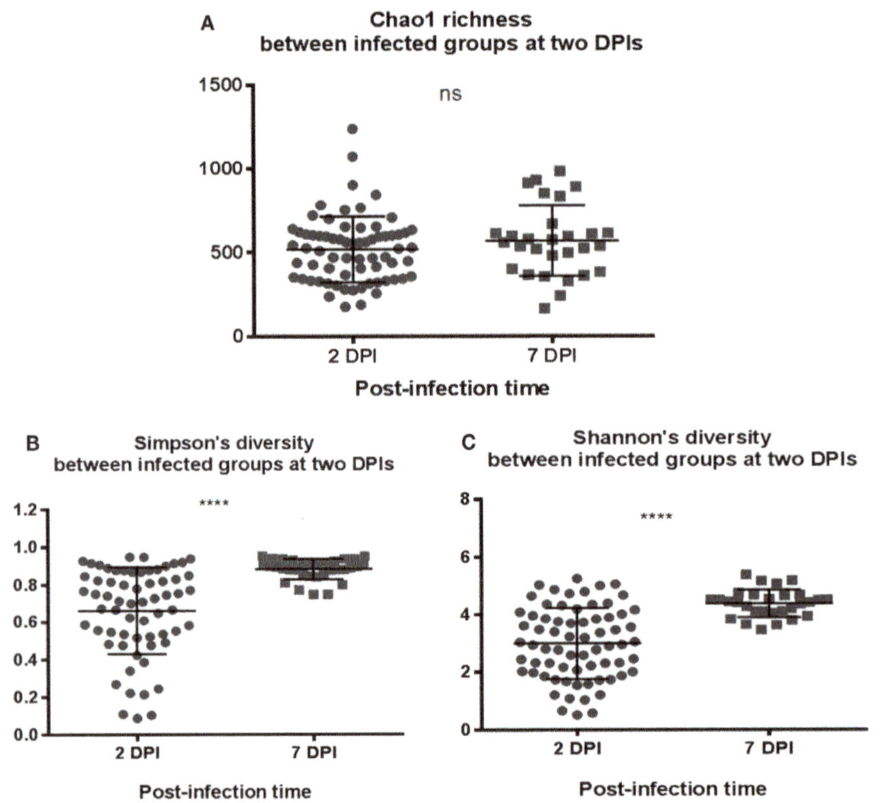

FIGURE 4 | Comparison of the diversity indices of *S.* Enteritidis-infected chicks at different time-points of post infection periods at 2 and 7 DPI. **(A)** Chao1 richness estimate, **(B)** Simpson's diversity, and **(C)** Shannon's diversity index were analyzed. **(B,C)** Simpson and Shannon's diversity showed significant difference in microbial diversity between two infected groups of chicks with increased diversity in microbiota composition at 7 DPI compared to 2 DPI. Both diversity metrics were evaluated using Mann–Whitney *U* test. ****p value < 0.0001.

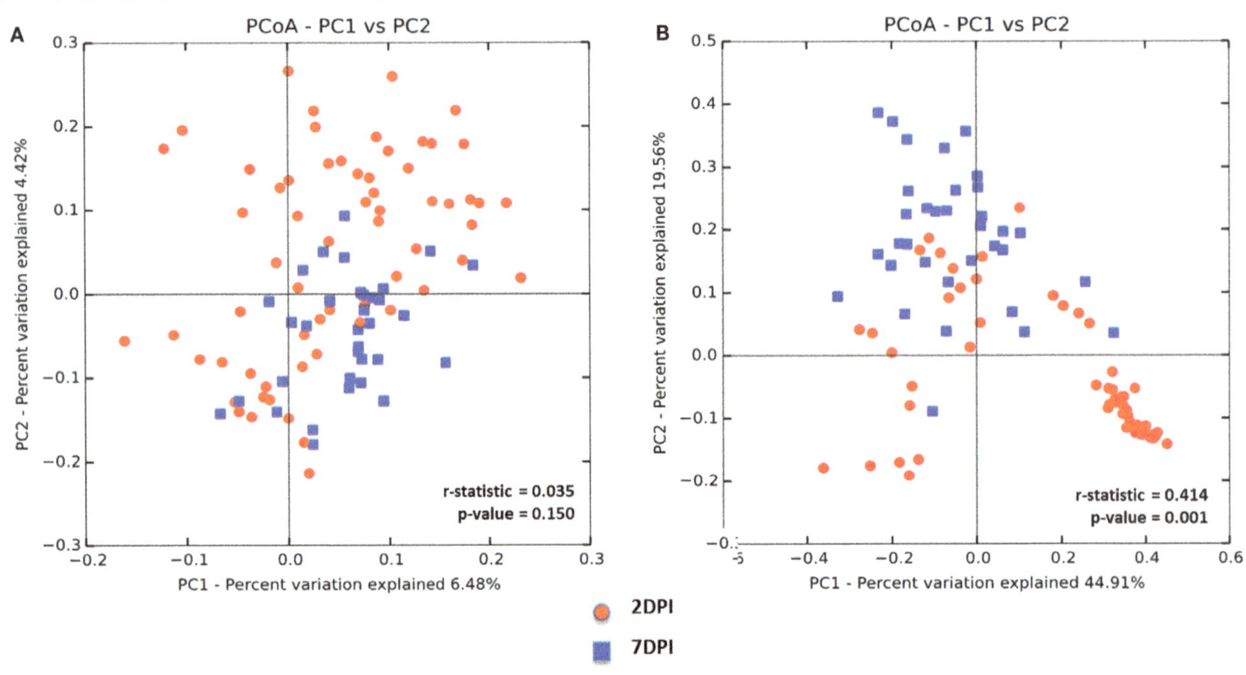

FIGURE 5 | Principal coordinate analysis (PCoA) based on (A) unweighted and (B) weighted UniFrac distances was analyzed for two age groups of infected chicks. ANOISM with 999 permutations was used to detect the statistical significant difference between microbial communities of different groups, where both r and p value is reported. Abbreviations: 2 DPI, 2 days post infection; 7 DPI, 7 days post infection.

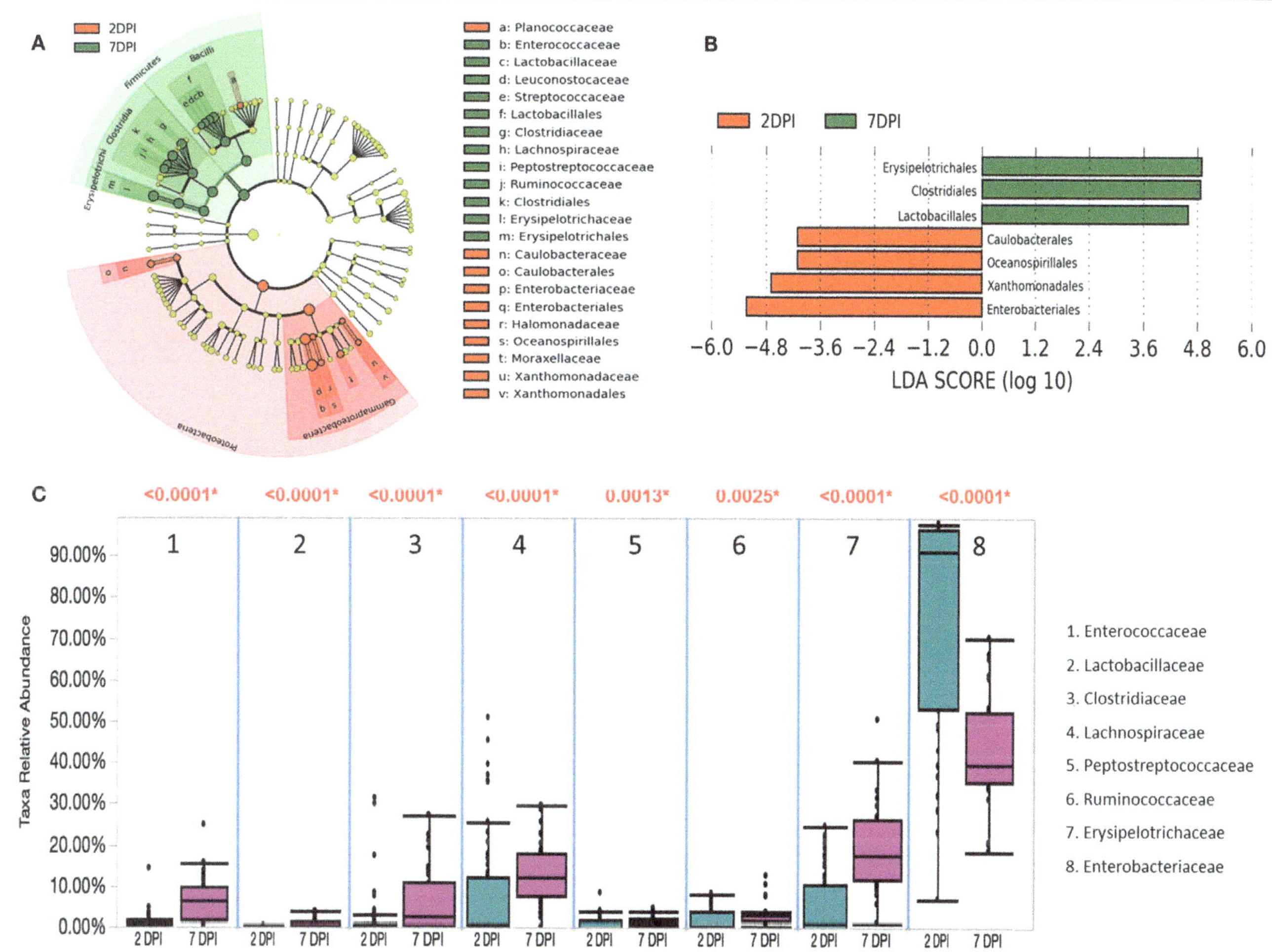

FIGURE 6 | Differential abundances of cecal microbial communities between two postinfection times of *S.* Enteritidis-infected chicks. **(A)** Taxonomic cladogram generated from LefSe analysis showing significant difference in microbiota profile of 2 DPI (red) and 7 DPI (green). **(B)** Differently abundant taxa detected with cut-off value of linear discriminant analysis (LDA) score >2.0. Enriched taxa in 2 DPI group are indicated with negative LDA score (red) and taxa enriched in 7 DPI have positive LDA score (green). **(C)** Comparison of relative abundance levels of cecal microbiota at family level in *S.* Enteritidis-infected chicks between two postinfection times was evaluated. The boxplot shows the quartiles above and below the median with dark line at center of the box denoting median, black dots showing the outlier. The respective *p* value for each family group is reported using Wilcoxon rank sum test. Abbreviations: 2 DPI; 2 days post infection, 7 DPI; 7 days post infection.

DISCUSSION

Maintenance of intestinal microbiota homeostasis is a key determinant for overall health and nutrition state of the host. Development of gut microbiota in the chick begins immediately after the hatch where a number of external factors such as environment, feed, and contact with chick handler could influence the overall microbial community structure (27). In addition, the host genotype is another important factor in affecting the composition of the gut microbiota (7, 9, 11). Early encounter with diverse enteric pathogens present in the environment during posthatch period also poses great risk for newly hatched chicks. This early host–pathogen interaction could potentially impact the further colonization of other microbes and shape the overall structure of gut microbiota. In this study, we therefore address this dominant potential of early pathogen exposure on shaping the microbiota composition by using 1-day-old chickens from two genetically distinct lines as infection model.

Chicken MHC and its association with resistance to avian disease, such as Marek's disease, infectious bronchitis virus (IBV), avian influenza virus, ectoparasite, and *Staphylococcus aureus* had been documented in several studies (14, 15, 17, 20). However, the role of MHC on the resistance to *S.* Enteritidis infection had been contradictory. Study by Cotter et al. (13) suggested an association of MHC B haplotype with resistance to *S.* Enteritidis infection in a neonatal chick infection model of 12 MHC-congenic chicken lines. On the other hand, another study by the Bumstead and Barrow (12) stated that there was no evidence to support strong association of MHC haplotypes with resistance to *Salmonella typhimurium* in newly hatched chicks. Our findings in the current study indicated that MHC haplotype had significant effects only on early stage of systemic infection of *S.* Enteritidis

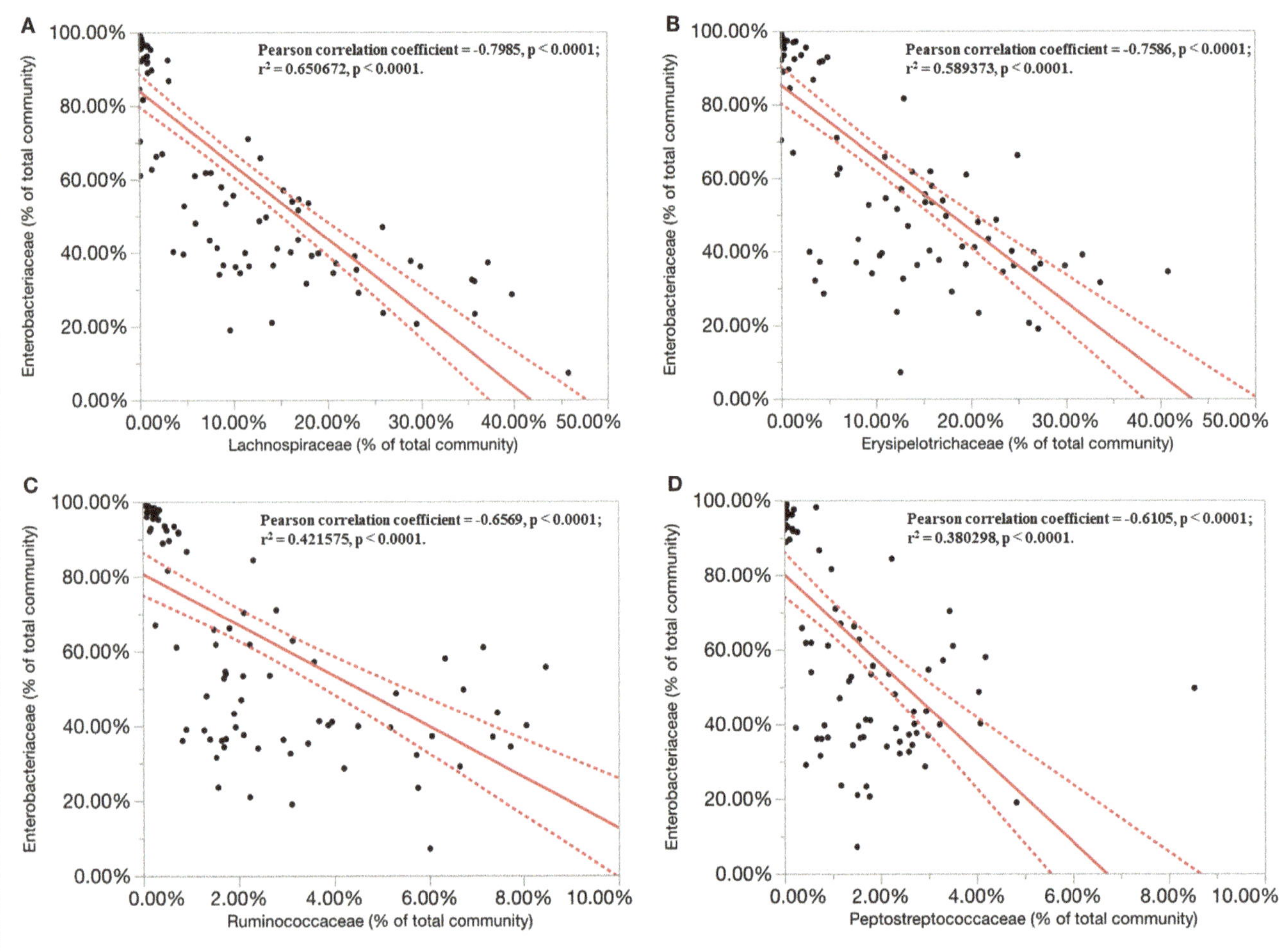

FIGURE 7 | Inverse correlation between relative abundance of members of *Enterobacteriaceae* family with other four major family groups. Dashed line indicated 95% confidence intervals. **(A)** Linear regression plots of relative abundance of bacteria (% of total community) belonging to *Enterobacteriaceae* family and *Lachnospiraceae* family in *S.* Enteritidis-infected group. **(B)** Linear regression plots of relative abundance of bacteria belonging to *Enterobacteriaceae* family and *Erysipelotrichaceae* family in *S.* Enteritidis-infected group. **(C)** Linear regression plots of relative abundance of bacteria belonging to *Enterobacteriaceae* family and *Ruminococcaceae* family in *S.* Enteritidis-infected group. **(D)** Linear regression plots of relative abundance of bacteria belonging to *Enterobacteriaceae* family and *Peptostreptococcaceae* family in *S.* Enteritidis-infected group.

(splenic bacterial burden difference at 2 DPI) and on late stage of local infection of *S.* Enteritidis (cecal bacterial burden difference at 7 DPI). However, in general, MHC genetic background had a limited effect on resistance to *S.* Enteritidis infection.

Developmental stage can have a significant impact on the microbiota composition in the GI tract. The early inoculum challenged to young chickens in this study could be a possible driving force in potentially rendering the microbiota composition of chickens of late stage. Without pathogen infection, microbiota diversity and complexity often increase with age of the chick (28, 29). Temporal changes in the chicken gut microbiota with aging could have important consequences on susceptibility to pathogen infection. The use of very young chickens as infection model is important for the current study as chickens are often exposed to *Salmonella* at very young age in natural setting. However, the immaturity of the immune system as well as non-establishment of complex microbiota in young chickens could have a significant effect on the outcome of the infection (30). Beaumont et al. (31) showed that increased resistance to *Salmonella* at adult chickens was negatively correlated to genetic resistance at the young age. Therefore, MHC haplotype effect on microbiota profile could be different by the use of different age infection model. Although it is beyond the scope of the current study, challenging at 2 weeks of age instead of 1-day-old chicks could provide additional insights of host genetic background impact on microflora composition and warranted further investigation.

In the non-infected chickens, Firmicutes followed by Proteobacteria phylum dominated the microbiota composition. Temporal fluctuation in the microbial community structure at the family level was observed as chick aged (from 3 to 8 D). *Enterobacteriaceae* family was significantly enriched in younger chickens, while *Lachnospiraceae* and *Ruminococcaceae* families were more abundant with a reduction in *Enterobacteriaceae* family in older chickens. The overall bacterial diversity in early life stage of chick host (both age groups) in the current study was low with a few members predominantly occupying the GI tract, which was in agreement with other studies (28, 29). Similar to another study, the non-infected chickens at 3 days old had high abundance of

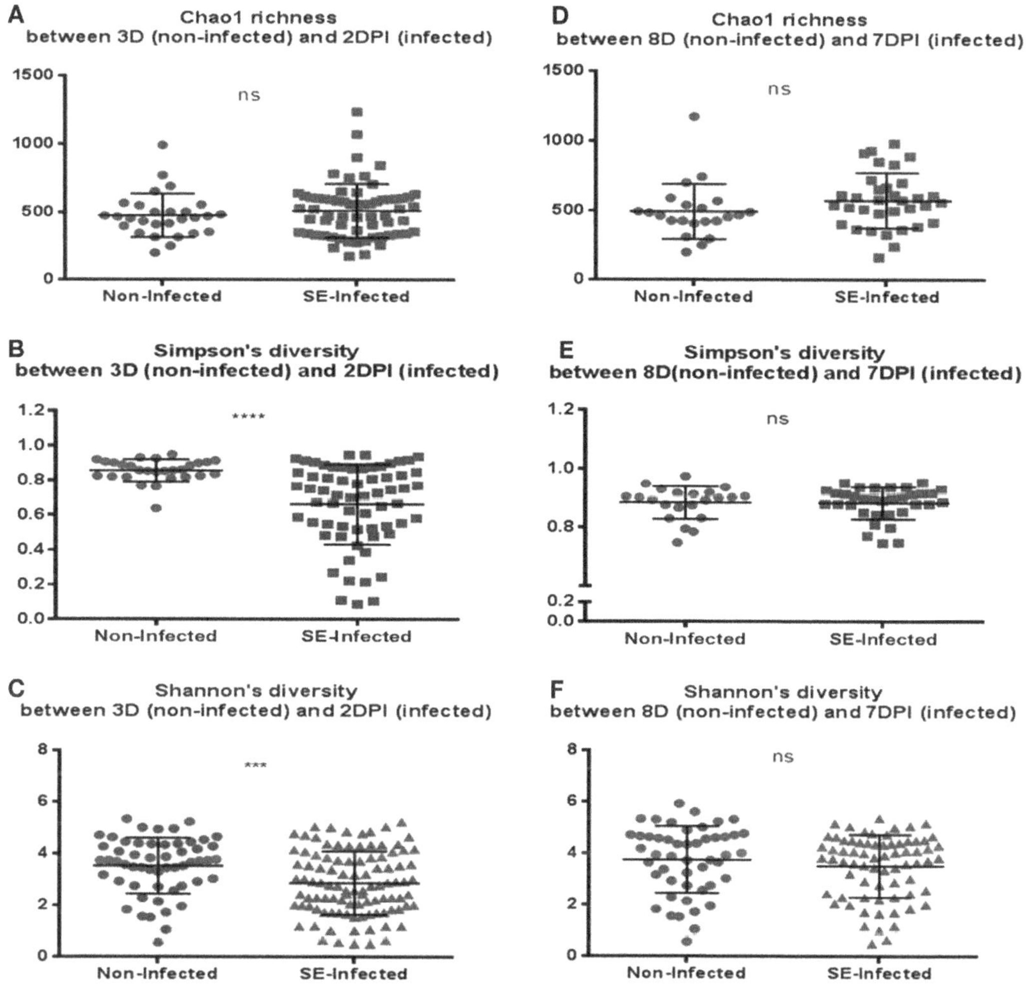

FIGURE 8 | Comparison of the diversity indices between the non-infected chicks and *S.* Enteritidis-infected chicks at 2 and 7 DPI: (A,D) Chao1 richness estimate, (B,E) Simpson's diversity, and (C,F) Shannon's diversity. At 2 DPI, there was significant reduction in microbial diversity of the *S.* Enteritidis-infected chicks compared to non-infected chicks for measurement of both Simpson and Shannon's diversity indices. Diversity metrics were evaluated using Mann–Whitney *U* test. ***p value <0.001, ****p value <0.0001, and ns = non-significant.

Enterobacteriaceae (32). Members of the *Enterobacteriaceae* family including bacterial pathogens like *Salmonella*, *Escherichia coli*, and *Shigella* are known enteric pathogens in the GI tract. Harboring high level of *Enterobacteriaceae* in young chickens could potentially increase their susceptibility to infection by related enteric pathogens. Indeed, studies in mouse model have shown that increased susceptibility to related enteric pathogen infections were observed in host whose microbiota composition was dominated by the presence of *E. coli* belonging to *Enterobacteriaceae* family (33, 34). The concept of "like will to like" was proposed by the Stecher et al. to help explain the bloom of closely related bacterial species in the GI tract that result in dysbiosis of microbiota in the disease host (33). It had been suggested that high prevalence of certain bacterial species in the microbiota community could alter the conditions within the gut that selectively confer the fitness advantage upon other related species within the same phylogenetic group (35, 36). We speculate that early colonization by members of *Enterobacteriaceae* family in GI tract of the newly hatched chickens could potentially precondition the intestinal tract of the chick host to allow easy colonization by enteric pathogens. Thus, depletion of certain bacteria taxa from *Enterobacteriaceae* family during the early posthatch period could potentially enhance the host resistance to enteric pathogen infection. This may be how growth promoters work in poultry feed as antibiotics in the growth promoters can eliminate certain members of *Enterobacteriaceae* family.

Once successful invasion by pathogen like *S.* Enteritidis is established within the niche of the GI tract, pathogen-associated alteration in microbial community structure occurred (37–39). Our results revealed that *S.* Enteritidis infection resulted in significant reduction in bacterial diversity specifically at early postinfection period. Reduction in bacterial diversity in the infected birds was partially attributed by the presence of the *Enterobacteriaceae* family that dominated the microbial community. Major phylum shift was observed in infected group at 2 DPI where there was expansion of Proteobacteria with concomitant reduction in Firmicutes phyla. This sudden shift in microbial population structure due to *S.* Enteritidis infection changed the ratio

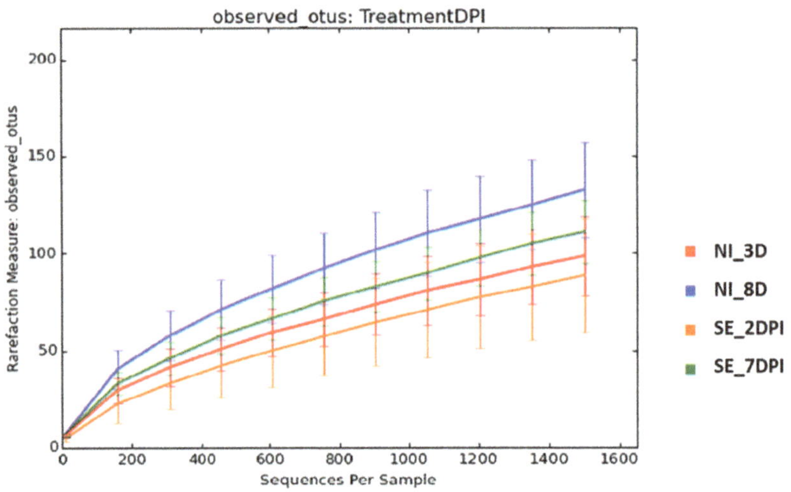

FIGURE 9 | Rarefaction curves of number of observed OTUs based on 97% sequence similarities for treatment group at different time points. Abbreviations: NI_3 D, non-infected chicks at 3 days old; NI_8 D, non-infected chicks at 8 days old; SE_2 DPI, *S.* Enteritidis-infected chicks at 2 days post infection; SE_7 DPI, *S.* Enteritidis-infected chicks at 7 days post infection.

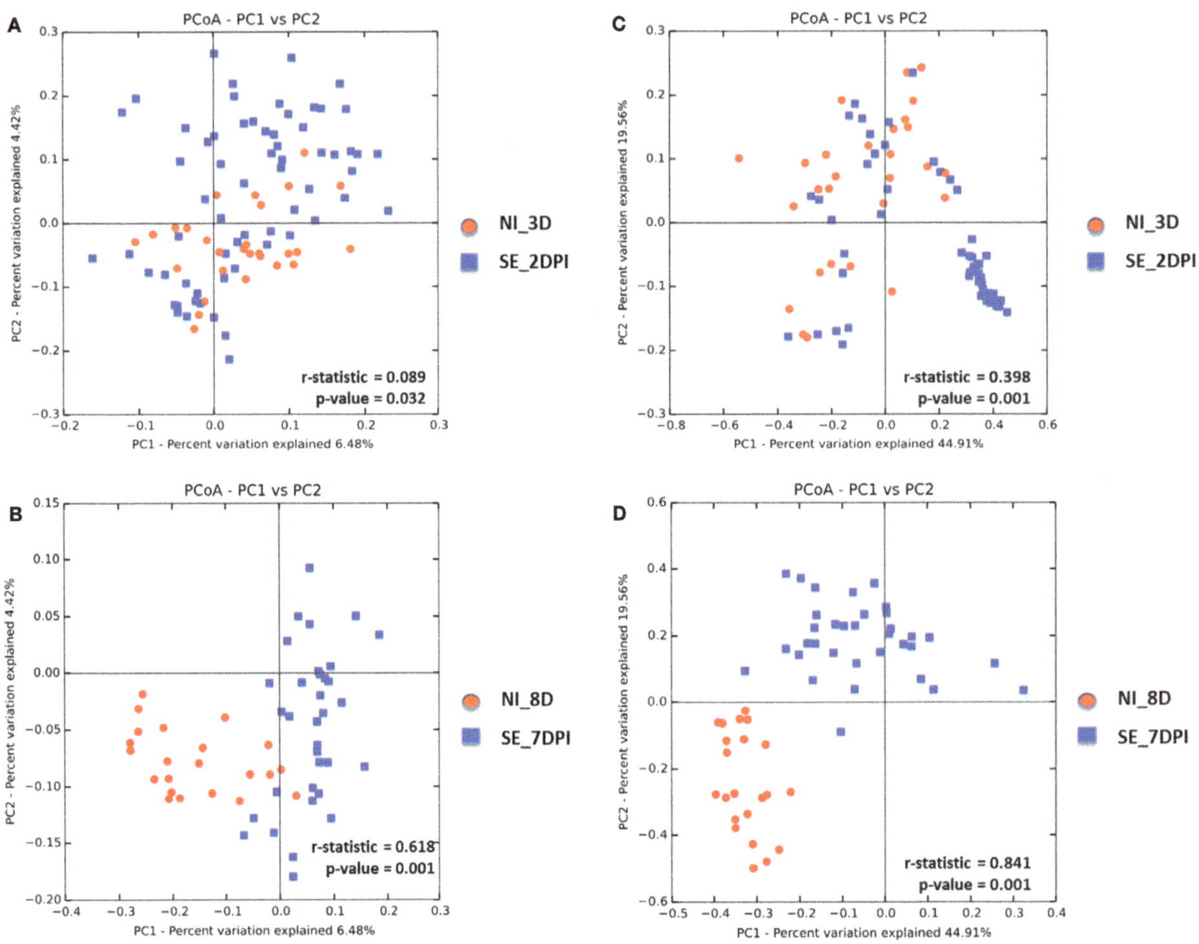

FIGURE 10 | Principal coordinate analysis (PCoA) based on (A,B) unweighted and (C,D) weighted UniFrac distances was analyzed for same-age group comparison between non-infected and infected chicks. ANOISM with 999 permutations was used to detect the statistical significant difference between microbial communities of different groups, where both *r* and *p* value is reported. Abbreviations: NI_3 D, non-infected chicks at 3 days old; SE_2 DPI, *S.* Enteritidis-infected chicks at 2 days post infection; NI_8 D, non-infected chicks at 8 days old; SE_7 DPI, *S.* Enteritidis-infected chicks at 7 days post infection.

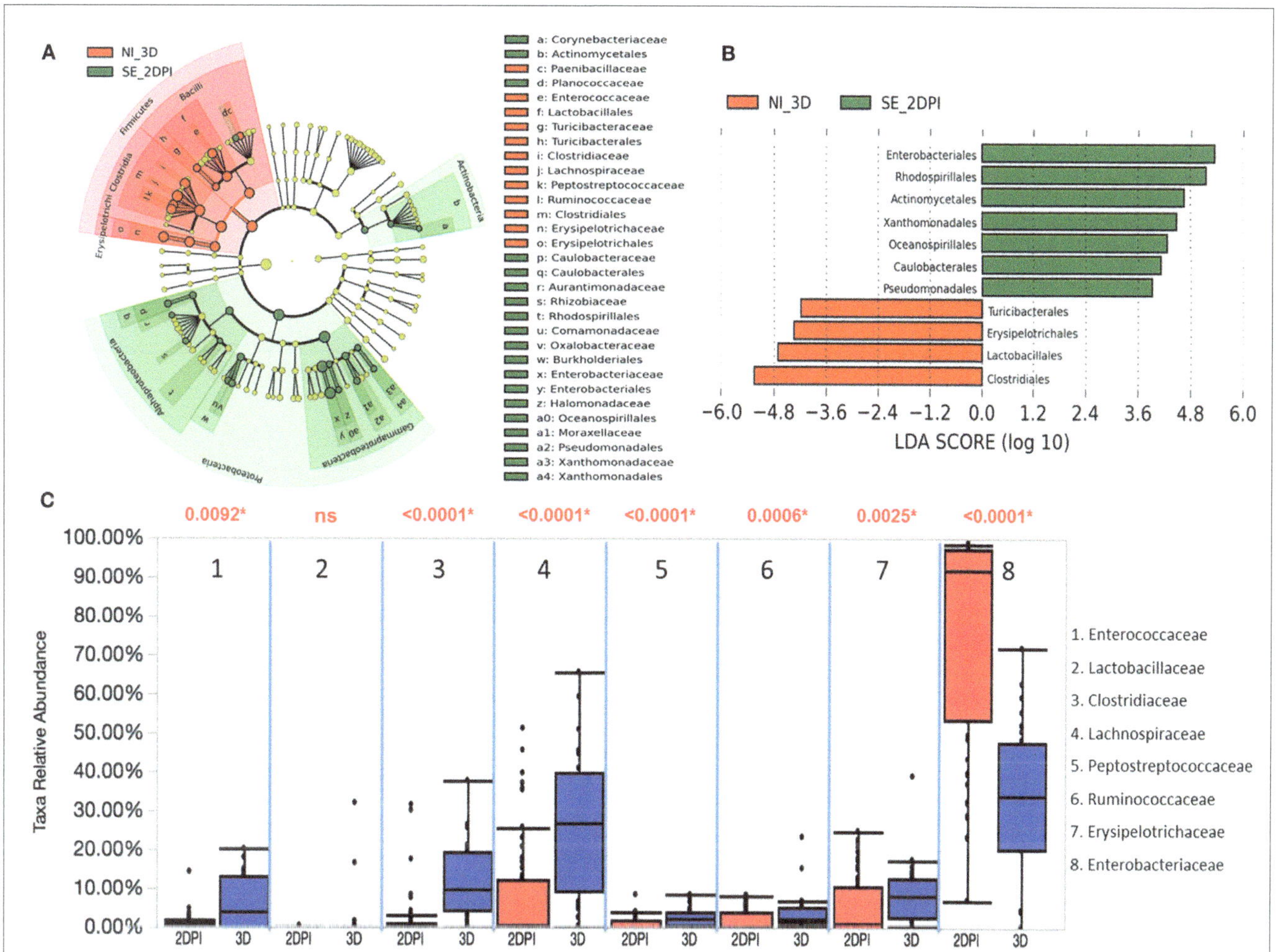

FIGURE 11 | Differential abundances of cecal microbial communities between infected and non-infected group at 2 DPI. (A) Taxonomic cladogram generated from LefSe analysis showing significant difference in microbiota profile of non-infected (red) and *S.* Enteritidis-infected (green) at early days post infection (2 DPI). **(B)** Differently abundant taxa detected with cut-off value of linear discriminant analysis (LDA) score >2.0. Non-infected enriched taxa are indicated with negative LDA score (red) and taxa enriched in *S.* Enteritidis-infected have positive LDA score (green). **(C)** Comparison of relative abundance levels of cecal microbiota at family level in treatment group was evaluated. The boxplot shows the quartiles above and below the median with dark line at center of the box denoting median, black dots showing the outlier. The respective *p* value for each family group is reported using Wilcoxon rank sum test. Abbreviation: NI_3 D, non-infected chicks at 3 days old; SE_2 DPI, *S.* Enteritidis-infected chicks at 2 days post infection.

of two major phyla groups, which is the hallmark indicator of intestinal microbiota dysbiosis in disease host (40, 41). *Salmonella* associated alteration of the gut microbiota could be a result of either pathogen-commensal microbiota interaction or host mucosal immune response to the pathogen or even a combination of both (38). Host-mediated inflammation response triggered by the presence of the pathogen could also change the conditions within the GI tract to favor and support the growth of specific member of the microorganisms. Studies in mouse colitis models have showed that inflammation allow facultative anaerobes like *Salmonella* or other members of the *Enterobacteriaceae* family to utilize anaerobic respiration as alternative growth pathway to gain competitive advantage over resident microbes that are mostly obligate anaerobe (34, 38, 40, 42–44). The underlying mechanism that is driving the bloom of Proteobacteria phylum in chick host following *Salmonella* infection is not yet known. Whether similar route of respiration pathway is being utilized by *Salmonella* to gain growth advantage in inflamed chicken gut is the hypothesis that we are currently investigating.

Comparisons between microbial communities of non-infected and infected groups showed that the community structure of the two groups appeared to be more similar initially at an early development stage (3 D vs. 2 DPI). However, as time progresses with *S.* Enteritidis infection, a significant difference in community structure between the two groups was apparent, with clear separation in the group's clustering pattern on PCoA plots (8 D vs. 7 DPI). This result suggests that the impact of *S.* Enteritidis infection on microbial communities was more substantial in late stage than in early stage. A study by Videnska et al. (45) found that members of the families *Lachnospiraceae* and *Ruminococcaceae* are predominantly present in the 2-week-old laying chickens, and likely play an important role in the overall development of the gut microbial community. Further analysis at the family level found that two core members of the gut microbiota belonging to

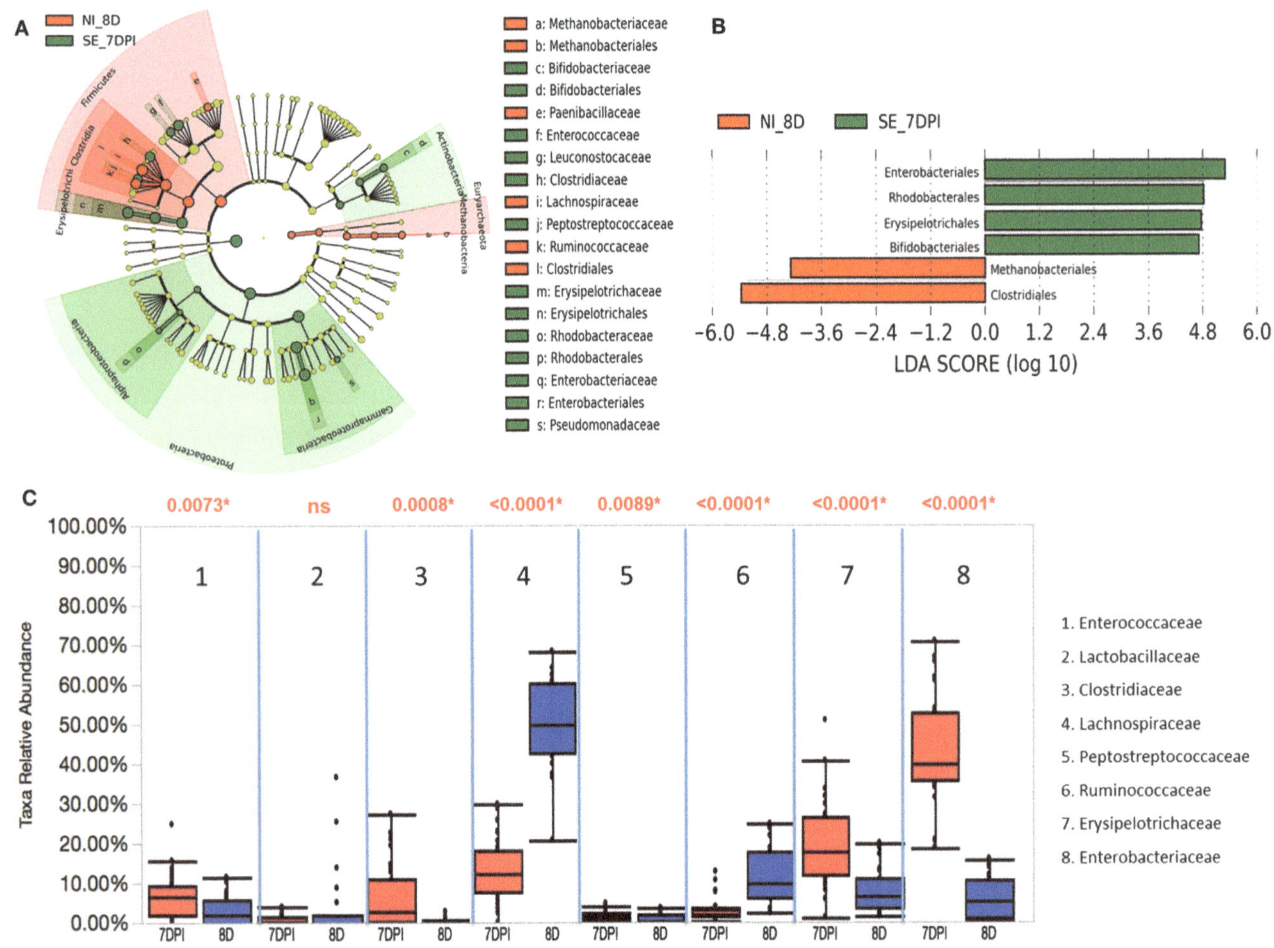

FIGURE 12 | Different abundances of cecal microbial communities between infected and non-infected group at 7 DPI. (A) Taxonomic cladogram generated from LefSe analysis showing significant difference in microbiota profile of non-infected (red) and *S.* Enteritidis-infected (green) at 7 DPI. (B) Differently abundant taxa detected with cut-off value of linear discriminant analysis (LDA) score >2.0. Non-infected enriched taxa are indicated with negative LDA score (red) and taxa enriched in *S.* Enteritidis-infected have positive LDA score (green). **(C)** Comparison of relative abundance levels of cecal microbiota at family level in treatment group was evaluated. The boxplot shows the quartiles above and below the median with dark line at center of the box denoting median, black dots showing the outlier. Abbreviation: NI_8 D, non-infected chicks at 8 days old; SE_7 DPI, *S.* Enteritidis-infected chicks at 7 days post infection.

Lachnospiraceae and *Ruminococcaceae* families were significantly reduced in the infected groups. Our findings suggested that with *S.* Enteritidis infection, selective reduction of these bacterial genera could negatively impact gut microbial diversity and development. Although long-term impact of *S.* Enteritidis infection on microbiome development in adult chickens was not possible to be evaluated in the current study, further investigation in this regard could provide important insights on it.

Interestingly, a strong inverse correlation between *Enterobacteriaceae* and *Lachnospiraceae* was observed in both the non-infected and infected birds, suggesting a possible antagonistic interaction between the two members of these taxa that could influence the prevalence of different microbial populations in the gut. In addition, the abundance of members belonging to *Lachnospiraceae* family was significantly decreased with *S.* Enteritidis infection. Contrary to our findings, Videnska et al. (37) observed only minor modification in chicken gut microbiota with no significant changes in *Lachnospiraceae* family following *S.* Enteritidis infection. The discrepancies observed between this study and our findings may be attributed to different age of infection model, samples collected on different days of postinfection and different genetic background of chickens. *Lachnospiraceae* as well as another family, *Ruminococcaceae*, that also show significant reduction in the infected group, belong to the Clostridium clusters IV and XIVa (45). Members of these groups generate butyric acid, short chain fatty acids (SCFAs) that are produced as end products of fermentation of carbohydrate by anaerobic intestinal microbes. There is complex interplay between diet, SCFAs concentration, and microbiota composition that regulate the colonization level of members of the Proteobacteria phylum (36, 46). Depending on the type of SCFAs being produced and its concentration level in the gut, it can affect different members of microbial community in a different way. Specifically for *Salmonella*, high concentration of acetate production was found to increase the invasion gene expression of *Salmonella* Pathogenicity Island 1 (SPI1) (47). High concentration level of butyric acid, on the other hand, down-regulated the SPI1 gene expression level, which can reduce invasion capability of bacteria in the host (48). In the poultry industry, addition of butyric acid in feed has been shown to reduce both colonization and shedding of *Salmonella* in chickens (49, 50). Taken together, reduction in butyric acid producing bacteria such as *Lachnospiraceae* and *Ruminococcaceae* families with *S.* Enteritidis infection may implied that both producers and its products may have a potential protective role in providing colonization resistance against *Salmonella* infection or reducing the members of *Enterobacteriaceae* family in gut microbiota to maintain homeostasis. A novel *Salmonella* preventive strategies that implement combined approach of competitive exclusion bacteria with SCFAs should be explored to eliminate enteric pathogens and improve overall gut health of the chicken host.

In conclusion, our findings indicated that early exposure in young chickens to *Salmonella* influences and shape the overall microbiota composition. Microbial diversity was significantly reduced in *S.* Enteritidis-infected host compared to same-age non-infected group. Overall perturbation of microbiota community was found to be associated with expansion of *Enterobacteriaceae* family at early postinfection period. Decrease in butyrate producing bacteria belonging to *Lachnospiraceae* family was found to have a negative correlation with high prevalence of *Enterobacteriaceae* family, suggesting possible competitive interaction between the two bacterial taxa in the gut. Additionally, increased susceptibility to *Salmonella* infection in young chickens could be contributed by highly relative abundance of *Enterobacteriaceae* family in the gut. Predominance of this bacterial taxa could potentially confer competitive growth advantage upon its related species over resident microbiota during enteric infection via altering the environmental conditions of the GI tract of the host, which further promote the imbalance state of the young chick's gut microbiota. This study provided a preliminary insight into the contributing role of early host–pathogen interaction that influences the composition makeup of gut microbiota.

AUTHOR CONTRIBUTIONS

KM performed the experiment, analyzed the sequencing data, and drafted the manuscript. HZ designed the experiment, provided the concept of the analysis, and was involved in critical revision of the manuscript. PS and MH ran the scripts for sequencing data and help revised the manuscript. GC and HC helped with animal trials, sample collection and DNA extraction of samples. LG and EM provided primers, contributed ideas for analyzing the data and helped in revising the manuscript. All authors submitted comments, read and approved the final manuscript.

ACKNOWLEDGMENTS

This project was partially supported by the California Agricultural Experimental Station (HZ), United States Department of Agriculture, National Institute of Food and Agriculture, Multistate Research Project NC1170, NRSP8, and NE1334 (HZ) and partially supported by the USDA Agriculture and Food Research Initiative Competitive Grant no. 2015-67015-22930. Dr. Matthias Hess provided helpful comments on analyzing results.

REFERENCES

1. Apajalahti JK, Kettunen A, Graham H. Characteristics of the gastrointestinal microbial communities, with special reference to the chicken. *Worlds Poult Sci J* (2004) **60**(2):223–32. doi:10.1079/WPS20040017
2. Crhanova M, Hradecka H, Faldynova M, Matulova M, Havlickova H, Sisak F, et al. Immune response of chicken gut to natural colonization by gut microflora and to *Salmonella enterica* serovar enteritidis infection. *Infect Immun* (2011) **79**(7):2755–63. doi:10.1128/IAI.01375-10
3. Awad WA, Aschenbach JR, Khayal B, Hess C, Hess M. Intestinal epithelial responses to *Salmonella enterica* serovar enteritidis: effects on intestinal permeability and ion transport. *Poult Sci* (2012) **91**(11):2949–57. doi:10.3382/ps.2012-02448
4. Gantois I, Ducatelle R, Pasmans F, Haesebrouck F, Gast R, Humphrey TJ, et al. Mechanisms of egg contamination by *Salmonella* enteritidis. *FEMS Microbiol Rev* (2009) **33**(4):718–38. doi:10.1111/j.1574-6976.2008.00161.x
5. Jinu Manoj MKS, Singh YP. The role of poultry in food borne salmonellosis and its public health importance. *Adv Anim Vet Sci* (2015) **3**(9):485–90. doi:10.14737/journal.aavs/2015/3.9.485.490
6. Hu J, Bumstead N, Barrow P, Sebastiani G, Olien L, Morgan K, et al. Resistance to salmonellosis in the chicken is linked to NRAMP1 and TNC. *Genome Res* (1997) **7**(7):693–704.
7. Meng H, Zhang Y, Zhao LL, Zhao WJ, He C, Honaker CF, et al. Body weight selection affects quantitative genetic correlated responses in gut microbiota. *PLoS One* (2014) **9**(6):e89862. doi:10.1371/journal.pone.0101401
8. Rinttila T, Apajalahti J. Intestinal microbiota and metabolites-implications for broiler chicken health and performance. *J Appl Poult Res* (2013) **22**(3):647–58. doi:10.3382/Japr.2013-00742
9. Schokker D, Veninga G, Vastenhouw SA, Bossers A, de Bree FM, Kaal-Lansbergen LMTE, et al. Early life microbial colonization of the gut and intestinal development differ between genetically divergent broiler lines. *BMC Genomics* (2015) **16**:418. doi:10.1186/S12864-015-1646-6
10. Stanley D, Geier MS, Denman SE, Haring VR, Crowley TM, Hughes RJ, et al. Identification of chicken intestinal microbiota correlated with the efficiency of energy extraction from feed. *Vet Microbiol* (2013) **164**(1–2):85–92. doi:10.1016/J.Vetmic.2013.01.030
11. Zhao LL, Wang G, Siegel P, He C, Wang HZ, Zhao WJ, et al. Quantitative genetic background of the host influences gut microbiomes in chickens. *Sci Rep* (2013) **3**:1163. doi:10.1038/Srep01163
12. Bumstead N, Barrow PA. Genetics of resistance to *Salmonella typhimurium* in newly hatched chicks. *Br Poult Sci* (1988) **29**(3):521–9. doi:10.1080/00071668808417078
13. Cotter PF, Taylor RL, Abplanalp H. B-complex associated immunity to *Salmonella* enteritidis challenge in congenic chickens. *Poult Sci* (1998) **77**(12):1846–51. doi:10.1093/ps/77.12.1846
14. Banat GR, Tkalcic S, Dzielawa JA, Jackwood MW, Saggese MD, Yates L, et al. Association of the chicken MHC B haplotypes with resistance to avian coronavirus. *Dev Comp Immunol* (2013) **39**(4):430–7. doi:10.1016/J.Dci.2012.10.006
15. Cotter PF, Taylor RL Jr, Abplanalp H. Differential resistance to *Staphylococcus aureus* challenge in major histocompatibility (B) complex congenic lines. *Poult Sci* (1992) **71**(11):1873–8. doi:10.3382/ps.0711873
16. Dalgaard TS, Hojsgaard S, Skjodt K, Juul-Madsen HR. Differences in chicken major histocompatibility complex (MHC) class Ialpha gene expression between Marek's disease-resistant and -susceptible MHC haplotypes. *Scand J Immunol* (2003) **57**(2):135–43. doi:10.1046/j.1365-3083.2003.01207.x

17. Hunt HD, Jadhao S, Swayne DE. Major histocompatibility complex and background genes in chickens influence susceptibility to high pathogenicity avian influenza virus. *Avian Dis* (2010) **54**(1 Suppl):572–5. doi:10.1637/8888-042409-ResNote.1
18. Lamont SJ. The chicken major histocompatibility complex and disease. *Rev Sci Tech* (1998) **17**(1):128–42.
19. Liu W, Miller MM, Lamont SJ. Association of MHC class I and class II gene polymorphisms with vaccine or challenge response to *Salmonella* enteritidis in young chicks. *Immunogenetics* (2002) **54**(8):582–90. doi:10.1007/S00251-002-0495-Z
20. Owen JP, Delany ME, Mullens BA. MHC haplotype involvement in avian resistance to an ectoparasite. *Immunogenetics* (2008) **60**(10):621–31. doi:10.1007/s00251-008-0314-2
21. Caporaso JG, Lauber CL, Walters WA, Berg-Lyons D, Lozupone CA, Turnbaugh PJ, et al. Global patterns of 16S rRNA diversity at a depth of millions of sequences per sample. *Proc Natl Acad Sci U S A* (2011) **108**(Suppl 1):4516–22. doi:10.1073/pnas.1000080107
22. Caporaso JG, Kuczynski J, Stombaugh J, Bittinger K, Bushman FD, Costello EK, et al. QIIME allows analysis of high-throughput community sequencing data. *Nat Methods* (2010) **7**(5):335–6. doi:10.1038/nmeth.f.303
23. DeSantis TZ, Hugenholtz P, Larsen N, Rojas M, Brodie EL, Keller K, et al. Greengenes, a chimera-checked 16S rRNA gene database and workbench compatible with ARB. *Appl Environ Microbiol* (2006) **72**(7):5069–72. doi:10.1128/AEM.03006-05
24. Grice EA, Kong HH, Renaud G, Young AC, Program NCS, Bouffard GG, et al. A diversity profile of the human skin microbiota. *Genome Res* (2008) **18**(7):1043–50. doi:10.1101/gr.075549.107
25. Lozupone C, Knight R. UniFrac: a new phylogenetic method for comparing microbial communities. *Appl Environ Microbiol* (2005) **71**(12):8228–35. doi:10.1128/AEM.71.12.8228-8235.2005
26. Segata N, Izard J, Waldron L, Gevers D, Miropolsky L, Garrett WS, et al. Metagenomic biomarker discovery and explanation. *Genome Biol* (2011) **12**(6):R60. doi:10.1186/gb-2011-12-6-r60
27. Stanley D, Geier MS, Hughes RJ, Denman SE, Moore RJ. Highly variable microbiota development in the chicken gastrointestinal tract. *PLoS One* (2013) **8**(12):e84290. doi:10.1371/journal.pone.0084290
28. van Dongen WF, White J, Brandl HB, Moodley Y, Merkling T, Leclaire S, et al. Age-related differences in the cloacal microbiota of a wild bird species. *BMC Ecol* (2013) **13**:11. doi:10.1186/1472-6785-13-11
29. Tanikawa T, Shoji N, Sonohara N, Saito S, Shimura Y, Fukushima J, et al. Aging transition of the bacterial community structure in the chick ceca. *Poult Sci* (2011) **90**(5):1004–8. doi:10.3382/ps.2010-01153
30. Calenge F, Beaumont C. Toward integrative genomics study of genetic resistance to *Salmonella* and *Campylobacter* intestinal colonization in fowl. *Front Genet* (2012) **3**:261. doi:10.3389/fgene.2012.00261
31. Beaumont C, Chapuis H, Protais J, Sellier N, Menanteau P, Fravalo P, et al. Resistance to *Salmonella* carrier state: selection may be efficient but response depends on animal's age. *Genet Res (Camb)* (2009) **91**(3):161–9. doi:10.1017/S0016672309000135
32. Videnska P, Faldynova M, Juricova H, Babak V, Sisak F, Havlickova H, et al. Chicken faecal microbiota and disturbances induced by single or repeated therapy with tetracycline and streptomycin. *BMC Vet Res* (2013) **9**:30. doi:10.1186/1746-6148-9-30
33. Stecher B, Chaffron S, Kappeli R, Hapfelmeier S, Freedrich S, Weber TC, et al. Like will to like: abundances of closely related species can predict susceptibility to intestinal colonization by pathogenic and commensal bacteria. *PLoS Pathog* (2010) **6**(1):e1000711. doi:10.1371/journal.ppat.1000711
34. Haag LM, Fischer A, Otto B, Plickert R, Kuhl AA, Gobel UB, et al. Intestinal microbiota shifts towards elevated commensal *Escherichia coli* loads abrogate colonization resistance against *Campylobacter jejuni* in mice. *PLoS One* (2012) **7**(5):e35988. doi:10.1371/journal.pone.0035988
35. Winter SE, Baumler AJ. Why related bacterial species bloom simultaneously in the gut: principles underlying the 'Like will to like' concept. *Cell Microbiol* (2014) **16**(2):179–84. doi:10.1111/cmi.12245
36. Spees AM, Lopez CA, Kingsbury DD, Winter SE, Baumler AJ. Colonization resistance: battle of the bugs or Menage a Trois with the host? *PLoS Pathog* (2013) **9**(11):e1003730. doi:10.1371/journal.ppat.1003730
37. Videnska P, Sisak F, Havlickova H, Faldynova M, Rychlik I. Influence of *Salmonella enterica* serovar enteritidis infection on the composition of chicken cecal microbiota. *BMC Vet Res* (2013) **9**:140. doi:10.1186/1746-6148-9-140
38. Barman M, Unold D, Shifley K, Amir E, Hung K, Bos N, et al. Enteric salmonellosis disrupts the microbial ecology of the murine gastrointestinal tract. *Infect Immun* (2008) **76**(3):907–15. doi:10.1128/IAI.01432-07
39. Juricova H, Videnska P, Lukac M, Faldynova M, Babak V, Havlickova H, et al. Influence of *Salmonella enterica* serovar enteritidis infection on the development of the cecum microbiota in newly hatched chicks. *Appl Environ Microbiol* (2013) **79**(2):745–7. doi:10.1128/AEM.02628-12
40. Stecher B, Robbiani R, Walker AW, Westendorf AM, Barthel M, Kremer M, et al. *Salmonella enterica* serovar typhimurium exploits inflammation to compete with the intestinal microbiota. *PLoS Biol* (2007) **5**(10):2177–89. doi:10.1371/journal.pbio.0050244
41. Carding S, Verbeke K, Vipond DT, Corfe BM, Owen LJ. Dysbiosis of the gut microbiota in disease. *Microb Ecol Health Dis* (2015) **26**:26191. doi:10.3402/mehd.v26.26191
42. Thiennimitr P, Winter SE, Winter MG, Xavier MN, Tolstikov V, Huseby DL, et al. Intestinal inflammation allows *Salmonella* to use ethanolamine to compete with the microbiota. *Proc Natl Acad Sci U S A* (2011) **108**(42):17480–5. doi:10.1073/pnas.1107857108
43. Lupp C, Robertson ML, Wickham ME, Sekirov I, Champion OL, Gaynor EC, et al. Host-mediated inflammation disrupts the intestinal microbiota and promotes the overgrowth of Enterobacteriaceae. *Cell Host Microbe* (2007) **2**(3):204. doi:10.1016/j.chom.2007.06.010
44. Winter SE, Winter MG, Xavier MN, Thiennimitr P, Poon V, Keestra AM, et al. Host-derived nitrate boosts growth of E. coli in the inflamed gut. *Science* (2013) **339**(6120):708–11. doi:10.1126/science.1232467
45. Khan CMA. The dynamic interactions between *Salmonella* and the microbiota, within the challenging niche of the gastrointestinal tract. *Int Sch Res Notices* (2014) **2014**:1–23. doi:10.1155/2014/846049
46. den Besten G, van Eunen K, Groen AK, Venema K, Reijngoud DJ, Bakker BM. The role of short-chain fatty acids in the interplay between diet, gut microbiota, and host energy metabolism. *J Lipid Res* (2013) **54**(9):2325–40. doi:10.1194/jlr.R036012
47. Lawhon SD, Maurer R, Suyemoto M, Altier C. Intestinal short-chain fatty acids alter *Salmonella typhimurium* invasion gene expression and virulence through BarA/SirA. *Mol Microbiol* (2002) **46**(5):1451–64. doi:10.1046/j.1365-2958.2002.03268.x
48. Gantois I, Ducatelle R, Pasmans F, Haesebrouck F, Hautefort I, Thompson A, et al. Butyrate specifically down-regulates *Salmonella* pathogenicity island 1 gene expression. *Appl Environ Microbiol* (2006) **72**(1):946–9. doi:10.1128/AEM.72.1.946-949.2006
49. Van Immerseel F, Boyen F, Gantois I, Timbermont L, Bohez L, Pasmans F, et al. Supplementation of coated butyric acid in the feed reduces colonization and shedding of *Salmonella* in poultry. *Poult Sci* (2005) **84**(12):1851–6. doi:10.1093/ps/84.12.1851
50. Fernandez-Rubio C, Ordonez C, Abad-Gonzalez J, Garcia-Gallego A, Honrubia MP, Mallo JJ, et al. Butyric acid-based feed additives help protect broiler chickens from *Salmonella* enteritidis infection. *Poult Sci* (2009) **88**(5):943–8. doi:10.3382/ps.2008-00484

Conflict of Interest Statement: The authors declare that the research was conducted in the absence of any commercial or financial relationships that could be construed as a potential conflict of interest.

27

Blurred lines: pathogens, commensals, and the healthy gut

*Paul Wigley**

Institute for Infection and Global Health, University of Liverpool, Liverpool, UK

Keywords: chicken, microbiome, gut health, probiotics, commensal, *Campylobacter*, *Clostridium perfringens*, *Escherichia coli*

Edited by:
Michael Kogut,
United States Department of Agriculture, Agricultural Research Service, USA

Reviewed by:
Haiqi He,
United States Department of Agriculture, Agricultural Research Service, USA
Bradley L. Bearson,
United States Department of Agriculture, Agricultural Research Service, USA
Rami A. Dalloul,
Virginia Tech, USA

Correspondence:
Paul Wigley
paul.wigley@liverpool.ac.uk

The Chicken Microbiome and Health

Detailed studies of the chicken microbiome have emerged in recent years, largely due to the impact of next-generation sequencing (NGS). We increasingly understand how the microbiome is important in health, in development of the gut and the immune system, and in maintenance of homeostasis. Manipulation of the microbiota directly through probiotics or antimicrobials or indirectly through feed and feed additives has long been used by the poultry industry to increase growth rates and feed conversion, to improve gut health, and to reduce the burden of pathogens and, in particular, to reduce the load of foodborne zoonotic pathogens such as *Salmonella* and *Campylobacter*. We can now begin to mechanistically determine how these treatments affect the microbiota and the wider host, and this understanding will allow us to use more targeted approaches in the future. In terms of food security, increasing yield is clearly a good thing. However, it is far from clear what represents a "healthy" microbiome, and the lines between what is a "harmless" commensal and what is a pathogen are often blurred. As such an understanding of the microbial ecology of the gut and how this is affected by manipulation of the microbiome or indeed treatment of "pathogens" is essential in ensuring that treatments intended to improve health and productivity do not in fact cause more problems.

Is it a Pathogen or a Commensal?

The chicken microbiome consists of around 1,000 bacterial species, though the composition varies over time, between breeds and lines of birds, between flocks, individuals, and at different sites within the gut (1–5). Proteobacteria make up a relatively small amount of species in the microbiome, but among these species are a number that may cause disease in the chicken, notably *Escherichia coli* and *Clostridium perfringens*, and as such are often considered pathogens (4–6). In contrast, the foodborne zoonotic pathogen *Campylobacter jejuni* is also found frequently as a component of the cecal microbiome but is often considered to be a "harmless commensal." However, in reality, these species can have the properties of either pathogen or commensal depending on the bacterial pathotype, host immune status, diet, and coinfection.

Of these three exemplars, *E. coli* has perhaps the least direct impact on gut health. However, extraintestinal infections are a considerable health problem in both broiler and layer chicken production. Isolates associated with disease are termed avian pathogenic *E. coli* or APEC. Much effort has been directed at understanding the virulence factors and pathogenesis of APEC, and there are clearly a number of pathotypes that can cause disease (7, 8). However, wider analysis of isolates associated with systemic infection or colibacillosis of broiler chickens and those associated with a healthy gut show that disease may be caused by isolates that harbor few, if any, APEC-associated virulence factors while apparently "commensal" isolates carry numerous virulence factors (9). The implication is that in many clinical cases of colibacillosis, commensal bacteria act as an opportunistic pathogen due to host factors, environmental stress, poor management, or as a secondary infection.

As such infections are rarely investigated in detail such as genotyping of isolates; the more generic term of APEC has become associated with all *E. coli* isolated from diseased chickens rather than those *E. coli* isolates that are primary pathogens *per se.*

Campylobacter jejuni is the most common cause of foodborne human gastrointestinal infection worldwide. Chicken is the main reservoir of infection with around 70% of UK retail chicken contaminated in recent surveys (10, 11). *C. jejuni* colonizes the lower gastrointestinal tract of the chicken to a high level and has been considered to be a commensal due to the absence of clinical disease in experimental infection studies (12). However, in recent years, we have begun to reassess this paradigm. Experimental infection of broiler breeds with *C. jejuni* leads to an inflammatory response and changes to gut structure (13–16). Generally, it would appear that this inflammation is regulated by IL-10-producing cells, but in some broiler breeds, regulation appears to be dysfunctional and infection may lead to prolonged inflammation, damage, and diarrhea. Does this mean that *C. jejuni* is truly a pathogen of the chicken or more a reflection of dysregulation of mucosal immune regulation? Indeed, poor gut health is often considered as a problem for broiler chickens. Wet litter, due to loose feces mixed with the bedding substrate, and dysbacteriosis are frequent problems in broiler production that affect productivity and animal welfare both directly and through resulting problems such as pododermatitis and hock burn (17–19). Modern broiler chickens have been successfully bred to efficiently convert grain into protein and grow rapidly, reaching slaughter weight at 6–7 weeks of age and we increasingly understand the genetic basis for this (20, 21). This, however, may have consequences; well-documented musculoskeletal problems are being addressed, but problems with gut health may be less obvious and harder to deal with. One may pose the question to what extent are these problems related to the composition of the microbiota and development of a healthy gut or more a consequence of a defect in their gut physiology or immune function? Additionally, to what extent could inappropriate or poorly regulated responses to the "normal" microbiota be contributing to poor gut health? The example of *C. jejuni* illustrates how the balance in maintaining a healthy gut is likely to be influenced by a large number of both host and microbial factors.

Clostridia are a major component of the proteobacteria in the chicken microbiome (5). Of these species, *C. perfringens* is the most important in poultry health. Variants of *C. perfringens* are associated with the gut of many species, and it can be generally considered as a commensal. Yet, it may produce toxins associated with disease including human food poisoning or in necrotic infections of the gut or deep tissue. In the chicken, the *C. perfringens* toxin group A has become most associated with necrotic enteritis (NE), these isolates producing alpha and particularly netB toxins (22). Despite *C. perfringens* producing these toxins being closely associated with NE, it had proved very difficult to fulfill Koch's postulates as such isolates are frequently found in healthy birds and reliable experimental infection models for NE based on *C. perfringens* infection alone have proved hard to develop. This is largely due to most clinical disease being multifactorial involving predisposing factors such as coinfection particularly with species of the apicomplexan protozoan parasite *Eimeria* or due to dietary factors such as diets high in non-starch polysaccharides (NSPs; wheat, rye, and barley) or animal proteins that provide favorable conditions for the growth of *C. perfringens* A and stress on birds in production (23). Again it is difficult to define *C. perfringens* as a true gut pathogen, but more of an opportunist that frequently makes up part of the microbiome.

Manipulation of the Microbiome: Past and Future Implications for Gut Health

Historically, currently and likely into the future, the chicken microbiome has been manipulated perhaps more than any other vertebrate species through the use of growth-promoting antimicrobials, prebiotic and probiotic treatments, and dietary additives (24–27). Feed additives such as enzymes have been used to increase productivity. For example, the use of phytases to allow the breakdown of plant phytates to be utilized in diet (28). Other additives such as plantain NSPs have been proposed to reduce the burden of infections such as *Salmonella* (29). The use of growth-promoting antimicrobials has been banned in the European Union since 2006 and their use in the USA is under increasing pressure due to their role in development of antimicrobial resistance. Not unexpectedly, the use of antimicrobial growth promoters affects the composition of the microbiota (30, 31), and equally the withdrawal of both growth-promoting and anticoccidial drugs will lead to change in the microbiota composition in commercial flocks. Interestingly, a recent study on drug-free broiler production systems in Canada showed an increase in *C. perfringens* (32). Anecdotally, the increased prevalence of both NE and colibacillosis in Europe has been blamed, at least in part, on the withdrawal of growth promoters. While the overriding problems associated with the emergence of antimicrobial resistance rightly mean that growth-promoting antibiotics have been or are being withdrawn, it clearly illustrates how the manipulation of microbiota can have positive effects on health of the chicken. Equally, we need to be aware that changing the microbiota or modulating host responses that are affected by or effect changes upon the microbiome may have undesirable effects. In the case of growth promoters, this was their role in the development of resistant bacteria and potential drug residues in the food chain. As such a better understanding of microbial ecology and how interventions impact on the microbiota and the host is needed before we adopt such changes wholesale. Manipulation of the microbiome may be used to improve productivity, although the consequences of removing "detrimental" or enriching "beneficial" taxa are likely to go beyond improving feed conversion. A perturbed microbiome may reveal commensals as having pathogenic potential and lead to problems in development of the gut and immune system and poor gut homeostasis. Manipulation of the gut, the microbiome, and the immune response has all been proposed in reducing the burden of carriage of foodborne bacterial pathogens. Our work on feed supplementation with plantain NSP showed successful inhibition of *Salmonella* invasion (29), but rather unexpectedly lead to increased colonization of the intestinal tract with *Salmonella gallinarum*. *S. gallinarum* has evolved with several defective metabolic pathways that make it a poor colonizer of the chicken gut, but supplementation with plantain NSP increased colonization either through a direct nutritional source or more likely utilization of breakdown products of microbiota components (33). Equally immunological manipulation may have unexpected consequences. Both colonization of *Salmonella* and *Campylobacter* are accompanied by regulation of innate responses to these bacteria in the gut (13, 34, 35). It has been proposed that depletion of the regulatory $CD4^{+}$ $CD25^{+}$ T-cell population will enhance clearance and thereby reduce the public health risk due to these pathogens (36, 37). A downside of this may be increased inflammation and more significantly loss of regulation to components of the microbiome, again blurring lines between pathogen and commensal and leading to poor gut and poor health.

Conclusion

Ultimately, the "take-home" message in this article is that the power of NGS and metagenomic approaches allow us to understand the composition of microbiomes in multiple individuals of a livestock species quickly and relatively easily. We can associate individual taxa and species with good or poor outcomes in productivity or health. Yet, this power needs to be tempered with (often substantial) gaps in our understanding of microbial ecology within the gut. Can changing the microbiota lead to perturbation of gut regulation? As we have seen, there are blurred lines between pathogens and commensals, and so can changes to remove apparent pathogens have negative consequences on other aspects of gut health or could the promotion of "good bacteria" lead to emergence of "new pathogens." The historical example of growth-promoting antimicrobials illustrates the point. Their use was successful in increasing productivity yet almost certainly has contributed to antimicrobial resistance (38). Their subsequent withdrawal is now resulting in problems in our faster growing modern broiler chickens. Our understanding of the microbiome and its manipulation offers a wealth of opportunities, though may not be without risk.

Funding

This work was supported by the Biotechnology and Biological Science Research Council though grant number BB/J017353/1.

References

1. Oakley BB, Buhr RJ, Ritz CW, Kiepper BH, Berrang ME, Seal BS, et al. Successional changes in the chicken cecal microbiome during 42 days of growth are independent of organic acid feed additives. *BMC Vet Res* (2014) **10**:282. doi:10.1186/s12917-014-0282-8
2. Schokker D, Veninga G, Vastenhouw SA, Bossers A, de Bree FM, Kaal-Lansbergen LM, et al. Early life microbial colonization of the gut and intestinal development differ between genetically divergent broiler lines. *BMC Genomics* (2015) **16**:418. doi:10.1186/s12864-015-1646-6
3. Stanley D, Hughes RJ, Moore RJ. Microbiota of the chicken gastrointestinal tract: influence on health, productivity and disease. *Appl Microbiol Biotechnol* (2014) **98**:4301–10. doi:10.1007/s00253-014-5646-2
4. Stanley D, Geier MS, Hughes RJ, Denman SE, Moore RJ. Highly variable microbiota development in the chicken gastrointestinal tract. *PLoS One* (2013) **8**:e84290. doi:10.1371/journal.pone.0084290
5. Oakley BB, Lillehoj HS, Kogut MH, Kim WK, Maurer JJ, Pedroso A, et al. The chicken gastrointestinal microbiome. *FEMS Microbiol Lett* (2014) **360**:100–12. doi:10.1111/1574-6968.12608
6. Stanley D, Geier MS, Chen H, Hughes RJ, Moore RJ. Comparison of fecal and cecal microbiotas reveals qualitative similarities but quantitative differences. *BMC Microbiol* (2015) **15**:51. doi:10.1186/s12866-015-0388-6
7. Dziva F, Hauser H, Connor TR, van Diemen PM, Prescott G, Langridge GC, et al. Sequencing and functional annotation of avian pathogenic *Escherichia coli* serogroup O78 strains reveal the evolution of *E. coli* lineages pathogenic for poultry via distinct mechanisms. *Infect Immun* (2013) **81**:838–49. doi:10.1128/IAI.00585-12
8. Guabiraba R, Schouler C. Avian colibacillosis: still many black holes. *FEMS Microbiol Lett* (2015) **362**(15). doi:10.1093/femsle/fnv118
9. Kemmett K, Humphrey T, Rushton S, Close A, Wigley P, Williams NJ. A longitudinal study simultaneously exploring the carriage of APEC virulence associated genes and the molecular epidemiology of faecal and systemic *E. coli* in commercial broiler chickens. *PLoS One* (2013) **8**:e67749. doi:10.1371/journal.pone.0067749
10. FSA welcomes retailers' efforts to reduce *Campylobacter* on chickens. *Vet Rec* (2015) **176**:639. doi:10.1136/vr.h3270
11. FSA survey puts pressure on retailers to reduce *Campylobacter* in chickens. *Vet Rec* (2015) **176**:243. doi:10.1136/vr.h1187
12. Hermans D, Pasmans F, Heyndrickx M, Van Immerseel F, Martel A, Van Deun K, et al. A tolerogenic mucosal immune response leads to persistent *Campylobacter jejuni* colonization in the chicken gut. *Crit Rev Microbiol* (2012) **38**:17–29. doi:10.3109/1040841X.2011.615298
13. Humphrey S, Chaloner G, Kemmett K, Davidson N, Williams N, Kipar A, et al. *Campylobacter jejuni* is not merely a commensal in commercial broiler chickens and affects bird welfare. *Mbio* (2014) **5**:e1364–1314. doi:10.1128/mBio.01364-14
14. Awad WA, Smorodchenko A, Hess C, Aschenbach JR, Molnár A, Dublecz K, et al. Increased intracellular calcium level and impaired nutrient absorption are important pathogenicity traits in the chicken intestinal epithelium during *Campylobacter jejuni* colonization. *Appl Microbiol Biotechnol* (2015) **99**:6431–41. doi:10.1007/s00253-015-6543-z
15. Awad WA, Aschenbach JR, Ghareeb K, Khayal B, Hess C, Hess M. *Campylobacter jejuni* influences the expression of nutrient transporter genes in the intestine of chickens. *Vet Microbiol* (2014) **172**:195–201. doi:10.1016/j.vetmic.2014.04.001
16. Awad WA, Molnár A, Aschenbach JR, Ghareeb K, Khayal B, Hess C, et al. *Campylobacter* infection in chickens modulates the intestinal epithelial barrier function. *Innate Immun* (2015) **21**:151–60. doi:10.1177/1753425914521648
17. Dumas MD, Polson SW, Ritter D, Ravel J, Gelb J Jr, Morgan R, et al. Impacts of poultry house environment on poultry litter bacterial community composition. *PLoS One* (2011) **6**:e24785. doi:10.1371/journal.pone.0024785
18. Taira K, Nagai T, Obi T, Takase K. Effect of litter moisture on the development of footpad dermatitis in broiler chickens. *J Vet Med Sci* (2014) **76**:583–6. doi:10.1292/jvms.13-0321
19. van der Hoeven-Hangoor E, Paton ND, van de Linde IB, Verstegen MW, Hendriks WH. Moisture content in broiler excreta is influenced by excreta nutrient contents. *J Anim Sci* (2013) **91**:5705–13. doi:10.2527/jas.2013-6573
20. Davis RV, Lamont SJ, Rothschild MF, Persia ME, Ashwell CM, Schmidt CJ. Transcriptome analysis of post-hatch breast muscle in legacy and modern broiler chickens reveals enrichment of several regulators of myogenic growth. *PLoS One* (2015) **10**:e0122525. doi:10.1371/journal.pone.0122525
21. Godoy TF, Moreira GC, Boschiero C, Gheyas AA, Gasparin G, Paduan M, et al. SNP and INDEL detection in a QTL region on chicken chromosome 2 associated with muscle deposition. *Anim Genet* (2015) **46**:158–63. doi:10.1111/age.12271
22. Timbermont L, Haesebrouck F, Ducatelle R, Van Immerseel F. Necrotic enteritis in broilers: an updated review on the pathogenesis. *Avian Pathol* (2011) **40**:341–7. doi:10.1080/03079457.2011.590967
23. Moran ET Jr. Intestinal events and nutritional dynamics predispose *Clostridium perfringens* virulence in broilers. *Poult Sci* (2014) **93**:3028–36. doi:10.3382/ps.2014-04313
24. Kerr AK, Farrar AM, Waddell LA, Wilkins W, Wilhelm BJ, Bucher O, et al. A systematic review-meta-analysis and meta-regression on the effect of selected competitive exclusion products on *Salmonella* spp. prevalence and concentration

in broiler chickens. *Prev Vet Med* (2013) **111**:112–25. doi:10.1016/j.prevetmed.2013.04.005

25. Nava GM, Bielke LR, Callaway TR, Castaneda MP. Probiotic alternatives to reduce gastrointestinal infections: the poultry experience. *Anim Health Res Rev* (2005) **6**:105–18. doi:10.1079/AHR2005103
26. Babu US, Raybourne RB. Impact of dietary components on chicken immune system and *Salmonella* infection. *Expert Rev Anti Infect Ther* (2008) **6**:121–35. doi:10.1586/14787210.6.1.121
27. Pedroso AA, Hurley-Bacon AL, Zedek AS, Kwan TW, Jordan AP, Avellaneda G, et al. Can probiotics improve the environmental microbiome and resistome of commercial poultry production? *Int J Environ Res Public Health* (2013) **10**:4534–59. doi:10.3390/ijerph10104534
28. Ptak A, Bedford MR, Swiatkiewicz S, Zyla K, Jozefiak D. Phytase modulates ileal microbiota and enhances growth performance of the broiler chickens. *PLoS One* (2015) **10**:e0119770. doi:10.1371/journal.pone.0119770
29. Parsons BN, Wigley P, Simpson HL, Williams JM, Humphrey S, Salisbury AM, et al. Dietary supplementation with soluble plantain non-starch polysaccharides inhibits intestinal invasion of *Salmonella typhimurium* in the chicken. *PLoS One* (2014) **9**:e87658. doi:10.1371/journal.pone.0087658
30. Pourabedin M, Guan L, Zhao X. Xylo-oligosaccharides and virginiamycin differentially modulate gut microbial composition in chickens. *Microbiome* (2015) **3**:15. doi:10.1186/s40168-015-0079-4
31. Lin J, Hunkapiller AA, Layton AC, Chang YJ, Robbins KR. Response of intestinal microbiota to antibiotic growth promoters in chickens. *Foodborne Pathog Dis* (2013) **10**:331–7. doi:10.1089/fpd.2012.1348
32. Gaucher ML, Quessy S, Letellier A, Arsenault J, Boulianne M. Impact of a drug-free program on broiler chicken growth performances, gut health, *Clostridium perfringens* and *Campylobacter jejuni* occurrences at the farm level. *Poult Sci* (2015) **94**:1791–801. doi:10.3382/ps/pev142
33. Parsons BN, Campbell BJ, Wigley P. Soluble plantain nonstarch polysaccharides, although increasing caecal load, reduce systemic invasion of *Salmonella gallinarum* in the chicken. *Lett Appl Microbiol* (2015) **60**:347–51. doi:10.1111/lam.12377
34. Shanmugasundaram R, Selvaraj RK. Regulatory T cell properties of chicken CD4+CD25+ cells. *J Immunol* (2011) **186**:1997–2002. doi:10.4049/jimmunol.1002040
35. Withanage GS, Wigley P, Kaiser P, Mastroeni P, Brooks H, Powers C, et al. Cytokine and chemokine responses associated with clearance of a primary *Salmonella enterica* serovar Typhimurium infection in the chicken and in protective immunity to rechallenge. *Infect Immun* (2005) **73**:5173–82. doi:10.1128/IAI.73.8.5173-5182.2005
36. Shanmugasundaram R, Selvaraj RK. In ovo injection of anti-chicken CD25 monoclonal antibodies depletes CD4+CD25+ T cells in chickens. *Poult Sci* (2013) **92**:138–42. doi:10.3382/ps.2012-02593
37. Shanmugasundaram R, Selvaraj RK. Effects of in vivo injection of anti-chicken CD25 monoclonal antibody on regulatory T cell depletion and CD4+CD25− T cell properties in chickens. *Dev Comp Immunol* (2012) **36**:578–83. doi:10.1016/j.dci.2011.09.015
38. Soulsby L. Antimicrobials and animal health: a fascinating nexus. *J Antimicrob Chemother* (2007) **60**(Suppl 1):i77–8. doi:10.1093/jac/dkm358

Conflict of Interest Statement: The author declares that the research was conducted in the absence of any commercial or financial relationships that could be construed as a potential conflict of interest.

28

Pharmacokinetic–Pharmacodynamic Modeling of Enrofloxacin Against *Escherichia coli* in Broilers

KaNa Sang[1,2†], HaiHong Hao[1,2†], LingLi Huang[1,2], Xu Wang[3] and ZongHui Yuan[1,2,3*]*

[1] National Reference Laboratory of Veterinary Drug Residues (HZAU), Huazhong Agricultural University, Wuhan, China, [2] MAO Key Laboratory for Detection of Veterinary Drug Residues, Huazhong Agricultural University, Wuhan, China, [3] MOA Laboratory for Risk Assessment of Quality and Safety of Livestock and Poultry Products, Huazhong Agricultural University, Wuhan, China

Edited by:
Guillermo Tellez,
University of Arkansas, USA

Reviewed by:
Sherry Layton,
Vetanco, Argentina
Vivek A. Kuttappan,
University of Arkansas, USA

***Correspondence:**
Lingli Huang
huanglingli@mail.hzau.edu.cn;
ZongHui Yuan
yuan5802@mail.hzau.edu.cn

†KaNa Sang and HaiHong Hao have contributed equally to this work.

The purpose of the present study was to establish a pharmacokinetic/pharmacodynamic (PK/PD) modeling approach for the dosage schedule design and decreasing the emergence of drug-resistant bacteria. The minimal inhibitory concentration (MIC) of 929 *Escherichia coli* isolates from broilers to enrofloxacin and ciprofloxacin was determined following CLSI guidance. The MIC_{50} was calculated as the populational PD parameter for enrofloxacin against *E. coli* in broilers. The 101 *E. coli* strains with MIC closest to the MIC_{50} (0.05 μg/mL) were submitted for serotype identification. The 13 *E. coli* strains with O and K serotype were further utilized for determining pathogencity in mice. Of all the strains tested, the *E. coli* designated strain Anhui 112 was selected for establishing the disease model and PK/PD study. The PKs of enrofloxacin after oral administration at the dose of 10 mg/kg body weights (BW) in healthy and infected broilers was evaluated with high-performance liquid chromatography (HPLC) method. For intestinal contents after oral administration, the peak concentration (C_{max}), the time when the maximum concentration reached (T_{max}), and the area under the concentration-time curve (AUC) were 21.69–31.69 μg/mL, 1.13–1.23 h, and 228.97–444.86 μg h/mL, respectively. The MIC and minimal bactericidal concentration (MBC) of enrofloxacin against *E. coli* (Anhui 112) in Mueller–Hinton (MH) broth and intestinal contents were determined to be similar, 0.25 and 0.5 μg/mL respectively. In this study, the sum of concentrations of enrofloxacin and its metabolite (ciprofloxacin) was used for the PK/PD integration and modeling. The *ex vivo* growth inhibition data were fitted to the sigmoid E_{max} (Hill) equation to provide values for intestinal contents of 24 h area under concentration-time curve/MIC ratios (AUC0–24 h/MIC) producing, bacteriostasis (624.94 h), bactericidal activity (1065.93 h) and bacterial eradication (1343.81 h). PK/PD modeling was established to simulate the efficacy of enrofloxacin for different dosage regimens. By model validation, the protection rate was 83.3%, demonstrating that the dosage regimen of 11.9 mg/kg BW every 24 h during 3 days provided great therapeutic significance. In summary, the purpose of the present study was to first design a dosage regimen for the treatment *E. coli* in broilers by enrofloxacin using PK/PD integrate model and confirm that this dosage regimen presents less risk for emergence of floroquinolone resistance.

Keywords: enrofloxacin, *Escherichia coli*, PK/PD modeling, broiler, intestinal content

INTRODUCTION

Antimicrobial resistance is a principal threat to both animals and humans, the main reason for the increasing bacterial resistance is the overuse and misuse of antibiotics. Optimizing the dosage schedules is essential for achieving clinical cures and minimizing the emergence of antimicrobial drug resistance (1, 2). Currently, the optimal dose regimen should be calculated according to the relationship between pharmacokinetics (PKs) and pharmacodynamics (PD) (3). PK/PD modeling can reflect the relationship between the drug, the bacteria, and the animals. It has been demonstrated in many studies that the integration and modeling of the relationship between PK and PD can quantify the potency and efficacy of antimicrobials against target pathogens and provide a basis for the dose optimization (4–7).

PK/PD modeling can be used to evaluate the clinical efficacy of antimicrobial agents (4, 8). The most widely used PK parameters are the area under the plasma concentration-time curve (AUC) and the maximum plasma concentration (C_{max}). The most commonly used PD parameters include minimal inhibitory concentration (MIC) and time-kill curve. The integration of PK and PD establishes a mathematical and theoretical link between them. The three PK/PD parameters are AUC/MIC ratio, C_{max}/MIC ratio, and the percentage of a 24-h time period that the unbound drug concentration exceeds the MIC (T > MIC) (7, 9, 10). Fluoroquinolones are classified as typical concentration-dependent drugs, the initially reported AUC/MIC and C_{max}/MIC are better predictors than T > MIC for the antibacterial effect (11, 12). Therefore, it is very important to determine the AUC/MIC value of enrofloxacin against *Escherichia coli* in broilers.

Escherichia coli is a Gram-negative facultative anaerobe, it is a frequent cause of septicemia, Enterocolitis, and diffuse peritonitis. Colibacillosis has caused great economic losses to the poultry industry and commonly fluoroquinolones are used for the treatment (13–15). At the same time, the serious abuse of fluoroquinolones in clinical settings has been implicated in treatment dissatisfaction or even treatment failure, it also contributes to the emergence of bacterial antibiotic resistance.

Pharmacokinetics of enrofloxacin has already been studied in many species, including calves, turkeys, horses, goats, sheep and pigs (16–21); however, studies on the PK of enrofloxacin in infected animals are quite few even though the PK parameters in infected animals are more close to the clinical conditions (22). The metabolism of enrofloxacin to ciprofloxacin in broilers is limited to 5 and 10% (23, 24). There is some research on the PK of enrofloxacin in intestinal contents (25, 26), but limited data are available regarding the PK/PD in broiler intestinal contents.

The objectives of the study were to: (1) investigate the population MIC and select clinical strains with higher pathogenicity for establishing bacterial infected model, (2) determine the PK of enrofloxacin orally administrated in healthy and infected broilers, (3) determine the PD of enrofloxacin against clinical *E. coli* pathogenic strains, (4) use the PK/PD model to optimize the dosage regimen of enrofloxacin against colibacillosis in broilers, and (5) validate the model to verify the clinical efficacy of the resulting dosage regimen.

MATERIALS AND METHODS

Animals

Broilers

Thirty-day-old healthy KeBao broilers obtained from a commercial poultry farm in Jiang Xia were utilized for this experiment ($n = 160$), the broilers were mixed sex (50:50) with weights ranging between 0.9 and 1.2 kg. The broilers were randomly distributed into two treatment groups ($n = 80$/treatment group) Group 1 served as the non-infected healthy controls animals and Group 2 the *E. coli*-infected disease animals. All broilers were allowed 7 days for acclimation before the experiments began. All broilers were housed in a climate control environment under identical conditions with standard commercial diet and water supplied.

Mice

Four-week-old healthy Kunming mice (SPF grand, kw: 18 ± 2 g, $n = 120$, half male and half female) were obtained from the Center of Experimental Animal of Hubei, and housed in SPF animal room in our lab [Licence# SCXK(E) 2008-0005].

All experimental procedures in this study were performed according to the guidelines of the committee on the use and care of the laboratory animals in Hubei province, China. The study was approved by the Animal Care Center, Hubei Science and Technology Agency in China (SYXK 2013–0044). All the animals were monitored throughout the study for any signs of adverse effects.

Chemicals and Reagents

The Enrofloxacin reference standard (98% purity) and Ciprofloxacin Hydrochloride reference standard (95% purity) were purchased from Dr. Ehrenstorfer (Augsburg, Germany). The Enrofloxacin API (98% purity) used for PKs study was acquired from a local distributor (Wuhan Midland Chemical Co., Ltd.), the supplied powder was dissolved in 5% sodium carboxymethyl cellulose (CMC) to allow for oral administration. Acetonitrile (ACN), formic acid and methanol (MeOH) were provided by TEDIA (USA). All chemicals used in this experiment were analytical grade or higher and dissolved or diluted using de-ionized water (Milli-Q Millipore Corp.).

Bacteria

The clinical *E. coli* pathogenic strain designated Anhui112 was previously isolated from broiler chickens with colibacillosis. This strain was used for the PD study and the *E. coli* infection model. The commonly used quality control standard *E. coli* strain ATCC 25922 was purchased from Chinese Veterinary Culture Collection. All strains were stored at −80°C until use. Before each experiment, these bacteria cultures were sub-cultured on Mueller–Hinton agar and incubated at 37°C for 18–24 h.

Determining the MIC of Enrofloxacin Against Clinical *E. coli* Isolates

A total of 929 clinical isolates collected from five provinces in central China and stored in the laboratory were studied in this experiment. The determination of MIC for enrofloxacin and ciprofloxacin against all clinical *E. coli* strains was determined by the microdilution broth method, using the *E. coli* ATCC 25922 as the experimental control strain and following CLSI (Clinical and Laboratory Standards Institute, 2009, M07-A9) protocol. MICs were found to be in the range between 0.04 and 64 μg/mL. Using SPSS 16.0, the 50% minimum inhibitory concentration (MIC_{50}) 0.50 μg/mL and 90% minimum inhibitory concentration (MIC_{90}) 16.21 μg/mL were determined to represent the population PD of enrofloxacin against clinical *E. coli*.

Serotype Identification

The clinical *E. coli* strains, approximately 101 strains, with the MIC closest to MIC_{50}, were further tested for determining which strains were serotype O or K positive. The O and K anti-serum was purchased from China Institute of Veterinary Drug Control (IVDC). Serotype was determined by traditional slide agglutination test using the commercialized antigen diagnostic serum following previously published methods (27).

Pathogenicity Experiment on Mice

The strains previously identified as either serotype O or K ($n = 13$) were used in a pathogenicity experiment on mice. Each of the 13 strains were administered intra-peritoneally (200 ul) to a separate group of mice ($n = 9$/group) at three different doses [1×10^8, 1×10^7, and1×10^6 colony forming units (CFU)/mL, $n = 3$/dose] to establish the infection model; additionally there was a none treated control group for a total of 14 groups. All mice were closely observed for the first 6 h and then once every 2 h for the remainder of the day. Any behavioral changes observed were noted and recorded by time and group. At the conclusion of this experiment, the data were analyzed and the most virulent strain was selected to conduct PD study and establish the *E. coli* infection model.

Establishing *E. coli* Infection Model in Broilers

After a 7-day acclimation period, 160 broilers were randomly selected and distributed into one of two experimental groups ($n = 80$/group). Each of the 80 broilers in the infection group was inoculated by oral gavage with 8 mL of *E. coli* culture (previously determined to be the most virulent) containing 1.2×10^9 CFU/mL. Birds were observed after inoculation for clinical symptoms and pathological changes. After 12 h, sterile tissue (liver) samples were collected by necropsy from dead broilers and cultured to confirm that mortality was caused by the inoculated strain.

Pharmacokinetic Experiment

After a 7-day acclimation period, 160 broilers were randomly divided into two groups ($n = 80$/group): the *E. coli* infection model and healthy control model. On the morning of the eighth day, enrofloxacin was orally administered at a dose of 10 mg/kg to all broilers. At the following time points after oral administration of enrofloxacin: 0, 0.25, 0.5, 0.75, 1, 1.5, 2, 3, 4, 8, 12, 24, and 48 h, six broilers per group were humanly killed to collect blood samples (2 mL) and intestinal contents (2 mL).

Blood samples collected with anticoagulant were centrifuged for 10 min at 3000 rpms to obtain plasma. The plasma was removed to a clean sterile tube and stored at −20°C until analysis. At a later time point, 1 mL of plasma was added to a 10 mL tube, 2 mL of ACN was then added to precipitate proteins. The tube was vortexed for 2 min and centrifuged at 4000 rpms for 10 min, the aqueous phase was transferred to a clean tube and dried under nitrogen. One milliliter of 14% ACN was used to reconstitute the dried pellet. The sample was filtered through a 0.22 μm membrane into the high-performance liquid chromatography (HPLC) detection vial.

Intestinal content (1 g) was homogenized for 1 min in a 50 mL tube, 2 mL of 0.5 M EDTA (pH 7.0) was then added to the homogenate followed by 15 mL of dichloromethane. The mixture was vortex-mixed for 1 min and centrifuged at 5000 rpms for 5 min. This extraction procedure was repeated twice and then dried under nitrogen. The dried pellet was reconstituted using 1 mL 12% ACN then centrifuged at 12,000 rpm for 5 min before analysis. The supernatant was removed and filtered through a 0.22 μm membrane, into the HPLC detection vial.

The concentration of enrofloxacin and ciprofloxacin in plasma and intestinal content were determined by the HPLC method with UV (UltraViolet) detector (28) under the following conditions: UV detection 278 nm, column temperature 30°C, mobile phase water with 0.1% formic acid and ACN, and sample size 40 μL injected into the HPLC (Waters 2695) system with a flow rate 1 mL/min.

The concentration–time data variables and Pharmacokinetics parameters of enrofloxacin and ciprofloxacin were derived from the Winnonlin program (version 5.2.1, Pharsight Corporation, Mountain View, CA, USA). The plasma concentration determined data were analyzed with compartmental method. The linear trapezoidal rule was used to calculate the AUC.

Determination of MIC, MBC, MPC, and PAE

The MIC of Anhui112 was determined using the previous detailed method.

The minimal bactericidal concentration (MBC) was determined after MIC reading, 100 μL bacteria suspension from each well of the 96 microwell plate was spread on MH agar plates and incubated at 37°C for 24 h for bacterial counting. MBC in broth and intestine were determined as the lowest concentration at which bacteria numbers were reduced by 99.9%.

The mutant prevention concentration (MPC) of enrofloxacin was determined using the agar method (29). The 10^{10} CFU/mL *E. coli* strains were inoculated on the agar plates containing serial concentration of enrofloxacin (1 × MIC, 2 × MIC, 4 × MIC, 8 × MIC, 16 × MIC, and 32 × MIC) and cultured at 37°C for 72 h. The MPC was defined as the lowest concentration of enrofloxacin on agar plates without bacterial growth.

For the post-antibiotic effect (PAE) determination, the bacterial was exposed to three different concentrations (1 × MIC, 2 × MIC and 4 × MIC) of enrofloxacin for 1 or 2 h. The media containing enrofloxacin was removed by centrifuge at 12000 × g for 5 min. The bacterial was re-grew in fresh media without enrofloxacin for another 24 h. The bacterial numbers were determined at different time points. The PAE was the time difference (in hours) for antimicrobial-treated bacterial to increase in number by 1 $\log_{10}$ minus the same determination for non-treated cultures of the same test bacterial.

Drawing *In vitro* and *Ex Vivo* Bacterial Killing Curves

In vitro bacterial killing curves were determined in MH broth. Different concentrations of enrofloxacin: 1/2MIC, 1MIC, 2MIC, 4MIC, 8MIC, 16MIC, and 32MIC were prepared in MH broth, the tubes were then inoculated with *E. coli* Anhui112 (10^6CFU/mL) and incubated at 37°C. The bacterial count (CFU/mL) was determined for each tube after 1, 2, 4, 6, 8,12, and 24 h of incubation. Briefly, 100 μL culture was obtained for each time point, serially diluted with sterile saline plated and the colonies counted the next morning. The limit of detection was 10 CFU/mL. Each concentration test was performed in triplicate.

The *Ex vivo* bacterial killing curves were determined in intestinal content samples obtained from broilers at different time points after oral administration with enrofloxacin following the method as described earlier for the *in vitro* study. The tubes containing bacterial culture and intestinal content were incubated at 37°C and then viable bacteria counts were determined at 1, 2, 4, 8, 12, and 24 h time points. The limit of detection was 10 CFU/mL. Each concentration test was performed in triplicate.

PK and PD Integration and Modeling

All PK parameters were calculated by WinNonlin 5.2 software, including T > MIC, C_{max}, $T_{1/2}$, AUC, etc. PK analysis was performed with one-compartmental model. Using *in vitro* MIC and *in vivo* PK parameters, the surrogate parameters (C_{max}/MIC, AUC/MIC, and T > MIC) of intestinal content were determined after oral administration of enrofloxacin. The relationship between the *ex vivo* AUC_{24h}/MIC ratio and the bacterial count after 24 h of incubation in intestinal content was determined by using the sigmoid inhibitory E_{max} model. This model is described by the following equation:

$$E = E_{max} - \frac{(E_{max} - E_0) \cdot C^N}{C^N + EC_{50}{}^N}$$

In which, E is the antibacterial effect measured as the change in the bacterial count ($\log_{10}$CFU/mL) in the serum sample after 24 h of incubation compared to the initial $\log_{10}$CFU/mL; E_{max} is the maximum antibacterial effect determined as the difference of $\log_{10}$CFU/mL in sample incubated between 0 and 24 h time point; E_0 is the $\log_{10}$ difference of bacterial count in the control sample containing tylosin after 24 h of incubation; EC_{50} is the AUC/MIC producing 50% of the maximum antibacterial effect; C is the AUC/MIC in the effect compartment (the *ex vivo* site, that is serum); and N is the Hill coefficient, which describes the steepness of the AUC/MIC-effect curve.

To investigate the effect of different dosage regimens, the PD model describing bacterial growth rate in function of enrofloxacin concentration was combined with the PK model and simulations were performed with mlxplore software (version-1.1.0, Lixoft, Orsay, France).

Dosage Regiment

Four levels of antibacterial effect of enrofloxacin were quantified from the sigmoid E_{max} equation by determining AUC/MIC required for bacteriostatic action (no change in bacterial count after 24 h of incubation, E = 0), a 50% reduction of the bacterial count, bactericidal action (a 99.9% decrease in the bacterial count, E = 3), and bacterial elimination (the lowest AUC/MIC that produce a 99.99% reduction in the count, E = 4) in each intestinal content. The calculation of potential optimal dosage can use the following equation:

$$X = d \times \frac{AUC_{\text{ex vivo}} / MIC_{\text{tested}}}{AUC_{\text{in vivo}} / MIC_{\text{target}}}$$

where *d* is the projected dosage (mg/kg), 10 mg/kg was used in this study. The value of the *ex vivo* AUC_{24}/MIC obtained from intestinal content represents bacteriostatic activity, bactericidal activity, and elimination of organisms, respectively. The *in vivo* AUC is obtained from the PK using MIC_{50} as the target MIC in this study.

Risk Assessment of *E. coli* Resistance

The concentration of enrofloxacin was adjusted to 0, 0.125, 0.25, 0.5, 1, 2, 4, and 8 μg/mL with MH broth and 10^9 CFU/mL of bacteria were added to each tube; after 2, 4, 6, 8,12, 18, 24,36, and 48 h of incubation 100 μL was removed from each tube and plated on MH agar plates which contained 1 μg/mL enrofloxacin. Any plate containing 100 CFUs or less were not considered to be a drug induced mutation.

Model Validation of the Dosage Regiment

In order to verify the clinical efficacy of the resulting suggested dosage regimen, 24 broilers with artificially induced colibacillosis were divided into two groups randomly (n = 12/group), and administered saline or antibiotic at a previously determined dosage regimen. Clinical symptoms and pathological changes were observed and recorded for 48 h.

Ethical Statement

All the experimental procedures in this study were performed according to the guidelines of the laboratory care and use committee in Hubei province, China. The study was approved by Animal Ethics Committee of Huazhong Agricultural University and the Animal Care Center, Hubei Science and Technology Agency in China (SYXK 2013-0044). All the animals were monitored throughout the study for any adverse effect signs. This experiment is in line with national regulations regarding animal welfare ethics. Ethical approval number is hzauch 2014-002.

RESULTS

MIC Distribution of the Clinical *E. coli* Strains

The MIC distribution of the 929 *E. coli* strains to enrofloxacin and ciprofloxacin is shown in **Figure 1**. The MIC for enrofloxacin and ciprofloxacin exhibited a trimodel distribution, indicating that

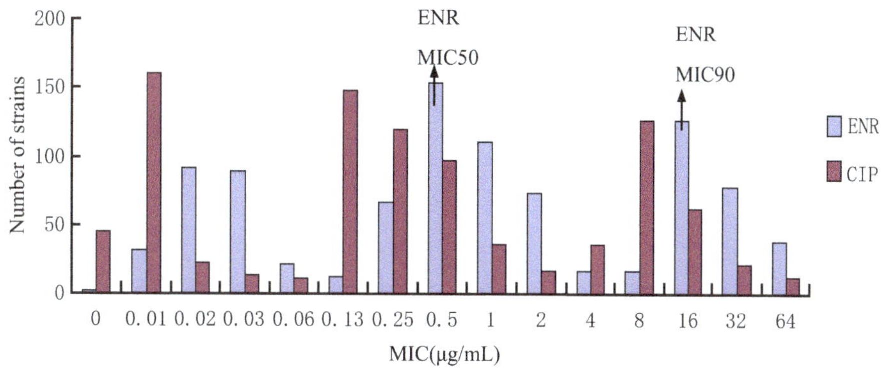

FIGURE 1 | Enrofloxacin and ciprofloxacin MIC distribution of 929 *Escherichia coli* strains isolated from broiler farms. The *X*-axis was the MIC values and *Y*-axis was the strain number in each MIC value.

TABLE 1 | MIC and serotype distribution of clinical isolates (microgram per milliliter).

Bacteria	MIC	O	K	Death/total[a]		
				1 × 10[8] CFU[b]	1 × 10[7] CFU[b]	1 × 10[6] CFU[b]
Zhengzhou379	0.25	O75	987P	1/3	0/3	0/3
Zhengzhou384	0.125	O40	K99	1/3	0/3	0/3
Zhengzhou389	0.125	O9	K88	0/3	0/3	0/3
Zhengyang113	0.125	O18	K99	0/3	0/3	0/3
Jingzhou9	0.25	O93	K88	3/3	2/3	1/3
Jingzhou77	0.06	O138	K88	2/3	0/3	0/3
Xinzhou18	0.25	O139	K99	2/3	1/3	0/3
Xinzhou52	0.25	O101	K88	2/3	1/3	1/3
Xinzhou54	0.25	O80	K99	1/3	0/3	0/3
Xinzhou100	0.25	O40	K99	1/3	0/3	0/3
Anhui112	0.25	O2	K88	3/3	3/3	2/3
Zhengzhou16	0.25	O18	K88	1/3	0/3	0/3
Zhengyang18	0.25	O20	K88	0/3	0/3	0/3
Control group				0/3	0/3	0/3

[a]*Represents the death number of mice and the ratio of the total.*
[b]*Number of colonies to each mice by intraperitoneal injection.*

there may be some resistant strains. The MIC_{50} and MIC_{90} for enrofloxacin were 0.05 and 16 μg/mL, respectively.

Serotype and Pathogenicity of the Selected *E. coli* Strains

Approximately, 101 *E. coli* strains; which were closest to MIC_{50} (0.05 μg/mL) were selected for further analysis by serotyping specifically selecting for serotypes O and K. Only 13 *E. coli* isolates were identified as O or K serotype. And these 13 *E. coli* isolates were used for a pathogenicity experiment in mice. From the results (**Table 1**), we were able to identify the most virulent strain, Anhui 112. Therefore, *E. coli* Anhui 112 was selected to conduct the PD study and to establish the infection model.

E. coli Infection Model

Using *E. coli* Anhui 112, we were able to successfully reproduce an *E. coli* infection model in commercial broiler chickens, within 12 h after challenge with Anhui 112, broilers exhibited typical clinical signs of colibacillosis, such as the elevated temperature, loss of appetite, and white loose droppings. Lesions examined by necropsy showed a layer of white cellulose pseudo-membranous covering the surface of the liver and heart consistent with classical colibacillosis, clearly seen in **Figure 2**.

Pharmacokinetics of Enrofloxacin

The intestinal content concentrations of enrofloxacin and ciprofloxacin were determined after oral administration of the antibiotics to the healthy and infected broilers (**Figure 3**). After oral administration, plasma and intestinal content concentration of enrofloxacin was best fitted with a one-compartment model, all PK parameters were calculated by WinNonlin 5.2. The PK parameters of enrofloxacin in intestinal content are illustrated in **Table 2**. In the healthy model, the AUC, C_{max}, and T_{max} were 228.97 μg mL^{-1} h, 21.69 μg mL^{-1}, and 1.23 h, respectively. In the

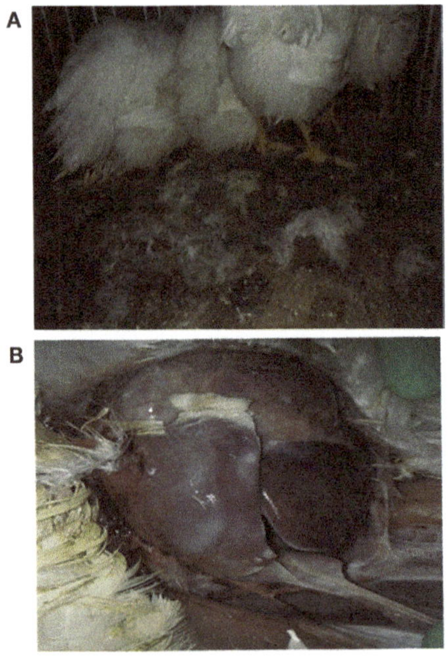

FIGURE 2 | Broilers infected with *E. coli* Anhui112 strains. After infection by E.coli, the broilers had serious Diarrhea **(A)** and liver lesions **(B)**.

infected model the AUC, C_{max}, and T_{max} were 444.86 μg mL^{-1} h, 31.69 μg mL^{-1}, and 1.13 h, respectively.

MIC, MBC, MPC, and PAE of Enr and Cip Against Anhui 112

The MIC and MBC of enrofloxacin in MH broth and intestinal contents were similar 0.25 and 0.5 μg/mL, respectively. The MPC value of enrofloxacin and ciprofloxacin against Anhui 112 were 7 and 0.625 μg/mL, respectively. The PAE showed strong concentration-dependent tendencies. These results are presented in **Table 3**.

In vitro and *Ex Vivo* Antimicrobial Activity

According to the MIC values, a series of varying concentrations of enrofloxacin and ciprofloxacin were prepared in MH broth (1/2–32MIC) to ascertain the *in vitro* bactericidal curve against Anhui 112 (**Figure 4**). The curves are characteristically typical for concentration-dependent antibiotic activity. When exposed to the higher concentration (≥1 × MIC) of enrofloxacin or ciprofloxacin for 6 h, the bacterial CFUs were significantly decreased to undetectable level (<30 CFU). When the bacterial was exposed to 1 × MIC of the two drugs, the growth of bacterial was inhibited at the first 8 h but was rebounded during 8–24 h.

The results showed that in an *ex vivo* environment enrofloxacin is typically concentration dependent (**Figure 5**), consistent with

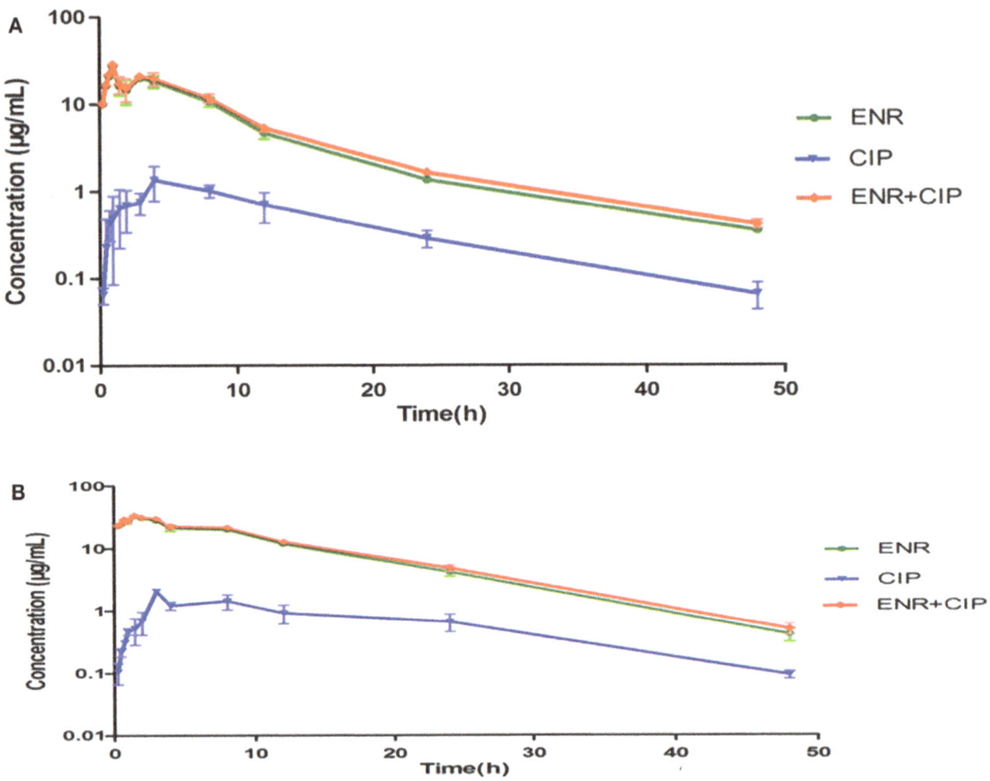

FIGURE 3 | Concentration-time curves of enrofloxacin and ciprofloxacin in the intestinal contents from healthy chicken (A) and bacterial infected chicken (B). The *X*-axis was the time point and *Y*-axis was the drug concentrations. The ciprofloxacin was the metabolite of enrofloxacin in chicken intestinal contents.

TABLE 2 | Pharmacokinetic parameters of enrofloxacin and ciprofloxacin in intestinal contents after oral administration of enrofloxacin at 10 mg/kg BW to broilers.

PK parameters (units)	Healthy model			Infected model		
	ENR	CIP	ENR + CIP	ENR	CIP	ENR + CIP
AUC (μg h/mL)	206.30	18.63	228.97	406.74	31.39	444.86
T_{max} (h)	1.18	5.50	1.23	1.06	6.09	1.13
C_{max} (μg mL^{-1})	21.07	1.11	21.69	30.88	1.46	31.69
V/F (mL/kg)	413.02	4967.17	403.45	296.59	4392.84	289.02
Cl/F (mL/h/kg)	48.47	536.84	43.67	24.58	318.52	22.48
Ka (h^{-1})	2.79	0.28	2.72	3.66	0.31	3.43
Ke (h^{-1})	0.12	0.11	0.11	0.08	0.07	0.08
$T_{1/2e}$ (h)	5.91	6.41	6.40	8.36	9.56	8.91
T > MIC	39.29	30.08	42.79	49.89	43.59	49.95

TABLE 3 | Antibacterial activity of enrofloxacin and ciprofloxacin against *E. coli in vitro*.

Drug	MIC (μg/mL)	MBC (μg/mL)	MPC (μg/mL)	PAE		
	Broths and intestinal	Broths and intestinal	Broths	Concentration (μg/mL)	Expose (1 h)	Expose (2 h)
ENR	0.25	0.5	7	MIC (0.25)	0.2 h	0.4 h
				2 MIC (0.5)	0.8 h	1.2 h
				4 MIC (1)	1.4 h	1.6 h
CIP	0.125	0.25	0.625	MIC (0.125)	0.2 h	0.4 h
				2 MIC (0.25)	0.8 h	1.4 h
				4 MIC (0.5)	1.5 h	1.6 h

the *in vitro* antibacterial curve. In the high concentration group, the enumerated CFUs changed significantly. After 4-h and 8-h cultures, there were no detectable bacteria in infected broilers.

PK/PD Integration and Analysis

The integration of *in vivo* PK and *in vitro* PD data of enrofloxacin in intestinal contents showed AUC/MIC_{50} ratios for healthy and infected broilers to be 455.20 and 884.41 h, respectively. The C_{max}/MIC ratios were 43.38 and 63.38, respectively. Sigmoid E_{max} model was utilized to simulate the relationships between C_{max}/MIC, AUC/MIC, and *ex vivo* antimicrobial efficacy.

Dosage Determination

According to the dosage equation $X = d \times \frac{AUC_{ex\ vivo} / MIC_{tested}}{AUC_{in\ vivo} / MIC_{target}}$, the optimal dose X (mg/kg/d) was calculated. The d was the projected dosage (10 mg/kg) in this study. The $AUC_{in\ vivo}/MIC_{target}$(0.5 μg/mL, the MIC_{50} of enrofloxacin against clinical strains) for infected broilers were 455.20 and 884.41 h, respectively. See **Table 4** of *ex vivo* parameters, when $E = 0$, the $AUC_{ex\ vivo}/MIC_{test}$ (0.25 μg/mL, MIC of enrofloxacin to *E. coli* Anhui112) for healthy and infected broiler were 258.73 and 624.94 h, respectively. When $E = -3$, the $AUC_{ex\ vivo}/MIC_{test}$ for healthy and infected broiler were 451.35 and 1065.93 h, respectively. When $E = -4$, the $AUC_{ex\ vivo}/MIC_{test}$ for healthy and infected broiler were 567.39 and 1343.81 h, respectively. Therefore, see **Table 5**, the doses calculated for bacteriostatic action ($E = 0$) in healthy and infected broilers were 5.6 and 7 mg/kg BW. The doses calculated for bactericidal action ($E = -3$) in healthy and infected broilers were 9.8 and 11.9 mg/kg BW. The calculated for bacterial eradication ($E = -4$) in healthy and infected broilers were 12.4 and 15.1 mg/kg BW. Ultimately, for treatment *E.coli* infection in broiler, the preventive, therapeutic, and bacterial eradication dose of enrofloxacin were chosen as 7.0, 11.9, and 15.1 mg/kg BW.

Due to intensive broiler rearing practices, a mixed feeding dosage regimen was also calculated in our study. According to the groups feeding dosing formula $D = d \times n/W$, for 21-day-old broilers, the value of W is approximately 120 g/kg/d, n is the daily dosing frequency and D is group mixed feeding dosage. When the MIC_{50} against clinical strains is 0.5 μg/mL, the optimum dose is 99 mg/kg for mixed feeding.

Using the PK/PD model with the PD parameters derived from *ex vivo* antimicrobial activity, three selected doses (7.0, 11.9, 15.1 mg/kg BW) were separately simulated. As shown in **Figure 6**, after single dose treatment for 24 h, higher dose (11.9 and 15.1 mg/kg BW) played bactericidal or eradication action during 0–18 h, but the bacteria rebound phenomenon was occurred under the lower dose (7 mg/kg BW) treatment. As shown in **Figure 7**, after daily-treatment of the three selected doses (7.0, 11.9, 15.1 mg/kg BW) for 3 days, the higher doses (11.9, 15.1 mg/kg BW) exhibited great bactericidal and eradication action; however, the bacterial was not inhibited under lower 3-day treatment of lower dose (7 mg/kg BW).

Assessment of Bacterial Resistance

Results in **Table 6** show that when the drug concentration is higher than 8 μg/mL, drug-resistant strains do not appear;

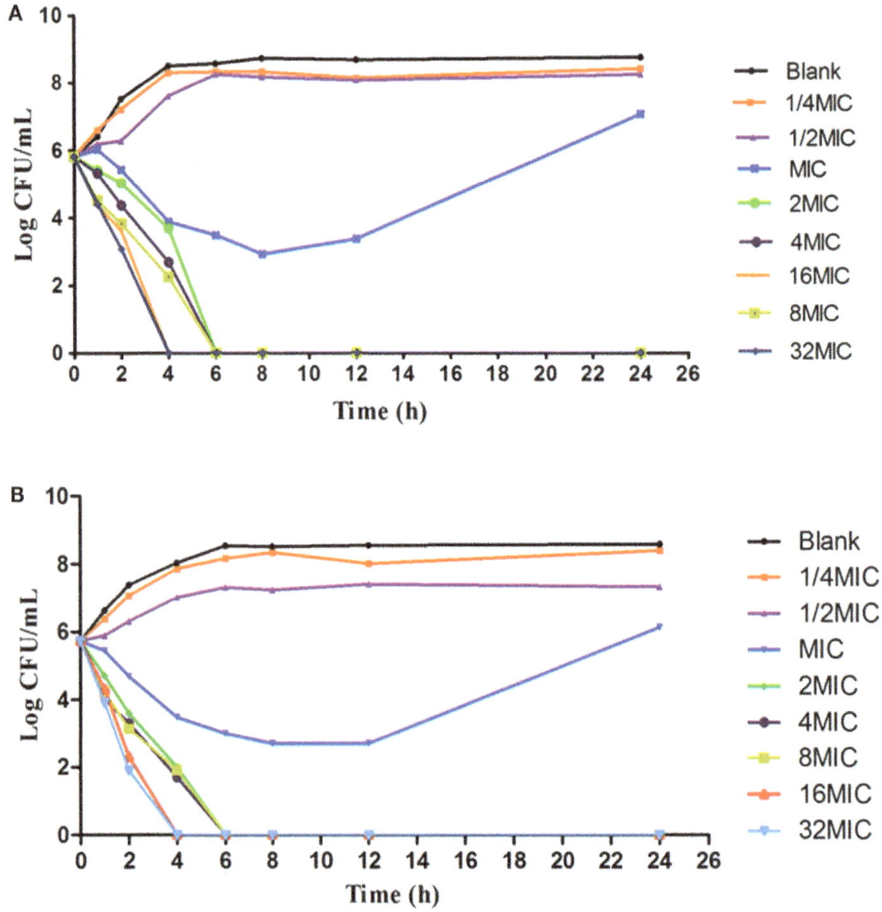

FIGURE 4 | The *in vitro* kill bacteria curve of enrofloxacin (A) and ciprofloxacin (B) against *E.coli* Anhui112. The *X*-axis was the time point during the 24-hours incubation and *Y*-axis was the bacterial number under exposure to deferent concentration (1/4 × MIC, 1/2 × MIC....0.32 × MIC) of drug.

however, when the drug concentration is 2–4 μg/mL, drug resistance strains appear after 36 h. Resistance strains are most easily achieved when the drug concentrations are between 0.25 and 1 μg/mL after 24 h. Similar results were observed between the blank samples (without drug) and the samples whose concentration is 0.125 μg/mL or less. The data indicate resistant strains generally appear after 24 h; therefore, the dosing interval was chosen to be 24 h.

Model Validation

Results show that the protection rate of control group was 8.3%, while the protection rate of the experiment group was 83.3%. These data indicate that the dosage regimen chosen has a significant therapeutic effect, suitable for clinical treatment (**Table 7**).

DISCUSSION

In this investigation, enrofloxacin was orally administered at a clinical recommended effective dose (10 mg/kg BW) in healthy and infected broilers. Although the PK of enrofloxacin in the serum of goats, pigs, calves, horses, and sheep after administration has already been investigated many times (16–19, 30), reports concerning the PK in the intestinal contents are quite few. In this study, enrofloxacin concentrations in intestinal contents were calculated to be 0.35~28.05 μg/mL. These concentrations were much higher than the concentration of enrofloxacin in plasma of healthy broilers, which were between 0.04 and 2.01 μg/mL. According to Slana et al. (24) enrofloxacin concentrations in manure samples, after 15 mg/kg BW orally administered, ranged between 39.2 and 55.0 μg/g. Moraru et al. (31) detected enrofloxacin concentrations in excreta samples ranged between 40.5 and 50.7 μg/g after 3 days orally treatment with 10 mg enrofloxacin/kg BW. Devreese et al. (26) found enrofloxacin concentrations in cloacal samples ranged between 20.1 and 55.7 μg/g after orally treatment of 10 mg enrofloxacin/kg BW. In this study, we found the enrofloxacin concentrations in the intestinal contents were significantly less than previously reported concentrations that maybe due to sample and dosage differences.

The PKs of enrofloxacin in the infected and healthy models were quite different. Higher AUC was obtained in infected broilers (406.7 μg h/mL) when compared to healthy (206.3 μg h/

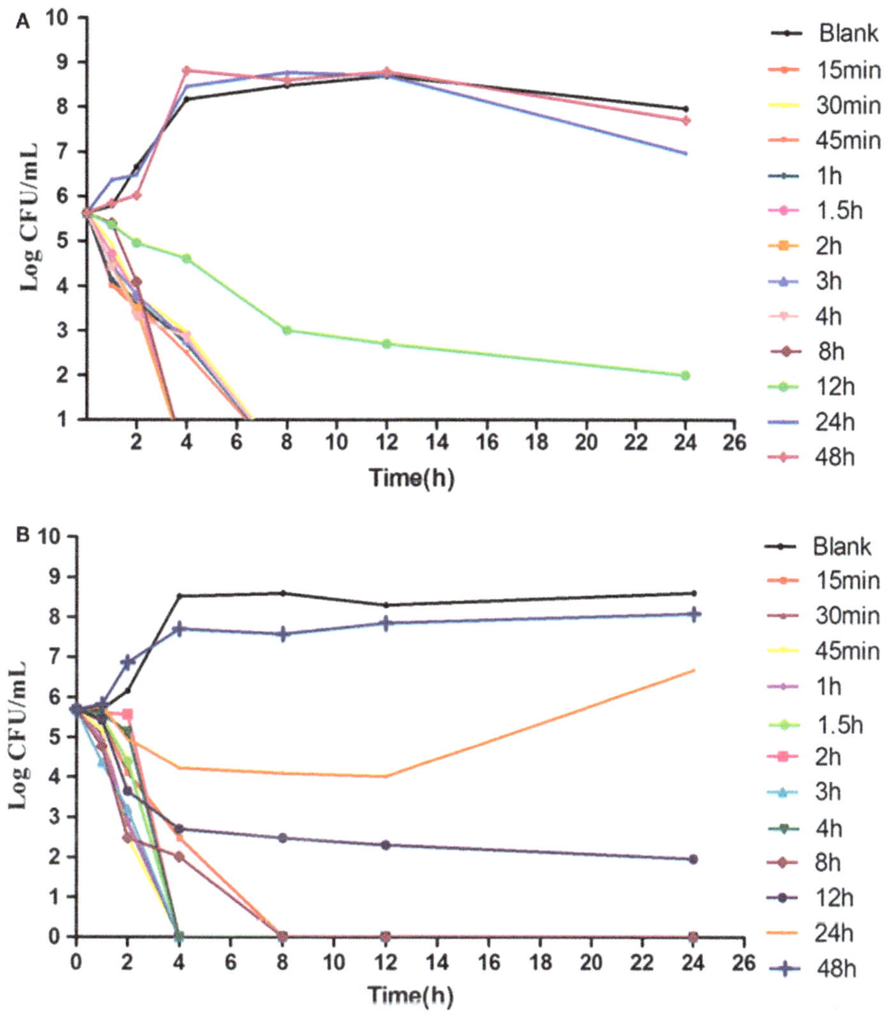

FIGURE 5 | TheEx *vivo* inhibition curve in the intestinal content from healthy chicken (A) and infected chicken (B). The *X*-axis was the time point during the 24-hours incubation and *Y*-axis was the bacterial number under exposure to intestinal samples collected from different time point in the PK study.

TABLE 4 | PK/PD parameter of *ex vivo* data after oral administration enrofloxacin in chicken.

Parameter	Unit	Healthy	Infected
E_{max}	Log10CFU/mL	2.35	2.91
E_0	Log10CFU/mL	−5.62	−5.69
E_{max}−E_0	Log10CFU/mL	7.97	8.60
EC_{50}	h	348.51	802.26
Slope (N)	–	2.85	2.72
AUC_{24}/MIC for bacteriostatic action (E = 0)	h	258.73	624.94
AUC_{24}/MIC for bactericidal action (E = −3)	h	451.35	1065.93
AUC_{24}/MIC for bacterial eradication (E = −4)	h	567.39	1343.81

mL) broilers. The differences of the PKs in healthy and infected broilers maybe due to the changes of the physiological and bio-chemical indexes, such as the change in their body temperature,

TABLE 5 | The different dosages (milligram per kilogram) when MIC of enrofloxacin is 0.5 μg/mL.

Effect (E)	Healthy dosage	Infected dosage
Bacteriostatic action (E = 0)	5.6	7.0
Bactericidal action (E = −3)	9.8	11.9
Bacterial eradication (E = −4)	12.4	15.1

the decrease of the protein in plasma, decline of blood pressure, anemia, liver dysfunction by acetylation, and so on. The PK parameter in diseased animals is much similar to clinical conditions. As previous research has shown, the metabolic conversion of enrofloxacin to ciprofloxacin is quite different in different animal species for example: 59% in dairy cows, 36% in sheep, 47% in buffalo calves, and 64% in beef steers (32–34).

In this study, the ratio of ciprofloxacin AUC (31.39) and enrofloxacin AUC (406.74) is 7.71% after oral administration in infected broilers. Differing from other animal species, the

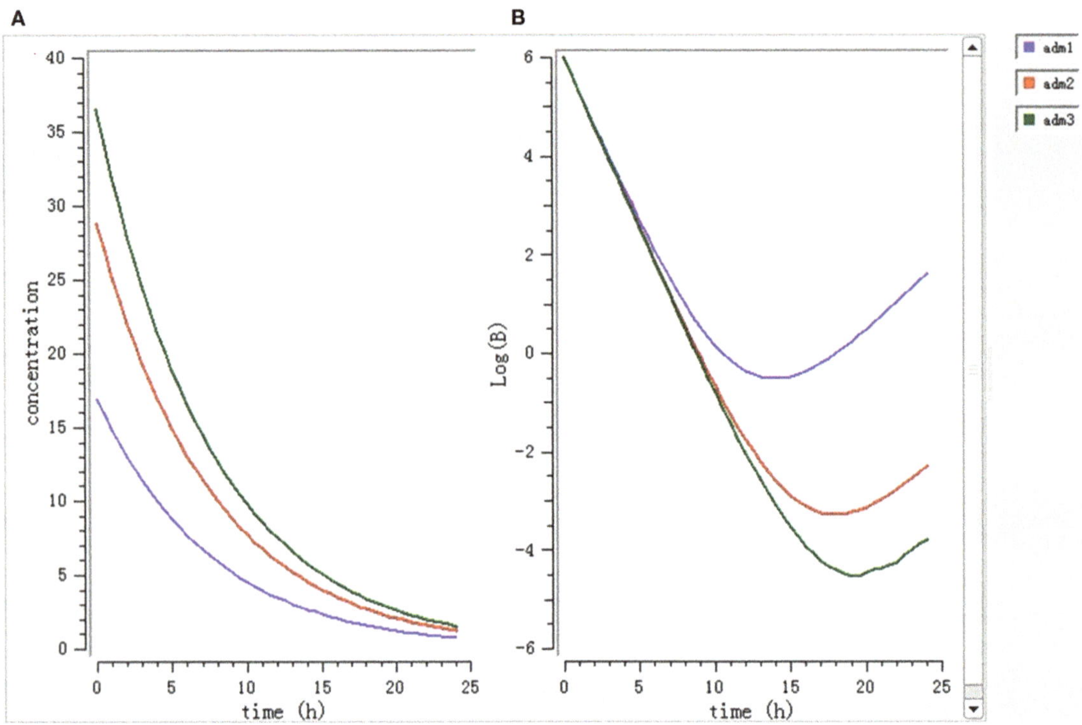

FIGURE 6 | The pharmacokinetic change (A) and pharmacodynamic change (B) under 1-day single treatment simulated by mlxplore software. Adm1, 2, and 3 represented 1-day single treatment with 7.0, 11.9, and 15.1 mg/kg enrofloxacin, respectively.

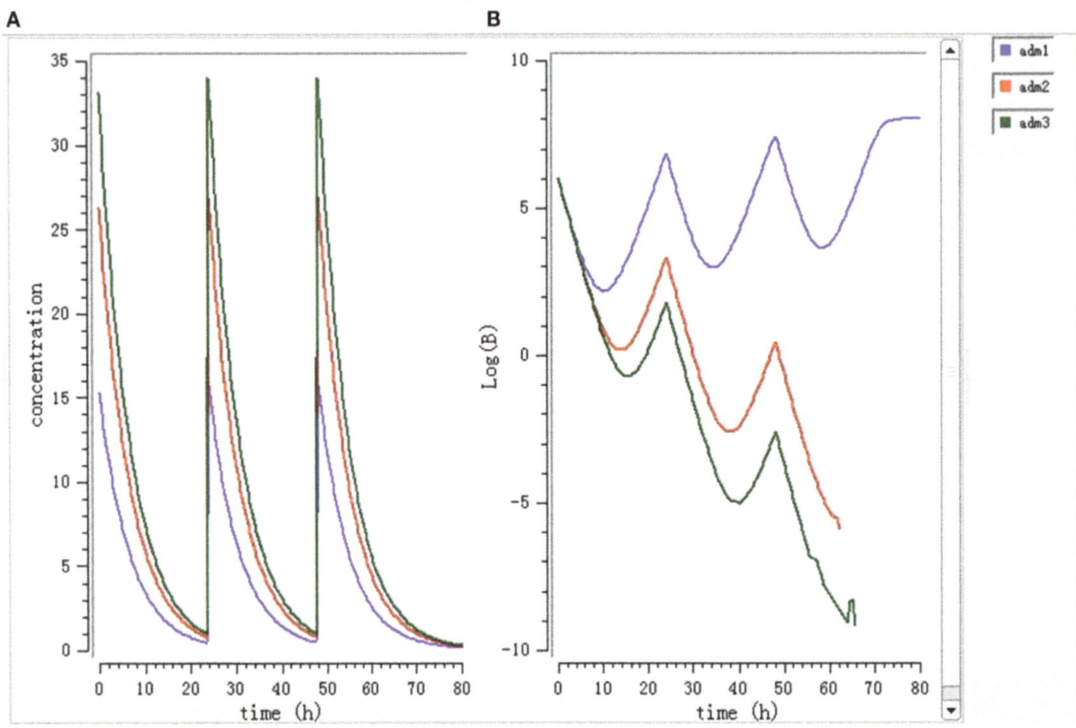

FIGURE 7 | The pharmacokinetic change (A) and pharmacodynamic change (B) under 3-day treatment simulated by mlxplore software. Adm1, 2, and 3 represented 3-day daily-treatment with 7,11.9, and 15.1 mg/kg enrofloxacin, respectively.

TABLE 6 | The growth of resistant strains after exposed to different drug concentrations.

Time (h)	B	0.125	0.25	0.5	1	2	4	8
2	N	N	N	N	N	N	N	N
4	N	N	N	N	N	N	N	N
6	N	N	N	N	N	N	N	N
8	+	N	+	N	N	N	N	N
12	+	+	N	N	+	N	N	N
18	+	N	+	N	+	+	N	N
24	++	++	+	++	N	+	N	N
36	++	++	++	+	N	++	++	N
48	++	++	++	++	+	++	++	N

B, the blank group.
N, colony number below 10 CFU/mL.
+, colony number between 10 and 100 CFU/mL.
++, colony number beyond 100 CFU/mL.

TABLE 7 | The therapeutic effect of enrofloxacin against colibacillosis.

Group	Bacterial	Concentration	Sum chickens	Dead chickens	Protection rate
Test	8 mL,10^9 CFU/mL	11.9 mg/kg BW	12	2	83.3%
Control	8 mL,10^9 CFU/mL	No treatment	12	11	8.3%

biotransformation of enrofloxacin to ciprofloxacin in poultry is limited to only 5–10%, and the ciprofloxacin concentrations are always below the LOQ. (23, 35, 36). The metabolite ciprofloxacin usually has antimicrobial activity, so it is quite important to evaluate the combined action of the enrofloxacin and ciprofloxacin (37). As such, the sum of the concentrations of two drugs should be evaluated by the PK/PD integration and modeling.

The MIC results suggest a bimodal distribution and the 349 strains with MIC ranging between 1 and 64 μg/mL indicates the high increase of antibiotic resistance. Compared to other studies on APEC and AFEC strains (38), 28.5% strains with MIC between 0.5 and 1 μg/mL were considered intermediately resistant, confirming the trend of increasing resistance. In recent years, it has been suggested that the optimization of dosing regimen not only for the treatment but also for reducing antimicrobial resistance development. MIC is used as an *in vitro* reference value to predict the antimicrobial efficacy and potency of a drug. The MIC values in broth and biological fluids reported in previous research (39) shows that the serum inhibitory activity is reduced for most fluoroquinolones. In this study, the MIC values of the pathogen *E. coli* (Auihui 112) for enrofloxacin in intestinal contents and broth both are 0.25 μg/mL, which indicates that enrofloxacin has the same antimicrobial activity in broth and intestinal contents. In our study, the *in vitro* and *ex vivo* time-kill curves indicate that enrofloxacin rapidly eliminates *E. coli*. Rapid inhibition and killing of bacteria exhibited by *ex vivo* inhibition curves is consistent with *in vitro* time-kill data and the previous studies published for danofloxacin and marbofloxacin (39, 40). The time-kill curves seem to indicate that enrofloxacin is concentration dependent. The data from the current study show that bacterial counts will increase after 24-h incubation a time when the antibiotic concentration is lower. These data confirms findings in previous publications stating that MIC alone does not offer enough information about the efficacy of therapy (21).

Enrofloxacin shows a concentration-dependent killing activity like other fluoroquinolone drugs (41). The main PK/PD parameters for concentration-dependent antimicrobials are C_{max}/MIC and AUC/MIC, the AUC/MIC ratio is a more important surrogate for the PK/PD analysis (42).

The breakpoint of $C_{max}/MIC \geq 10$ and $AUC_{24}/MIC \geq 125$ is an indicator for the success of therapy and preventing the emergence of resistance of fluoroquinolones (43). *In vivo* AUC_{24}/MIC_{50} are 455.20 and 887.41, respectively, for healthy and infected broilers at the dosage of 10 mg/kg. The values of *ex vivo* AUC/MIC obtained for bactericidal action in intestinal contents from healthy and infected broilers is 451.35 and 1065.93, respectively. The enrofloxacin concentrations in intestine are detected in much higher concentrations than in plasma; which would potentially lead to an eradication of the *E. coli* in intestine. In this study, based on the $MIC_{50} = 0.5$ μg/mL, values of C_{max}/MIC (43.12) and AUC_{24}/MIC (455.20) both values exceed the predictive effective values. These values are comparable with the values of C_{max}/MIC (38) and AUC_{24}/MIC (293) obtained from buffalo calves (44).

Pharmacokinetic/pharmacodynamic modeling serves as a bridge between PK and PD and has been considered as a promising approach (4, 8, 20). Results obtained from this study based on the PK/PD integration suggest that when the MIC_{50} of enrofloxacin is 0.5 μg/mL, for bacteriostasis, bactericidal, and bacterial eradication in infected broilers, the dosage should be 7.0, 11.9, and 15.1 mg/kg BW., respectively. Results from professional software used to simulate different dosage regimens for treatment show that a 3-day treatment of 11.9 mg/kg every 24 h should be efficient against *E. coli* (Anhui 112) in broilers. Therefore, the dose of 11.9 mg/kg BW. should be effective for treating colibacillosis when the $MIC \leq 0.5$ μg/mL.

Antimicrobial resistance is a principal threat for both animals and humans. Using PK/PD modeling choosing an appropriate therapeutic schedule is a suitable strategy to reduce antimicrobial resistance without influencing the treatment effect. Previous studies show that both AUC/MIC and C_{max}/MIC were related to emergence of resistance in *Pseudomonas aeruginosa* (45). In recent years, the drug resistance risk steadily increases rapidly. However, when the MIC is above the MPC in a wild population, the probability that it will undergo two resistant mutations is very low. It has been proposed that the AUC_{24}/MPC ratio could help as an indicator of drug exposure that stops the selection of drug-resistant mutants (46, 47). It has been proven that an AUC/MPC ratio that in the range of 9 and 12 could prevent the selection of resistant mutants for marbofloxacin in *E. coli* when the inoculum sizes was 10^5 and 10^7 CFU/mL (48). In this study, the AUC/MPC of enrofloxacin in healthy and infected broilers was 29.4 and 58.1, respectively. Indicating that the dosage used in this study potentially can prevent the selection of enrofloxacin resistant mutants.

FUNDING

This article is financially supported by Grants from National Basic Research program of China (2013CB127206), Fundamental Research Funds for the Central Universities (2662015PY035), project supported by the morning program of Wuhan in China (2015070404010191), National Natural Science Foundation of China (31101856/31302143), National Key Technology R&D Program (2012BAK01B00), and the identification of unknown risk factors and the tracking-assessment of known risk factors in livestock product (GJFP2015008).

REFERENCES

1. Toutain P, Lees P. Integration and modelling of pharmacokinetic and pharmacodynamic data to optimize dosage regimens in veterinary medicine. *J Vet Pharmacol Ther* (2004) **27**:467–77. doi:10.1111/j.1365-2885.2004.00613.x
2. Ambrose PG, Bhavnani SM, Rubino CM, Louie A, Gumbo T, Forrest A, et al. Pharmacokinetics-pharmacodynamics of antimicrobial therapy: it's not just for mice anymore. *Clin Infect Dis* (2007) **44**:79–86. doi:10.1086/510079
3. McKellar Q. How can knowledge of Pk/Pd interactions help limit the selection of antibiotic resistance. *International Conference on Antimicrobial Agents in Veterinary Medicine (AAVM)*. Helsinki (2002). p. 28–9.
4. AliAbadi FS, Lees P. Antibiotic treatment for animals: effect on bacterial population and dosage regimen optimisation. *Int J Antimicrob Agents* (2000) **14**:307–13. doi:10.1016/S0924-8579(00)00142-4
5. Toutain P. Pharmacokinetics/pharmacodynamics integration in dosage regimen optimization for veterinary medicine. *J Vet Pharmacol Ther* (2003) **26**:1–8. doi:10.1208/ps040438
6. Drusano GL. Antimicrobial pharmacodynamics: critical interactions of 'bug and drug'. *Nat Rev Microbiol* (2004) **2**:289–300. doi:10.1038/nrmicro862
7. Mouton JW, Dudley MN, Cars O, Derendorf H, Drusano GL. Standardization of pharmacokinetic/pharmacodynamic (PK/PD) terminology for anti-infective drugs: an update. *J Antimicrob Chemother* (2005) **55**:601–7. doi:10.1093/jac/dki079
8. Toutain P-L, Del Castillo JR, Bousquet-Mélou A. The pharmacokinetic-pharmacodynamic approach to a rational dosage regimen for antibiotics. *Res Vet Sci* (2002) **73**:105–14. doi:10.1016/S0034-5288(02)00039-5
9. Craig WA. Pharmacokinetic/pharmacodynamic parameters: rationale for antibacterial dosing of mice and men. *Clin infect Dis* (1998) **26**:1–10. doi:10.1086/516284
10. Andes D, Craig W. Animal model pharmacokinetics and pharmacodynamics: a critical review. *Int J Antimicrob Agents* (2002) **19**:261–8. doi:10.1016/S0924-8579(02)00022-5
11. Schentag JJ, Gilliland KK, Paladino JA. What have we learned from pharmacokinetic and pharmacodynamic theories? *Clin Infect Dis* (2001) **32**:S39–46. doi:10.1086/319375
12. Ball P, Baquero F, Cars O, File T, Garau J, Klugman K, et al. Antibiotic therapy of community respiratory tract infections: strategies for optimal outcomes and minimized resistance emergence. *J Antimicrob Chemother* (2002) **49**:31–40. doi:10.1093/jac/49.1.31
13. Webber M, Piddock LJ. Quinolone resistance in *Escherichia coli*. *Vet Res* (2001) **32**:275–84. doi:10.1051/vetres:2001150
14. Chansiripornchai N, Sasipreeyajan J. Efficacy of sarafloxacin in broilers after experimental infection with *Escherichia coli*. *Vet Res Commun* (2002) **26**:255–62. doi:10.1023/A:1016078222398
15. Fiorentin L, Soncini RA, Da Costa JLA, Mores MA, Trevisol IM, Toda M, et al. Apparent eradication of *Mycoplasma synoviae* in broiler breeders subjected to intensive antibiotic treatment directed to control *Escherichia coli*. *Avian Pathol* (2003) **32**:213–6. doi:10.1080/0307945021000071641
16. Kaartinen L, Salonen M, Älli L, Pyörälä S. Pharmacokinetics of enrofloxacin after single intravenous, intramuscular and subcutaneous injections in lactating cows. *J Vet Pharmacol Ther* (1995) **18**:357–62. doi:10.1111/j.1365-2885.1995.tb00604.x
17. Giguere S, Sweeney R, Belanger M. Pharmacokinetics of enrofloxacin in adult horses and concentration of the drug in serum, body fluids, and endometrial tissues after repeated intragastrically administered doses. *Am J Vet Res* (1996) **57**:1025–30.
18. Anadon A, Martinez-Larra Aga M, Diaz M, Fernandez-Cruz M, Martinez M, Frejo M, et al. Pharmacokinetic variables and tissue residues of enrofloxacin and ciprofloxacin in healthy pigs. *Am J Vet Res* (1999) **60**:1377–82.
19. Elmas M, Tras B, Kaya S, Bas AL, Yazar E, Yarsan E. Pharmacokinetics of enrofloxacin after intravenous and intramuscular administration in Angora goats. *Can J Vet Res* (2001) **65**:64.
20. McKellar Q, Sanchez Bruni S, Jones D. Pharmacokinetic/pharmacodynamic relationships of antimicrobial drugs used in veterinary medicine. *J Vet Pharmacol Ther* (2004) **27**:503–14. doi:10.1111/j.1365-2885.2004.00603.x
21. Haritova AM, Rusenova NV, Parvanov PR, Lashev LD, Fink-Gremmels J. Integration of pharmacokinetic and pharmacodynamic indices of marbofloxacin in turkeys. *Antimicrob Agents Chemother* (2006) **50**:3779–85. doi:10.1128/AAC.00711-05
22. Levison ME. Pharmacodynamics of antimicrobial drugs. *Infect Dis Clin North Am* (2004) **18**:451–65. doi:10.1016/j.idc.2004.04.012
23. Garcia Ovando H, Gorla N, Luders C, Poloni G, Errecalde C, Prieto G, et al. Comparative pharmacokinetics of enrofloxacin and ciprofloxacin in chickens. *J Vet Pharmacol Ther* (1999) **22**:209–12. doi:10.1046/j.1365-2885.1999.00211.x
24. Slana M, Pahor V, Cvitkovič Maričič L, Sollner-Dolenc M. Excretion pattern of enrofloxacin after oral treatment of chicken broilers. *J Vet Pharmacol Ther* (2014) **37**:611–4. doi:10.1111/jvp.12130
25. Wiuff C, Lykkesfeldt J, Aarestrup FM, Svendsen O. Distribution of enrofloxacin in intestinal tissue and contents of healthy pigs after oral and intramuscular administrations. *J Vet Pharmacol Ther* (2002) **25**:335–42. doi:10.1046/j.1365-2885.2002.00430.x
26. Devreese M, Antonissen G, De Baere S, De Backer P, Croubels S. Effect of administration route and dose escalation on plasma and intestinal concentrations of enrofloxacin and ciprofloxacin in broiler chickens. *BMC Vet Res* (2014) **10**:289. doi:10.1186/s12917-014-0289-1
27. Blanco J, Blanco M, Alonso MP, Blanco JE, Garabal JI, Gonzale EA. Serogroups of *Escherichia coli* strains producing cytotoxic necrotizing factors CNF1 and CNF2. *FEMS Microbiol Lett* (1992) **75**:155–9. doi:10.1111/j.1574-6968.1992.tb05409.x
28. Haritova A, Urumova V, Lutckanov M, Petrov V, Lashev L. Pharmacokinetic-pharmacodynamic indices of enrofloxacin in *Escherichia coli* O78/H12 infected chickens. *Food Chem Toxicol* (2011) **49**(7):1530–6. doi:10.1016/j.fct.2011.03.044
29. Pasquali F, Manfreda G. Mutant prevention concentration of ciprofloxacin and enrofloxacin against *Escherichia coli*, *Salmonella typhimurium* and *Pseudomonas aeruginosa*. *Vet Microbiol* (2007) **119**(2):304–10. doi:10.1016/j.vetmic.2006.08.018
30. McKellar Q, Gibson I, Monteiro A, Bregante M. Pharmacokinetics of enrofloxacin and danofloxacin in plasma, inflammatory exudate, and bronchial

secretions of calves following subcutaneous administration. *Antimicrob Agents Chemother* (1999) **43**:1988–92.
31. Moraru R, Pourcher A-M, Jadas-Hecart A, Kempf I, Ziebal C, Kervarrec M, et al. Changes in concentrations of fluoroquinolones and of ciprofloxacin-resistant in chicken feces and manure stored in a heap. *J Environ Qual* (2012) **41**:754–63. doi:10.2134/jeq2011.0313
32. Mengozzi G, Intorre L, Bertini S, Soldani G. Pharmacokinetics of enrofloxacin and its metabolite ciprofloxacin after intravenous and intramuscular administrations in sheep. *Am J Vet Res* (1996) **57**:1040–3.
33. Kumar N, Singh SD, Jayachandran C. Pharmacokinetics of enrofloxacin and its active metabolite ciprofloxacin and its interaction with diclofenac after intravenous administration in buffalo calves. *J Vet Pharmacol Toxicol* (2003) **165**:302–6. doi:10.1016/S1090-0233(02)00248-4
34. Idowu O, Peggins J, Cullison R, Von Bredow J. Comparative pharmacokinetics of enrofloxacin and ciprofloxacin in lactating dairy cows and beef steers following intravenous administration of enrofloxacin. *Res Vet Sci* (2010) **89**:230–5. doi:10.1016/j.rvsc.2009.12.019
35. Carreras I, Castellari M, Regueiro JG, Guerrero L, Esteve-Garcia E, Sarraga C. Influence of enrofloxacin administration and α-tocopheryl acetate supplemented diets on oxidative stability of broiler tissues. *Poult Sci* (2004) **83**:796–802. doi:10.1093/ps/83.5.796
36. Dimitrova D, Lashev L, Yanev S, Pandova B. Pharmacokinetics of enrofloxacin in turkeys. *Res Vet Sci* (2007) **82**:392–7. doi:10.1016/j.rvsc.2006.09.004
37. Prescott JF, Yielding KM. In vitro susceptibility of selected veterinary bacterial pathogens to ciprofloxacin, enrofloxacin and norfloxacin. *Can J Vet Res* (1990) **54**:195.
38. Ozawa M, Baba K, Shimizu Y, Asai T. Comparison of in vitro activities and pharmacokinetics/pharmacodynamics estimations of veterinary fluoroquinolones against avian pathogenic *Escherichia coli* isolates. *Microb Drug Resist* (2010) **16**:327–32. doi:10.1089/mdr.2010.0024
39. Aliabadi FS, Lees P. Pharmacokinetic-pharmacodynamic integration of danofloxacin in the calf. *Res Vet Sci* (2003) **74**:247–59. doi:10.1016/S0034-5288(03)00005-5
40. Sidhu P, Landoni M, Aliabadi M, Toutain P-L, Lees P. Pharmacokinetic and pharmacodynamic modelling of marbofloxacin administered alone and in combination with tolfenamic acid in calves. *J Vet Pharmacol Ther* (2011) **34**:376–87. doi:10.1111/j.1365-2885.2010.01247.x
41. Meinen J, Mcclure J, Rosin E. Pharmacokinetics of enrofloxacin in clinically normal dogs and mice and drug pharmacodynamics in neutropenic mice with *Escherichia coli* and staphylococcal infections. *Am J Vet Res* (1995) **56**:1219–24.
42. Anadon A, Martınez-Larranaga M, Iturbe J, Martınez M, Dıaz M, Frejo M, et al. Pharmacokinetics and residues of ciprofloxacin and its metabolites in broiler chickens. *Res Vet Sci* (2001) **71**:101–9. doi:10.1053/rvsc.2001.0494
43. Forrest A, Nix DE, Ballow CH, Goss TF, Birmingham M, Schentag J. Pharmacodynamics of intravenous ciprofloxacin in seriously ill patients. *Antimicrob Agents Chemother* (1993) **37**:1073–81. doi:10.1128/AAC.37.5.1073
44. Balaje RM, Sidhu PK, Kaur G, Rampal S. Mutant prevention concentration and PK/PD relationships of enrofloxacin for *Pasteurella multocida* in buffalo calves. *Res Vet Sci* (2013) **95**:1114–24. doi:10.1016/j.rvsc.2013.07.019
45. Blaser J, Stone BB, Groner MC, Zinner SH. Comparative study with enoxacin and netilmicin in a pharmacodynamic model to determine importance of ratio of antibiotic peak concentration to MIC for bactericidal activity and emergence of resistance. *Antimicrob Agents Chemother* (1987) **31**:1054–60. doi:10.1128/AAC.31.7.1054
46. Zhao X, Drlica K. Restricting the selection of antibiotic-resistant mutants: a general strategy derived from fluoroquinolone studies. *Clin Infect Dis* (2001) **33**:S147–56. doi:10.1086/321841
47. Olofsson SK, Marcusson LL, Lindgren PK, Hughes D, Cars O. Selection of ciprofloxacin resistance in *Escherichia coli* in an in vitro kinetic model: relation between drug exposure and mutant prevention concentration. *J Antimicrob Chemother* (2006) **57**:1116–21. doi:10.1093/jac/dkl135
48. Ferran A, Dupouy V, Toutain P-L, Bousquet-Mélou A. Influence of inoculum size on the selection of resistant mutants of *Escherichia coli* in relation to mutant prevention concentrations of marbofloxacin. *Antimicrob Agents Chemother* (2007) **51**:4163–6. doi:10.1128/AAC.00156-07

Conflict of Interest Statement: The authors declare that the research was conducted in the absence of any commercial or financial relationships that could be construed as a potential conflict of interest.

Permissions

All chapters in this book were first published in FVETS, by Frontiers; hereby published with permission under the Creative Commons Attribution License or equivalent. Every chapter published in this book has been scrutinized by our experts. Their significance has been extensively debated. The topics covered herein carry significant findings which will fuel the growth of the discipline. They may even be implemented as practical applications or may be referred to as a beginning point for another development.

The contributors of this book come from diverse backgrounds, making this book a truly international effort. This book will bring forth new frontiers with its revolutionizing research information and detailed analysis of the nascent developments around the world.

We would like to thank all the contributing authors for lending their expertise to make the book truly unique. They have played a crucial role in the development of this book. Without their invaluable contributions this book wouldn't have been possible. They have made vital efforts to compile up to date information on the varied aspects of this subject to make this book a valuable addition to the collection of many professionals and students.

This book was conceptualized with the vision of imparting up-to-date information and advanced data in this field. To ensure the same, a matchless editorial board was set up. Every individual on the board went through rigorous rounds of assessment to prove their worth. After which they invested a large part of their time researching and compiling the most relevant data for our readers.

The editorial board has been involved in producing this book since its inception. They have spent rigorous hours researching and exploring the diverse topics which have resulted in the successful publishing of this book. They have passed on their knowledge of decades through this book. To expedite this challenging task, the publisher supported the team at every step. A small team of assistant editors was also appointed to further simplify the editing procedure and attain best results for the readers.

Apart from the editorial board, the designing team has also invested a significant amount of their time in understanding the subject and creating the most relevant covers. They scrutinized every image to scout for the most suitable representation of the subject and create an appropriate cover for the book.

The publishing team has been an ardent support to the editorial, designing and production team. Their endless efforts to recruit the best for this project, has resulted in the accomplishment of this book. They are a veteran in the field of academics and their pool of knowledge is as vast as their experience in printing. Their expertise and guidance has proved useful at every step. Their uncompromising quality standards have made this book an exceptional effort. Their encouragement from time to time has been an inspiration for everyone.

The publisher and the editorial board hope that this book will prove to be a valuable piece of knowledge for researchers, students, practitioners and scholars across the globe.

List of Contributors

Artur Summerfield and Nicolas Ruggli
Institute of Virology and Immunology - IVI, Bern, Switzerland

Ganapathi Raj Murugesan and Chasity Pender
BIOMIN America Inc., San Antonio, TX, USA

Basharat Syed
BIOMIN Holding GmbH, Getzersdorf, Austria

Sudipto Haldar
Department of Animal Nutrition, West Bengal University of Animal and Fishery Sciences, Kolkata, India

Timm Konold, Anthony Duarte and Hugh A. Simmons
Animal Sciences Unit, Animal and Plant Health Agency Weybridge, Addlestone, UK

Stephen A. C. Hawkins
Pathology Department, Animal and Plant Health Agency Weybridge, Addlestone, UK

Lisa C. Thurston
Surveillance and Laboratory Services, Animal and Plant Health Agency Penrith, Penrith, UK

Ben C. Maddison
ADAS UK, School of Veterinary Medicine and Science, University of Nottingham, Sutton Bonington, UK

Kevin C. Gough
School of Veterinary Medicine and Science, University of Nottingham, Sutton Bonington, UK

Juxing Chen, James D. Richards and Jeffery Escobar
Novus International, Inc., St. Charles, MO, USA

Guillermo Tellez
Department of Poultry Science, University of Arkansas, Fayetteville, AR, USA

Susanna Sternberg Lewerin
Department of Biomedical Sciences and Veterinary Public Health, Swedish University of Agricultural Sciences (SLU), Uppsala, Sweden

Ayuub A. Ayoola, Ramon D. Malheiros, Jesse L. Grimes and Peter R. Ferket
Prestage Department of Poultry Science, North Carolina State University, Raleigh, NC, USA

Nobuko Mori, Yuki Okada, Naoto Tsuchida, Yutaka Hatano, Makoto Habara, Shingo Ishikawa, Ichiro Yamamoto and Toshiro Arai
Department of Basic Veterinary Medicine, School of Veterinary Medicine, Nippon Veterinary and Life Science University, Tokyo, Japan

Michael H. Kogut and Ryan J. Arsenault
Southern Plains Agricultural Research Center (SPARC), Agricultural Research Service (ARS), United States Department of Agriculture (USDA), College Station, TX, USA

Jessica L. Danzeisen, Jonathan B. Clayton and Shivdeep S. Hayer
Department of Veterinary and Biomedical Sciences, University of Minnesota, Saint Paul, MN, USA

Hu Huang
Department of Biomedical Informatics and Computational Biology, University of Minnesota, Minneapolis, MN, USA

Dan Knights
Department of Biomedical Informatics and Computational Biology, University of Minnesota, Minneapolis, MN, USA
Department of Computer Science and Engineering, University of Minnesota, Minneapolis, MN, USA
Biotechnology Institute, University of Minnesota, Saint Paul, MN, USA

Brian McComb
Willmar Poultry Company, Willmar, MN, USA

Timothy J. Johnson
Department of Veterinary and Biomedical Sciences, University of Minnesota, Saint Paul, MN, USA
Mid-Central Research and Outreach Center, University of Minnesota, Willmar, MN, USA

Pietro Celi
DSM Nutritional Products, Animal Nutrition and Health, Columbia, MD, USA
Faculty of Veterinary and Agricultural Sciences, The University of Melbourne, Parkville, VIC, Australia

Gianfranco Gabai
Department of Comparative Biomedicine and Food Science, University of Padova, Legnaro, Italy

Nancy W. Shappell
USDA-ARS Animal Metabolism-Agricultural Chemicals Research, Fargo, ND, USA

Michael D. Flythe and Glen E. Aiken
USDA-ARS Forage-Animal Production Research Unit, Lexington, KY, USA

Joshua J. Jackson, Merlin D. Lindemann, James A. Boling and James C. Matthews
Department of Animal and Food Sciences, University of Kentucky, Lexington, KY, USA

Lonneke Onrust, Richard Ducatelle, Karolien Van Driessche, Celine De Maesschalck, Karen Vermeulen, Freddy Haesebrouck, Venessa Eeckhaut and Filip Van Immerseel
Department of Pathology, Bacteriology and Avian Diseases, Ghent University, Merelbeke, Belgium

David González-Barrio, Isabel G. Fernández-de-Mera and Francisco Ruiz-Fons
Health and Biotechnology (SaBio) Group, Spanish Wildlife Research Institute IREC (CSIC, Universidad de Castilla-La Mancha, Junta de Comunidades de Castilla-La Mancha), Ciudad Real, Spain

José Antonio Ortiz
Medianilla S. A., Benalup-Casas Viejas, Spain

João Queirós
Health and Biotechnology (SaBio) Group, Spanish Wildlife Research Institute IREC (CSIC, Universidad de Castilla-La Mancha, Junta de Comunidades de Castilla-La Mancha), Ciudad Real, Spain
Centro de Investigacão em Biodiversidade e Recursos Genéticos (CIBIO), InBio Laboratório Associado, Universidade do Porto, Vairão, Portugal
Departamento de Biologia, Faculdade de Ciências da Universidade do Porto, Porto, Portugal

Muhammad J. Uddin and Willy W. Suen
School of Veterinary Science, University of Queensland, Gatton, QLD, Australia

Natalie A. Prow
QIMR Berghofer Medical Research Institute, Brisbane, QLD, Australia

Roy A. Hall
Australian Infectious Diseases Research Centre, University of Queensland, St Lucia, QLD, Australia
School of Chemistry and Molecular Biosciences, University of Queensland, St Lucia, QLD, Australia

Helle Bielefeldt-Ohmann
School of Veterinary Science, University of Queensland, Gatton, QLD, Australia
Australian Infectious Diseases Research Centre, University of Queensland, St Lucia, QLD, Australia
School of Chemistry and Molecular Biosciences, University of Queensland, St Lucia, QLD, Australia

Star A. Schnell, Yasunaga Yoshikawa, Kiyotaka Watanabe and Koichi Orino
Laboratory of Veterinary Biochemistry, School of Veterinary Medicine, Kitasato University, Towada, Japan

Hiromichi Ohtsuka
Large Animal Clinical Sciences, School of Veterinary Medicine, Rakuno Gakuen University, Ebetsu, Japan

Seiichi Kakinuma
Kakinuma Veterinary Hospital, Honjou, Japan

Juan D. Latorre, Vivek A. Kuttappan, Amanda D. Wolfenden, Lisa R. Bielke, Billy M. Hargis and Guillermo Tellez
Department of Poultry Science, University of Arkansas, Fayetteville, AR, USA

Xochitl Hernandez-Velasco
Departamento de Medicina y Zootecnia de Aves, Facultad de Medicina Veterinaria y Zootecnia, Universidad Nacional Autonoma de Mexico, Mexico City, Mexico

Ross E. Wolfenden and Jose L. Vicente,
Pacific Vet Group-USA, Inc., Fayetteville, AR, USA

Omar F. Prado-Rebolledo
Facultad de Medicina Veterinaria y Zootecnia, Universidad de Colima, Colima, Mexico

Eduardo Morales
Departamento de Produccion Agricola y Animal, Universidad Autonoma Metropolitana, Mexico City, Mexico

Stephanie M. Roto, Peter M. Rubinelli and Steven C. Ricke
Department of Food Science, Center for Food Safety, University of Arkansas, Fayetteville, AR, USA

Corliss A. O'Bryan, Sean J. Pendleton, Philip G. Crandall and Steven C. Ricke
Department of Food Science, Center for Food Safety, University of Arkansas, Fayetteville, AR, USA

Rebecca J. Tokach, Flavio R. B. Ribeiro and Bradley J. Johnson
Department of Animal and Food Sciences, Texas Tech University, Lubbock, TX, USA

Ki Yong Chung
Hanwoo Research Institute, National Institute of Animal Science, Rural Development Administration, Kangwon, South Korea

Whitney Rounds
Kemin Animal Nutrition and Health North America, Des Moines, IA, USA

Parthiban Rajasekaran
NanoScience Technology Center, University of Central Florida, Orlando, FL, USA

Swadeshmukul Santra
NanoScience Technology Center, University of Central Florida, Orlando, FL, USA
Department of Chemistry, University of Central Florida, Orlando, FL, USA
Department of Materials Science and Engineering, University of Central Florida, Orlando, FL, USA
Burnett School of Biomedical Sciences, University of Central Florida, Orlando, FL, USA

Kelsy Robinson and Zhuo Deng
Department of Animal Science, Oklahoma State University, Stillwater, OK, USA

Yongqing Hou
Hubei Key Laboratory of Animal Nutrition and Feed Science, Wuhan Polytechnic University, Wuhan, China

Guolong Zhang
Department of Animal Science, Oklahoma State University, Stillwater, OK, USA
Hubei Key Laboratory of Animal Nutrition and Feed Science, Wuhan Polytechnic University, Wuhan, China

Ryan J. Arsenault
Department of Animal and Food Sciences, University of Delaware, Newark, DE, USA

Michael H. Kogut
United States Department of Agriculture, Agricultural Research Service, Southern Plains Agricultural Research Center, College Station, TX, USA

Nilusha Malmuthuge and Le Luo Guan
Department of Agricultural, Food and Nutritional Science, University of Alberta, Edmonton, AB, Canada

Philip J. Griebel
Vaccine and Infectious Disease Organization, University of Saskatchewan, Saskatoon, SK, Canada
School of Public Health, University of Saskatchewan, Saskatoon, SK, Canada

Vivek A. Kuttappan, Eduardo A. Vicuña, Juan D. Latorre, Amanda D. Wolfenden, Guillermo I. Téllez, Billy M. Hargis and Lisa R. Bielke
Department of Poultry Science, University of Arkansas, Fayetteville, AR, USA

Khin K. Z. Mon, Perot Saelao, Michelle M. Halstead, Ganrea Chanthavixay, Huai-Chen Chang, Lydia Garas, Elizabeth A. Maga and Huaijun Zhou
Department of Animal Science, University of California Davis, Davis, CA, USA

Paul Wigley
Institute for Infection and Global Health, University of Liverpool, Liverpool, UK

KaNa Sang, HaiHong Hao and LingLi Huang
National Reference Laboratory of Veterinary Drug Residues (HZAU), Huazhong Agricultural University, Wuhan, China
MAO Key Laboratory for Detection of Veterinary Drug Residues, Huazhong Agricultural University, Wuhan, China

Xu Wang
MOA Laboratory for Risk Assessment of Quality and Safety of Livestock and Poultry Products, Huazhong Agricultural University, Wuhan, China

ZongHui Yuan
National Reference Laboratory of Veterinary Drug Residues (HZAU), Huazhong Agricultural University, Wuhan, China
MAO Key Laboratory for Detection of Veterinary Drug Residues, Huazhong Agricultural University, Wuhan, China
MOA Laboratory for Risk Assessment of Quality and Safety of Livestock and Poultry Products, Huazhong Agricultural University, Wuhan, China